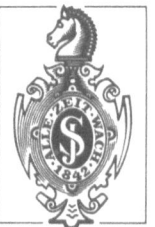

Springer-Verlag France S.A.R.L

Pierre Bret,
Christine Cuche and Gérard Schmutz

Radiology of the small intestine

Preface by Igor Laufer

Foreword by Henri Nahum

With 550 illustrations

Springer-Verlag France S.A.R.L

Pierre Bret
2, quai Augagneur
69003 Lyon
France

Christine Cuche
28, avenue Foch
07300 Tournon
France

Gérard Schmutz
Hospices civils de Strasbourg
Service de Radiologie — Clinique médicale B
1, place de l'Hôpital
67091 Strasbourg Cedex
France

Translation supervised by
Alan Barkun

© Springer-Verlag France 1989
Originally published by Springer-Verlag France, Paris in 1989
Softcover reprint of the hardcover 1st edition 1989

The use of registred names, trademarks, etc. in this publications does not imply, even in the absence of a specific statement, that such names are exempt from the relevant protective laws and regulations and therefore free for general use.
Product Liability ; The publisher can give no guarantee for information about drug dosage and application there of contained in this book. In every individual case the respective user must check its accuracy by consultinf other pharmaceutical literature.

ISBN 978-2-8178-0893-2   ISBN 978-2-8178-0891-8 (eBook)
DOI 10.1007/978-2-8178-0891-8

2918/3917/543210 - Printed on Acid-free paper.

Preface

There is a tradition behind the current radiologic examination of the small bowel. Many of the great names in gastrointestinal radiology have established their reputations on the basis of their work in the small bowel. This is an area which is assuming ever greater importance for radiologists as its mucosal surface continues to elude the endoscopist. Moreover, it is an aspect of radiology which calls for the greatest technical and interpretative skill.

It is a great pleasure to welcome the English language version of this beautiful work on *Radiology of the Small Intestine*. English-speaking physicians are frequently not as familiar with the large body of work published in French as they should be. Tant pis ! Dr. Bret and his co-workers have been pioneers in the pursuit of excellence in gastrointestinal radiology. During all the years that I have been involved in this field, I have admired their work.

This volume on the small bowel is typical of their approach to gastrointestinal radiology. It combines the best elements of radiological art and science. It is a pleasure to leaf through this book just to glance at the pictures. The text is also clear and gives much valuable advice regarding the diagnosis of diseases in the small bowel. I am sure that all physicians will find this book of value since it relies not on any single technique but on the entire range of imaging modalities that apply to the small bowel. Nevertheless, the emphasis is clearly on barium studies and I am sure that this volume will serve as an inspiration to all physicians who work in this area.

Igor Laufer, M.D.

Foreword

Gastrointestinal radiology has been at the forefront of French Radiology for decades: the technical perfection of the examinations and the sophisticated precision of their analysis are part of our heritage. Endoscopy first challenged and quickly, it must be said, replaced the radiological examination.

But the radiologists stand firm and double-contrast techniques have since continued to improve the performance of conventional Radiology; we must realise though that today, in the late 1980 s, this effort has yielded only a moral victory.

Yet one area remains unchallenged: the small bowel. Up to now, this mass of innumerable superimposed loops had remained an enigma for contrast Radiology. Unfamiliar with the organ's pathology and uncomfortable with the imaging techniques required, the radiologists had long abandoned this field, thus limiting its diagnostic work-up to physiological testing.

All the credit belongs to Pierre Bret for having deciphered this riddle. Pierre Bret is a complete radiologist, both conventional and innovative, he is a practicioner and a teacher. Technically demanding, analytically rigorous and clinically superb, he is one of the great masters of gastrointestinal Radiology.

He was the first in France to use double contrast techniques, to opacify directly the biliary ducts, and perform radiologically guided biopsies. He is today the undisputed national leader in digestive Radiology.

Limiting himself to the practical and the useful, Pierre Bret has fathered a simple and reproducible technique of examination of the small bowel. He has perfected an analytical model which is easily learned. From the constellation of signs he describes, stems a reliable and brilliant diagnostic precision based on a rigorous methodology.

This book is both the product and the essence of a man and his School.

Translated from Henri Nahum's preface
to the French version of this textbook

Introduction

The small intestine is the longest part of the gastrointestinal tract. It ensures digestion and absorption of food and plays an important part in immunity. Direct endoscopic exploration is confined to its extremities. The small bowel is the privileged domain of Radiology. It provides the only technique that allows for the morphological study of all its loops. Complementary studies include ultrasound, computed tomography and angiography.

Today's radiologists can use a reliable technique based on the continuous opacification and palpation of all intestinal loops under fluoroscopic monitoring. The films thus obtained must be studied methodically. This book contains the description of technical requirements and of a method of analysis needed to obtain and interpret the films. They are followed by radiological descriptions of small bowel pathology. We have thus attempted to include all the elements needed to carry out and interpret the radiological examination of the small intestine. We base this work on our personal experience as well as the published literature. As the bibliography of such a book cannot be complete, we have had to choose the references we found most useful and have listed them at the end of each chapter.

The authors wish to thank:

- Alain Chayvialle, who reviewed the «clinical notes» in this book,

- Pierre Bensimon, who reviewed the anatomicopathological notes in this book,

- all our colleagues who contributed to illustrating this book:
Jean-Pierre Barbut, Françoise Berger, Michel Bretagnolle, Alain Fond, Denis Gauthier, Gérard Gay, Guy Jeannot, Jean-Pierre Moiroud, Jean-Marie Pouillaude,

- the members of GERMAD (research group on the radiological study of digestive pathology): Jean-Michel Bigot, Patrice Bret, Jean-Michel Bruel, Jean-Baptiste Carcy, Jean De Toeuf, Louis Engelholm, Christian Garcin, Claude Guien, Louis Jourde, Claude L'herminé, Pierre Mahieu, Yves Menu, Maurice Piante, Jacques Pringot, Denis Régent, Pierre-Jean Valette

- Alan Barkun for his help with the english version of this textbook.

References works

Dünndarmradiologie : Einführung und Atlas (1988) Antes G, Eggemann F. Springer-Verlag Berlin

Gastro-entérologie (1986) Bernier JJ. Flammarion, Paris

Gastroenterolgy (1985) Bockus H. Saunders, Philadelphie (4e édition)

Radiologie de l'intestin grêle et du colon : technique et sémiologie (1981) Bret P. SIMEP, Lyon

L'intestin grêle normal et pathologique (étude clinique et radiologique) (1957) Chérigié E, Hillemand P, Proux CH, Bourdon R. Expansion scientifique française, Paris

Précis des maladies du tube digestif (1977) Sous la direction de CH Debray et Y Geffroy. Masson, Paris

Encyclopédie médico-chirurgicale (1988) Éditions Séguier, Paris

Radiologic examination of the small intestine (1959) Golden R. Lippincott, Philadelphie (2e édition)

Double contrast gastro-intestinal radiology (1979) Laufer I. Saunders , Philadelphie

Alimentary Tract Roentgenology (1973) Margulis AR, Burhenne HJ. Mosby

Radiology of the small intestine (1976) Marshak RH, Lindner AE. Saunders, Philadelphie

Traité de radiodiagnostic (1982) :
— Tome IV — *Urgences abdominales, grêle et colon* Nahum H, Geindre M, Bigot JM, Monnier JM, Stérin P. Masson, Paris
— Tome XVIII — *Radiopédiatrie : appareil digestif et urinaire* Lefebvre S, Fauré C, Sauvegrain J, Nahum H, Fortier-Beaulieu M, Hassan M. Masson, Paris

Radiologie clinique de l'intestin grêle (1954) Porcher P, Buffard P, Sauvegrain J. Masson, Paris

Radiology of the small bowel. Modern enteroclysis — Technique and atlas (1982) Sellink JL, Miller RE. Martinus Nijhoff

Contents

Clinical and technical aspects

General review

For radiologists, the small intestine is defined as the part of the small bowel located between the duodenum and the colon, including both the jejunal and ileal segments.

Embryology

The primitive intestinal loop, located in the midsagittal plane, communicates with the umbilical vesicle anteriorly through the vitelline or omphalomesenteric duct and is attached to the posterior abdominal wall by the mesentery. The terminal part of the duodenum, the jejunum and most of the ileum develop from the previtelline segment, and the distal 80 cm of ileum and right colon from the postvitelline portion of the primitive intestinal loop.

The axis of the primitive intestinal loop is the superior mesenteric artery. The loop undergoes first a lengthening and a 90° counterclockwise rotation followed by a further 270° rotation, so that the ileocecal junction comes to lie in the right iliac fossa.

While the duodenum and the right colon are contiguous to the posterior abdominal wall, the small intestine is free in the abdominal cavity and tethered to its posterior aspect by the widely extended mesentery.

Anatomy (fig. 1)

The small intestine is made up of loops that are relatively mobile within the abdominal cavity between two segments attached to the posterior abdominal wall: the duodenum and the right colon. The small intestine is approximately 3 m long in living humans, and up to twice as long after death as its walls lose their tone.

The duodenum and the jejunum join at the ligament of Treitz located to the left of the spine at the level of the L1-L2 intervertebral space. The jejunal loops are 2.5 cm wide and lie in the left abdomen. They lead to the ileal loops, which lie partly in the pelvic cavity, where the terminal ileum courses obliquely and cephalad into the right iliac fossa as the ileocolic valve connects it to the medial aspect of the right colon. The width of the ileal loops is slightly narrower than that of the jejunal loops, measuring 2 cm in their terminal portion. The opening of the ileocecal valve is 1 cm wide and delimited by two more or less prominent lips, the upper one being up to 3 cm thick. There is wide anatomical variability in the location of the small bowel loops.

The small intestine is attached to the posterior parietal peritoneum by the mesentery. The root of the mesentery stretches obliquely, caudally and to the right, from the ligament of Treitz to the ileocecal valve over about 15 cm. The mesentery is about 20 cm wide between its root and its free edge. It contains fat, blood vessels, lymphatics and nerves. The free edge of the mesentery ends in the tunica serosa, the outermost layer of the intestinal wall. Each intestinal loop thus has both a mesenteric and a free antimesenteric aspect.

The vascular supply is provided for by the superior mesenteric artery, the branches of which anastomose into arches which increase in number from the jejunum to the ileum. These arches give rise to

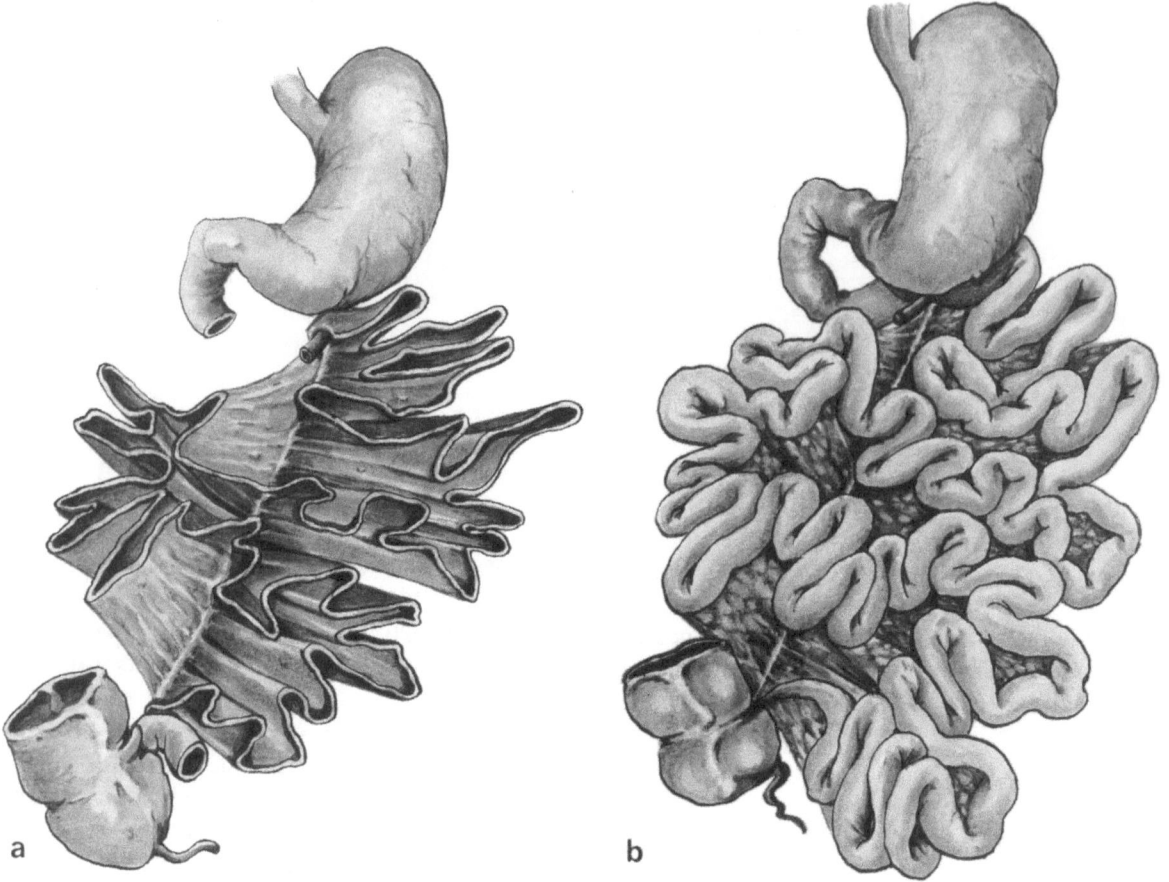

a   b

Fig. 1. a,b . Schematic drawing of **a** the mesentery and **b** the small intestine (Courtesey of D Gauthier)

straight vessels that are perpendicular to the bowel lumen. These are all of equal length and anastomose densely as they surround the intestinal loops. The lymphatics follow the course of the arteries and finally reach the lumbar and left paraaortic chains. The extrinsic innervation of the small bowel is made up of sympathetic fibres along the prevertebral nerves and of parasympathetic fibres along both vagus nerves. These fibres are monosynaptic and end in the bowel wall within the plexuses of Meissner and Auerbach.

Histology (fig. 2)

The walls of the small intestine appear macroscopically as dense folds. These are known as the valvulae conniventes or Kerkring's folds and are about 5 mm high. They are numerous in the jejunum, but progressively decrease in number as they disappear completely in the terminal ileum. The folds are covered with many little projections or villi, which are initially 0.5 mm high and 0.2 mm wide; these become progressively smaller from the jejunum to the ileum. The small intestine contains an estimated 10 million such villi.

The histological study of the intestinal wall shows that it is made up of 4 layers, the mucosa with its lamina propria, the submucosa, the muscularis and the serosa. Kerkring's folds include the first 2 layers; their axis is formed by the submucosa.

The mucosa includes the villi and the crypts of Lieberkühn. Each of the villi is made up of connective, vascular and lymphatic tissue (the lamina propria) with an epithelial margin that includes enterocytes, goblet cells and rare neuroendocrine cells. Every enterocyte carries a brush border comprised of about 1700 microvilli, each about one micron in length. Lymphocytes migrating from the lamina propria are found between the enterocytes. The epithelium is separated from the lamina propria by a basement membrane. The lamina propria con-

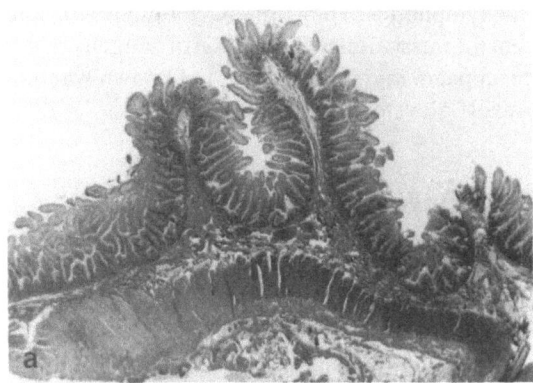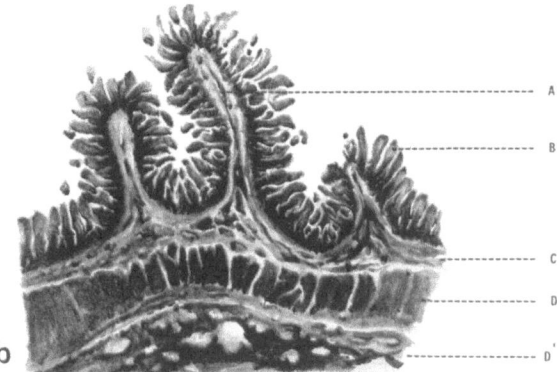

Fig. 2. a Photomicrograph of a section through the wall of the small intestine, **b** corresponding drawing : A : Kerkring's folds or valves, B: mucosa with villous folds, C : submucosa containing blood and lymph vessels and Meissner's plexus, D and D' : circular (D) and longitudinal (D') layers of the muscularis

tains lymphoid follicles (which if grouped are called Peyer's patches), plasmocytes, macrophages and eosinophils. The openings of the crypts of Lieberkühn lie between the villi. The crypts are also lined with epithelium; it is here where the enterocytes arise and where argentaffin endocrine cells and Paneth cells are found. The muscularis mucosae separating the mucosa and the submucosa is made up of an elastic network of smooth muscle cells.

The submucosa contains connective tissue and is rich in elastic fibres, blood vessels, lymphatics, nonmyelinated nerve fibres and ganglia which compose Meissner's plexuses. Lymphocytes and other immunological cells are also found in this layer.

The muscularis is made up of two layers of smooth muscle, a thick internal layer of circular fibres and an external layer of longitudinal fibres. Sympathetic and parasympathetic nerve fibres form the Auerbach's plexuses found between these two layers.

The serosa is in continuity with the mesentery.

Physiology

Motility

The motility of the small intestine is completely autonomous. A contraction arises in endogenous small bowel pace-maker cells. The rate of propagation of the impulse among the cells of the muscular layers is one to two centimeters per second. Segmental contractions occur in the circular muscular layer in order to mix the intestinal contents, which are forwarded

by peristaltic contractions originating in both muscular layers. Measurement of electric activity shows that muscular cells have a fluctuating resting membrane potential, while the intermittent action potential spikes cause contraction of the circular fibres and emptying of the intestine.

Activity in the postprandial period is characterized by propulsive contractions. Distention at one point causes active contraction upstream and relaxation downstream. During all other periods, a cyclical peristaltic activity is observed from the duodenum to the ileum, forming the migrating motor complex which propagates at a rate of a few centimeters per minute.

The motor activity of the small intestine is modulated by the sympathetic nervous system, which has an inhibiting action and contracts the sphincters, and by the usually excitatory parasympathetic system, through neuromediators (norepinephrine, acetylcholine, serotonin, VIP, substance P...) and several hormonal factors (gastrin, secretin, CCK-PZ, insulin, motilin, neurotensin, glucagon, thyroxin, serotonin, prostaglandins...).

Absorption

The absorptive surface is very large, as the total surface of the folds, villi and microvilli reaches 300 to 500 m². Absorption occurs mainly in the epithelial enterocytes of the jejunum. These cells have a very short life span, and turn over every 48 h.

Absorption occurs passively for water and some vitamins, yet involves active processes for most other nutrients, such as electrolytes, sugars, aminoacids and lipids. Almost all these elements are taken up by the capillaries. Long-chain fatty acids, triglycerides and cholesterol are taken up by lymphatics because of their large volume.

The site of absorption differs according to the nutrients: sugars, lipids, aminoacids, folate and most vitamins are absorbed in the duodenum and the jejunum; calcium is taken up in the duodenum and the proximal jejunum in presence of vitamin D. Iron absorption occurs in the duodenum, and vitamin B12 and biliary salts absorption in the ileum. Electrolytes and water are absorbed throughout the small intestine.

Secretion

Several intracellular enzymes active in protein, carbohydrate and lipid digestion are released into the intestinal lumen by cell desquamation. Moreover, epithelial cells secrete enterokinase and invertin, to which are added the enzymatic secretions of the normal microbial flora. Other substances are secreted hormonally, including enteroglucagon, which may have a trophic effect on the intestinal epithelium, histamine (secreted by mast cells), serotonin (secreted by enterochromaffin cells), villikinin, and perhaps also secretin, CCK-PZ, VIP and motilin.

Immune function

The walls of the small intestine contain many immune cells, mainly B lymphocytes but also T lymphocytes, macrophages, polymorphonuclear and mast cells. These cells are mainly found in the lamina propria and the submucosa, more specifically in the Peyer's patches of the terminal ileum, and in the epithelium. The macrophages phagocyte antigens, and inform the lymphocytes about their configuration. The T lymphocyte maturation takes place in the thymus; these play a cytotoxic role in tissue immunity. The more numerous B lymphocytes are formed in the bone marrow and participate in humoral immunity. They differentiate into plasmocytes responsible for the secretion of immunoglobulins. These are polypeptides made up of two heavy chains (divided into 5 classes, A, G, M, D and E), and two light chains according to their structure. The immunoglobulins found in the gut are mainly IgA (composed of two heavy alpha chains and two light chains) and, to a lesser extent, IgM and IgG. The IgA molecules are secreted into the intestinal lumen, the blood vessels and the lymphatics. They limit bacterial growth, and prevent the intracellular penetration of antigens. Their action appears regional, and it is not known whether they exert a systemic effect.

Clinical findings

The importance and diversity of functions of the small intestine account for its varied pathological phenomena. The contribution of the radiologist depends on the indication for the examination:
- In the case of a partial occlusion, of Koenig's syndrome, or of a malabsorption syndrome, the small bowel follow-through is abnormal in 50% of cases.
- Gastrointestinal bleeding involves the small bowel in only 5 to 10% of cases. Barium studies should be performed only when gastroduodenal and colonic examinations are found to be negative. In these instances, however, radiologists should be especially vigilant as the origin of the hemorrhage is most often found in the small intestine.
- Only 5% of small bowel follow-through for indications of a palpable abdominal mass or abdominal pain yield positive findings.

Physiologic testing

Some relatively simple tests point to disease in the small intestine:
- Stool examination:
    . weight (usually less than 400 g/day, or 1% of body weight),
    . stool fat quantification (normally less than 2.5 g/day): steatorrhea of over 5g/day signals pancreatic, biliary or jejunoileal dysfunction;
    . fecal nitrogen excretion: creatorrhea begins at 1.5 g/day in pancreatic insufficiency and malabsorption;
    . fecal sodium loss in excess of 15 meq/day usually signals disease of the small intestine.
- Transit time is measured by the carmine red test; the dye is usually eliminated within 24 h.
- The D-xylose test specifically studies jejunal malabsorption in the absence of hepatic or renal insufficiency. The patient ingests 25 g of D-xylose dissolved in 500 ml of water. Malabsorptive states are associated with 5-h urine excretion less than 2.5 g (normal excretion should exceed 4 g).
- Lack of absorption of labelled vitamin B12 bound to the intrinsic factor (Schilling's test) indicates ileal disease or intestinal bacterial overgrowth. In these

cases, the 24-h urine excretion is less than 7% of the ingested dose.
- The various deficiencies that can be seen in malabsorptive states are assessed by measurements of the serum protein, iron, vitamin B12, calcium, and folic acid levels, as well as the red blood cell count and the prothrombin time. The decrease in the level of folic acid is a sign of duodenojejunal involvement. The decrease in proteins due to loss in the gut (protein-losing enteropathy) can be assessed by the measurement of the excretion of labelled albumin over 6 days, which is normally lower than 1% of the absorbed quantity, or by the more recent technique of alpha-1-antitrypsin clearance.
- Immunoelectrophoresis is useful in diseases affecting the immune system.
- Intestinal bacterial overgrowth is determined by quantifying the bacterial content after a protected jejunal intubation. The colony counts normally number less than 10^5/ml. Another method is a respiratory test based on the decarboxylation of labelled biliary salts which measures the expired CO_2 after the ingestion of labelled glycocholic acid.

Endoscopic studies

Endoscopic examination of the small intestine is usually confined to the first jejunal loop and to the terminal ileum. Besides direct visualisation, the intubation of the small bowel makes it possible to collect aspirates which may be useful for diagnosis. Biopsies of the jejunum allow for the assessment of the height and number of villi, and the presence of pathological cells in the lamina propria. These also permit enzymatic and immunological studies, as well as the identification of parasites (giardia). Biopsies of the terminal ileum can yield a diagnosis of Crohn's disease, tuberculosis, lymphoma, carcinoid tumour, etc.

Radionuclide scanning

The measurement of radioactivity in stools following the injection of Chromium[51] tagged red blood cells indicates the presence and extent of even a minute GI bleed.

The injection of Technetium labelled red blood cells allows for localization of the origin of a GI bleed in 25 to 45% of cases. The uptake of radioactivity at the point of bleeding is pinpointed by a camera within one hour following the injection. Delayed scanning (up to 24 h after the injection) can be useful in intermittent hemorrhage. Although this method provides less precise localization than arteriography, it is twice as sensitive and produces less ionizing radiation (about 1 rad).

The use of technetium scanning in Meckel's diverticulum is discussed in chapter II.

Plain film of the abdomen (figs. 3 to 5)

Plain films of the abdomen are always taken before a small bowel examination. They are recorded on a 36 x 43 size film with a low penetration (60 to 70 kV) with the patient lying in the supine position. A small quantity of air is generally visible within the small bowel loops. Greater quantities of air are not always pathological, especially in elderly or bedridden patients. Various abnormal patterns of gas distribution may be noted by the radiologist:
- Distension of a gas-filled bowel loop beyond 3 cm should initiate a careful search for air-fluid levels on upright or lateral decubitus films. This appearance suggests obstruction, but air-fluid levels without gaseous distension can also be observed in diarrhea.
- Thickened folds seen due to gas contrast point to inflammatory or ischemic diseases.
- An abnormal opacity in the abdomen in association with the displacement of gas-filled intestinal loops suggests a tumor mass or a fluid collection (abscess or cyst). Calcifications are sometimes visible within a tumour mass.
- The appearance of a gas collection with festooned contours, displacing neighbouring loops of bowel, sometimes located within an abnormal opacity, may be seen with lymphomas, leiomyosarcomas or metastases.
- A localized and heterogeneous opacity with a striped or mottled appearance may indicate a phytobezoar or a residual postoperative foreign body. If the image contains small air bubbles, it may also represent an abscess. Intraluminal serpiginous densities amidst intestinal gas suggest the diagnosis of ascariasis.
- A round calcification located in the usual course of the small intestine with proximal dilatation suggests gallstone ileus, especially when it is associated with pneumobilia. In the absence of the latter finding, it

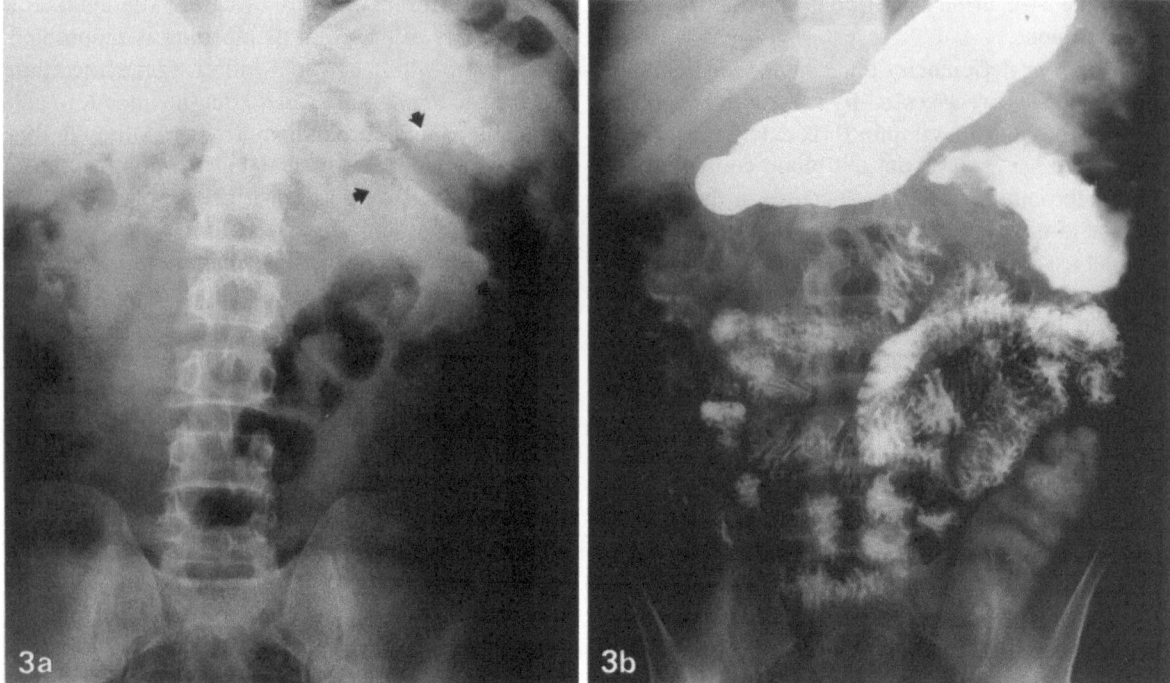

Fig. 3. a,b Plain abdominal film. **a** gas in the left hypochondrium forms a lucency with irregular contours. **b** The corresponding lesion is outlined after barium administration (lymphoma)

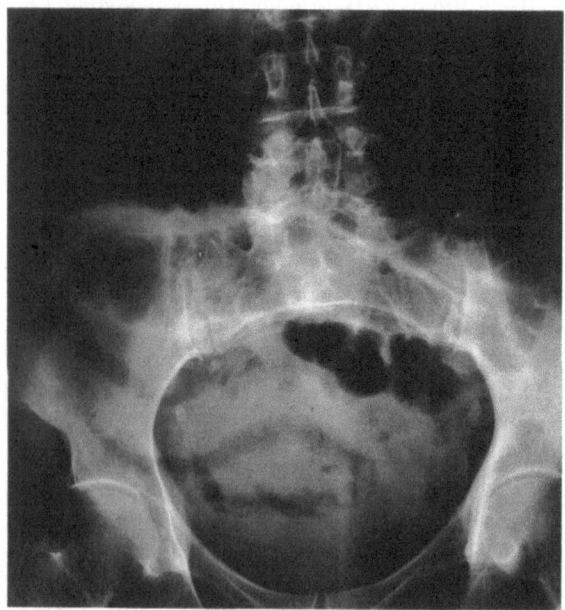

Fig. 4. Plain abdominal film. Gas has distended the jejunum because of a long ribbon stenosis of an ileal loop within a pelvic opacity: this is an intrumural hematoma caused by anticoagulant therapy

may be caused by another type of foreign body (a fruit pit for instance).

- The scattered calcifications of a vascular malformation or the string of gas bubbles seen in pneuma-

tosis cystoides intestinalis are only rarely observed.
- Lastly, plain radiographs can show vascular or nodal calcifications, hepatomegaly, splenomegaly or ascites. It also allows for the study of bony structures.

In practice, any abnormal lucency or density should be noted; and, if the other abdominal organs appear uninvolved, the radiologist should proceed with the small bowel follow-through.

Barium studies of the small intestine
Barium studies remain the cornerstone of the radiology of the small intestine.

History

Small quantities of barium suspension were formerly used for fear of having the opacified loops superimposed on each other. In 1927, Pansdorf advocated «fractional meals», a method consisting of having the patient drink 30 ml of a Barium solution every 10 mn during 1 h. On the other hand, Cherigié preferred a «short index», consisting of 3 to 4 teaspoons full of a concentrated solution of barium sulfate. These techniques have the disadvantage of lasting several hours (6 to 8) and of yielding a discontinuous

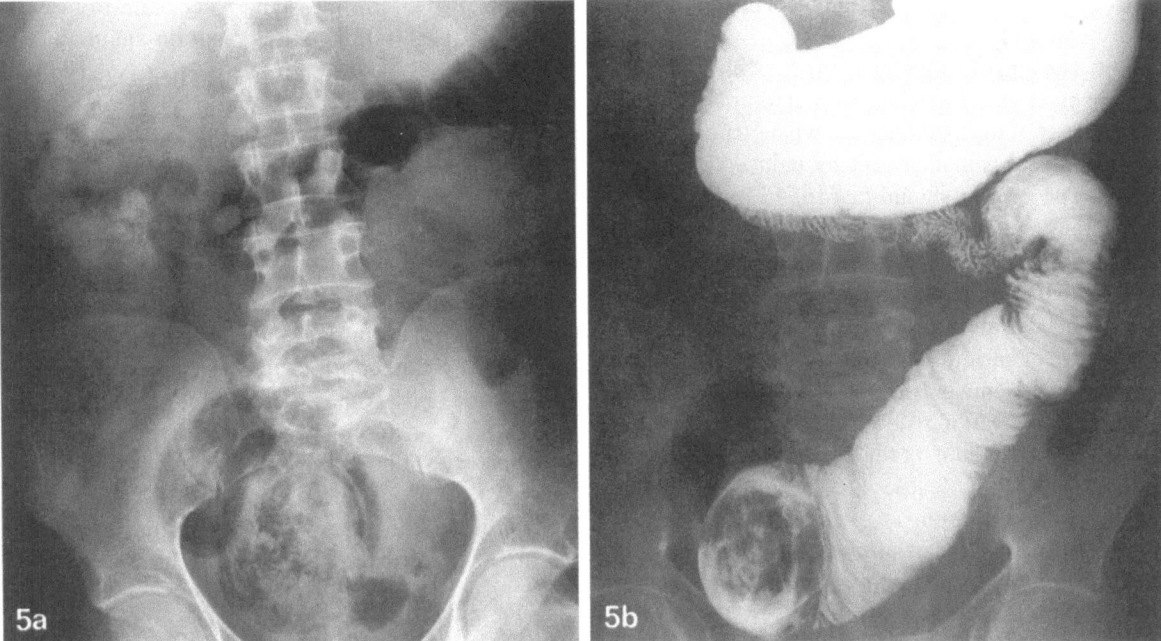

Fig. 5 a, b. Plain abdominal film. **a** The round, heterogeneous pelvic density with a fibrillar structure represents a residual postoperative sponge having migrated into the small intestine, **b** small bowel follow through (SBFT) showing jejunal dilatation proximal to the obstruction

view of the small intestine. Flocculation attributable to the small quantity of barium used and to the duration of the examination accounts for defects in the casting of the intestinal walls, which deprives the technique of much of its reliability.

These insufficiencies led the practicioners to increase the doses of barium ingested. As early as 1937, Weltz used 200 ml of barium, followed by 30 ml every 5 minutes. Prévost and De Busscher had their patients ingest 3 doses of 80 ml of barium each hour and Naumann two doses of 200 ml every half-hour. In the United States, Golden advocated a single dose of 280 ml. Marshak went one step further, recommending doses of 400 to 600 ml of a 50% barium solution. This technique was adopted and made popular in Europe by Bodart.

Several techniques have also been suggested to accelerate intestinal transit time. Weintraub and Williams resorted to the ingestion of 120 g of barium sulfate diluted in 120 ml of isotonic solution, followed by 250 ml of ice-cold saline twice 5 minutes apart. Porcher and Caroli added 30 g of Sorbitol to the barium solution. For his cineradiographic views, Morin used cholecystokinin. Grivaux and Kreel accelerated the duodenojejunal transit time by also administering parenteral metoclopramide, Margulis used the enterokinetic effect of neostigmine.

In 1929, Pesquera brought forth a new imaging technique by advocating an opaque small bowel enema after duodenal intubation. The interest for enteroclysis grew as evidenced by the works of Gershon-Cohen en 1939, Schatzki en 1943, and Tavernier in France. In 1950, Friedmann used a modified Miller-Abbott tube with an inflatable balloon to perform a double-contrast study of the small intestine. After a certain latent period, the technique of enteroclysis became popular again as evidenced in 1976 by the publications of Sellink, who advocated the infusion of a contrast medium after intubation of the small bowel to the ligament of Treitz by a Dotter-Bilbao tube. He aslo defined more precisely the indications for this study. Several French authors have since adopted a similar approach, including Clément and Burelle, Fournier, Loubière, Vidal, Schmutz, etc.

Present techniques

The current barium examinations of the small intestine are based on two principles : filling and palpation of all the intestinal loops in a relatively short time.

Filling is aimed at obtaining a continuous and simultaneous image of the entire small intestine. It can be obtained either by small bowel follow-through or by enteroclysis.

The aim of palpation is to dissociate, collapse, and displace each intestinal loop. It represents the essential part of the examination, whatever the method of filling, and is made easier by induced hypotonia.

The subject should fast for 12 h after having taken four 5 mg tablets of bisacodyl (Contalax). The contrast medium is a solution (weight-volume 100/100) of Micropaque diluted in water (40 % Micropaque, 60 % water). The only two contraindications for the use of barium sulfate are intestinal perforation and colonic stenosis because of the risks of barium plugging (the latter risk being absent in the small intestine). Iodinated products provide insufficient contrast and may cause electrolytic imbalances, especially in children.

In France, the examination is usually performed on a "universal" remote-controlled table fitted with an undertable image intensifyer. Palpation is ensured by a Holzknecht manual compression device. The radiographs are exposed at 125 KV tension with a 0,6 mm focus. Image intensifyer photographs, if available, are a good substitute for the 24 x 30 films divided in 2 or 4, as discussed later.

Small bowel follow-through

The contrast medium is distributed into 3 glasses, each one containing 300 ml of the suspension. Once the patient has ingested the contents of the first glass and as soon as duodenal opacification occurs, a radiograph of the stomach 24 x 30 and one or two sets of duodenal images (24 x 30 films divided in 4) are taken in the prone position under compression by a partly inflated rubber balloon. Additional views are taken if required in the absence of previous gastroduodenal examinations.

The patient then drink the contents of the second glass and lies in the right lateral decubitus position to improve gastric emptying. A 24 x 30 radiograph of the first jejunal loops is taken 5 min later with the patient lying in the supine position slighty on the right. The patient then resumes the right lateral decubitus position.

The first overhead view, labelled D1 (30 x 40, 35 x 35 or 36 x 43 according to the patient's build) is taken at the 10 th minute, preferably in the supine position to prevent the lower edge of the stomach from concealing the proximal jejunal loops. If the ileum is not yet opacified, the patient ingests the contents of the third glass and places him-or herself in the right lateral decubitus position again.

Overhead radiographs (labelled D2, D3 and D4) are taken in the prone position at the 20th, 30th and if need be, the 60 th minute. Light compression is ensured by an incompletely inflated 20 cm rubber balloon, which spreads apart the intestinal loops. Beetwen radiographs, the loops are palpated under fluoroscopic monitoring. Any abnomality is recorded on spot films (24 x 30 size divided in 2 or 4). As soon as the terminal ileum is opacified, a set of radiographs is taken with appropriate compression in both prone and supine positions. This latter examination prior to the injection of the hypotonic agent is necessary : although hypotonia does provide more information, if the terminal ileum is at the stage of evacuation at the time of injection, it may thereafter be difficult to obtain satisfactory filling.

Hypotonia is induced by the intravenous injection of 15 mg of tiemonium (3 ampoules of Viscéralgine®) or, if this is contraindicated (glaucoma, urinary retention), 1mg of glucagon. Other sets of radiographs of the terminal ileum are taken in the same manner as previously described. The entire small intestine is then palpated under fluoroscopic monitoring, following the winding course of the loops with the Holzknecht device as would a surgeon, letting the segments slide between the fingers. Each loop should be separated from the neighbouring ones by the Holzknecht device, which assesses its flexibility and mobility and ensures a balanced compression of its contents - essential for the proper visualization of the mucosal pattern. Once the course of the small intestine has been examined from the ligament of Treitz to the ileocecal valve, its entire path should be retraced to make sure that no bend has escaped palpation. A number of radiographs are taken during this operation (24 x 30 size divided in 2 or 4) to confirm that the examination is carried out properly.

Several difficulties may arise during the examination :
- The reluctance of nauseated patients to ingest the contrast medium is usually overcome by persuasion. Gastric stasis requires the administration of two spoonfuls of metoclopramide syrup (Primperan®).
- Ileal stasis observed after the 30th minute can be overcome by inducing peristalsis again, either with the ingestion of a fourth dose of barium (with the addition of Primperan if the patient has not yet received any) or with the intravenous injection of 0,5 mg of neostigmine (one ampoule of Prostigmine®)

in the absence of any contraindications such as arterial hypertension or coronary insufficiency.

- If delayed transit is observed at the 60 th minute in spite of a neostigmine injection, the patient should be asked to swallow the contents of an additional glass of Micropaque® or, in some cases, of ice-cold water in order to avoid hyperconcentration and flocculation of the contrast medium.

- It is frequently impossible to dissociate or palpate the pelvic loops in the supine position in thin patients. These are better seen by studying the patient in the prone position under compression by a rather thick, well inflated rubber balloon, with the patient in forced expiration and in the Trendelenburg position. For greater efficiency, inclination in this position ought to be more than 20°. If this fails, filling of the bladder, accomplished by the intravenous injection of 20 mg of furosemide (one ampoule of Lasilix®) usually frees the pelvic loops. A shoot-through lateral view is sometimes needed to visualize a loop lying behind the bladder.

- It is sometimes interesting to resort to retrograde insufflation of the ileum by air with a rectal tube. This complements the examination, requires only a couple of minutes to perform, and is usually well tolerated by the patients. It provides good double contrast images of the terminal ileum.

These ancillary techniques should be used only when they are necessary. Intestinal transit acceleration, specifically, may cause functional, motor and· secretory disorders. These are usually not a major problem as they are suppressed by the injection of tiemonium ; the important aim is opacification of the ileocecal region in less than one hour.

When necessary, a double contrast barium swallow can be carried out at the end of the examination with the ingestion of effervescent salts and high-density barium.

Enteroclysis

Enteroclysis consists in the regular, continous infusion of large quantities of opaque contrast medium (1000 to 1500 ml) into the distal duodenum or the proximal jejunum by means of a tube, in order to perform an opaque enema of the entire small intestine.

The duodenal enema is administered through a 120 cm long radioopaque Dotter-Bilbao tube with an outer diameter of 5 mm. Its distal end has 6 lateral holes and contains an opaque. sphere. A flexible, radioopaque guide can be inserted through the internal lumen to the distal end to stiffen the tube.

Brief explanations should be given to the patient about the procedure and its indication. With the patient lying in the supine position, the lubricated tube is inserted through a nare into the pharynx. The tube is then swallowed into the hypopharynx, and passes into the esophagus ans stomach. Under fluoroscopic monitoring, the tube and its guide are progressively pushed along the greater curvature of the stomach down to the pylorus. The guide is then pulled back one centimeter, and the patient is asked to perform exaggerated respiratory excursions with his/her abdominal muscles. The end of the tube then advances through the pylorus and the duodenal bulb. The guide is progessively withdrawn as the tube progresses in the duodenum and distally to the ligament of Treitz. With experience, the positioning of the tube requires only a few minutes.

The insertion may pose a number of problems:
- The oral route can be used in case of nasal obstruction, but is generally less well tolerated.
- If the tube is stopped by the posterior wall of the pharynx or goes down into the trachea, swallowing some water may make its passage into the esophagus easier.
- If the tube is curled in the fundus or body of the stomach and causes nausea, it must be made to slide along the greater curvature while the patient is standing in an upright position. To do so, the gastric air bubble may need to be aspirated.
- If the tube does not progress through the pylorus, administration of 20 to 40 ml of barium visualizes the axis of the pylorus and the duodenal bulb. The tube may thus be reorientated with the help of the palpating device, with the patient lying in the right posterior decubitus position. Alternatively, the repositioning may be done with the help of a properly placed compression balloon with the patient in the prone position. Similar manoeuvres can help the tube progress through the duodenum;all of these may be facilitated by tilting the examination table to a near-vertical position.
- Once the final position has been reached, it may be useful to pull the tube back a couple of centimeters before fixing it to the nare, in order to straighten out the gastric coil which may cause the tube to slip out of the duodenum during the examination.
- In case the tube should not go any further than the distal duodenum, the patient must not be displaced during the opacification and remains in the left posterior oblique supine position.

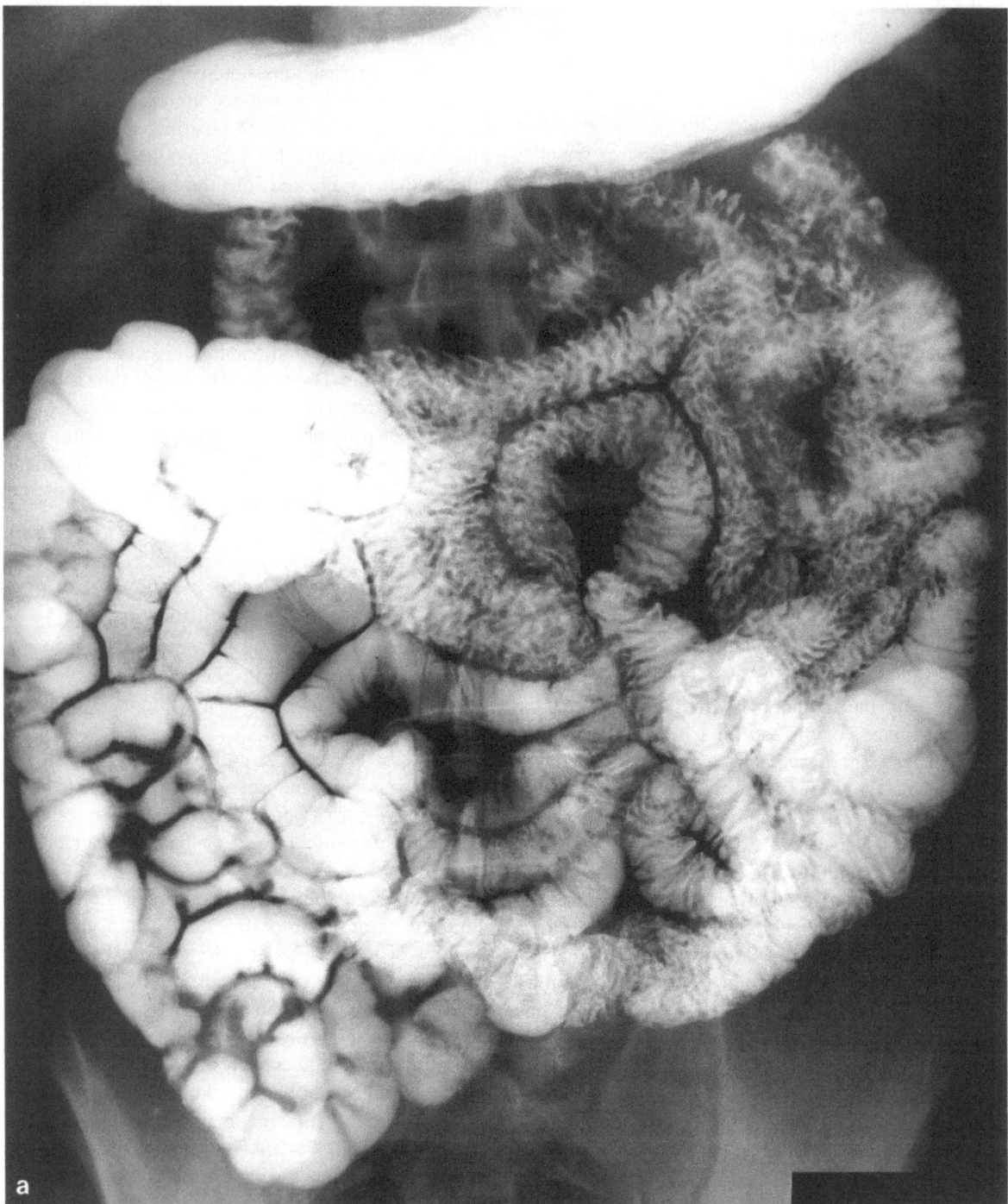

Fig. 6 a-e. Small bowell follow-through. **a** Overhead view of the small intestina, **b** normal jejunum, **c** normal ileum, **d** normal terminal ileum, ▶
e same segment after drug-induced hypotonia

Fig. 7 a, b. Advantages of induced hypotonia. **a** The terminal ileum in a young patient, **b** demonstration of lymphoid follicles in the terminal ▶
ileum of that same patient after drug-induced hypotonia

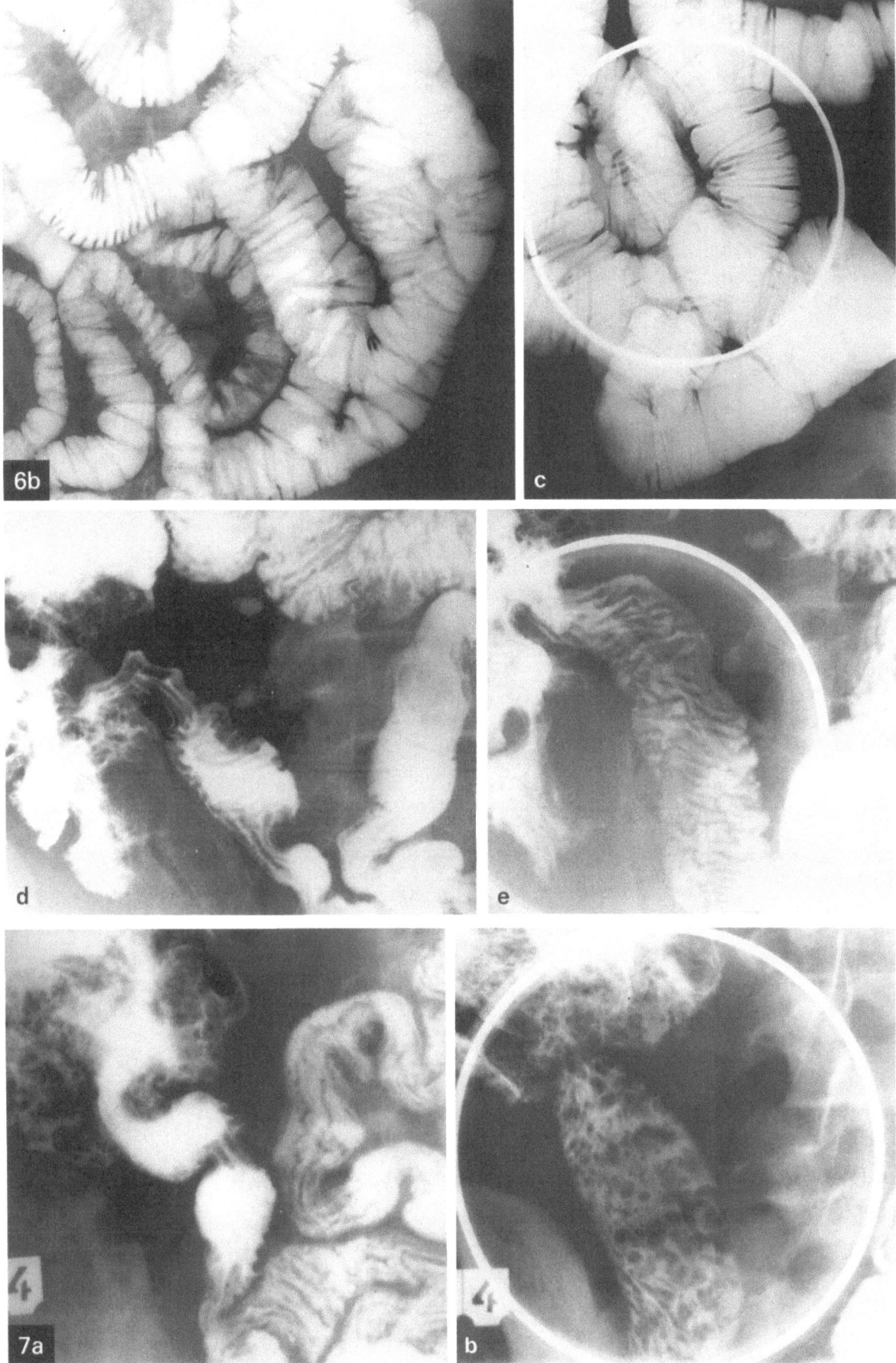

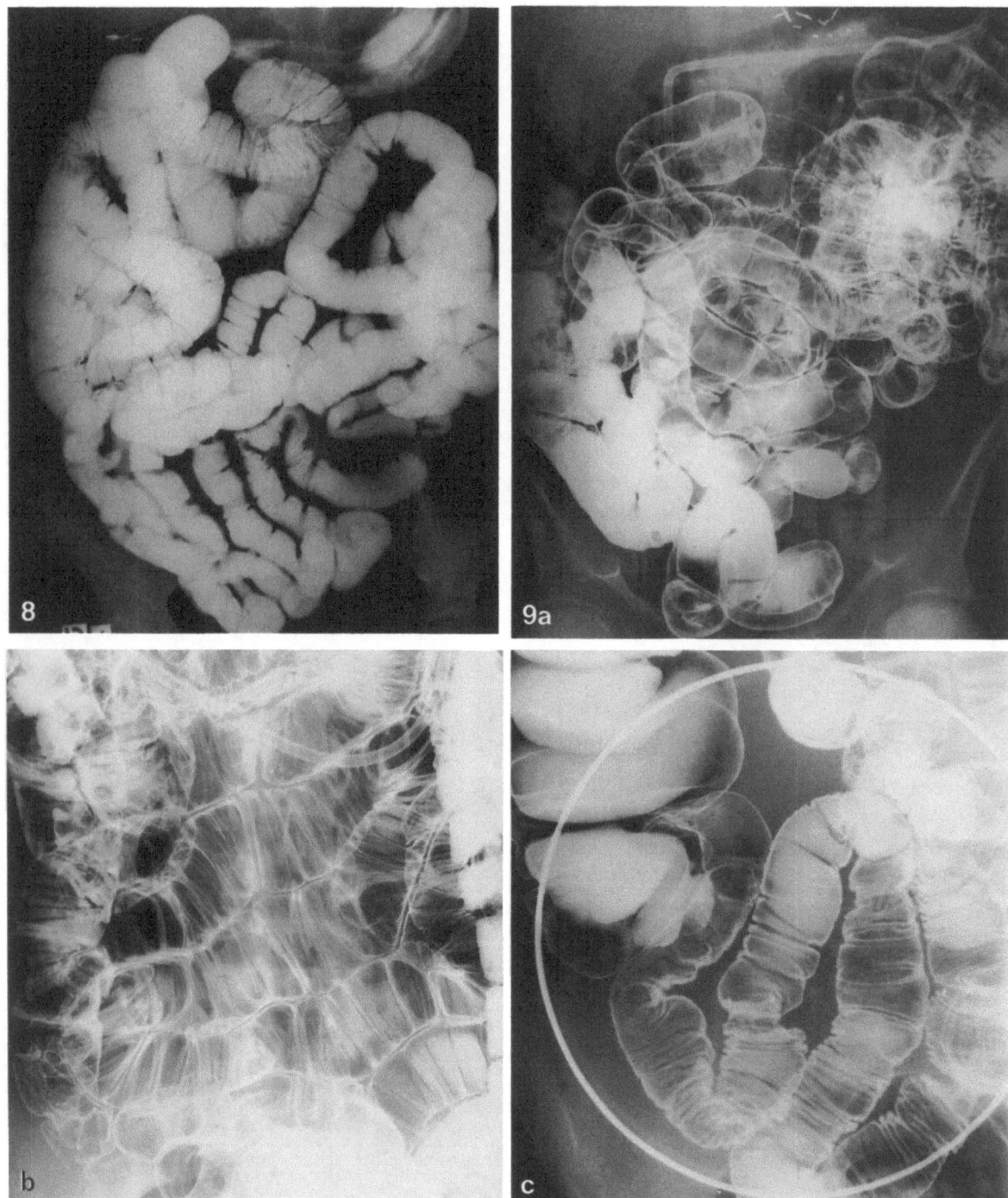

Fig. 8. Enteroclysis. Overhead view of the small intestine

Fig. 9 a-c. Double air contrast enteroclysis. **a** Overhead view, **b** normal jejunum, **c** normal ileum

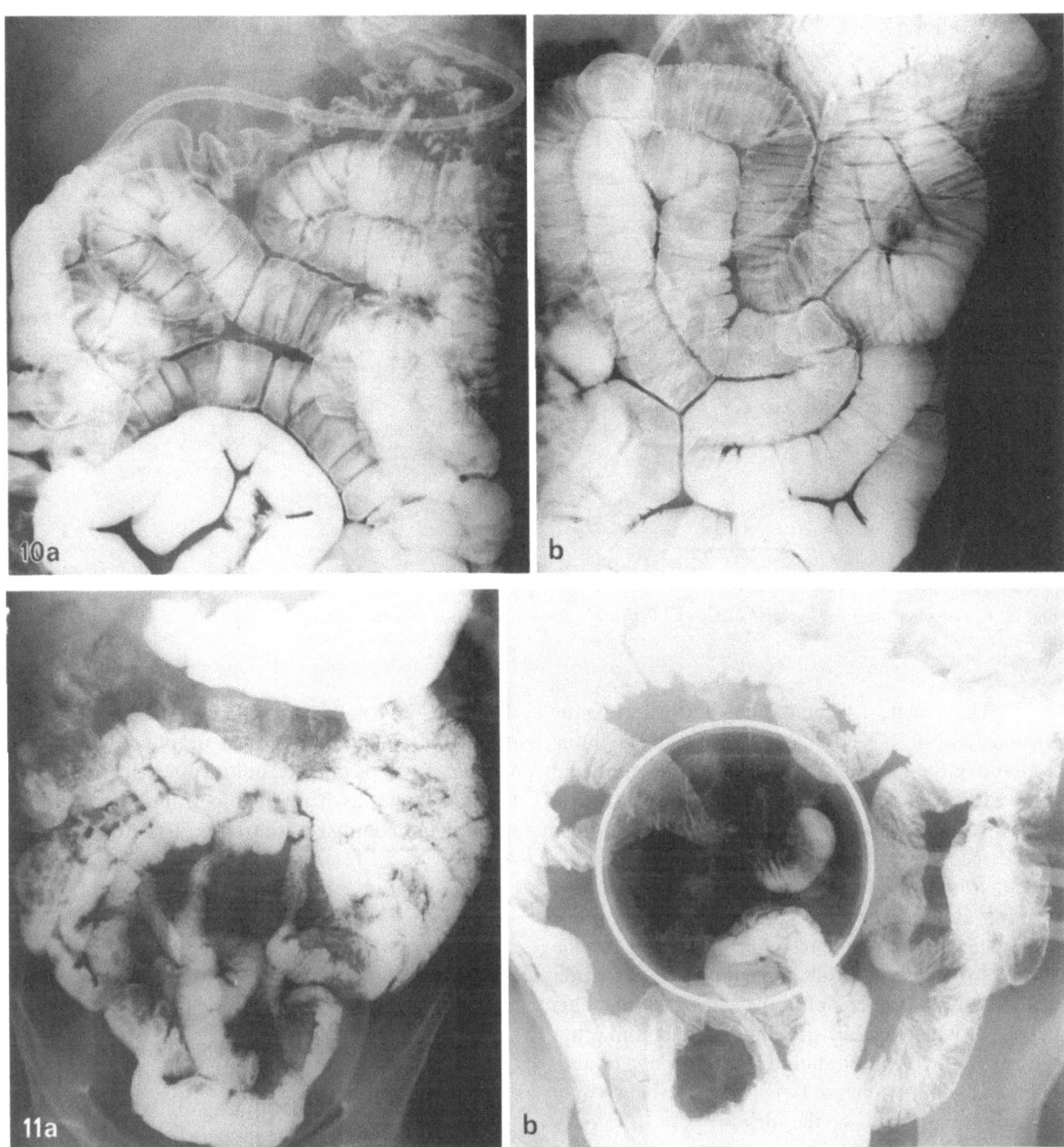

Fig. 10 a, b. Double contrast enteroclysis. **a** With water showing a normal jejunum, **b** with methylcellulose outlining a normal jejunum

Fig. 11 a, b. Results of compression. **a** Overhead view of apparently normal small intestinal loops, **b** spot film with compression demonstrating a Meckel's diverticulum

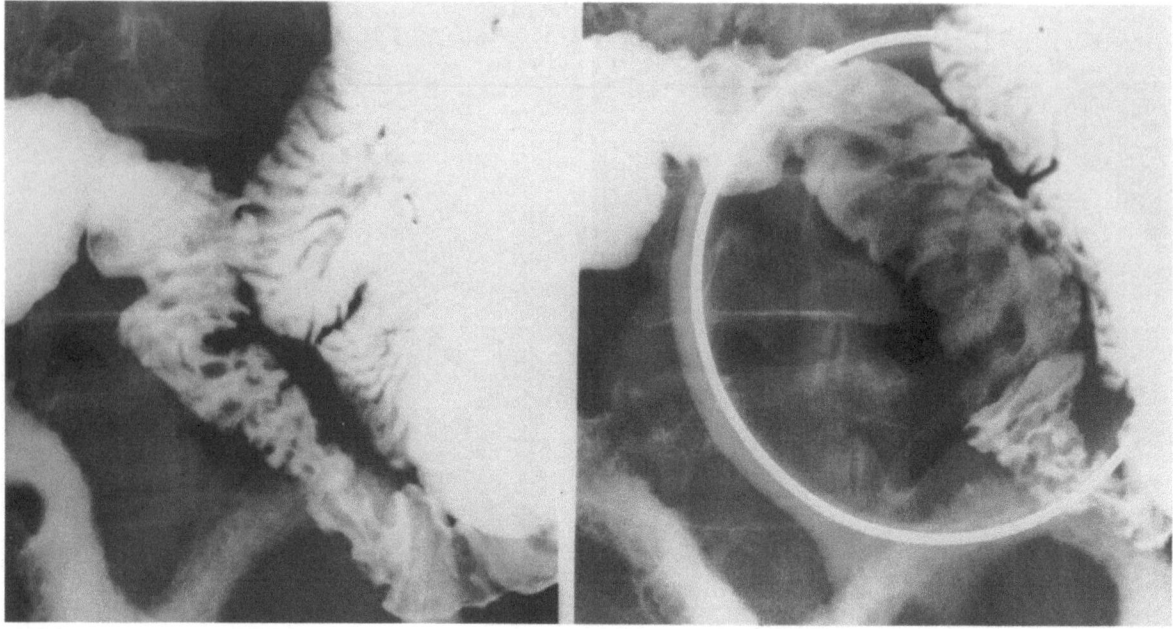

Fig. 12. Results of compression : aphtoid ulcerations in Crohn's disease (right) that were not otherwise visible (left)

The plastic bag containing the Micropaque suspension (40 % Micropaque, 60 % water) is hung 2 m above the floor and connected to the duodenal tube with a three-way valve. The rate of infusion ranges from 90 to 100 ml/mn. The caudal progress of the opacifier is followed by fluoroscopy, and the infusion is slowed down to 20 ml/mn when the terminal ileum is opacified. Radiographs are taken with and without compression as described for the small bowel follow-through technique, as palpation of the loops is carried out in the same fashion. This palpation is performed with induced hypotonia, but the hypotonic injection should be avoided if a double contrast examination is to be performed, since it may hamper the progress of the air.

The double contrast study is a complement to, and not a substitute for, the single contrast study. It can be performed by replacing the contrast medium in the container by water at an infusion of 120 ml/ mn. In order to prevent the water from quickly flushing the deposited opaque film along the walls needed for the double contrast, the administration of 150 ml of a high-density barium suspension (EZ-HD, Telebar or Micropaque H D) is performed before the infusion of water. Some authors achieve the same goal by adding a solution of methylcellulose to the water (10 g in 250 ml of hot water, topped up by cold water to a volume of 2 l). Most achieve double contrast by insufflating gas, either with a syringe with the use of a three-way valve that allows for easy injection of the 800 to 1000 ml of air, or simply with a pump. Air must never be injected before opacification of the terminal ileum, as it might block the forward progress of the contrast by moving distal to it.

Compared advantages of both procedures

Tolerance
Most patients prefer drinking 3 glasses of barium rather than undergo the insertion of a tube through their nose. However, it is often possible to gently convince a reluctant patient, especially in a hospital setting, of the merits of the procedure. Other patients are unwilling to ingest a large quantity of barium.

The patient receives a slightly greater amount of ionizing radiation in enteroclysis, as the progress of the barium meal is directed under fluoroscopic guidance. Accidents occuring during the insertion of the tube are very rare, since the tube is immediately withdrawn if it is mistakingly guided into the trachea.

Difficulty
The difficulty in inserting a duodenal tube decreases as the radiologist becomes more experienced, but the success of the operation may be made difficult or delayed by the patient's anxiety or anatomy.

Duration of the examination
In more than 80 % of cases, the terminal ileum can be opacified in less than one hour by small bowel follow-through, with the help of the tips provided above. Enteroclysis usually shortens the duration of the examination by an average 30 min, but it requires the continuous presence of the operator, who cannot simultaneously perform another examination in a neighbouring room as with a small bowell-through.

Results
Enteroclysis has a number of *advantages* :
- It ensures a better fluoroscopic follow-up of the forward progress of the contrast medium, so that diagnostically significant morphological abnormalities can be detected during filling.
- It also produces a continuous and homogeneous image of the jejunal loops ans sometimes of the ileal loops during filling. As the barium meal exerts a constant pressure on the intestine, it rids itself of most gastric secretions which are a cause of contrast heterogeneity.
- The best indication for enteroclysis is in cases of obstructive lesions. The pressure of the infusion ensures the progress of the barium and casting of the obstruction that is not easily achieved with small bowel follow-through due to stasis. Poorly mobile loops are more readily identified by enteroclysis.
- It also permits to complete the conventional examination with a double contrast study. When performed with water, the latter produces an excellent global image of the jejunal loops ; when performed with air, it helps to dissociate the pelvic loops, whose study may be difficult during filling as they are «coiled up» behind the bladder. As we stated above, the «aeration» of the pelvic loops can be achieved in a small bowel follow-through by retrograde insufflation of the colon. Double air contrast is more useful in the study of abnormalities observed during filling rather than at their initial detection.

Enteroclysis exhibits three *disadvantages* :
- The stomach and the duodenum cannot be examined. Although such a study is theoretically possible at the end of the examination by double contrast, it is often made difficult by the distension of the bowel, especially that of the transverse colon.
- Rapid transit time may limit adequate compression of questionable lesions involving the terminal ileum seen in repletion, and the search for small ileal lesions, prior to colonic filling which partly hides the loops of small intestine and hinders their proper compression.

- The pressure of the infusion tends to mask some functional diagnostically significant signs, such as those of intussusception in celiac disease.

Practical conclusions
The small bowell follow-through technique is most often chosen in private practice since enteroclysis is not readily performed. Hospital-based radiologist choose the technique they know best. However, the patient should be convinced to undergo enteroclysis in case of a suspected obstruction, for it is the best indication for this technique.

Pediatric techniques

The concentration of the contrast medium should be decreased with decreasing age :
1/4 Micropaque for 3/4 water for children aged less than 3, 1/3-2/3 for those less than 6. Enteroclysis with special pediatric equipment is the best solution, but it is not well accepted by the patient, and therefore difficult to perform. Because of this, the small intestine is most often opacified by barium ingestion only. The quantity of barium must be dosed according to the age and weight of the child :
200 ml for children aged 6 months to 3 years,
300 ml for those between 3 and 6,
and 400 ml if the child is 6 to 10 years of age.
The dose often has to be divided into several boluses because of the child's reluctance.
Persuasion has to be used to have child accept such a quantity of barium, and lesser doses lead to a high risk of flocculation because of stasis and the duration of the examination. The addition of Primperan® syrup should be avoided since the barium meal tends to be broken up into a discontinuous, heterogeneous column in small children. The administration of tiemonium at doses adjusted for the child's age and compression solve this problem and most often allow for an adequate examination of the intestinal loops.

Normal radiological images

The *transit time* is the time elapsed from the beginning of opacification of the small intestine to that of the ileocecal region. It varies according to the technique, averaging 10 min (5 to 15 min) with enteroclysis and 45 min with small bowel follow-through (5 min to 2h).

The transit time is determined by several physiological factors and may be quite different in the same subject from one day to the next.

Peristalsis and intestinal tone are assessed on overhead views. Fewer than 2/3 of the loops are normally contracted at the same time. The fluoroscopic examination is necessary to follow the progress of the barium meal, as well as the amplitude and rate of propagation of the peristaltic waves. Peristalsis is reduced by tiemonium and increased by metoclopramide and neostigmine, which may be administered during the examination. The latter drugs may induce the fragmentation of the barium column, especially in the ileum.

The position of the intestinal loops exhibits constant features. On radiographs, these lie between the liver, the stomach, and the spleen cranially (the anatomical limit being the transverse mesocolon, whose transverse margin can sometimes be approximated). The other surrounding structures include the colon (right and left) laterally, and the outline of the rectum and the bladder, caudally.

The mesentery is not visible on radiographs, but its root follows an oblique line stretching from the left edge of the 2nd lumbar vertebra to the right sacroiliac joint. The concavity of a loop relative to this line marks its mesenteric edge. The ligament of Treitz occupies a constant position, lying lateral and to the left of the L1-L2 disc space.

The first *jejunal* loops are stacked in the left hypochondrium and the distal jejunal loops in the midabdominal region, the left flank and often the right hypochondrium. The transition between jejunum and ileum is gradual. The ileal loops are located in the lower part of the abdomen and in the pelvic cavity. Their position varies much according to the subject's morphology and to the fullness of the bladder. The loops are located in the pelvis in thin subjects, especially when the bladder is not full, making their examination difficult, while they project into the periumbilical region in obese subjects. The course of the terminal ileum is an oblique one, oriented cranially and to the right, ending at the medial aspect of the cecum, or sometimes at its posterior or lateral margins. The ileocecal valve lies lateral to the superior part of the right sacroiliac joint, but its position is not constant as in some patients, the cecum may be found in the pelvis or under the liver.

The intestinal loops are arranged in regular congruous curves of short radii, which are superimposed with little space between them. The *interloop width* is measured between two contiguous loops filled with barium. This space is usually 2 to 3 mm wide, but may be more in obese subject. Normal anatomical imprints can be observed where the intestine abuts the spine, the bladder, and the sigmoid loops. The small intestine averages 3 m in length. Distances are difficult to measure when a lesion is to be pinpointed in view of surgery.

The density of the contrast medium is homogeneous and uniform over all segments during the examination. However, it may decrease at the head of the column of barium due to contact with digestive juices, food particles or air bubbles.

The width of a normal jejunal loop filled with barium ranges from 25 to 30 mm in a small bowel follow-through and reaches 40 mm during enteroclysis, although it usually decreases once the infusion of contrast has ceased. The ileal loops are 15 to 25 mm and 25 to 30 mm wide respectively for each technique. The width of the loops decreases naturally when contraction waves pass, and their average caliber increases after a hypotonic agent has been administered. The width of the terminal ileum tapers gradually and approximates 1 cm near the medial edge of the cecum (1)

The jejunal folds are oriented perpendicularly to the intestinal axis. They are narrowly spaced with parallel margins and although slightly curved, these appear almost straight with enteroclysis. They feel supple on palpation and are not flattened by moderate compression. The ileal folds are not as numerous and less well defined. With a tangential incidence, the folds form indentations becoming slightly broader towards the outer part of the loop. The folds become oriented longitudinally during contraction waves. The loops are sometimes seen during evacuation with single contrast technique. The folds intertwine to form a meshwork of curved lines with an average thickness of 2 mm, which disappear when compression is applied.
The folds are measured at the edge of the most prominent barium-filled loops. The folds are 1 to 2 mm thick in the jejunum and 0,5 to 1 mm thick in

---

(1) The figures quoted can be measured on images taken with «remote-controlled» floor stands producing a radiological magnification that is somewhat more than that of «conventional» tables.

the ileum. Their height is assessed by measuring the depth of the mucosal indentation and ranges from 2 to 5 mm for the jejunal and 0,5 to 3 mm for the ileal loops. The folds are 2 to 5 mm apart in the jejunum, though the distance can transiently vary between 1 and 10 mm. The ileal folds are more widely spaced with an average distance between two folds of 15 mm. The values obtained for the measurement of the folds are independent of the technique used.

The terminal ileum, especially in young subjects, often bears small round nodules, 1 to 2 mm in diameter, more or less regularly distributed over the last few centimeters of ileum (lymphoid follicles), with a density fo 3 to 4/cm³. These are sometimes found 3 or 4 cm from the ileocecal valve and may coalesce to form a fairly flat, 1 to 2 cm wide stripe (Peyer's patch). Accentuation of this nodularity indicates lymphoid hyperplasia, which most often is a reaction to common infections but may sometimes be due to a specific pathological process.

In children between the ages of 1 and 3, the diameter of the loops is under 16 mm. It is under 18 mm by age 4, 20 mm at age 5, 22 mm between ages 6 and 8, and under 23 mm by age 9, according to Haworth. The folds are not visible until 3 months of age. They are less than 1 mm in width until age 1 and reach 1,5 mm by age 6 (Smith). The lymphoid follicles in the terminal ileum are usually seen.

The outlines of the *normal villi* is not visible with the techniques described, and heralds disease if present. The use of high-density barium suspensions, as in gastroduodenal radiology (EZ HD, Telebar, Micropaque HD, etc.) often makes it possible to see the normal contour of villi in the duodenum and jejunum (Gelfand). The suspension used for the stomach must be diluted in 4 to 5 parts water in order to limit overlap of the jejunal loops. Radiographs are taken with a 0,6 mm focal spot (if no 0,3 mm focal spot is available). The films are exposed at 100 to 120 kv according to the patient's build. The contour of the villi appears as finely etched dots in the luminal space, with microspiculation of the edges. In suboptimal examinations, the edges are less well defined.

Approach to the analysis of abnormal radiological images

Abnormal radiological images need to be sought, and must be interpreted according to a strict analytic ap-

proach. They must not be described haphazardly. The analytical scheme consists in fragmenting the complex X-ray appearance into radiologically pathological units which must be systematically searched for according to a preset outline. Once these have been sorted out, they have to be compiled to try and recognize a syndrome. This radiological syndrome is then compared with the corresponding clinical and biological *syndromes* to arrive at a diagnosis.

We propose the following outline for the systematic analysis of small bowel X-rays ;
1 - recognizing the position of the lesions,
2 - the presence of functional abormalities,
3 - abnormalities in position and mobility,
4 - abnormal caliber,
5 - abnormal bowel wall expansion
6 - nodular images,
7 - ulcerations and fistulae,
8 - abnormal folds,
9 - abnormal villi.

First, bone and soft tissue abnormalities must be looked for on all the films. Large-size radiographs must be displayed close to one another on the viewer. This is made easier if the radiographs are numbered in the order in which they were taken (D1, D2, D3, D4). Large-size radiographs sometimes suggest a diagnosis. In practice, they are mainly used to help the radiologist in orienting the spot films. They also provide information about functional alterations and abnormalities in position, and highlight the presence of diffuse enteropathy. The normal appearance of overhead radiographs may conceal abnormalities seen only on spot films. Abnormal features may be detected during a first rapid examination of both types of radiographs. When such a finding is obvious, that particular abnormality should be «left aside», and the films studied for the presence of other abnormalities.

Position of the lesions

The analysis begins with the study of the position of the lesions, which can be diffuse, involving several loops, whether contiguous or not, or predominate in the jejunum or ileum. They can be localised, single or multiple.

Functional abnormalities

Functional abnormalities are partially overlooked on enteroclysis.

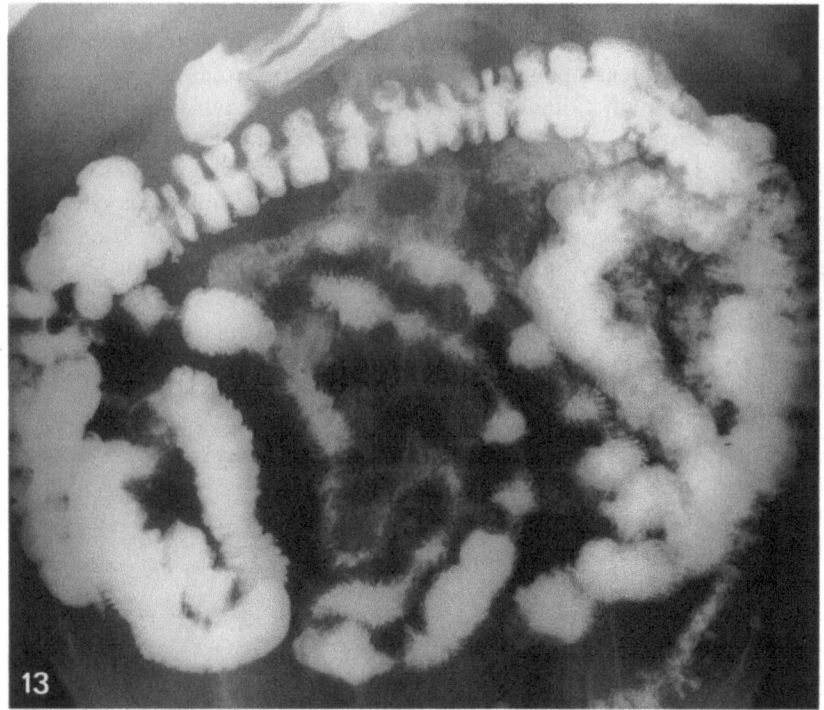

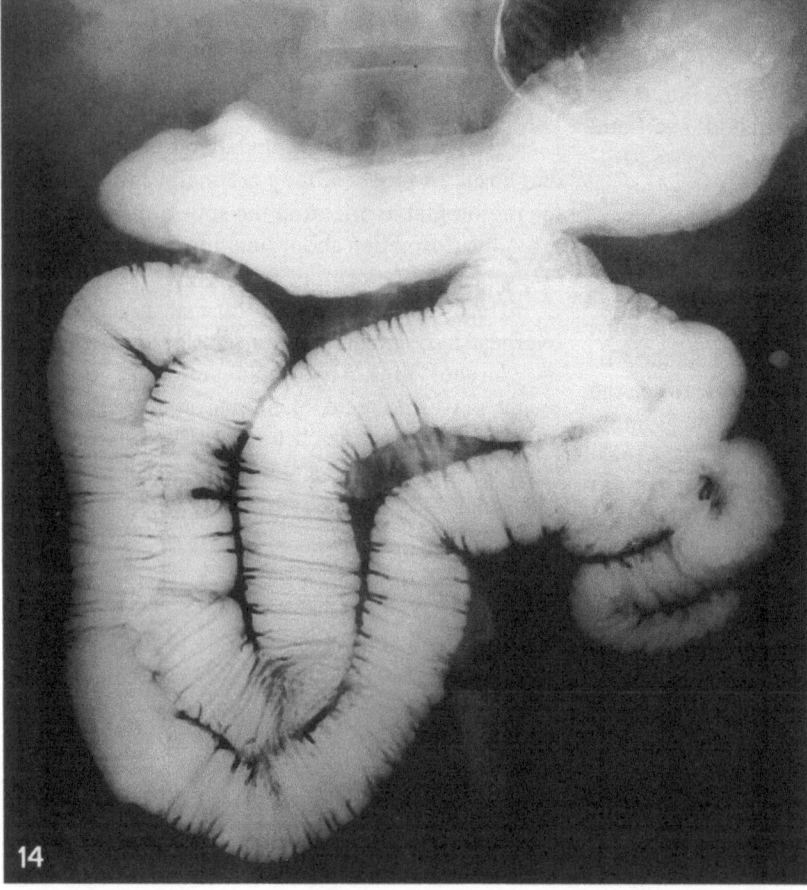

Fig. 13. Functional alterations : hyperperistalsis and diffuse hypertonia (carcinoid tumour)

Fig. 14. Functional alterations : jejunal atonia following vagotomy

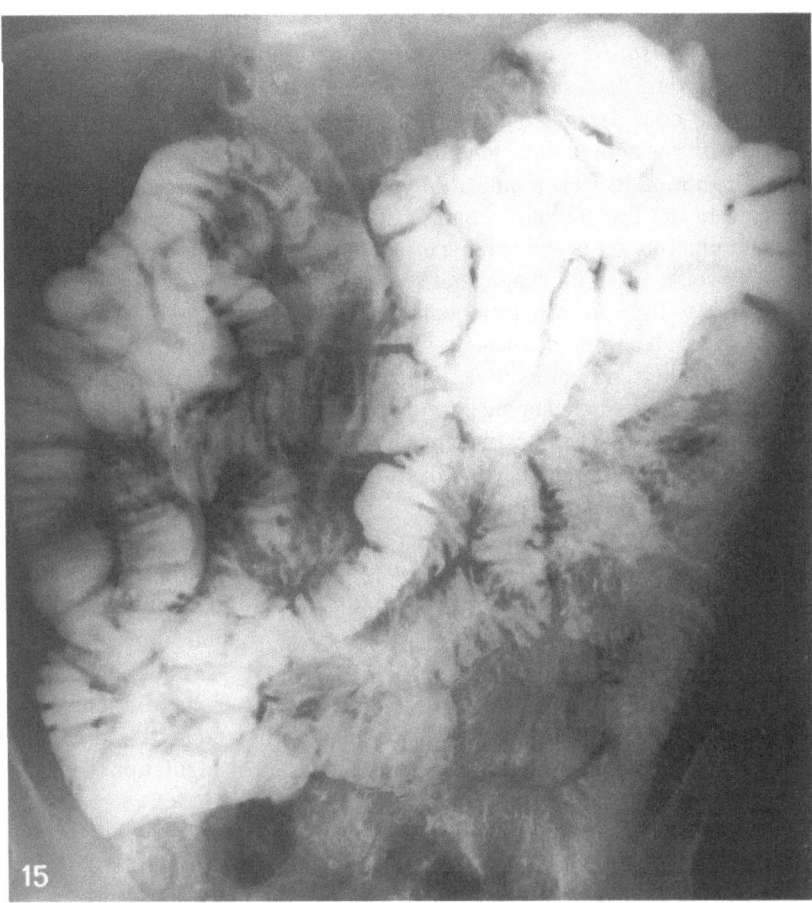

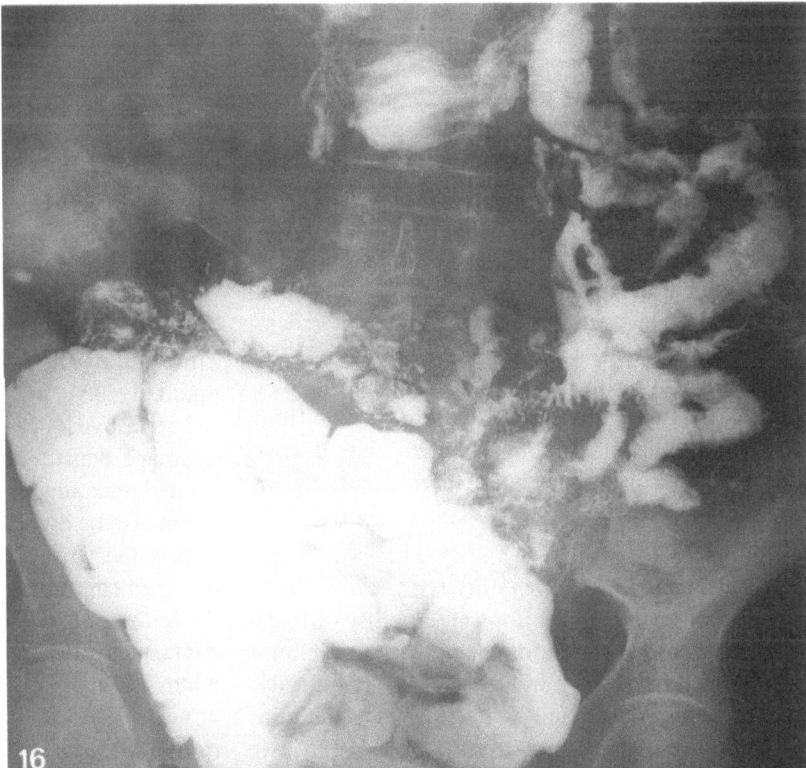

Fig. 15. Functional alterations : contrast medium dilution and disappearance of jejunal folds in celiac disease

Fig. 16. Functional alterations : contrast medium flocculation in jejunal loops during evacuation in a patient with celiac disease

Abnormal motility

Abnormal peristalsis is usually best seen under fluoroscopy during the examination. As physiological variation is considerable, only marked alterations of the transit time should draw attention. Frequent and ample contraction waves indicate hyperperistalsis, coupled to the fast forward progress of the barium train. If obstruction is present, hyperperistalsis may be observed with a blockage, and sometimes antiperistalsis will be present. Infrequent and very slow waves of small amplitude, usually with stasis of the column of barium, indicate a peristaltic defect. Overhead radiographs demonstrate these abnormalities more or less. The intestine appears segmented (carcinoid syndrome) or inert (celiac disease).

Abnormal tone usually accompanies abnormal peristalsis. Distortion in the caliber of the intestinal loops will vary from one film to another. It is usually best assessed under fluoroscopy. Hypertonia is differentiated from stenosis by the inconsistent and reversible appearance of the narrowed segment. Such an image often disappears when a hypotonic agent is administered. Hypotonia produces enlargement of one or several intestinal loops and is usually associated with stasis. It increased the juxtaposition of bowel wall and may account for misleading images appearing as defects (for example in celiac disease).

Abnormal secretion

Abnormalities in secretion are usually not a problem with the current techniques, as these used to be exaggerated with former methods utilizing smaller quantities of contrast medium.

Hypersecretion causes dilution of the contrast medium, a decrease in image density and defects in the casting of the opaque suspension along the intestinal walls. On post-evacuation films, hypersecretion is often associated with flocculation, i.e, the fragmentation of the contrast medium and the formation of small clusters of barium in the fluid. Flocculation becomes more prominent with decreasing amounts of barium, but seldom occurs during enteroclysis.

Abnormal position and mobility (figs. 17 to 19)

Abnormalities in the position and mobility of intestinal loops are sought before any other morphological anomalies, as they indicate either an extrinsic syndrome (tumour, liquid collection, metastatic infiltration of the mesentery, etc.) or the extrinsic component of an intestinal lesion (connective tumour developing whithin the subserosa, carcinoid tumour, etc.).

Abnormalities in position can be diffuse, for instance when the small intestine lies to the right of the midsagittal plane with a common mesentery, or segmental, for example when an intestinal loop courses into an internal or external hernia or an eventration. The following features must be searched for systematically :

- A *void* created by absent intestinal loops in a part of the abdomen. These images are characteristically associated with concavity of the bordering loops arranged in a circle indicating an extrinsic compression.

- A *gap larger than 3 mm* between two loops indicates either an extrinsic process (effusion, mesenteric sclerolipomatosis) or mucosal thickening (ischemia). These findings may occur normally in obese patient where fat disposition leads to parting of the intestinal loops.

- Abnormal curves within the loop must also be considered, including unfolding (when there is an increased radius of curvature within the loop) or angulation (where the loop is bent and forms an acute angle).

- *Loss of normal loop pliability* may be seen and represents loss of bowel wall flexibility during mobilization.

- *The loops may lose their mobility*. In this case resistance will be encountered on attempts at displacing these during palpation. It is normal though not to be able to mobilize deep pelvic loops located behind the bladder and seen on lateral views.

Abnormal caliber (figs. 20 to 24)

Abnormalities in caliber may appear as dilatation or narrowing (stenosis). Dilatation beyond 30 mm for a jejunal loop and 25 mm for an ileal loop after small bowel follow-through (or 40 and 35 respectively for enteroclysis) is pathological. It may involve a group of successive loops and be associated with a decrease in image density as the contrast medium becomes diluted, thus suggesting a postobstructive dilatation. It can also be discontinuous and transient, such as is seen if the bowel is atonic. Segmental ectasia with creviced contours associated with disappearance of the folds, indicates a tumor (lymphoma, leiomyosarcoma, metastasis, etc.). A stenosis may be of varying width and length ; it may be straight or not, in line or not in line with the normal lumen. The smooth or irregular appearance of its contour should be examined as well the presence or disappearance of normal

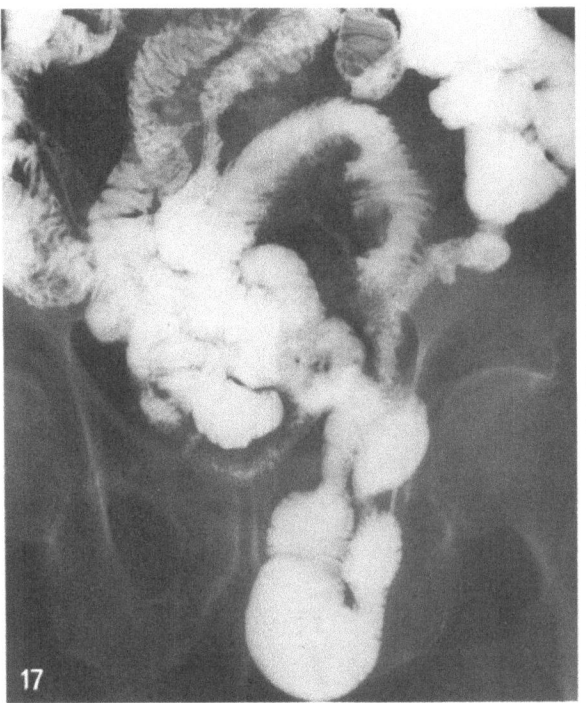

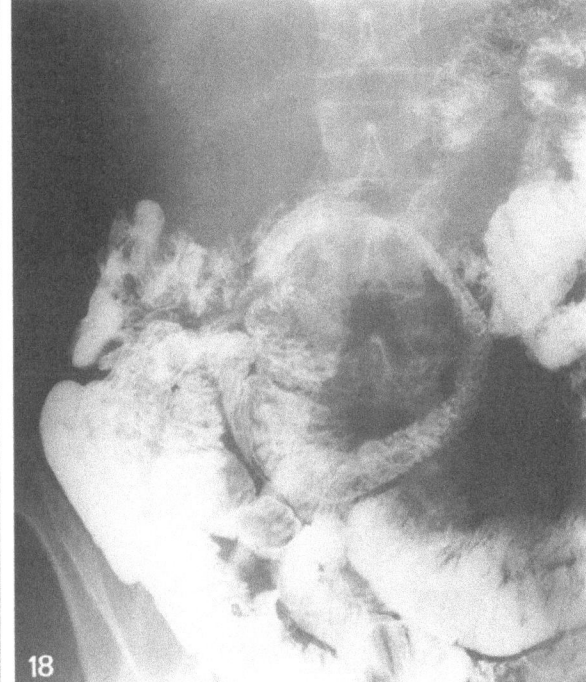

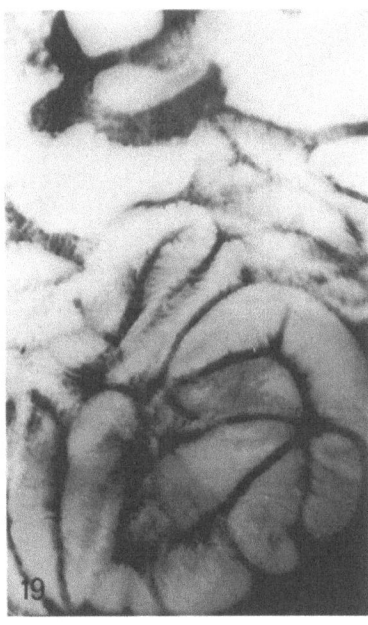

Fig. 17. Abnormal position : migration of an ileal loop into a left direct inguinal hernia

Fig. 18. Abnormal position : unfolding of a jejunal loop in contact with abnormal lymph node (malignant lymphoma)

Fig. 19. Abnormal position : discrete yet diffuse widening of the interloop gaps in ascites

folds in the narrowed segment and the transition of the segment with the bowel proximal and distal. This latter may be abrupt with an invaginated fold in an intrinsic malignant stenosis or infundibular in inflammatory or post-scar stenosis.

Abnormal bowel wall expansion (figs. 25 to 28)
An abnormal bowel wall expansion is observed along the edges of an intestinal loop and does not signifi-

cantly impinge on the lumen. It presents either as an addition image (diverticulum, sacculation), or a defect (notch), or causes retraction of one of the edges.

Diverticula are round or finger-like addition images connected to the wall of the intestine by a pedicle.

Sacculations appear as addition images similar to diverticula but without a pedicle. They are frequently located on the antimesenteric aspect of a

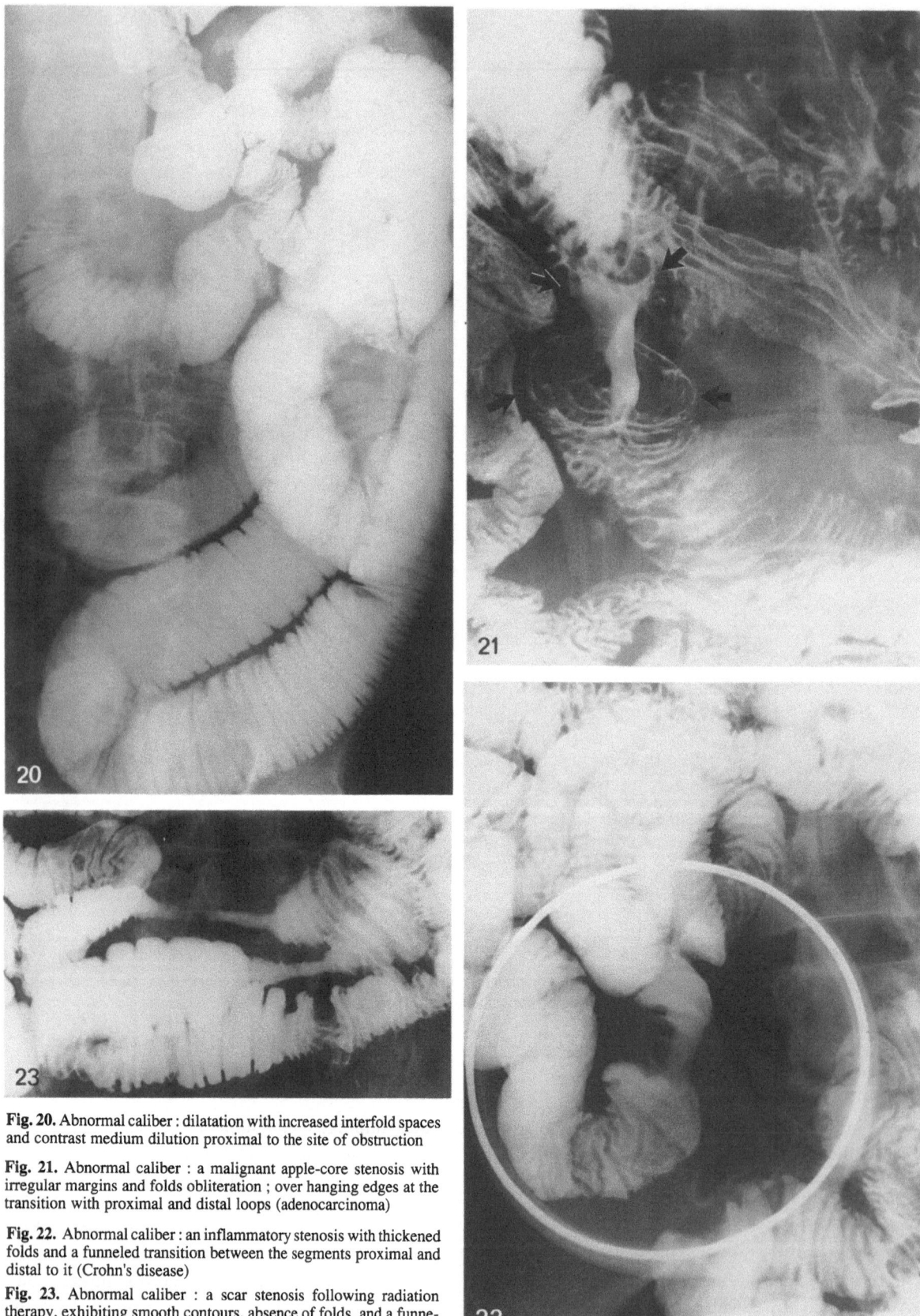

Fig. 20. Abnormal caliber : dilatation with increased interfold spaces and contrast medium dilution proximal to the site of obstruction

Fig. 21. Abnormal caliber : a malignant apple-core stenosis with irregular margins and folds obliteration ; over hanging edges at the transition with proximal and distal loops (adenocarcinoma)

Fig. 22. Abnormal caliber : an inflammatory stenosis with thickened folds and a funneled transition between the segments proximal and distal to it (Crohn's disease)

Fig. 23. Abnormal caliber : a scar stenosis following radiation therapy, exhibiting smooth contours, absence of folds, and a funne-led transition between the segments proximal and distal to it

loop, the mesenteric aspect of which usually shows retraction or a linear ulcer, to which it is connected by converging folds. Sacculations indicate the presence of excess tissue in front of retracted segment.

Notches are defined as curvilinear, variably deep and extended depressions, connected to the wall of the loop at broad angles, positioned at the edge of the intestinal wall. Seen on end, the notches can account for decreased opacification within a bowel loop. Marginal notches are often associated with a contiguous void image. They are distinguished from intramural nodules by their size which varies according to the incidence and the type of compression, as they are caused by extrinsic compression or local bowel wall coalescence.

Segmental retraction is indicated by local shortening of one edge and marginal *spiculation*. The spicules appear as small, dense, and sharp alternating addition and subtraction images (indentation). They can be caused by adhesions or recesses between nodules or folds. The microspicular appearance may be difficult to distinguish from microulcerations on tangential views.

Nodular images

Nodules (figs. 29 to 34) appear as subtraction images standing out in the intestinal lumen. Gas bubbles and lacunae formed by intraluminal foreign bodies, which are usally easily identified, are ruled out because of their mobility. The term polyp is reserved for pedunculated nodules.

Polyps are intraluminal nodules attached to the wall by a pedicle that is sometimes concealed by the projection of the head of the polyp, which is round or oval. Its contours are smooth or irregular, whithout folds. Polyps are relatively mobile and displaced by peristalsis or palpation. A depression generated by traction is often observed in the wall of the loop at the pedicular insertion site. Intussusception is a frequent complication of polyps. A round or punctate ulceration at the head of the polyp is not exceptional, but the radiological examination may fail to detect it. Polyps usually represent benign tumours of mucosal origin, typically adenomas or hamartomas as observed in Peutz-Jeghers syndrome.

Intraluminal nodules are sessile, round or oval with smooth or irregular contours and without mucosal folds. Tangential views show that they are attached to the wall at acute angles, their base being

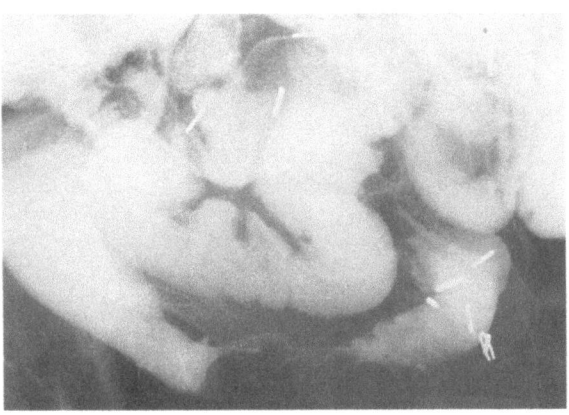

Fig. 24. Abnormal caliber : an excentered extrinsic stenosis, which follows an irregular course ; altered but preserved folds and an infundibular transition with the proximal and distal segments are seen (peritoneal metastases)

narrower than their equatorial diameter. Palpation should asses the relative mobility and malleability of the nodule. Invaginations or ulcerations are sometimes observed. Intraluminal nodules correspond to benign or malignant tumours originating most often in the mucosa (adenoma, hamartoma, adenocarcinoma), sometimes in the submucosa (lipoma, lymphoma, metastasis, carcinoid tumor).

Intramural nodules are sessile formations attached to the wall at obtuse angles, unlike the former, with the base representing their broadest diameter. They can be covered with apparently normal mucosa, which appears lifted by the nodule under the appropriate incidence. The top of the nodule may carry an umbilication or a punctate ulceration. Intramural nodules most often are due to tumors originating in the submucosa or the deeper layers of the mucosa, such as carcinoid tumors. They are not always readily differentiated from marginal notches, although the latter are usually modified by compression.

Intramural nodules may have a mainly *extraluminal* component. They produce void images, sometimes centered on a pool of barium attributable to central necrosis (connective tissue tumor, metastasis). Their implantation on an intestinal loop must be sought during palpation.

Some nodules exhibit *malignant* features such as an encased or an irregular base or nodular contour. Malignant nodules often present extensive ulceration with irregular contours (lymphoma, adenocarcinoma, metastases, etc.).

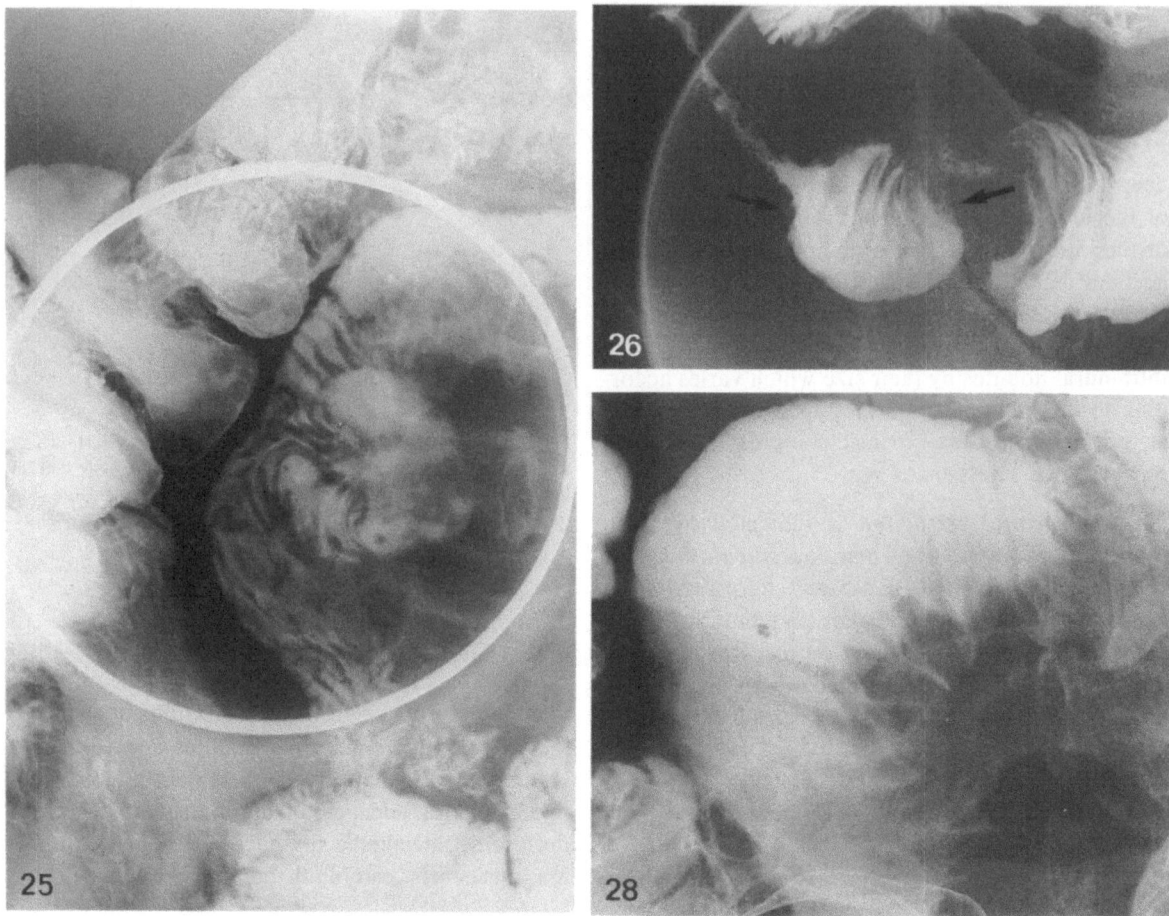

Fig. 25. Abnormal parietal expansion : a Meckel's diverticulum

Fig. 26. Abnormal parietal expansion : a saccule in Crohn's disease

Fig. 28. Abnormal parietal expansion : a marginal spiculation : adhesions

Nodulations (figs.35 to 38)

Nodulations are defined by the presence of several nodules. The image is variable according to the distribution and volume of the nodules. Nodulations can be made up of agglomerated, juxtaposed or scattered elements. When composed of agglomerated nodules, the nodulation consist of elements of variable sizes, which overlap, coalesce and are often entangled with prominent, thickened folds (lymphoma). Nodulations made of juxtaposed elements, often of similar size, are divided into prominent nodulations made up of protruding nodules, accounting for deep marginal indentations separated by spiculated recesses (lymphoma), and more flattened nodula-tions made up of sessile nodules, the tangential image of which does not significantly alter the margins of the loop. The meshes of such flattened nodulation are often produced by the intersection of longitudinal and transverse fissures isolating minimally protruding mucosa (cobblestoning in Crohn's disease). This forms an ulceronodular pattern that will be discussed later. The reticular pattern is formed by a network of 1 to 2 mm meshes isolating almost completely flat mucosal islands. Such images correspond either to the scar formation with re-epithelisation seen in Crohn's disease or to very superficial ulcerations delimitating flat mucosal nodules. The nodulations made up of scattered elements may be

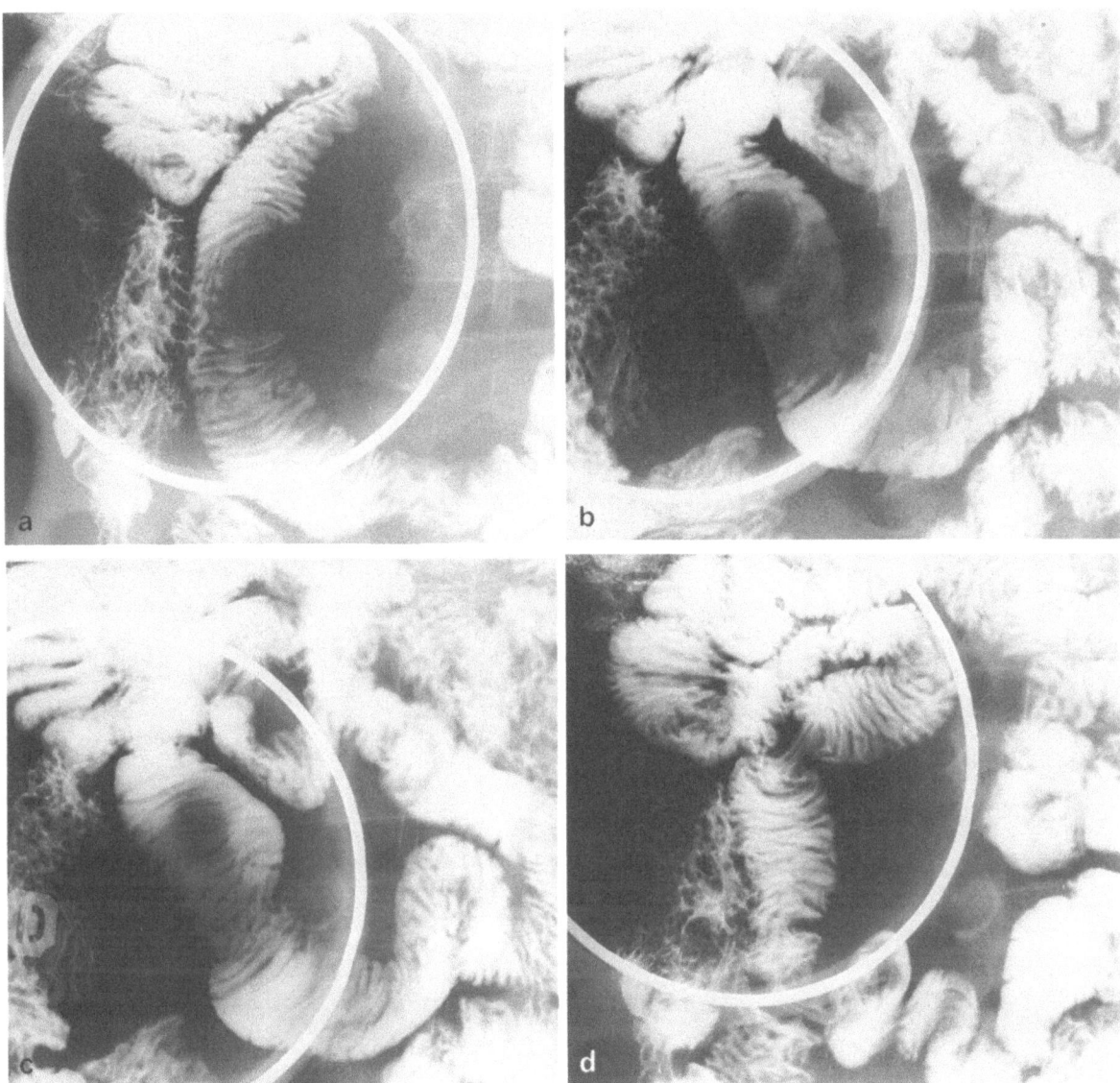

Fig. 27 a-d. Abnormal parietal expansion. **a** A marginal notch on side view is also visible in **b** frontal view, and **c, d** on compression as a plaque-like lesion with sloped contours progressively disappearing as compression decreases (mesenteric adenopathy)

composed of small, similar nodules regularly and densely distributed (lymphoid hyperplasia, such as observed in some immune deficits) or of varying sized nodules with or without pedicles, randomly distributed, such as in the Peutz-Jeghers syndrome, for instance.

Ulcerations and fistulae (figs. 39 to 46)
Ulceration is synonymous with mucosal involvement. Multiple ulcerations usually reflect the inflammatory nature of the disease process. Their appearance can suggest the etiology of the disease.

The typical ulcer is the peptic ulcer observed in a Meckel's diverticulum, or the postoperative peptic ulcer following gastrectomy. In frontal view, it appears round, oval, triangular, square or star-shaped, with an opaque center. On tangential views, it appears as a relatively large and deep pool of barium collection. It can be surrounded by radiating folds.

According to the extent and depth of the ulcer, microulcerations, geographic ulcerations and transmural ulcerations, which are perpendicular to the wall and are harbinger of fistulae formation, may occur.

The presence of *aphtoid ulcerations* suggest the diagnosis of Crohn's disease, although it may be observed in other conditions such as yersiniosis. This

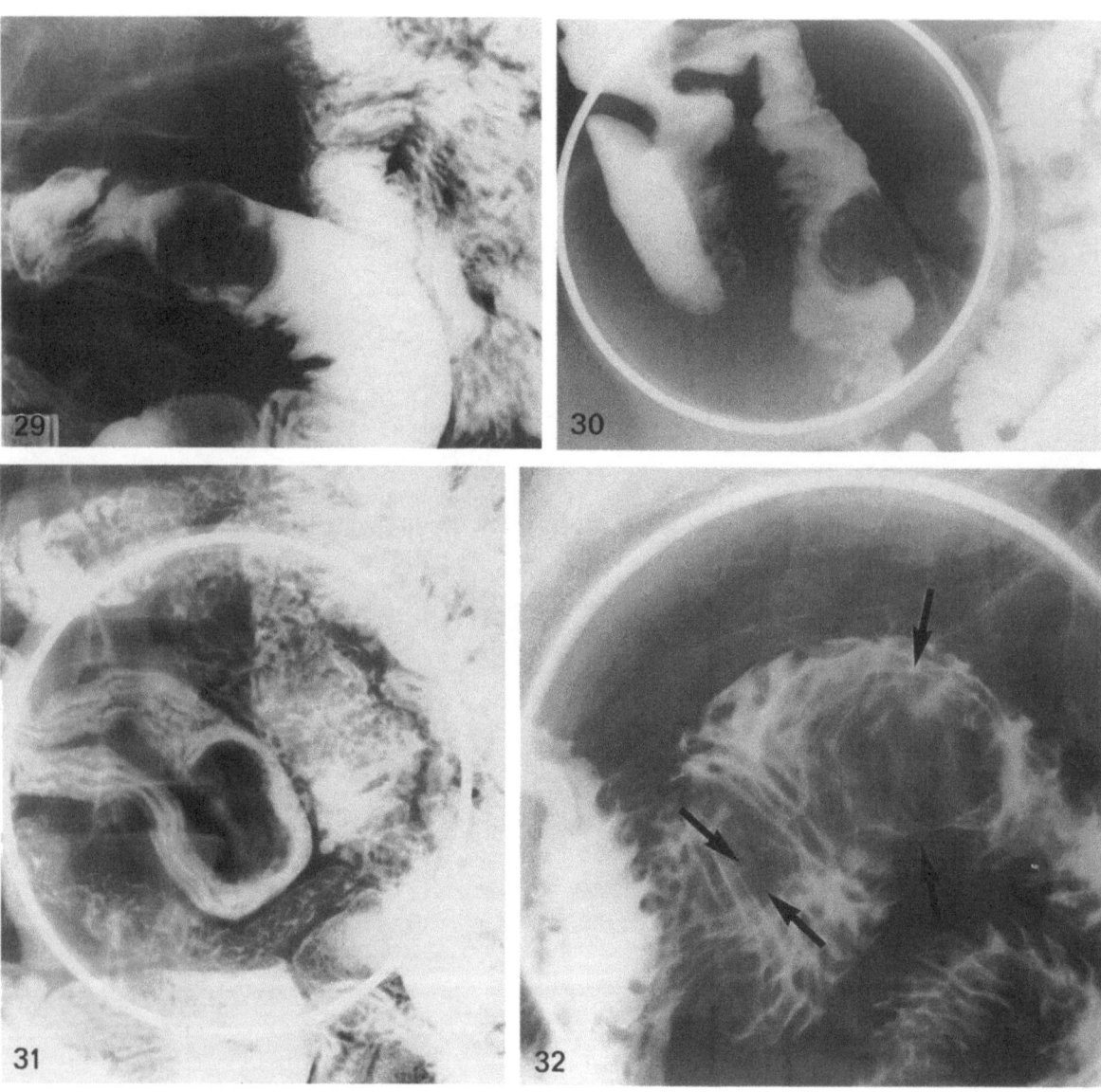

Fig. 29. Intraluminal nodule : a lipoma

Fig. 30. Intramural nodule : a carcinoid tumour

Fig. 31. Extramural nodule : a leiomyoma

Fig. 32. Polyp : a pediculated gangliocytic paraganglioma

pattern is caused by ulceration of submucosal lymphoid nodule. It appears as a 1 to 10 mm round, oval or polygonal opaque center with a more lucent rim representing the protruding lymphoid follicle. The latter is 1 to 5 mm wide with ill-defined and sloping margins that are sometimes outlined by radiating folds. Such features differentiate an aphtoid ulceration from an umbilicated benign nodule. The relative size of the diameters of the central spot and the peripheral ring are very variable, according to the presence of concomitant hypersecretion and the intensity of compression.

The transverse stripe or rhagade is pathognomonic for Crohn's disease, and indicated a relatively deep fissure in the mesenteric wall of an intestinal loop, forming an opaque line bordered by a more lucent rim and highlighted by radiating folds. This linear ulcer may sometimes be over 10 cm long and

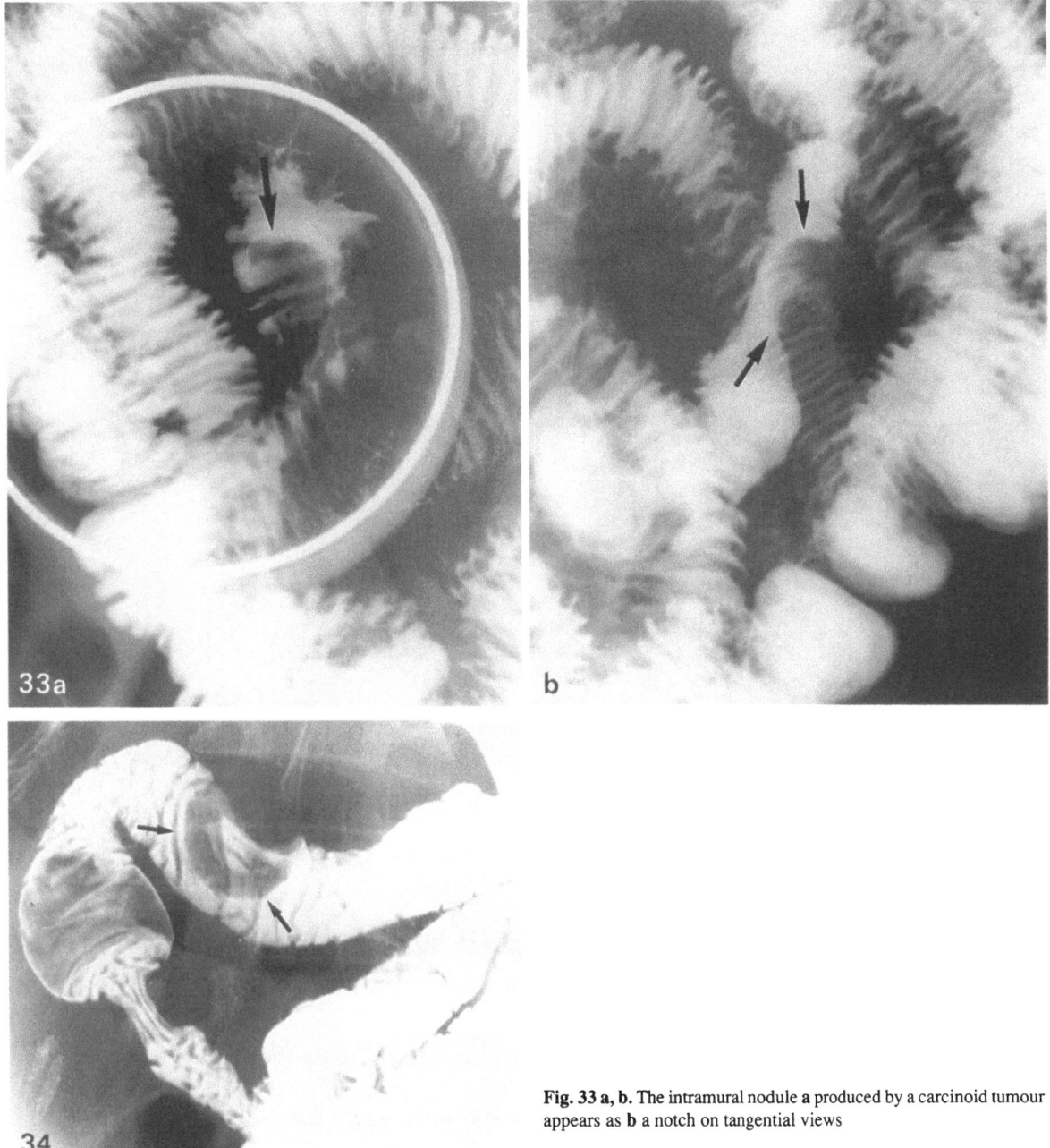

Fig. 33 a, b. The intramural nodule **a** produced by a carcinoid tumour appears as **b** a notch on tangential views

Fig. 34. Ulcerated nodule : a lymphoma (Courtesy of J P Moiroud)

is most evident on tangential views. The intensity of compression plays a vital role in detecting it as the image remains concealed by the opacified loop if compression is insufficient, and becomes obliterated if it is too intense.

A *stenosing ulcer* is frequently seen in the small intestine (Crohn's disease, tuberculosis, drug ulcer, etc.). The stenosis is usually short, so that a view of the ulceration may be difficult to show. An increase in the density of the barium column with a slight convexity of the edges should be sought within the stenosed segment.

The ulceronodular or "cobblestone" pattern described in the section on nodulations is specific for Crohn's disease. It is caused by the criss-crossing of longitudinal, transverse or serpiginous ulcerations along the wall.

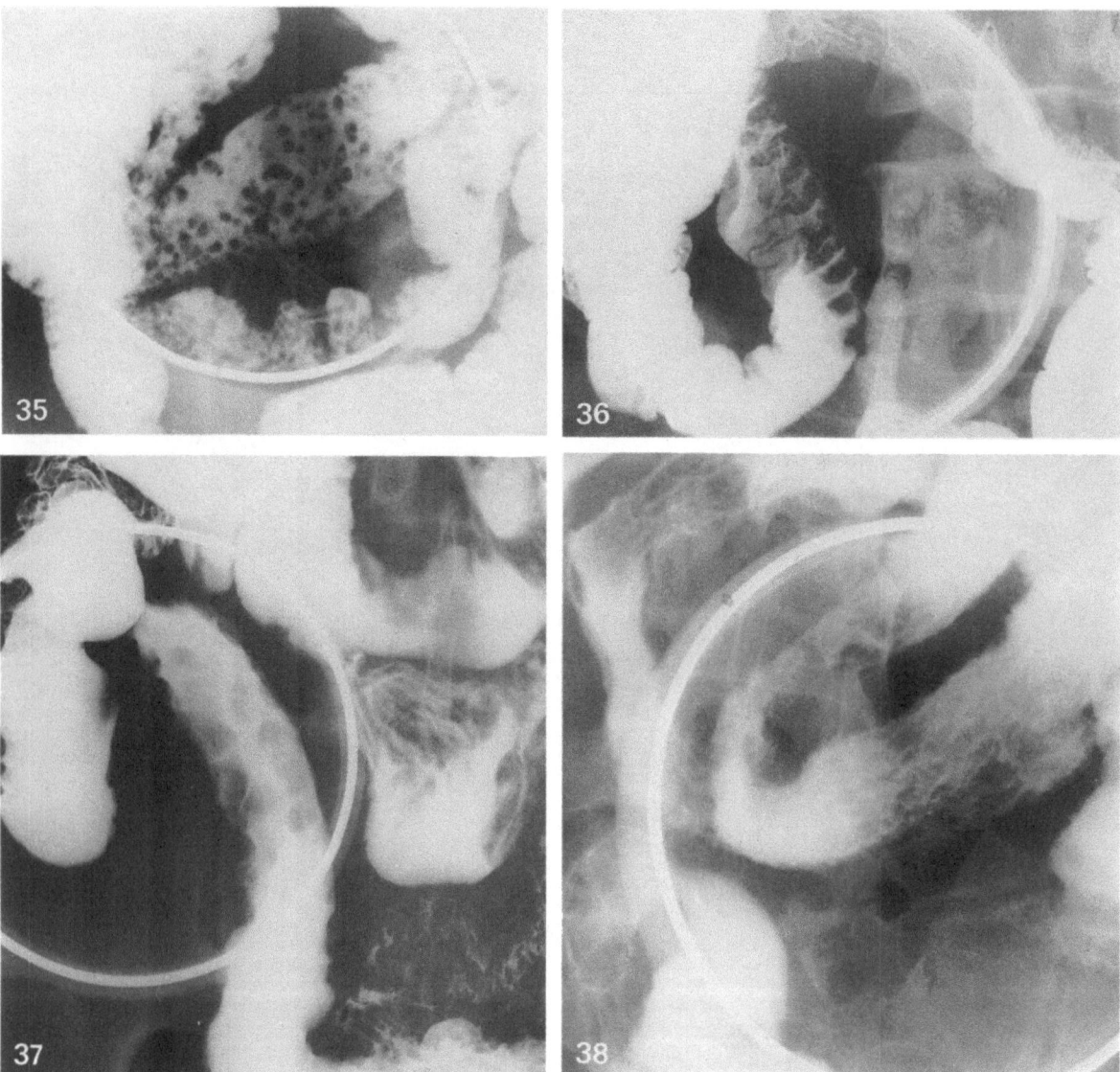

Fig. 35. Nodulation formed by scattered elements : lymphoid nodular hyperplasia

Fig. 36. Nodulation formed by juxtaposed protruded lesions : lymphoma

Fig. 37. Nodulation formed by juxtaposed flattened lesions : the ulceronodular pattern or cobblestoning seen in Crohn's disease

Fig. 38. Reticulation : network with flattened nodulation as seen in Crohn's disease

Fistulae are opaque, parallel or perpendicular to the intestinal loop, as they burrough through the wall, they may be long and wide, bunched together or ending blindly. They may also communicate with a neighbouring loop, the colon, the bladder, the vagina or the skin. They are especially frequent in Crohn's disease but are also observed after trauma, in the presence of postoperative foreign bodies and in cases of ischemia, tuberculosis, lymphoma, metastases or connective tissue tumors. All intermediate stages between transmural ulcerations and fistulae can be observed.

An irregular pool of contrast medium between displaced loops of small bowel may be in communication with a fistula in Crohn's disease, or may be an extensive extraluminal ulceration (connective tu-

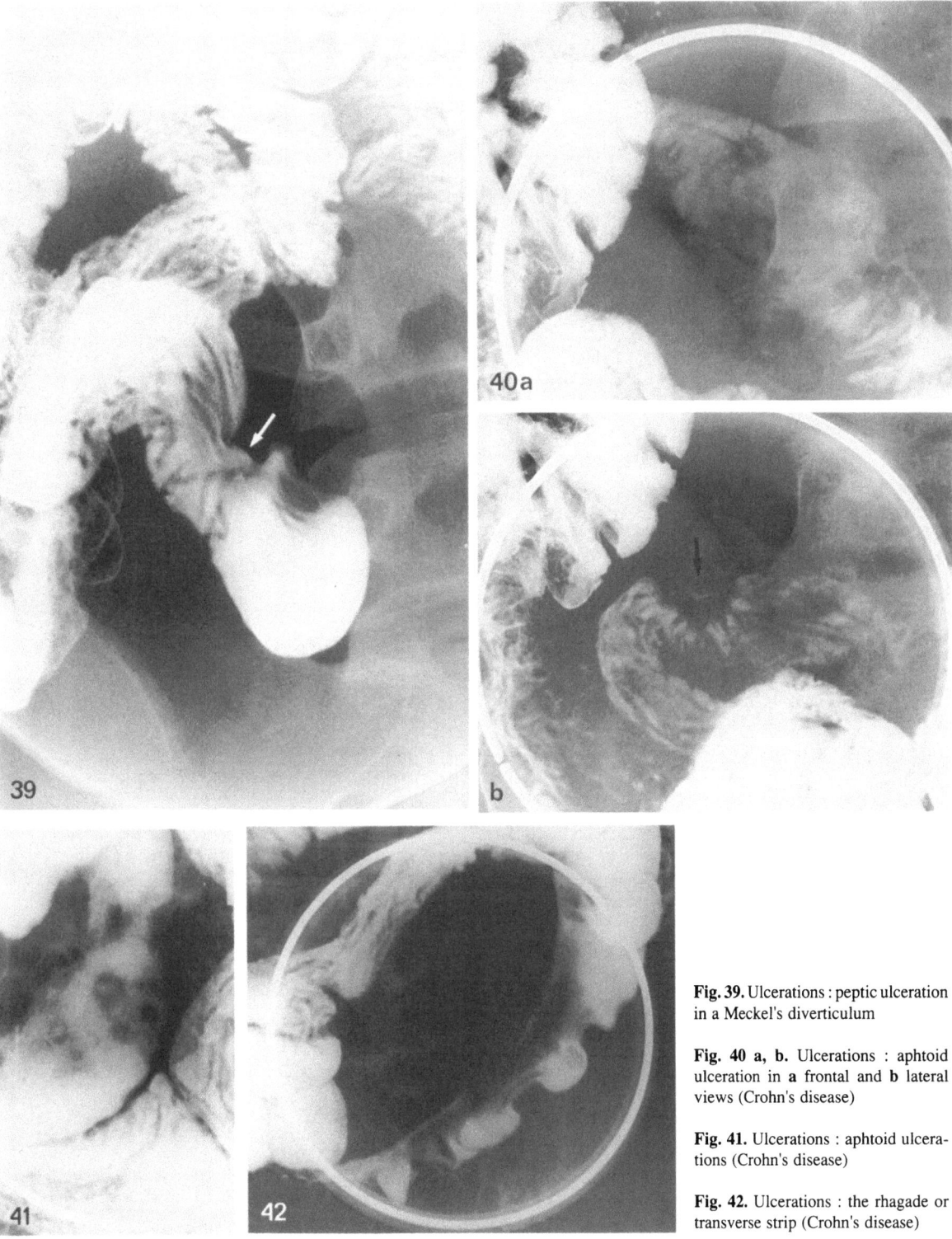

Fig. 39. Ulcerations : peptic ulceration in a Meckel's diverticulum

Fig. 40 a, b. Ulcerations : aphtoid ulceration in a frontal and b lateral views (Crohn's disease)

Fig. 41. Ulcerations : aphtoid ulcerations (Crohn's disease)

Fig. 42. Ulcerations : the rhagade or transverse strip (Crohn's disease)

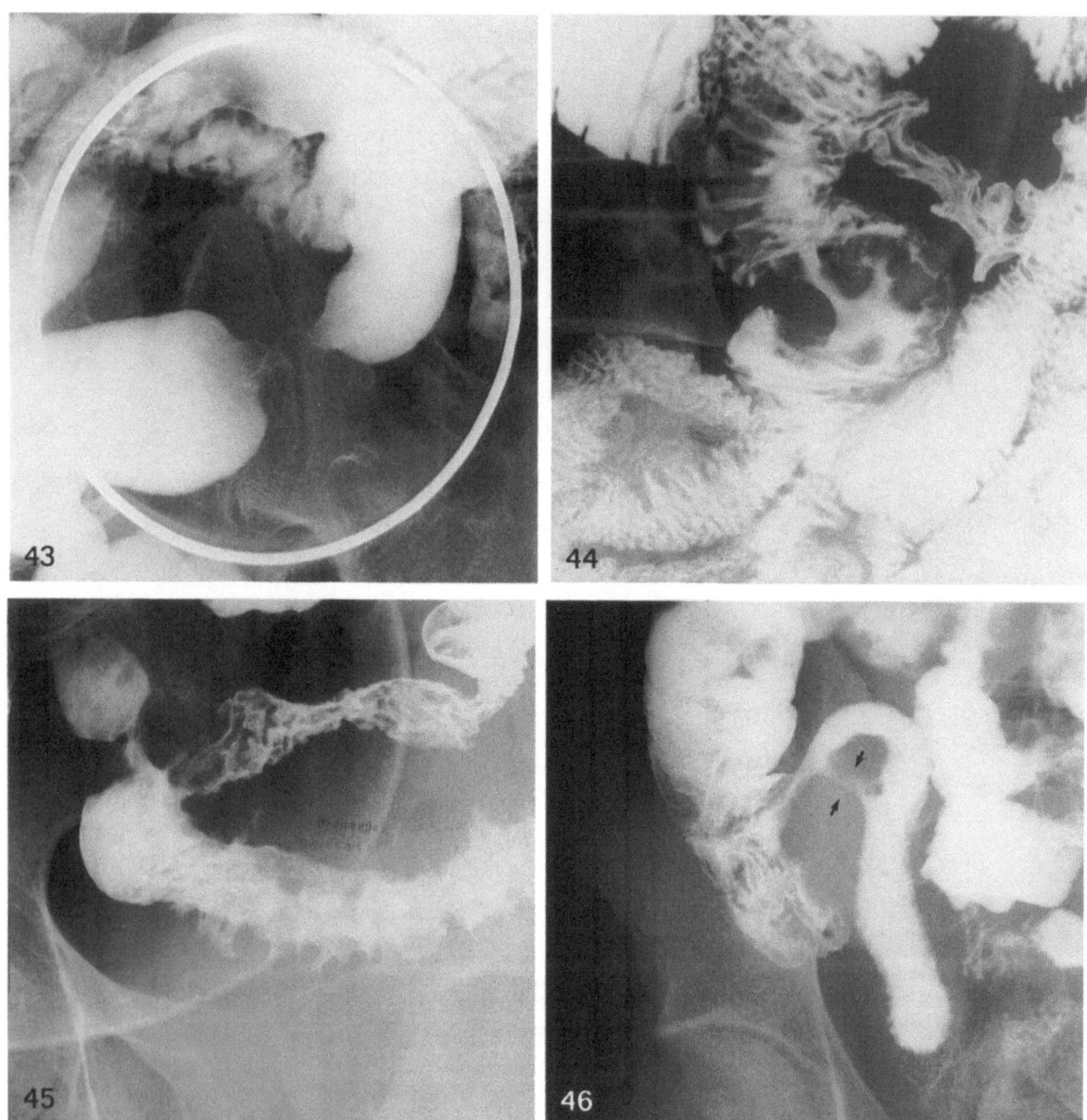

Fig. 43. Ulcerations : a stenosing ulceration (Crohn's disease)

Fig. 44. Ulcerations : a malignant ulceration with irregular contours and a nodular rim (adenocarcinoma)

Fig. 45. Ulcerations : Transmural ulcerations (Crohn's disease)

Fig. 46. An ileoileal fistula in a patient with Crohn's disease

mour, metastasis) or even an excentric segmental ectasia (lymphoma).
Abnormal folds (figs. 47 to 50)
Abnormalities in the structure of the folds may involve their number, width, height, course, shape or contour.

Number : A decrease in the number of folds produces an increase in the average distance between them, which should not exceed 5 mm in the jejunum. This is often associated with an increase in the loop diameter, which is moderate in celiac disease and more significant in poststenotic dilatation. This sign

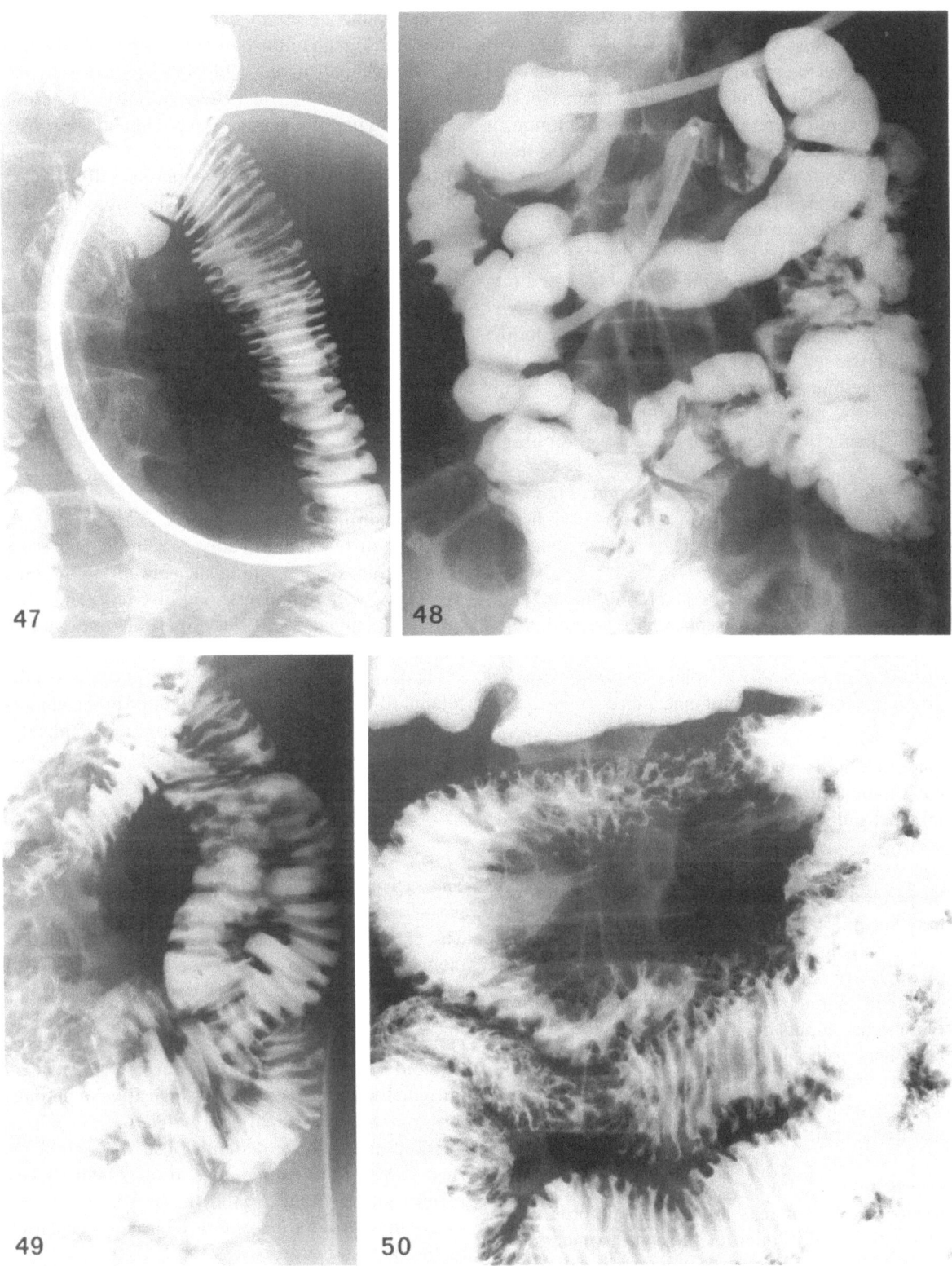

Fig. 47. Abnormal folds : The straight and closely spaced palisading folds of increased height of ischemia

Fig. 48. Abnormal folds : the sparse and flattened folds of celiac disease

Fig. 49. Abnormal folds : the broadened folds of celiac disease

Fig. 50. Abnormal folds : the nodular folds of alpha-chain disease

is more difficult to assess in the ileum as ileal folds are normally less numerous.

An increase in the number of folds may be associated with hypertonicity of the longitudinal fibers (for instance proximal to an obstruction). In the ileum, it may indicate functional adaptation if there is associated villous atrophy in the jejunum («inverted small intestine» in sprue). It is also seen in cases of intussusception and can be seen in ischemia.

Width : An increase in the width of the jejunal folds beyond 3 mm and of the ileal folds over 2 mm is pathological. It is usually associated with bowel wall thickening (more than 3 mm between the loops) and is observed in several diseases (hypoproteinemia, ischemia, lymphoma, Crohn's disease, Whipple's disease,etc.).
Folds thinner than 1 mm are practically never observed.

Height : An increase in the height of the folds over 5 mm is pathological : it is observed in hematomas and ischemia as well as in lymphedema, adhesion, etc.
A decrease in the height of jejunal folds under 1 mm, and all the more, their disappearance are pathological. These are observed in villous atrophy (celiac disease), inflammatory (Crohn's disease), parasitic diseases (giardasis), lymphomas, etc.

Course : A loss of flexibility of the folds causes their usual sinuous aspect to disappear. A pathological rectilinear pattern emerges with parallel «palisading» (hematoma) or converging folds (extrinsic syndrome).

Shape : The two edges of a fold can cease to be parallel. Their angle of incidence with the wall may become broader (wedge folds) or more acute, while the top of the folds becomes the site of a biconvex or nodular bulge. This appearance is observed in many diseases (Whipple's syndrome, lymphoma, alpha-chain disease, amyloidosis). A broadened fold with parallel contours is often associated with fluid infiltration (œdema, blood, etc.), whereas nodular contours suggest inflammatory or neoplastic infiltration.

Contours : The disappearance of the usual sharp contours of a fold, which become ill-defined or stopped, is generally associated with broadening of the fold and dilution of the contrast medium. It indicates inflammatory, infectious or parasitic involvement, or villous atrophy.

Abnormal villi (figs. 51 and 52)
The villous pattern observed, with our technique as

a finely punctate luminal space with a microspiculated appearance of the borders may be linked either to villous hypertrophy (Whipple's syndrome, hypertrophy as a reaction to extensive bowel resection, edema, hypoproteinemia, lymphangiectasia, Waldenström's disease, lactation, etc...) or to partial atrophy with larger and less numerous villi (Crohn's disease, ischemia, alpha-chain disease). It is not possible to differentiate both processes.

Radiological syndromes (fig. 53)

Once the elementary images have been recognised, they can be compiled into a radiological syndrome. This is the second step in analysing the radiographs.

The malabsorption syndrome

The malabsorption syndrome is characterized by signs of diffuse enteropathy : dilution and early flocculation of the contrast medium, hypotonia associated with a moderate and discontinuous dilatation of jejunal loops varying from one film to another ; there may be moderate and irregular increases in the interloop space and diffuse alteration of the jejunal folds, which may be thicker or in the contrary less prominent and even disappear completely. The malabsorption syndrome is most often observed in celiac disease but can accompany every diffuse disease of the small intestine, regardless of its nature.

The extrinsic syndrome (fig. 54)

The extrinsic syndrome consist of several different elementary images, the common feature of which is the fixed and asymmetric character of the lesions. Several patterns can be observed, and are sometimes concomitant ;
- a void image with one or several loops displaced, unfolded while arranged concentrically, sometimes with one or several marginal notches,
- a fixed angulation or radiation of several neighbouring loops, which sometimes form a star-shaped pattern with the folds forming the spokes of a wheel.
- a spiculation of the mesenteric edge and sacculation of the opposite edge,
- an enlargment of the gap between the loops, without enlargement of the folds.
The extrinsic syndrome can be associated with involvement of the small intestine in contiguous disease (effusion, sclerolipomatosis, peritoneal

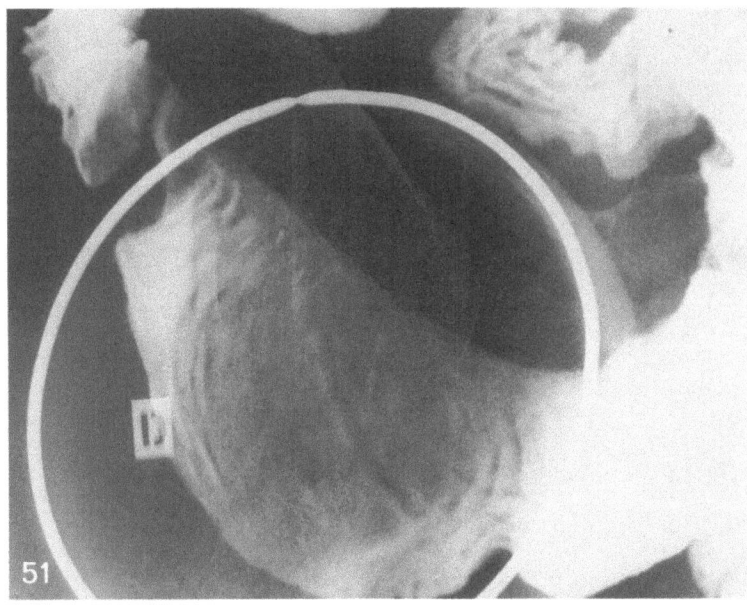

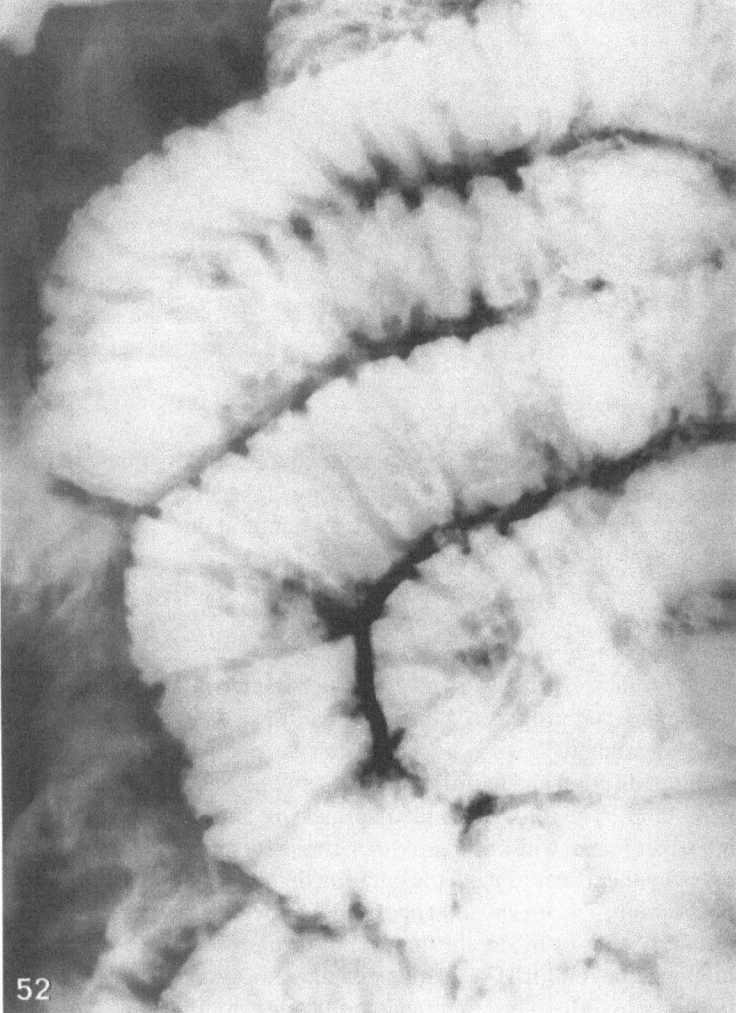

Fig. 51. Abnormal villi : the finely punctated luminal appearance seen in Crohn's disease

Fig. 52. Abnormal villi : Microspiculation of the mucosa in a patient with alpha-chain disease

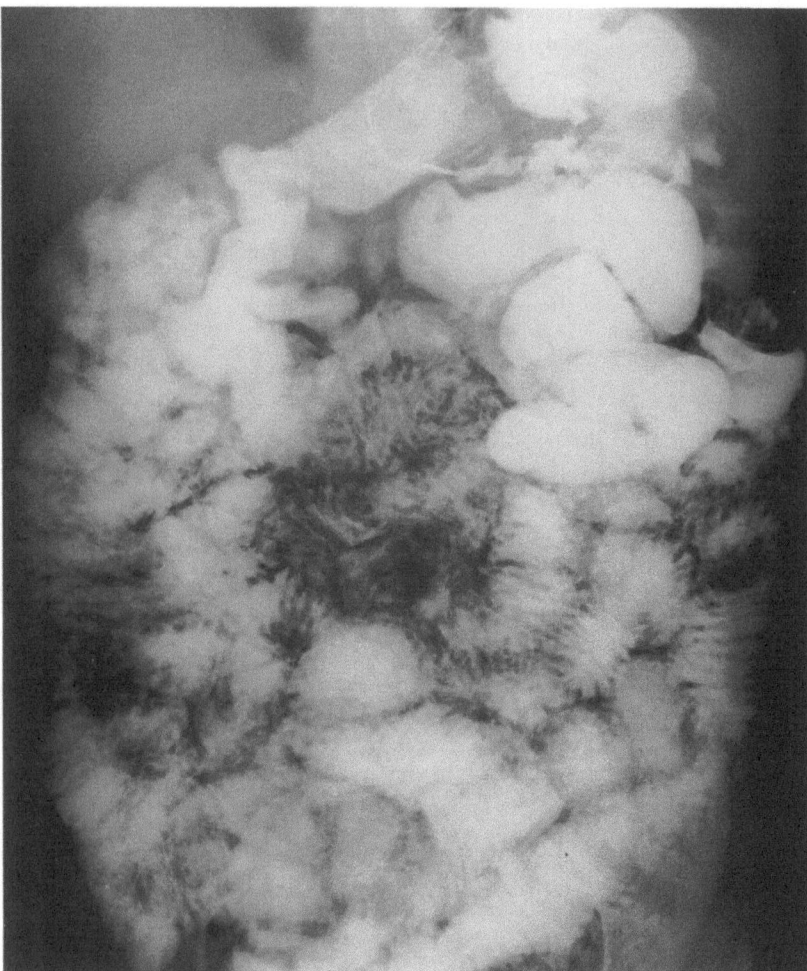

Fig. 53. The malabsorption syndrome : diffuse alterations with dilution, flocculation, and moderately widned folds . The appearance of the jejunum (moderate, discontinuous dilatation of the caliber and decrease in the number of folds) suggests a diagnosis of celiac disease

metastases, tumors, etc.), or with the extraintestinal development of small intestinal processes (abscess, fistula formation in Crohn's disease, extramural development of connective tissue tumors, etc.).

The chronic obstructive syndrome (fig. 55)

The chronic obstructive syndrome is characterized by the delayed progress of the barium meal , sometimes associated with hyperperistalsis, contrast medium dilution and uniform dilatation of one or several loops. The folds retain their normal size and are often rectilinear, with a decreased or increased distance between them according to the duration of the partial obstruction. The diagnosis is confirmed by detection of the stenosis or by the abrupt restoration of normal loop size beyond it. The features of the radiograph make it possible to differentiate chronic obstruction from other causes of intestinal dilatation, except in some (exceptional) cases of scleroderma, myopa-

thies or hereditary chronic pseudoobstruction syndrome.

Intussusception (fig. 56)

Intussusception is characterized by an enlarged loop, the lumen of which is not opacified by barium, bordered by straight, thinned and dense transverse folds. The "empty" loop is centred by a number of longitudinal folds belonging to the intussusceptum, sometimes preceded by the image of the lesion causing the intussusception (tumor nodule, Meckel's diverticulum). If seen along its axis, the image of the intussusception appears either as concentric circles or as a ring with a lucent center, the diameter of which is larger than that of the neighbouring loops: the"coil spring" appearance. Proximally, hyperperistalsis and antiperistalsis are frequently observed. Besides intussusception associated with an organic le-

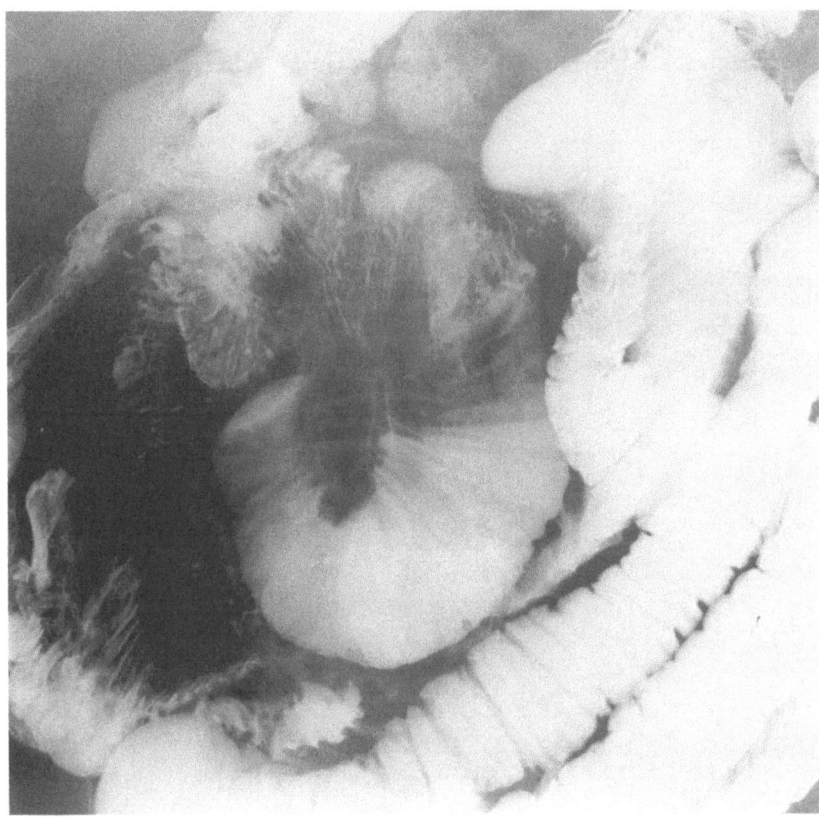

Fig. 54. The extrinsic syndrome : A fixed loop is arranged in a circle with spiculation along its concave edge and the presence of convergent folds ; this indicates mesenteric retraction and is due in this case to peritoneal metastases

sion, functional intussusception attributable to disorders of tone or peristalsis may be observed in celiac disease or in children.

The tumoral syndrome (fig. 57)

The tumoral syndrome is characterized by single or multiple segmental lesions.

The benign tumor syndrome appears as a nodule (or nodulation) with sharp margins. It may be pedunculated or ulcerated, yet without alteration of the folds or peristalsis (in the absence of intussusception or obstruction).

The appearance of the malignant tumor syndrome is more varied as it can present as a stenosis, a segmental ectasia, a nodule or nodulation that may be ulcerated, or an ulceration with heaped-up edges. Any may be seen in conjunction with an extrinsic syndrome. Even when the lesions are multiple, they exhibit sharp margins with no transition from the normal to the affected segments and usually no functional alterations except in the case of intussus-

ception or obstruction. The lesion is often fixed and rigid.

The inflammatory syndrome (fig. 58)

The inflammatory syndrome usually consist of the coexistence of functional, motor and secretory disorders, and of morphological alterations with ill-defined margins. It is characterized by a stenosis with a smooth and gradual transition with the segments proximal and distal to it, called "funneling". Nodulation with scalopped contours, and ill-defined, thickened or nodular folds may also be found. The presence of multiple ulcerations indicates the inflammatory character of a lesion, except in some cases of metastases.

Inflammatory and neoplastic diseases cannot always be differentiated : some lymphomas simulate malabsorption, while some types of stenoses caused by tumors resemble inflammatory stenoses (Crohn's disease, ischemia,etc.).

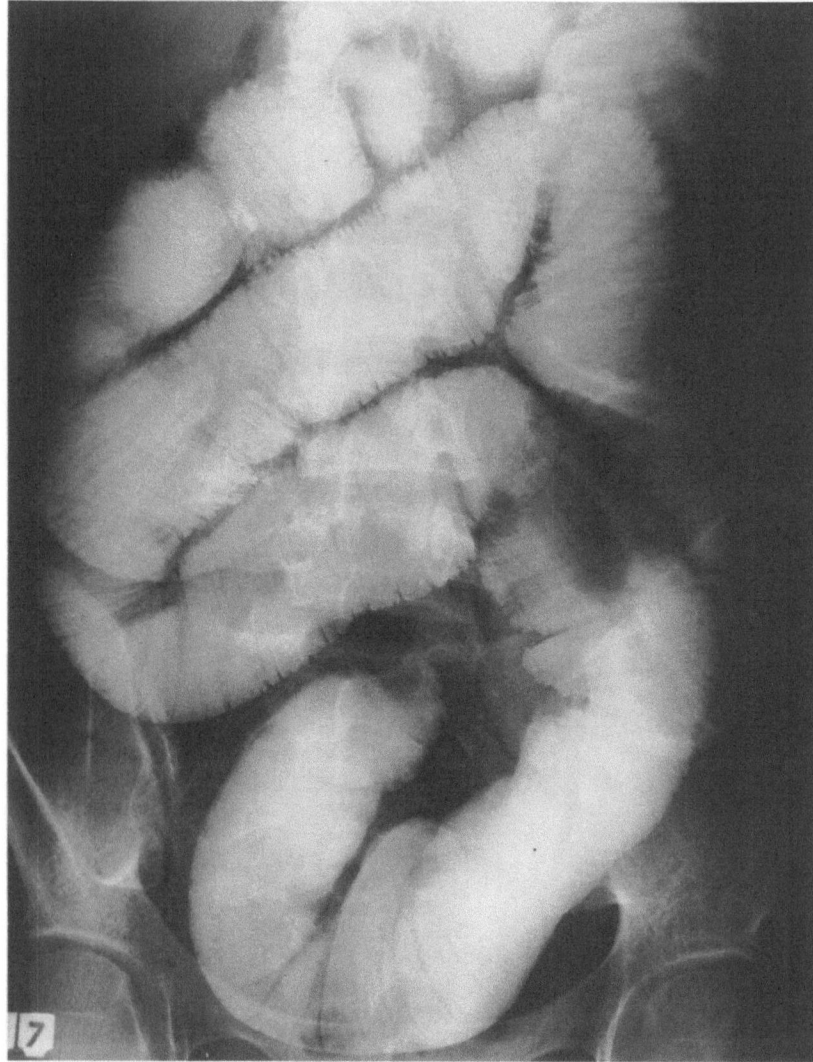

Fig. 55. The chronic obstructive syndrome : Continuous dilatation of the jejunal loops, dilution without flocculation, and increased interfold spaces near the stenosis

Other examinations with barium

Barium swallow

The first jejunal loops can be examined after a barium swallow. However, a study of the entire small bowel should be avoided after such an examination has been carried out with high-density barium, double contrast technique and drug-induced hypotonia. Hypotonia causes stasis and a considerable delay in transit time ; air breaks up the barium column and the high weight-to-volume ratio of the contrast medium is not suitable fot thin-layer coating of the intestinal loops. When both a barium swallow and a small bowel follow-through are required, a choice has to be made between performing the former examination with the same barium suspension as for the latter or performing both studies a few days apart. However, a proper double-contrast barium swallow may be carried out in some selected cases if high-density barium is delivered at the end of the small bowel follow-through, thus taking advantage of drug-induced hypotonia. The examination should therefore begin with examination of the small intestine.

Barium enema (figs. 59 and 60)

The reflux of a low density barium solution through the ileocecal valve is facilitated by drug-induced hypotonia, and allows for the retrograde opacification of the distal ileum by a barium enema. It is then

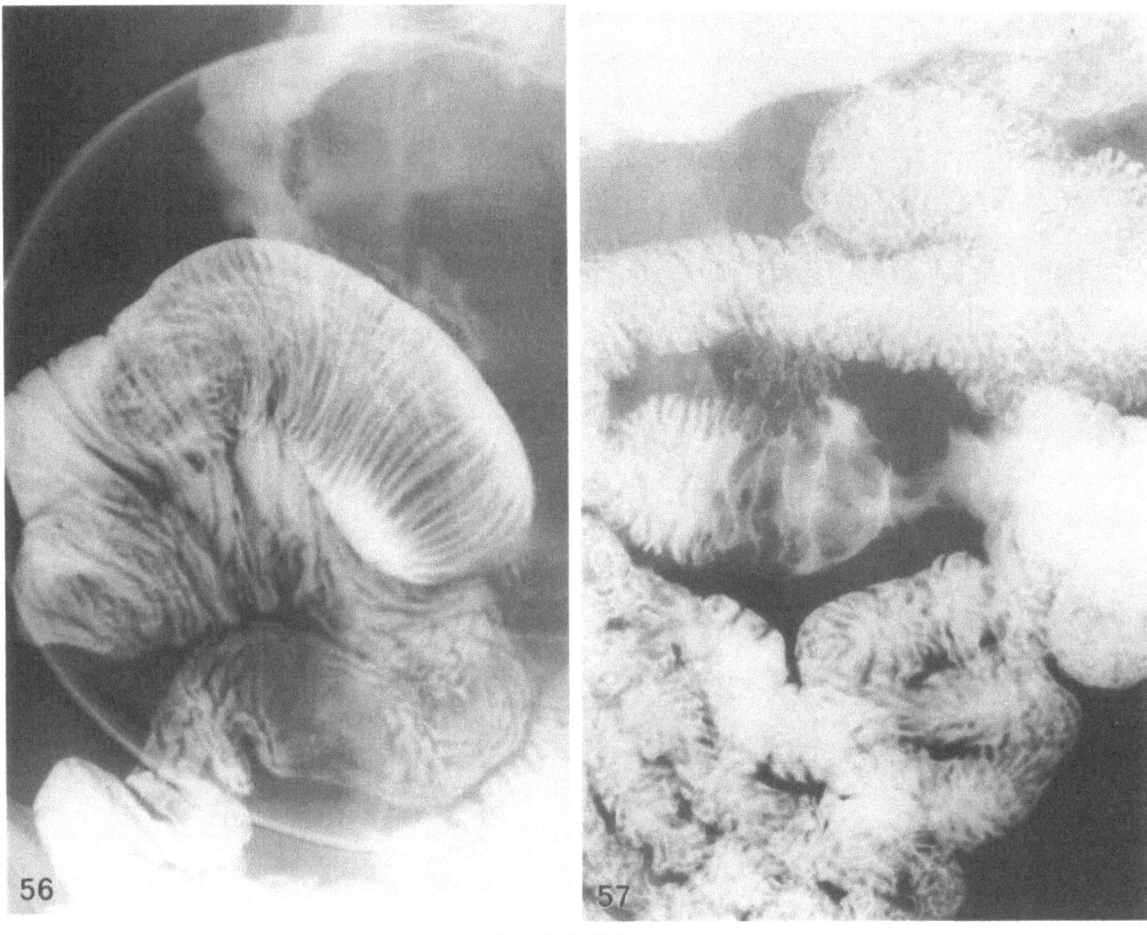

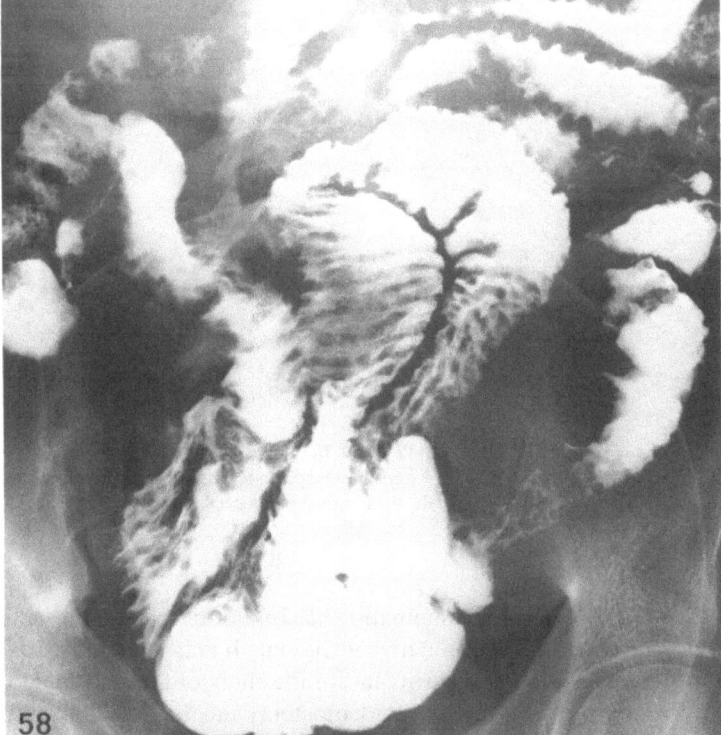

Fig. 56. Intussusception : A widened, empty loop is bordered by straight, narrow-spaced folds and with at the center longitudinal folds (celiac disease)

Fig. 57. The tumoral syndrome : a short stenosis with disappearing folds follows a nodulation, with abrupt transition distally. Note the normal appearance of the neighbouring parts of small intestine (lymphoma)

Fig. 58. The inflammatory syndrome: diffuse alterations with dilution, moderate flocculation and widened folds are seen in a patient with Crohn's disease

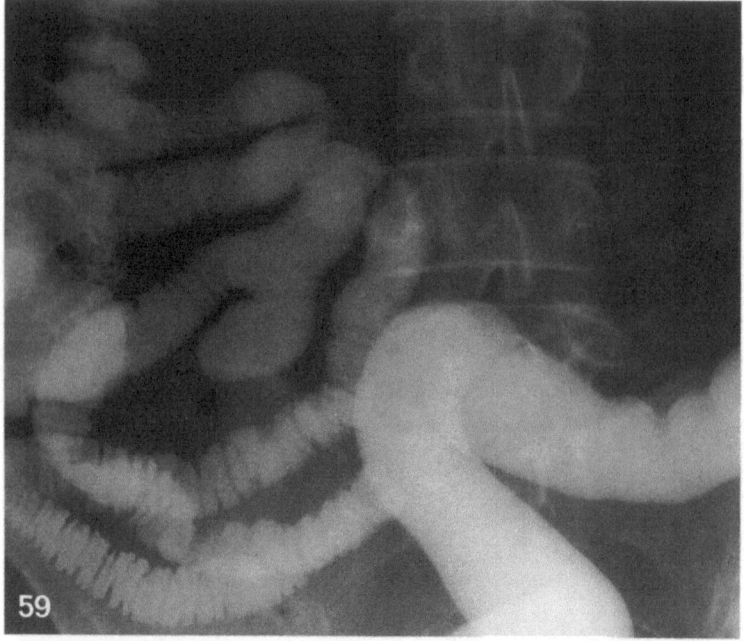

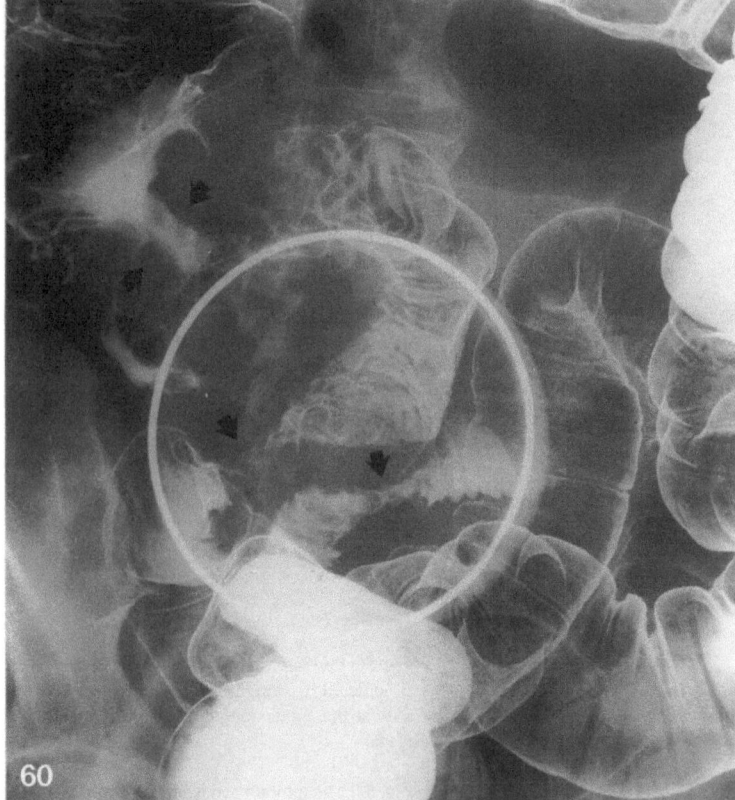

Fig. 59. Barium enema : demonstration of a Meckel's diverticulum

Fig. 60. Barium enema : double-contrast barium enema demonstrating two extrinsic stenoses of the terminal ileum caused by a cecal cancer metastasis

possible to detect ileal disease, for instance a Meckel's diverticulum. Good views of the terminal ileum are usually obtained during a double-contrast barium enema, so that neoplastic or inflammatory lesions located near the ileocecal valve can be seen. However, this examination has limitations, and represents only an adjunctive technique. It may nevertheless be useful, in particular for the study of the anastomotic loop following ileocolostomy and the early detection of recurrent Crohn's disease.

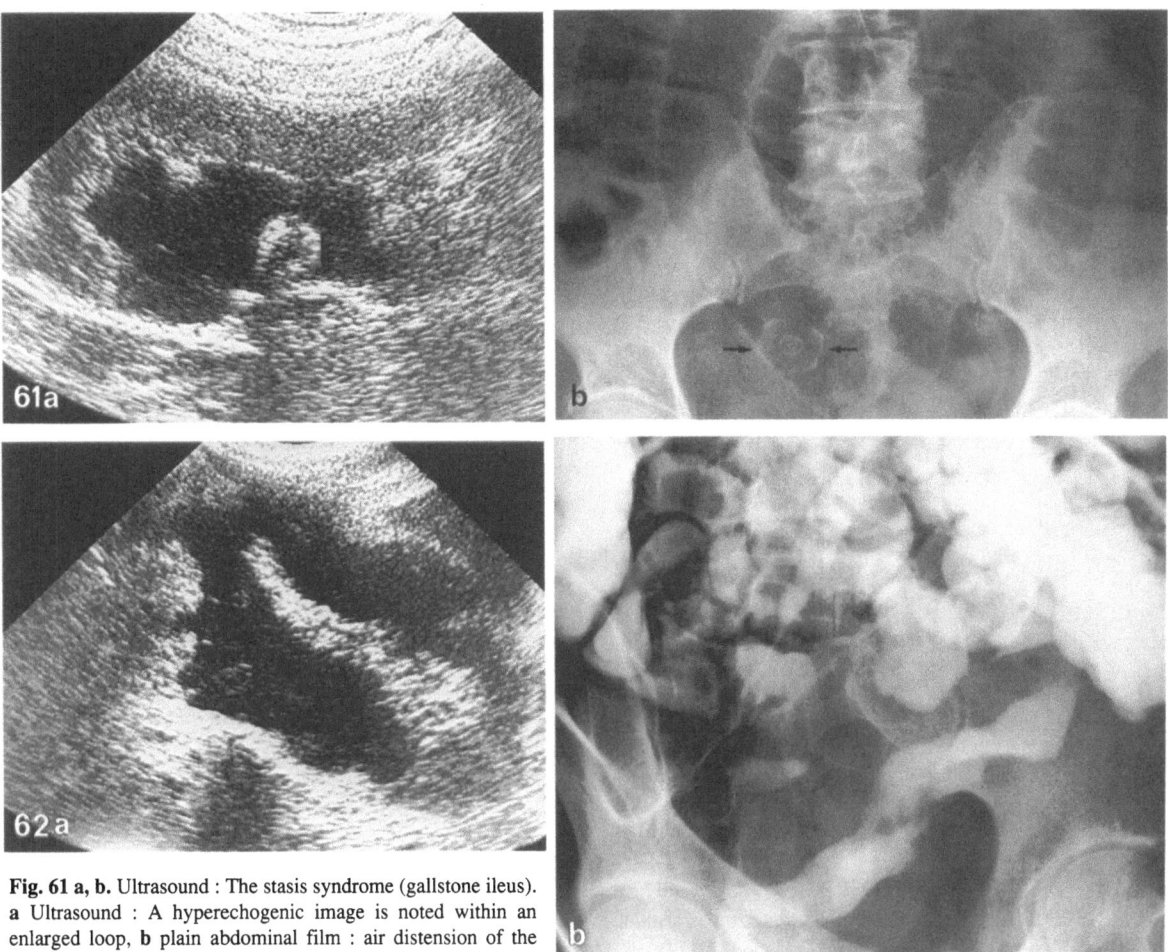

Fig. 61 a, b. Ultrasound : The stasis syndrome (gallstone ileus). **a** Ultrasound : A hyperechogenic image is noted within an enlarged loop, **b** plain abdominal film : air distension of the jejunum is seen proximal to the gallstone

Fig. 62 a, b. Ultrasound : the tumoral syndrome (lymphoma). **a** Ultrasound : irregularly thickened walls are noted in an ileal loop, **b** insert where SBFT is seen : stiffness and disappearance of the folds are demonstrated in an ileal loop with thickened walls

Ultrasound (figs. 61 to 64)

Ultrasound may be used for the study of the small intestine in the following two situations :
- while performing an abdominal ultrasound as a first-line investigation,
- or further work-up when a focal or segmental lesion is discovered on small bowel follow-through, in order to better assess the extraluminal extent of the lesion.

Technique

The exploration of the small intestine does not require any preparation except for a 12 h fast. The examination has to be performed with a high-definition «real-time» system with a 3,5 or 5 Mhz probe. A full

bladder makes pelvic exploration easier, and the image quality is improved by using a surface adapter or a water bag as the intestinal loops often lie in a superficial position. The air contained in the digestive tract makes it necessary to move the probe slowly and with continuous pressure in order to progressively expel it from the area under study. The barrier formed by air may be avoided by exploring the digestive structures with the help of organs with good ultrasound conductivity such as the liver, spleen, kidneys or bladder. The mobilisation of gas is also made easier by changes in the patient's position (left and right anterior oblique, upright position). Contiguous transverse sections are performed slowly and systematically, starting in the epigastric region and moving to the hypogastric area. Transverse scanning of the flanks is also carried out, as are longitudinal scanning from right to left of the hypochondrial

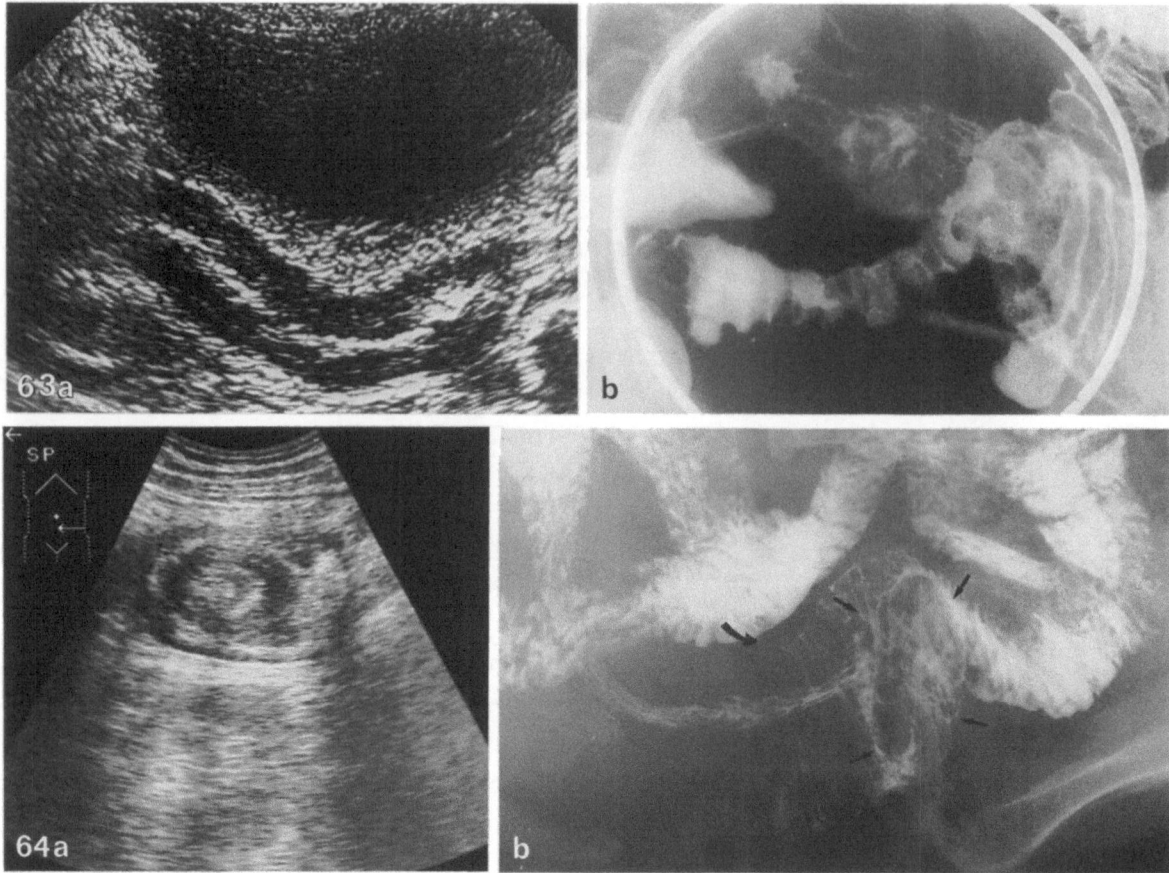

Fig. 63 a, b. Ultrasound : the inflammatory syndrome (Crohn's disease). **a** Ultrasound : regularly thickened walls are noted in an ileal loop, **b** SBFT : there is a stenosis and cobblestoning of the terminal ileum

Fig. 64 a, b. Ultrasound : Intussusception (lipoma). **a** Ultrasound : concentric image is seen within a jejunal loop, **b** SBFT : intussusception is demonstrated proximal to a tumor nodule

regions and the iliac fossae. The scanning needs to be performed very carefully. As soon as an echographic anomaly is detected, multiple sections must be obtained in all planes. Modifications of the ultrasound images during peristaltic waves and persistence of the anomaly in time must be noted. Such a study lasts twice as long as the usual abdominal ultrasound examination, and therefore is not carried out systematically but rather is only performed when the clinical findings require it.

Ultrasonographic interpretation

According to the patient's echogenicity and to the quantity of intestinal air, ultrasound images of the normal small intestine may be of different types. The loops most often appear as clusters of hyperechogenic nodules, either gathered or separated by hypo-echogenic stripes with ill-defined margins. Some of these nodules cause the posterior dispersion of the ultrasound beam. In the most favourable cases, a central echogenic area surrounded by a hypoechogenic rim can be identified within a loop. The central echo corresponds to the intestinal lumen with the gas and secretions it contains, and to the mucosa. The peripheral hypoechogenic ring is the ultrasound image of the wall (submucosa and muscularis). The diameter of the central echo ranges from 3 to 5 mm, and the thickness of the wall from 1 to 3 mm. The loop diameter is usually less than 10 mm. When the ultrasound beam is perpendicular to the cross-section of the loop, the image obtained is called a «target» image. A «sandwich» appearance is observed when the section is longitudinal. These images are continuously altered by peristalsis.

The ultrasound image is modified by pathological processes. The alteration is constant in time,

and the abnormal digestive structure is more easily distinguished from the rest of the digestive tract. Moreover, the elementary (target or sandwich) images are altered as follows :
- enlargement of the central echo,
- thickening of the hypoechogenic ring,
- increase in the caliber of one or several intestinal loops.

These observations allow for the identification of 3 types of syndromes :
- the stasis syndrome,
- the tumoral syndrome,
- the inflammatory syndrome.

The *stasis syndrome* appears as a dilatation of one or several loops, with no changes in the wall thickness. Kerkring's valves are clearly visible as linear hypoechogenic stripes across the intestinal lumen. The distension of the loops may be associated with some ascites. Intestinal obstruction is usually evidenced by the visualization of the valves, the only cause of falsenegative exam being due to the presence of massive ascites. Obstructive lesion should therefore be systematically searched for distally. Ultrasound signs of intestinal obstruction sometimes precede the appearance of air-fluid levels on radiography.

A particular form of obstruction is observed in intussusception. On transverse images, it appears as a target image formed by an enlarged loop, the lumen of which contains a round hypoechogenic nodule. In longitudinal sections, this appears as a central hypoechogenic stripe bordered on either side by hyperechogenic stripes with an outer hypoechogenic margin. A tumor should be sought if intussusception is observed in an adult. Ultrasound plays a capital role in the detection of intussusception in children.

The *tumoral syndrome* appears as a complete modification of the ultrasound image of a loop of small intestine. The lumen becomes, irregular and excentered, while the walls become thicker than 10 mm, multilobulated and asymmetric : this is the «pseudokidney» image. When extraluminal growth of the tumor predominates, the image consists of a round nodule of varying echogenicity and heterogeneity. The intestinal origin of the tumor is difficult to confirm initially. The intestinal origin of the tumor can be often determined by studying its relation to the other intraabdominal structures. It is not always possible to rule out an extrinsic lesion. A pseudokidney image almost always indicates a tumor, benign or malignant. However, benign non-neoplastic in-volvement, for instance an intramural hematoma or an abscess surrounding a gut lesion, may have the same appearance.

The *inflammatory syndrome* is different from the tumoral syndrome. The walls of the digestive tract are regularly and progressively thickened, while the lumen remains central and regular. Both intestinal walls are uniformly thickened ; the increase, ranging from 4 to 10 mm, produces a «target» image in transverse section and a «sandwich» image in longitudinal section ; both are easily differentiated from other intraabdominal structures. Peristaltic waves course through the area, which remains unchanged after the wave has passed. Such an image suggest principally an inflammatory process (often Crohn's disease, but also vascular or radiation-induced lesions). Some neoplastic or infiltrating processes (lymphoma) may have a similar appearance.

All these abnormalities can be confirmed by small bowel follow-through; a negative abdominal ultrasound is not sufficient to exclude abnormalities of small intestine. However, ultrasound is simple and easy to use ; it is thus indicated when intestinal pathology is suspected. Combined with a small bowel follow-through, it allows for the complete imaging of the small intestine since barium opacifies the intestinal lumen and ultrasound visualises the intestinal walls and the surrounding structures.

Computed tomography (figs. 65 to 69)

Computed tomography (CT) sometimes makes it possible to detect disease of the small intestine. It is most often used as an adjunct to the small bowell follow-through, since it provides information about the thickness of the intestinal wall and the extent of extramural lesions.

Technique

Abdominal CT, whatever its indication, requires previous opacification of the digestive tract with a water-soluble iodinated compound (25 to 30 ml of 30 to 40 % iodine solution diluted in 1 l of water) or with a 2 % weight-to-volume barium sulfate suspension. Ingestion of the contrast medium begins one hour before the examination and is continued until its beginning at a rate of one glass every 15 min. The filling of the small intestine may have to be completed during the examination, since ill-opacified

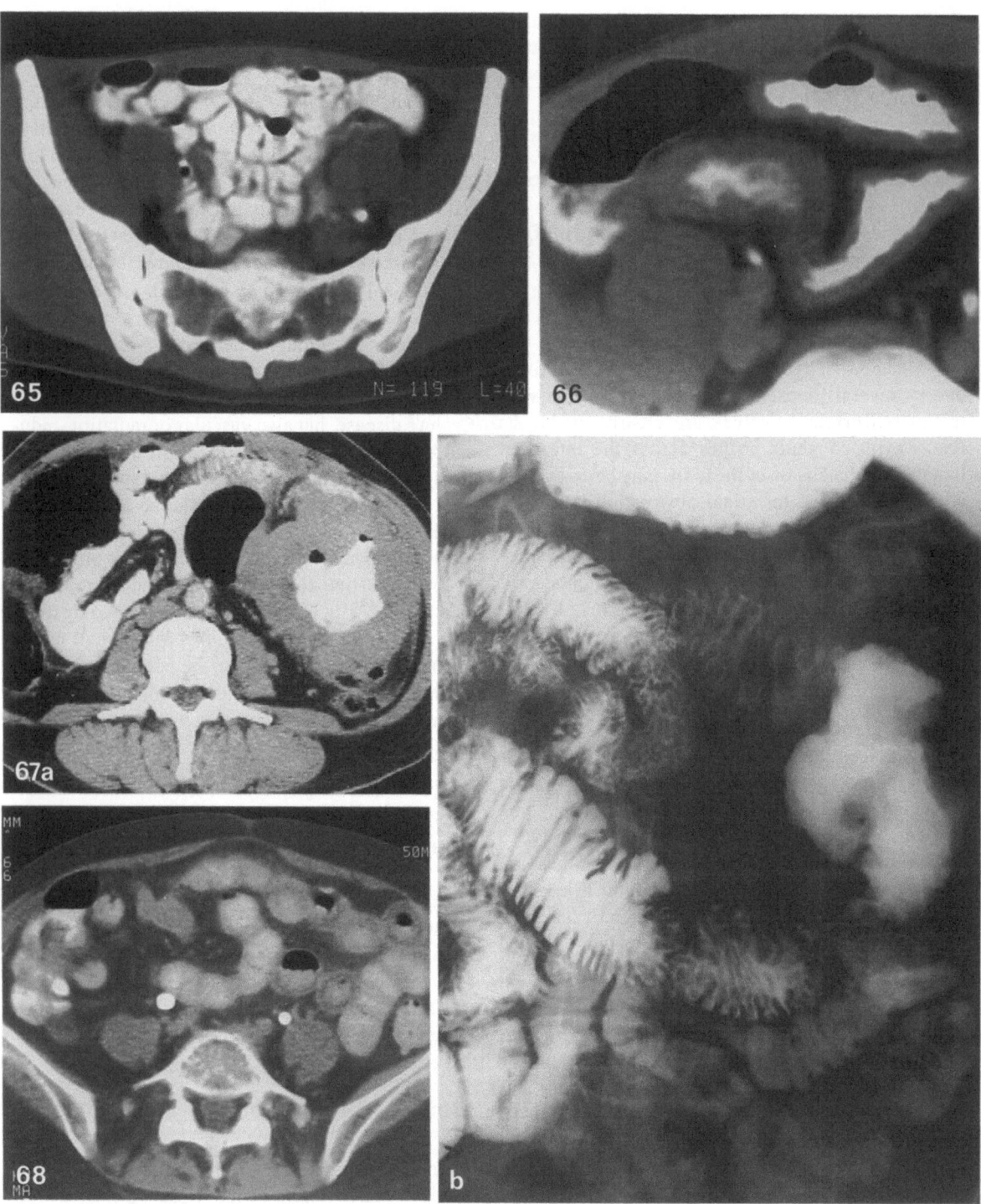

Fig. 65. Computed tomography : normal ileum

Fig. 66. Computed tomography : inflammatory thickening of th terminal ileal wall seen in Crohn's disease

Fig. 67. a Computed tomography : tumoral thickening of the wall of an enlarged jejunal loop caused by a lymphoma (Courtesy of D Régent), **b** SBFT: an image of ectasia is demonstrated

Fig. 68. Computed tomography : diffuse, regular thickening of the wall of ileal loops is shown in a patient with systemic lupus erythematosus

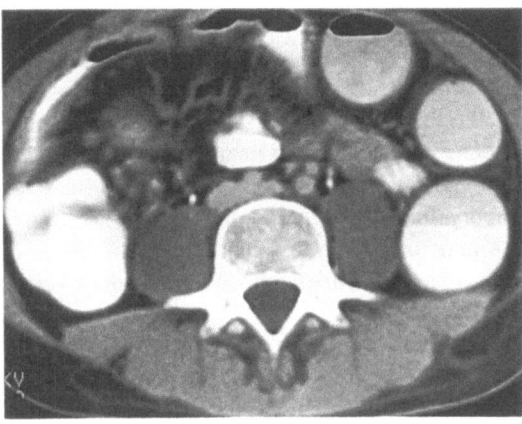

Fig. 69. Computed tomography : mesenteric sclerolipomatosis in Crohn's disease

loops cannot be studied and might be mistaken for intraabdominal masses. Insufflation of the colon is advisable for better localization. Exposure time should be short (3 to 5 s). Slices are taken every 10 mm before the contrast medium is injected. Other sections are taken in the area of concern after the rapid intravenous injection of 60 to 100 ml of contrast medium containing 30 to 40 % iodine. More sections are sometimes needed after a couple of minutes or after changing the patient's position (prone position, lateral decubitus) in order to dissociate the loops of small intestine. Drugs altering intestinal motility are sometimes used.

Normal appearance

The loops of small intestine appear as opacified segments of variable length, according to whether they are oriented tangentially or obliquely to the plane of section. They project as rings when their axis is perpendicular to the plane of section. The diameter of a fully opacified jejunal loop should not exceed 3 cm, that of an ileal loop being slightly less. The wall of a normal loop is 4 mm thick, but may be difficult to measure because of varying amounts of filling. The jejunal folds are not always visible. The upper mesenteric blood vessels are always clearly visible and make it possible to locate the mesentery. Normal mesenteric lymph nodes cannot be identified.

Interpretation

Computed tomography provides less information than a small bowel follow-through about small intestine yet provides details about the neighbouring lesions. Intestinal images should be interpreted carefully, since errors may be caused by variation in the position of the loop to be studied relative to the plane of section or by insufficient filling. It is necessary to study :

- The size of the lumen and the contours of the loop: dilatation of several contiguous loops with normal bowel wall thickness suggest a more distal obstruction. Segmental dilatation with irregular contours and mucosal thickening is seen with a malignant tumor (lymphoma or metastases for example). Stenosis is difficult to identify if a mass is not seen.
- The wall can be thickened in a diffuse, irregular fashion, with thickened folds. The thickening may be segmental and local, with or without the image of a mass. The intestinal lumen may be centred (hematoma) or not (Crohn's disease, malignant tumor). Thickening can also be segmental and multifocal (lymphoma, metastasis). The study of the CT density of the lesions (very low in lipomas), their homogeneity (possibly leading to the benign or malignant character of tumors), and their contrast enhancement after injection (none in ischemic lesions, moderate in lymphomas, more marked in Crohn's disease and metastase and very marked in connective tissue tumors) are helpful in reaching a diagnosis yet this remain difficult.

Intussusception has a characteristic appearance, consisting of two concentric images with tissue density centered on the intestinal lumen.

Other findings may include a mass with extraintestinal involvement. In this case, its relationships to the gut, as well as its density and contrast enhancement after injection must be considered. Masses with areas of water density or containing air bubbles may indicate a tumor with a necrotic center or an abscess near the small intestine. Such an image may also be observed with pancreatic pseudocysts.
- A fistula may appear as an extravasation of contrast medium, most often within a mass (tumor, abscess in Crohn's disease).
- Adenopathy is visible when the diameter of the lymph nodes exceeds 15 mm. The nodes may be large and scattered such as in lymphomas, thus allowing for determining the stage of the tumor. The adenopathy may result in masses as in carcinoid tumors, or may form smaller but more numerous clusters as is the case in Crohn's disease, Whipple's disease, etc.
- An abnormal mesentery caused by fibrosis or edema will increase the density of the mesenteric fat.

Retraction of the mesentery appears as CT dense linear images arranged in a star-shaped pattern.
- Pathological blood vessels, either disrupted or partially thrombosed, may also be visualized.
- Ascites or peritoneal metastases are detected.
- Hepatic metastases will appear hypodense and enhance after contrast injection.

Arteriography (figs.70 to 73)

The indications for arteriography are currently confined to unexplained intestinal hemorrhage, vascular pathology including vascular malformations and preoperative tumor imaging. It is also used following endoscopy, small bowel follow-through, radionuclide scanning, ultrasound and CT examinations. Moreover, it permits concomitant therapeutic modalities to be carried out, such as embolization, angioplasty, or the infusion of vasoconstrictors, vasodilators or antimitotic agents.

Technique

The examination is carried out according to the Seldinger method as an intra-arterial catheter is inserted through the femoral artery, sometimes under general anesthesia. The axillary approach is rarely used. In a suspected case of bowel ischemia, the examination includes aortography with both frontal and lateral views to evidence the origin of the major arteries. In cases of tumor or hemorrhage, arteriography of the superior mesenteric artery is performed first. It is followed by a celiac trunk arteriogram to study the hepatic vascularisation, and search for metastases. The inferior mesenteric artery sometimes has to be visualized if the radiologist is dealing with a large tumor or a vascular malformation. In cases of hemorrhage associated with a small lesion, intraoperative angiography sometimes helps the surgeon to detect the lesion. Contraindications for arteriography include patients with coagulopathes, renal failure and, those with previous allergic reactions to dye. Complications are observed in 0,5 % of all cases.

Anatomy

The superior mesenteric artery originates from the anterior aspect of the aorta at the level of the first lumbar vertebra, below the celiac artery, and forms a loop of caudal concavity, ending in the right iliac fossa where it gives off the appendiceal artery. From its media wall originate 12 to 15 branches perfusing the small intestine, which anastomose to form arches that become more numerous near the terminal ileum. The most distal arches branch into straight vessels that supply the walls of the small intestine. The veins are less numerous and follow the course of the arteries, draining eventually into the superior mesenteric vein.

Interpretation

Abnormalities in the caliber of the proximal trunk or the distal arteries consist of circumferential stenoses that are often excentred, luminal defects (e.g. atheromatous plaques), abrupt cut-offs (embolism or thrombosis), aneurysms (periarteritis nodosa), or alternating areas of stenosis and dilatation. Collaterals may also be seen.

Abnormalities in the course of an artery appear as a displacement, an angulation or a central tethering of the arteries, indicating an infiltration of the mesentery. These findings require that the radiologist search for postoperative adhesions, peritoneal metastases, a carcinoid tumour or sclerolipomatosis as seen in Crohn's disease.

Abnormal vascular patterns in the bowel wall are principally due to tumour neovascularization. This appears as a heterogeneous blush, often formed by short, winding vessels, sometimes with capillary stasis forming opaque pools or, on the contrary, early venous filling. The diagnosis of malignancy is difficult and based on abnormalities of vascular caliber, and the aberrant course of arterioles.

An increase in arteriolar caliber, coupled to early venous filling with or without a local tuft in the bowel wall may be caused by vascular malformations (angioma), which arteriography fails to differentiate from tumours.

Extravasated contrast appears as an opaque pool, either in the intestinal lumen or near the wall. Arteriography detects leakage only if the examination is performed during the hemorrhage and if bleeding is abundant (0,5 ml/mn). Late images make it possible to detect a thrombosis of the superior mesenteric vein when intestinal varices or unusual veins are observed.

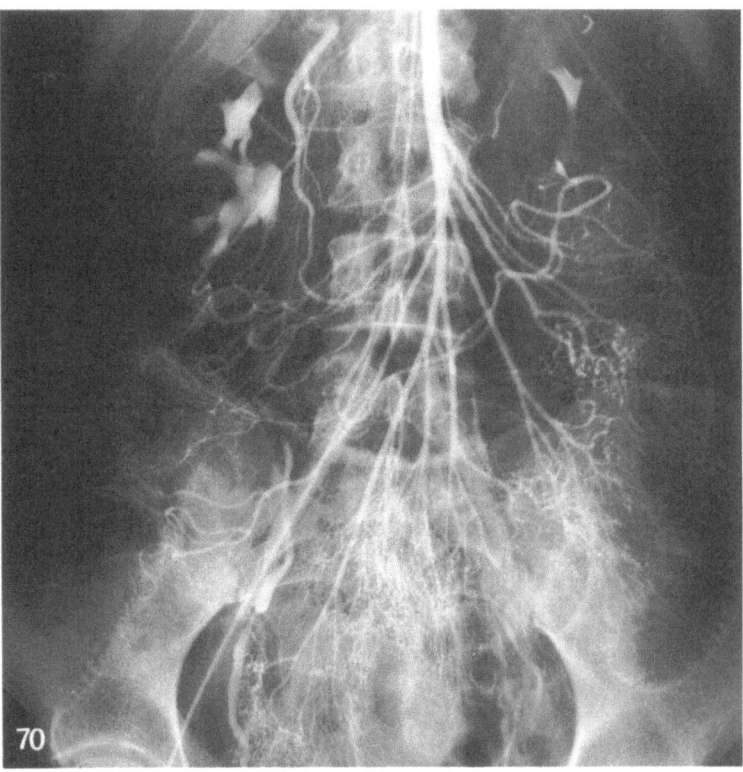

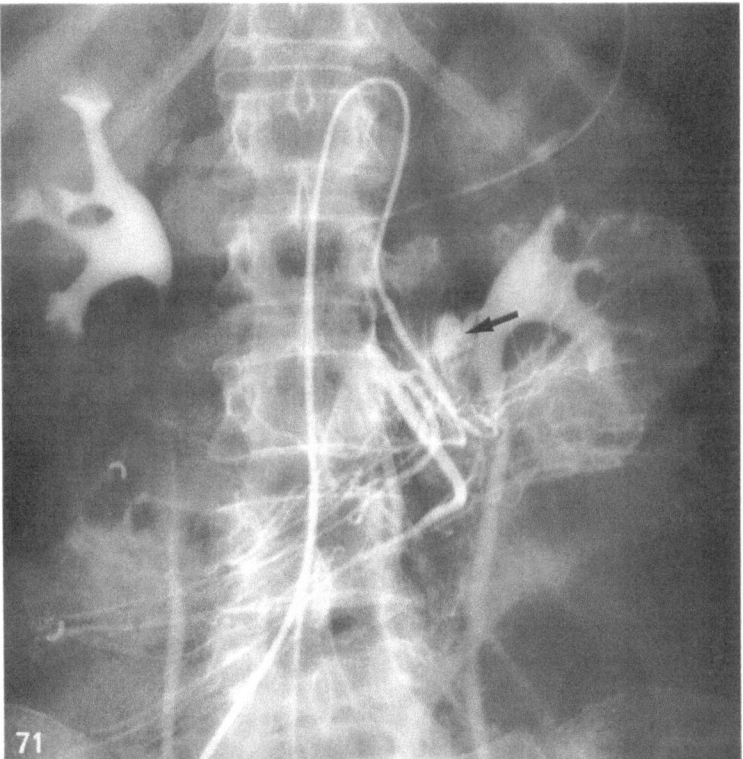

Fig. 70. Mesenteric arteriography : a normal arteriogram

Fig. 71. Mesenteric arteriography : extravasation has occured in one of the first jejunal loops (ulcerated jejunitis)

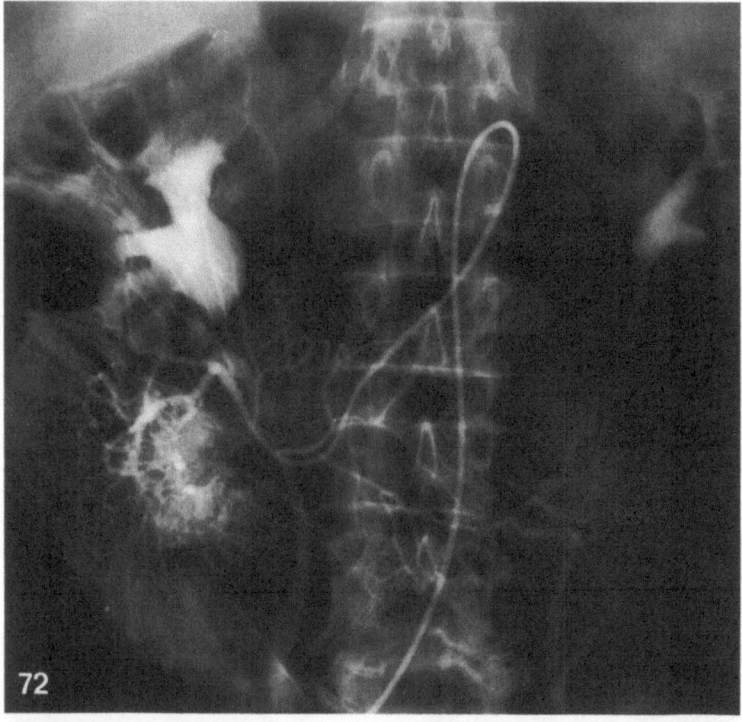

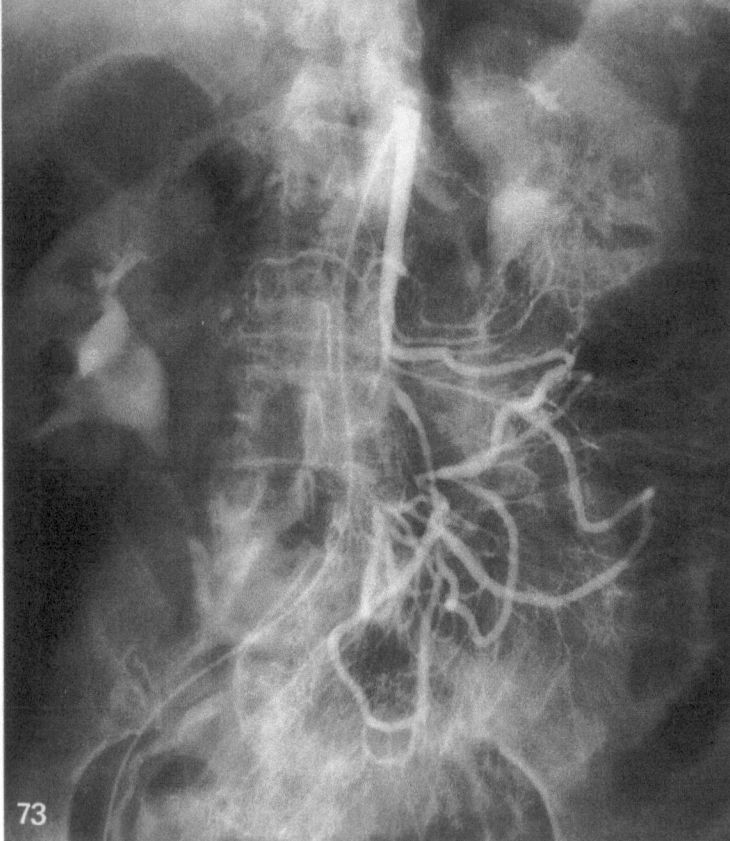

Fig. 72. Mesenteric arteriography : the tumorography of a carcinoid tumor of the ileum is shown

Fig. 73. Mesenteric arteriography : note the irregular course and caliber of the jejunal branches coupled to a stenosis of the superior mesenteric artery trunk (peritoneal metastases)

Practical conclusions

- Small bowel follow-through is the cornerstone of a small intestinal work-up. Its yield is good if its indication is appropriate.
- Whatever procedure is used to visualize the bowel (small bowel follow-through or enteroclysis), the goal is to obtain a continuous image of the whole small intestine and to carefully palpate each loop under fluoroscopy in order to detect all abnormalities.
- Analyzing an abnormal radiograph includes a standard search for its elementary abnormal images, a compilation of these to try and arrive at a radiological syndrome while comparing it to known clinical syndrome.
- Ultrasound, computed tomography and arteriography are complementary examinations that are often useful and sometimes necessary for the study of the area surrounding an intestinal lesion.

References

Physiology and clinic

André C, André F (1976) L'immunité intestinale. Lyon Méd 236 : 585-592

André C, Lambert R (1977) La fonction immunologique de l'intestin grêle. Concours Med, pp 14-18

Arnaud-Battandier F (1984) Le système lymphoïde intestinal : conceptions actuelles. Gastroenterol Clin Biol 8 : 632-640

Avouac B (1979) Physiologie de l'absorption intestinale. Gaz Med France 86 : 1359-1373

Bernier JJ (1979) Classification physiopathologique et anatomique des maladies de l'intestin grêle. Nouv Presse Med 8 : 1249-1341

Cattan D, Pappo E (1972) Que faire devant une diarrhée chez l'adulte. Masson, Paris

Cerf M (1979) Physiopathologie de la diarrhée. Ann Gastroenterol Hepatol 15 : 53-58

Fiorenza V, Yee YS, Zfass AM (1987) Small intestinal motility : normal and abnormal function. Am J Gastroent 82 : 1111-1114

Guerre J, Couturier D (1983) La motricité digestive et ses troubles. Ed Dacosta

Jarry A, Cerf-Bensussan N, Flejou JF, Brousse N (1986) Le système lymphoïde du tube digestif chez l'homme. Ann Pathol 6 : 265-275

Jerzy Glass GB (1970) Principes de physiologie gastrointestinale. Ed Hermann, Paris

Rabe FE, Becker GJ, Besozzi MJ, Miller RE (1981) Efficacy study of the small-boxel examination. Radiology 140 : 47-50

Touraine R, Sedel D (1975) Les syndromes cutanéo-intestinaux. Concours Med 97 : 5976-5997

Vuitton D, Ottignon Y, Seilles E, Zwaig J, Carayon P (1981) Fonctions immunitaires de l'intestin grêle normal. Ann Gastroenterol Hepatol 17 : 383-392

Radionuclide scanning

Alavi A (1980) Scintigraphic demonstration of acute gastrointestinal bleeding. Gastrointest Radiol 5 : 205-208

Atkins HL (1980) Radionuclide studies of the gastrointestinal tract. Gastrointest Radiol 5 : 193-194

Bunker SR, Brown JM, McAuley, Lull RJ, Jackson JH, Hattner RS, Huberty JP (1982) Detection of gastrointestinal bleeding sites : use of in vitro technetium. JAMA 237 : 789-792

Fischbach W, Becker W, Mössner J, Koch W, Reiners C (1987) Faecal alpha-1-antitrypsin and excretion of 111 Indium granulocytes in assessment of disease activity in chronic inflammatory bowel diseases. Gut 28 : 386-393

Markisz JA, Front U, Royal HD, Sacks B, Parker JA, Kolodny GM (1982) An evaluation of Tc-99 m labeled red blood cell scintigraphy for the detection and localization of gastrointestinal bleeding sites. Gastroenterology 83 : 394-398

Miskowiak J, Nielsen SL, Munck O, Burcharth F, Blicherttof M, Nadel MS (1979) Acute gastrointestinal bleeding detected with abdominal scintigraphy using technetium-99 m, labeled albumin. Scand J Gastroenterol 14 : 389-394

Simpson AJ, Previti FW (1982) Technetium sulfur colloid scintigraphy in the detection of lower gastrointestinal tract bleeding. Surg Gynecol Obstet 155 : 33-36

Small bowel follow-through

Antes G, Lissner J (1983) Double contrast small bowel examination with barium and methylcellulose, results in 300 cases. Radiology 148 : 37-40

Bilbao MK, Frische LH, Dotter CT, Rosch J (1967) Hypotonic duodenography. Radiology 89 : 438-443

Caldwell WL, Floch MH (1963) Evaluation of the small bowel barium motor meal with emphasis on the effect of volume of barium suspensions ingested. Radiology 80-3 : 383-391

Chabouis CF, Mordy M, Desoutter P, Baudet P, Cattini J (1982) Technique radiologique, nouvelle technique d'investigation radiologique du grêle. Ann Radiol 25 : 309-311

Clément JP, Burelle H, Corbeau A, Colleter JF (1977) Examen radiologique de l'intestin grêle en double contraste. J Radiol Electrol 58 : 231-236

De Busscher G (1954) Le transit accéléré non provoqué du grêle au cours de l'examen radiologique. Acta Gastroenterol Belg, pp 673-684

Ekberg O (1977) Double contrast examination of the small bowel. Gastrointest Radiology 1 : 349-353

Fisher JK (1982) Angled view of the distal small bowel. Radiology 144 : 417-418

Fournier AM, Cave P, Duval J (1979) Pour un grêle en double contraste... et en 6 mn. J Radiol 60 : 71-74

Fried AM, Poulos A, Hatfield DR (1981) The effectiveness of the incidental small-bowel series. Radiology 140 : 45-46

Friedmann J, Rigler LG (1950) A method of double-contrast roentgen examination of the small intestine. Radiology 54 : 365-379

Gelfand DW (1980) Complications of gastrointestinal radiologic procedures : I. Complications of routine fluoroscopic studies. Gastrointest Radiol 5 : 293-315

Gershon-Cohen J, Shay H (1939) Barium enteroclysis, a method for single and double contrast techniques. AJR 42-3 : 456-458

Gharemani GG, Turner MA, Port BB (1980) Iatrogenic intubation injuries of the upper gastro-intestinal tract in adult. Gastrointest Radiol 5 : 1-10

Goei R, Lamers RJS, Lamers JJH (1988) Enteroclysis. Improved performance using a flow inducer. Acta Radiol 29 : 665-668

Golden R (1959) Technical factors in the roentgen examination of the small intestine. AJR 82-6 : 965-972

Grivaux M, Cornet A, Wattez E (1964) Le métoclopramide en radiologie digestive. Sem Hop Paris 44 : 2338-2345

Grumbach K, Herlinger H, Laufer I, Levine MS (1985) Metoclopramide/ceruletide aided small bowel examination. Gastrointest Radiol 10 : 299

Herlinger H (1978) A modified technique for the double contrast small bowel enema. Gastrointest Radiol 3 : 201-207

Hudak A (1951) Le transit accéléré du grêle. Radiol Clin 20 : 148-154

Kreel L (1970) The use of metoclopramide in the barium meal and follow through examination. AJR 43 : 31-35

Loubière M, Grimaud A, Coussement A, Rampal P, Delmont J, Serres JJ (1977) L'étude radiologique en double contraste de l'intestin grêle sous intubation duodéno-jéjunale. J Radiol Electrol 58 : 75-79

Lura A (1951) Radiology of the small intestine enema of the small intestine with special emphasis on the diagnosis of tumors. Br J Radiol 24-281 : 264-271

Maglinte DDT, Burney BT, Miller RE (1982) Lesions missed on small-bowel follow-through : analysis and recommandations. Radiology 144 : 737-739

Maglinte DDT, Burney BT, Miller RE (1982) Technical factors for a more rapid enteroclysis. AJR 138 : 588-591

Maglinte DDT, Hall R, Miller RE, Chernish SM, Rosenak B, Elmore M, Burney BT (1984) Detection of surgical lesions of the small bowel by enteroclysis. Am J Surg 147 : 225-229

Maglinte DDT, Lappas JC, Chernish SM, Sellink JL (1986) Intubation routes for enteroclysis. Radiology 158 : 553-554

Maglinte DDT, Miller RE (1984) A comparison of pumps used for enteroclysis. Radiology 152 : 815

Maglinte DDT, Peterson LA, Vahey TN, Miller RE, Chernish SM (1984) Enteroclysis in partial small bowel obstruction. Am J Surg 147 : 325-329

Mandell GA, Teplick SK (1982) Glucagon, its application to childhood gastrointestinal radiology. Gastrointest Radiol 7 : 7-13

Margulis AR, Mandelstram (1961) The use of neostigmine in the roentgen study of the small bowel. Radiology 76 : 223-229

Miller RE, Sellink JL (1979) Enteroclysis : the small bowel enema how to succeed and how to fail. Gastrointest Radiol 4 : 269-283

Monod E (1964) Action enterokinétique de la Cécékine. Arch Mal App Dig 53 : 607-608

Morin G., Besançon F., Grall A., Jouve R., Debray C. (1965) Technique d'accélération du transit du grêle. Arch Mal App Dig 54 : 1285-1290

Morton JL (1961) Notes on a small bowel examination. AJR 86-1 : 76-85

Naumann W (1948) Funktionnelle Dünndarmdiagnostik im Röntgenbild. Thieme, Stuttgart

Nolan DJ (1979) Rapid duodenal and jejunal intubation. Clin Radiol 30 : 183-185

Nolan DJ, Cadman PJ, Jeffree MA (1985) Detailed per-oral small-bowel examination versus enteroclysis. Radiology 157 : 836-837

Ott DJ, Chen YM, Gelfand DW, Van Swearingen FV, Munitz HA (1985) Detailed per-oral small bowel examination vs, enteroclysis. Radiology 155 : 29-34

Ott DJ, Gelfand DW, Swearingen FV (1985) Peroral small bowel examinations vs, enteroclysis : expenditures and radiation exposure. Radiology 155 : 29-31

Pansdorf M (1937) Die fraktionierte Dünndarm-Füllung und ihre klinishe Bedeutung-Fortschr. Geb Röentgenstr

Pesquera GS (1929) A method for the direct visualization of lesions in the small intestines. AJR 22-3 : 254-257

Porcher P, Caroli S (1957) Un accélérateur inattendu du transit intestinal grêle et colique. Arch Mal App Dig 46 : 663-665

Pygott F, Street DF, Shellshear MF, Rhodes CJ (1960) Radiological investigation of the small intestine by small bowel enema technique. Gut 1 : 366-370

Schatzki R (1943) Small intestinal enema. AJR 50-6 : 743-751

Schmutz G, Jahn C, Benhaim M, Drape JL, Chapuis A, Vaxman F (1987) Intérêt du transit du grêle par entéroclyse dans les syndromes obstructifs de l'intestin grêle. A propos de 212 examens. J Radiol 68 : 23-30

Schmutz G, Zeller C, Riwer B, Kempf F (1981) Le transit du grêle en double contraste : techniques, indications et résultats, à propos de 300 examens. Ann Radiol 24 : 256-260

Scott-Harden WG, Hamilton HAR, McCall Smith S (1961) Radiological investigation of the small intestine. Gut 2 : 316-322

Skjennald A, Samset JH (1980) Duodeno-jejunal intubation in examination of the small bowel. Clin Radiol 31 : 221-224

Tavernier J, Comte B, Dilhuydy JM, Laraki D (1974) Transit du grêle par intubation duodénale. J Radiol Electrol 55 : 263-264

Vidal JL, Lestrade M, Joffre F, Fardou H, Carly JB (1975) Grêle en double contraste chez l'adulte. J Radiol Electrol 56 : 739-741

Weintraub S, Williams RG (1949) A rapid method of roentgenologic examination of the small intestine. AJR 61 : 45-55

Weltz GA (1937) Der kranke Dünndarm im Röntgenbild. Fortschritte R 55 : 20-40

Analysis of radiological images

Berk RN (1985) Classification radiologique simplifiée des maladies de l'intestin grêle. Arch Clin Imaging 1 : 42-48

Cherigie E, Deporte A, Tavernier C, Pradel-Raynal Mme (1959) Le grêle terminal de l'enfant, Etude anatomique, anatomo-pathologique et radiologique. Ann Radiol II : 319-374

Colleter JF (1977) La radiologie de l'intestin grêle en double contraste. Thèse, Marseille

Davis M, Siegel M, Parker T, Davis GS (1988) Small bowel edema : mosaic pattern. Gastrointest Radiol 13 : 219-220

Fanucci A, Cerro P, Fraracci L, Ietto F (1984) Small bowel length measured by radiography. Gastrointest Radiol 9 : 349-351

Gelfand DW, Ott DJ (1981) Radiographic demonstration of small intestinal villi on routine clinical studies. Gastrointest Radiol 6 : 21-27

Goldberg HI, Gould R, Rosenquist J, Royal S, Owens R, Silverman S (1982) In vivo demonstration of small intestinal villi in dogs and monkeys using radiographic magnification. Radiology 142 : 53-58

Goldberg HI, Sheft DJ (1976) Abnormalities in small intestine contour and caliber. Radiol Clin North Am 14 : 461-475

Haworth EM, Hodson CJ, Joyce CRB, Pringle EM, Solimano G, Young WF (1967) Radiological measurement of small bowel calibre in normal subjects according to age. Clin Radiol 18 : 417-421

Jones B, Hamilton SR, Rubesin SE, Bayless TM, Ravich WJ, Hendrix TR (1987) Granular small bowel mucosa : a reflection of villous abnormality. Gastrointest Radiol 12 : 219-225

Levesque M, Legmann P (1986) Exploration radiologique de l'intestin grêle, pourquoi, quand et comment ? Société Française de Radiologie ; Journées Francophones

Levesque M, Vallée C, Legman P (1983) Transit radiologique de l'intestin grêle, technique et sémiologie. Feuillets de Radiologie 23 : 269-298

Maglinte DDT, Lappas JC, Kelvin FM, Rex D, Chernish SM (1987) Small bowel radiography : how, when, and why ? Radiology 163 : 297-305

Meschan I (1984) An overview and summary of roentgen signs of diseases of the small intestine. Mount Sinai J Med 51 : 319-336

Meyers MA (1976) Clinical involvement of mesenteric and antimesenteric borders of small bowel loops. I — Normal pattern and relationships Gastrointest. Radiology 1 : 41-47

Meyers MA (1976) Clinical involvement of mesenteric and antimesenteric borders of small bowel loops. II — Radiologic interpretation of pathologic alteration. Gastrointest Radiology 1 : 49-58

Osborn AG, Friedland GW (1973) A radiological approach to the diagnosis of small bowel disease. Clin Radiol 24 : 281-301

Sanders DE, Ho CS (1976) The small bowel enema : experience with 150 examinations. AJR 127 : 743-751

Scherrer A, Nahum P, Nahum H (1977) La présence d'air dans le grêle est-elle pathologique ? J Radiol Electrol 58 : 199-202

Stevenson GW, Collins SM, Somers S (1988) Radiological appearance of migrating motor complex of the small intestine. Gastrointest Radiol 13 : 215-218

Tully TE, Feinberg SB (1974) A roentgenographic classification of diffuse disease of the small intestine presenting with malabsorption. AJR 121 : 283-290

Vallance R (1980) An evaluation ot the small bowel enema based on an analysis of 350 consecutive examinations. Clin Radiol 31 : 227-232

Zahnd G, Golmard JL, Curet Ph, Grellet J (1980) L'air dans le grêle chez l'adulte, résultats sur un groupe témoin de 827 sujets. J Radiol 61 : 759-762

Ultrasound

Bluth EI, Merritt CRB, Sullivan MA (1979) Ultrasonic evaluation of the stomach, small bowel and colon. Radiology 133 : 677-680

Bowerman RA, Silver TM, Jaffe MH (1982) Real time ultrasound diagnosis of intussusception in children. Radiology 143 : 527-529

Cholankeril JV, Ketyer S, Kessler MA, Kogan E (1982) Computerized tomography and ultrasonography in intussusception of the small bowel. CT 6 : 167-170

Derchi LE, Solbiati L, Rizzatto G, Depra L (1987) Normal anatomy and pathology changes of the small bowel mesentery : US appearance. Radiology 164 : 649-652

Dubbins PA (1984) Ultrasound demonstration of bowel wall thickness in inflammatory bowel disease. Clin Radiol 35 : 227-231

Fakhary JR, Berk RN (1981) The « target » pattern : characteristic sonographic feature of stomach and bowel abnormalities. AJR 137 : 969-972

Fleischer AC, Dowling AD, Weinstein ML, James AE Jr (1979) Sonographic patterns of distended fluid, filledbowel. Radiology 133 : 681-685

Fleischer AC, Muhletaler CA, James AE (1981) Sonographic assessment of the bowel wall. AJR 136 : 887-891

Fleischer AC, Muhletaler CA, James AE Jr (1980) Sonographic patterns arising from normal and abnormal bowel. Radiol Clin North Am 18 : 145-159

Frank VP, Menges V, Klein M (1978) Die Ultraschalldiagnostik bei wandinfiltrativen Prozessen des Intestinalteration. Fortschr Röntgenstr 129 : 90-98

Jenss H (1982) Bedeutung der Sonographie für Magen un Darmdiagnostik. Internist 23 : 541-547

Kremer H, Kellner E, Schierl W, Zollner N (1978) Sonographische Diagnostik beiden infiltrativen Magendarm-Erkrankungen. Dtsch Med Wochenschr 1903 : 965-966

Lutz HT, Petzoldt R (1976) Ultrasonic patterns of space occupying lesions of the stomach and the intestine. Ultrasound Med Biol 2 : 129-132

Montali G, Croce F, De Pra L, Solbiati L (1983) Intussusception of the bowel a new sonographic pattern. Br J Radiol 56 : 273-276

Morgan CL, Trought WS, Oddson TA, Clark WM, Rice RP (1980) Ultrasound patterns of disorders affecting the gastointestinal tract. Radiology 135 : 129-1345

Morin ME, Brumenthal DH, Tan A, Li YP (1981) The ultrasonic appearance of ileocolic intussusception. J Clin Ultrasound 9 : 516-518

Oliva L, Derchi LE, Giggi E, Cicio GR (1986) Echographie du tube digestif. JEMU 7 : 137-144

Peterson LR, Cooperberg PL (1978) Ultrasound demonstration of lesions of the gastrointestinal tract. Gastrointest Radiol 3 : 303-306

Schmutz G (1988) L'échographie du tube digestif. Feuillets de Radiologie 28 : 137-144

Schmutz G, Benhaim M, Hannequin F, Ridereau C, Drapé JL, Beigelman C (1988) L'échographie abdominale dans l'exploration morphologique de l'intestin grêle. JEMU 9 : 72-77

Weil F (1978) Ultrasonography of digestive diseases. Mosby éd, Paris

Weill F, Zeltnerf, Rottmer P, Bihr E, Tuetey JB (1979) Les images gastriques et intestinales en ultrasonographie abdominale, le signe du mouvement brownien. J Radiol 60 : 579-590

Computed tomography

Chambers SE, Best JJK (1984) A comparison of dilute barium and dilute water-soluble contrast in opacification of the bowel for abdominal computed tomography. Clin Radiol 35 : 463-464

Cholankeril JV, Ketyer S, Kessler MA, Kogan E (1982) Computerized tomography and ultrasonography in intussusception of the small bowel. CT 6 : 167-170

Curcio CM, Feinstein RS, Humphrey RL, Jones B, Siegelman SS (1982) Computed tomography of enteroenteric intussusception. J Comput Assist Tomogr 6 : 969-974

James S, Balfe DM, Lee JKT, Picus D (1987) Small bowel disease : categorization by CT examination. AJR 148 : 863-868

Lubat E, Balthazar EJ (1988) The current role of computerized tomography in inflammatory disease of the bowel. Am J Gastro Ent 83 : 107-113

Marks WM, Goldberg HI, Moss AA, Koehler FR, Federle MP (1980) Intestinal pseudotumors : a problem in abdominal computed tomography solved by directed techniques. Gastro-intest Radiol 5 : 155-160

Meyers M (1986) Computed tomography of the gastro-intestinal tract. Springer-Verlag New York

Schnyder P, Candardjis G (1983) CT detection of benign and malignant abnormalities of the small bowel. Eur J Radiol 3 : 33-38

Schnyder P, Candardjis G (1985) Evaluation de la pathologie de l'intestin grêle par tomographie numérisée, à propos de 34 cas. J Radiol 66 : 753-761

Seltzer SE (1984) Abnormal intraabdominal gas collections visualized on computed tomography : a clinical and experimental study. Gastrointest Radiol 9 : 127-131

Solomon A, Papo J, Pikielny S, Stern D (1987) Computed tomographic investigation of serosal and intramural gastrointestinal pathology. Gastrointest Radiol 12 : 13-17

Styles RA, Larsen CR (1983) CT appearance of adult intussusception. J Comput Assist Tomogr 7 : 331-333

Arteriography

Curet P, Waiss L, Wiart D, Grellet J (1983) Malabsorption et anomalies vasculaires mésentériques supérieures complexes. J Radiol 64 : 69-72

Fazio FW, Zelas P, Weakley FL (1980) Intraoperative angiography and the localization of bleeding from the small intestine. Surg Gynecol Obstet 151 : 637-640

Hines JR, Stryker SJ, Neiman HL, Larsen LR, Gottlieb J, Craig RM, Poticha SM (1981) Intraoperative angiography in intestinal angiodysplasia. Surg Gynécol Obstet 152 : 453-460

Lang EK (1979) Current and future applications of angiography in the abdomen. Radiol Clin North Am 17 : 55-75

Myllylä V, Päivänsalo M, Leinonen A (1984) Angiographic diagnosis at gastrointestinal hemorrhage. Diagn Imag Clin Med, 53 : 135-140

Nyman U, Boijsen E, Lindström C, Rosengren JE (1980) Angiography in angiomatous lesions of the gastrointestinal tract. Acta Radiol 21 : 21-31

Palmaz JC, Walter JF, Cho KJ (1984) Therapeutic embolization of the small-bowel arteries. Radiology 152 : 377-382

Rahn NH, Tishler JM, Han SY, Russinovich NAE (1982) Diagnostic and interventional angiography in acute gastrointestinal hemorrhage. Radiology 143 : 361-366

Ross JA (1952) Vascular patterns of small and large intestine compared. Br J Surg 39 : 330-333

Tillotson CL, Geller SC, Kantrowitz L, Eckstein MR, Waltman AC, Athanasoulis CA (1988) Small bowel hemorrage : angiographic localization and intervention. Gastrointest Radiol 13 : 207-211

Congenital pathology

Malformations of the small intestine appear either during the neonatal period (stenosis, atresia) or during life (malrotation of the primitive umbilical loop, segmental dilatation, congenital adhesions, hernias or eventrations, Meckel's diverticula, duplications, vascular malformations).

Stenosis and atresia of the small intestine (fig. 1)

Single or multiple stenosis and atresia or agenesis of the small intestine indicate a defect in the development of a segment of the gut. This kind of malformation has no site of predilection, and is often associated with malformations of other organs.

These present as cases of neonatal occlusion. Plain radiographs show gas distension proximal to the obstruction and, according to the degree of occlusion, the presence or absence of meconial densities distally to it.

The barium enema can flow up to the stenosis and demonstrate it, especially when the obstruction is localized to the ileum. Antegrade studies of the small bowel should be avoided.

Segmental dilatation (figs. 2 to 4)

Well-delimited segmental ectasia without peristalsis can be observed in jejunal or ileal loops in continuity with proximal and distal segments exhibiting normal peristalsis. Its pathogenesis is controversial: either it is due to temporary obstruction by the vitelline vessels during development, or to a real dysplasia, since heterotopic tissue (pulmonary, laryngeal,

œsophageal or gastric) is observed in 20% of cases. The disease is also associated with other malformations (omphalocele, Meckel's diverticulum, imperforate anus, myelomeningocele, etc.) in one third of cases.

Pathological examination demonstrates thinned muscular layers and, in some cases, lesions of the intramural neural plexuses. Ulcerations are observed in adults.

This abnormality is often asymptomatic. Symptoms, when present in neonates, are that of intestinal obstruction. In later life, affected subjects may develop bouts of partial bowel obstruction, hemorrhage, malabsorption, and bacterial overgrowth syndromes.

Plain radiographs may demonstrate the dilated area as an oval gas-filled structure which may contain an air-fluid level. Proximal dilatation may also be observed.

Barium studies opacify the aperistaltic pouch intercalated between two normal loops. The folds in the dilated segment may be normal or rarefied, and ulceration may occur.

Visceral myopathy and neuropathy (fig. 5)

These visceral myopathies and neuropathies are rare diseases, often familial. They may be associated with malformations such as intestinal malrotation, pyloric hypertrophy, and megabladder. The digestive signs are akin to those of scleroderma, from which these diseases differ by the absence of systemic involvement and by different histological features. In the visceral myopathies, the rarefaction and vacuolization of muscle cells is associated with fibrosis. Unlike scleroderma, the lesions are mainly found

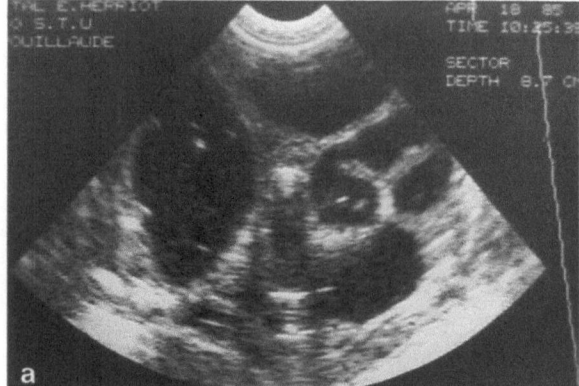

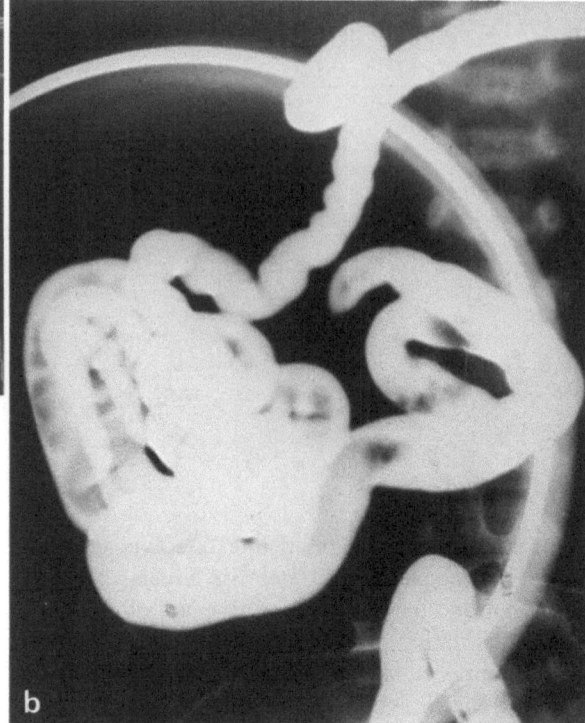

Fig. 1 a, b. Ileal atresia (Courtesy of J M Pouillaude) Neonatal occlusion. **a** Ultrasound : dilatation of loops, **b** Gastrografin enema : backwash into the small intestine stopped at 30 cm. Surgery showed atresia secondary to antenatal volvulus

in the longitudinal muscular layer. In the visceral neuropathies, the lesions involve the myenteric neural plexuses, where axonal degeneration and drop-out can be seen.

Such diseases appear in children and adults of both sexes equally, and present as intermittent bouts of partial intestinal obstruction. Other signs may include diarrhea paradoxically, as well as malabsorption or steatorrhea which may develop due to a bacterial overgrowth syndrome. The mortality is high in infants because of malnutrition or perforation. The disease is lethal in 50% of adults after a variably lengthy, relapsing course, often studded with multiple futile surgical procedures. No treatment is known other than antibiotic therapy, which is effective in bacterial overgrowth and may also reduce malabsorption.

Plain radiographs of the abdomen often demonstrate dilatation and air-fluid levels. Besides the multiple episodes of subocclusion, the clinician should suspect this diagnosis if there exists a discrepancy between the impressive radiological picture and the mild character of the clinical signs.

Barium studies demonstrate a slower transit time, atonia with mainly duodenal and jejunal dilatation, a decrease in peristalsis with ineffective contractions (sometimes occurring at random) and less often, a segmentation of the contrast medium with misleading spasms. The folds are normal, the interfold spaces are not decreased contrary to what is observed in scleroderma. Diverticula and pneumatosis cystoides intestinalis have been observed. The diagnosis may be suggested by a considerable duodenal dilatation proximal to the arterial mesenteric takeoff, an unusual sign seen in obstruction. Manometric and radiological abnormalities of the esophagus and of the colon are often present: esophageal atonia, usually without associated reflux unlike what is observed in scleroderma, and colonic atonia with dilatation, diverticular formations and rarefied haustrations are noted. The stomach is usually normal.

In summary, the clinical and radiological findings may sometimes make it possible to suspect a diagnosis of pseudo-obstruction in the case of an occlusion of the small intestine, and thus avoid inappropriate surgery.

Hirschsprung's disease

Along with the immaturity of the neural plexuses in newborn infants, which makes temporary parenteral

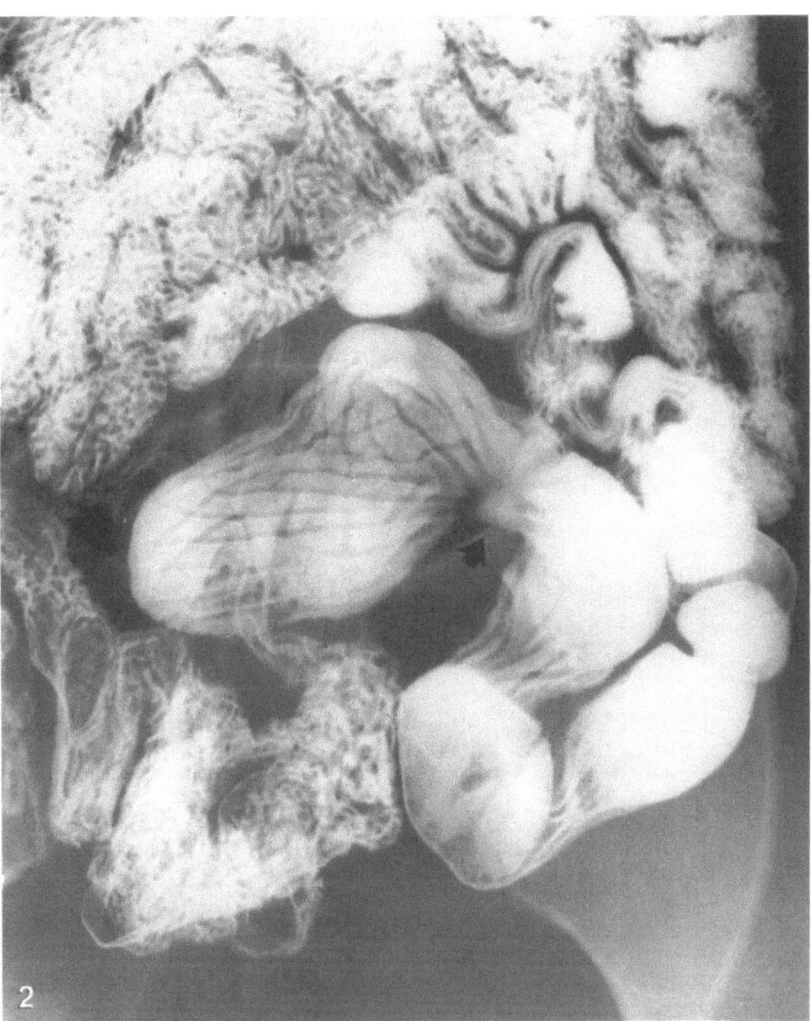

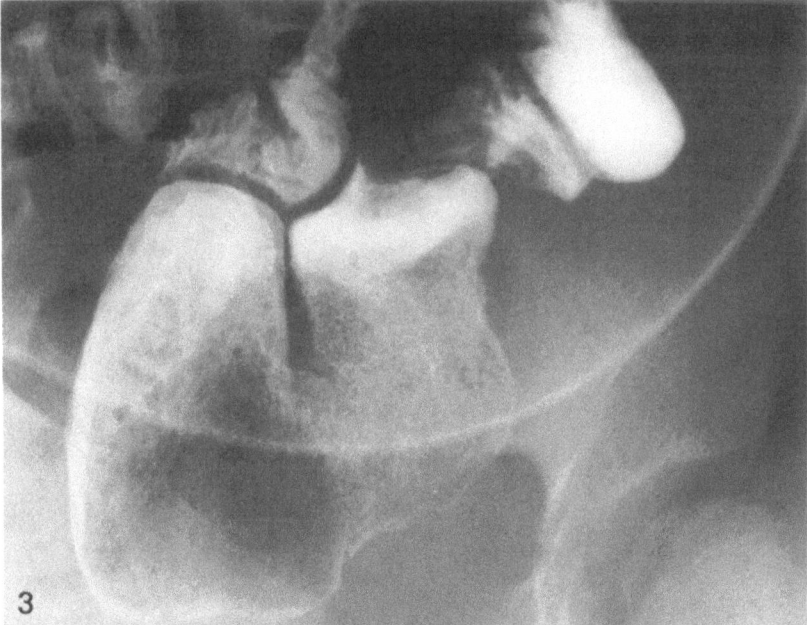

Fig. 2. Congenital segmental dilatation. This 39-year-old woman presented with a hypochromic anemia and a positive isotopic Weber test. The SBFT demonstrated a fusiform dilatation of a pelvic loop extending over 15 cm, with a medial ulceration outlined by radiating folds

Fig. 3. Congenital segmental dilatation. An 8-year-old girl presented with hypochromic anemia. The SBFT showed segmental dilatation of a pelvic loop

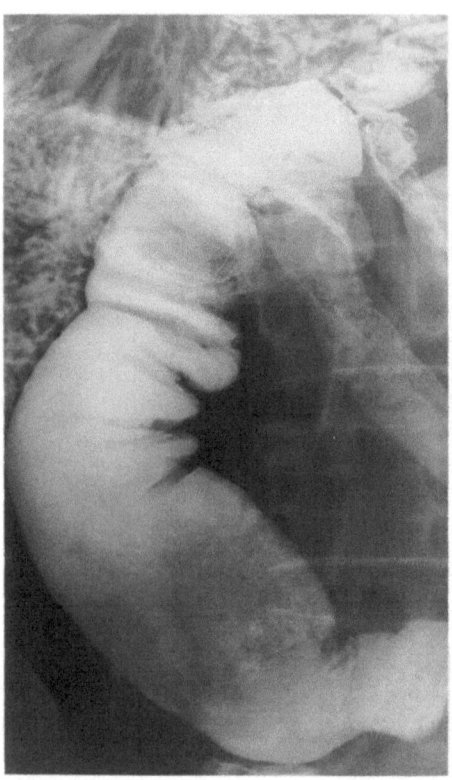

Fig. 4. Congenital segmental dilatation. A 39-year-old man complained of umbilical pain and bouts of melena. The SBFT showed segmental dilatation of an ileal loop

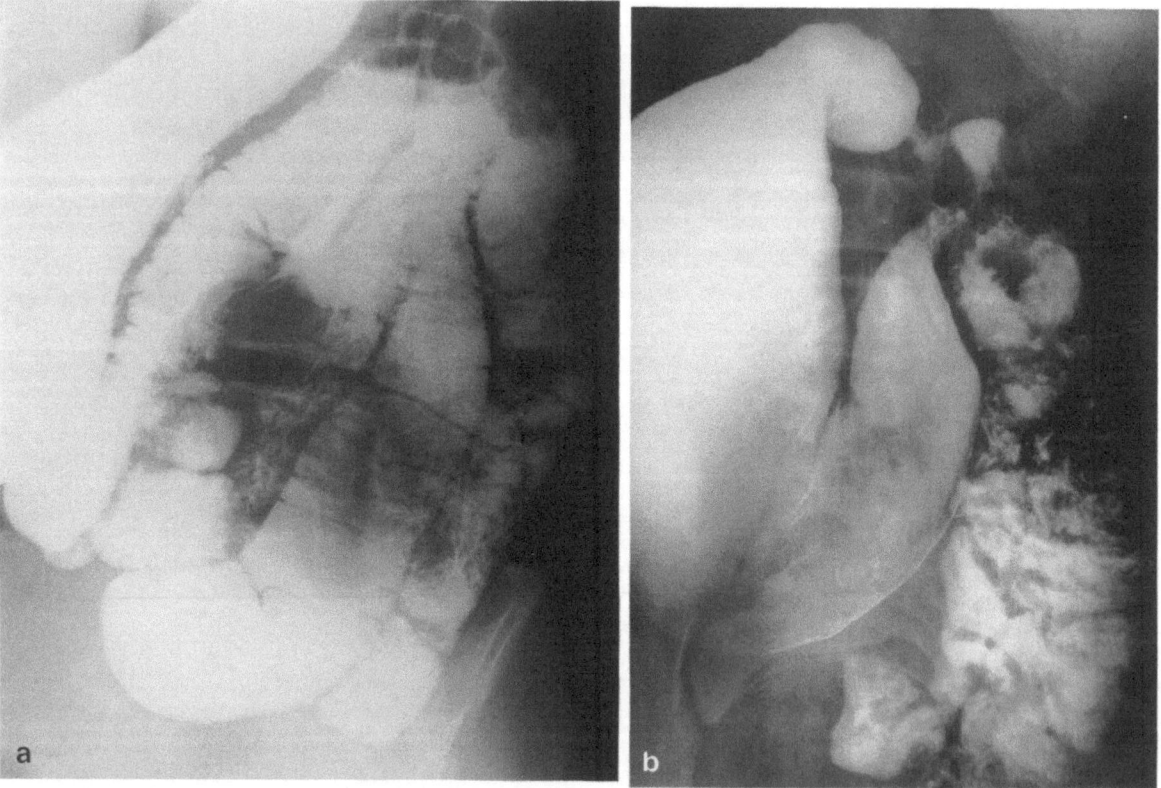

Fig. 5 a,b . Hereditary visceral myopathy. A 45-year-old constipated woman presented with a family history of intestinal obstruction. a Note the jejunal atony, b A megaduodenum was found in her daughter

nutrition necessary, aganglionosis can affect the entire colon and the terminal ileum. This presents as sub-occlusion or complete obstruction in newborns and infants. The small intestine is dilated proximal to the terminal ileum and the colon, which have a normal appearance. Intussusception often occurs in the area of transition. The prognosis is serious and complete colectomy is often necessary.

Adhesions, hernias, eventrations (fig. 6)

The diagnosis of eventration is based on clinical findings.

In the neonatal period, adhesions and hernias rarely cause acute obstruction, the etiological diagnosis of which is made at surgery. On the other hand, either may cause an obstructive syndrome during later life.

Congenital adhesions are less frequent in the small intestine than in the duodenum and are usually not very obstructive. Plain abdominal radiographs may demonstrate distension and air-fluid levels. Barium studies demonstrate dilatation of one or several loops proximal to a short stenosis, which does not move with palpation and sometimes causes angulation.

Congenital internal hernias are usually well tolerated and are almost never observed in children. They are discovered in adults after an acute accident, the severity of which depends on the extent of the ischemic insult of the herniated loops. Retroperitoneal internal hernias, are mainly paraduodenal or paracecal hernias with a sac and have to be distinguished from the less frequent hernias occurring through mesenteric or mesocolic openings.

The radiological diagnosis of an internal hernia on barium contrast can be based on the abnormal position of several loops, which form a mass with a circular or ovoid contour corresponding to the hernial sac. Intestinal dilatation may be observed either in the migrated loops or proximally, in contrast to the hernial pedicle which is made up of more or less narrowed loops. Computed tomography is sometimes useful to demonstrate the abnormal position of the loops.

One or several loops of small intestine may incarcerate in an external (inguinal, crural, umbilical) or diaphragmatic hernia or into an eventration.

Malrotations of the primitive loop (fig. 7)

These abnormalities remain usually silent and are often discovered accidentally, although some of them may favour the appearance of a volvulus, especially in neonates where the condition may be lethal unless the diagnosis is made rapidly on the basis of plain radiographs.

Absence of rotation is very rare. Inverted rotation leads to situs inversus, thus producing a mirror-image position of the abdominal organs, with or without dextrocardia. Rotation limited to 90° is the most frequent abnormality and is termed a common mesentery. On barium studies, the mobile duodenum and the loops of the small intestine are found to lie to the right of the midsagittal plane, and the colon on its left. The cecum is often mobile and in paramedian position. When rotation ceases at 180°, the cecum (erectum) and the terminal ileum are located under the liver. When rotation exceeds 270°, the mobile right colon (recurvatum) is followed by the cecum and the terminal ileum into the right iliac fossa. This mobility favours episodes of volvulus.

Suspicion of malrotation sometimes arises on the basis of plain abdominal radiographs, especially in infants. Malrotations are easily evidenced by a barium small bowel follow-through or enema. Computed tomography demonstrates the position of the small bowel loops relative to the superior mesenteric artery, but is not necessary for diagnosis.

Diverticula

Diverticulosis (fig. 8)

Congenital diverticula are mainly found on the antimesenteric aspect of the intestine, while acquired diverticula appear on the mesenteric aspect near the sites of penetration of blood vessels. Clinical signs are rare and due to complications: hemorrhage due to an ulcer, abscess formation, obstruction, which may be from a volvulus, perforation, or malabsorption due to bacterial overgrowth. Plain radiographs sometimes show an image mimicking an obstruction, with air-fluid levels on upright films. Calcified foreign bodies may be seen within the diverticula. If the diverticula are multiple, opacification of these with barium is superimposed on the image of the jejunal loops.

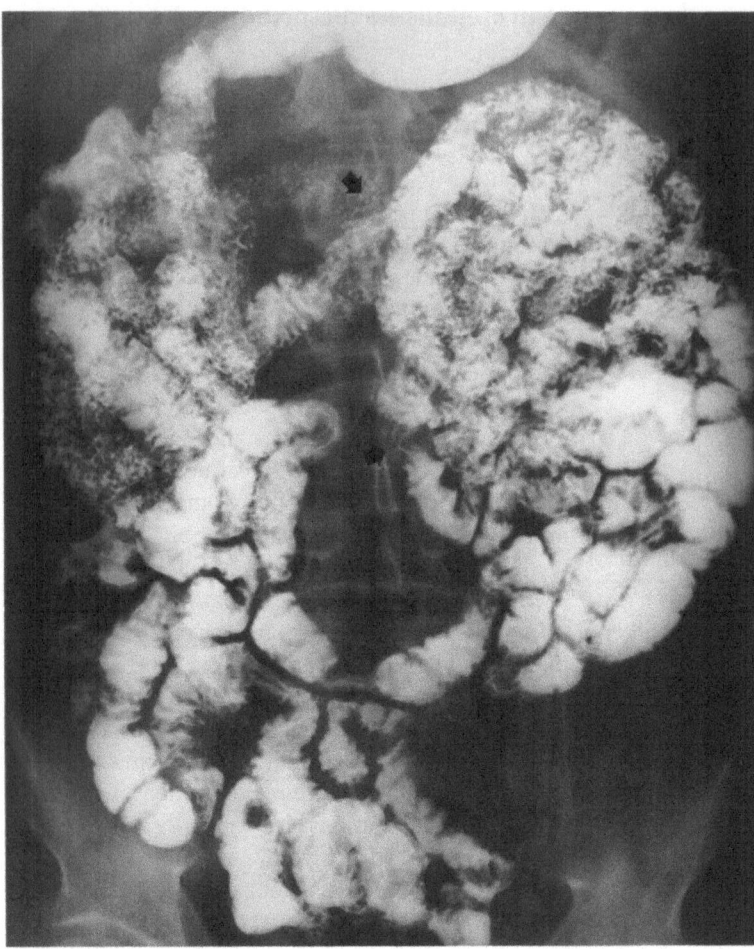

Fig. 6. Congenital internal hernia (Courtesy of D Régent). A 70-year-old man presented with periumbilical pain. The SBFT showed jejunal loops gathered in a circular cluster located in the left hypochondrium

Some reports on the presence of intraluminal diverticula of the small intestine, similar to the more frequent duodenal diverticula, have been published. The pathophysiology postulated is the same: the diverticulum is probably a sign of partial obstruction caused by a membrane, which is progressively displaced by peristalsis along the intestinal lumen. With a barium contrast it appears as a nodule or a pocket in the intestinal lumen.

Meckel's diverticulum (figs. 9 to 23)

A Meckel's diverticulum is an embryonic remnant produced by the incomplete involution of the vitelline duct. It is found in 1 to 2% of autopsy cases with equal prevalence in both sexes. It is more frequently detected in children and young adults and the patients are usually in their twenties at the time of

surgical excision. Some familial cases have been reported.

Pathology

The involution of the vitelline duct, which connects the upper part of the primitive intestinal loop to the umbilicus, is normally completed at the 3rd month of intrauterine life. A defect in the obliteration of the duct produces an umbilical fistula. The obliterated duct may remain as a fibrous tract linking the small intestine to the umbilicus. Incomplete obliteration accounts for the formation of a diverticulum protruding from the convex aspect of a loop of small intestine and with a free edge (84% of all cases) or extending to the umbilicus (15%). The diverticulum is usually found 20 to 90 cm from the ileocecal valve. Its shape is more often finger-like than saccular. Its free end sometimes carries projections. In 80% of

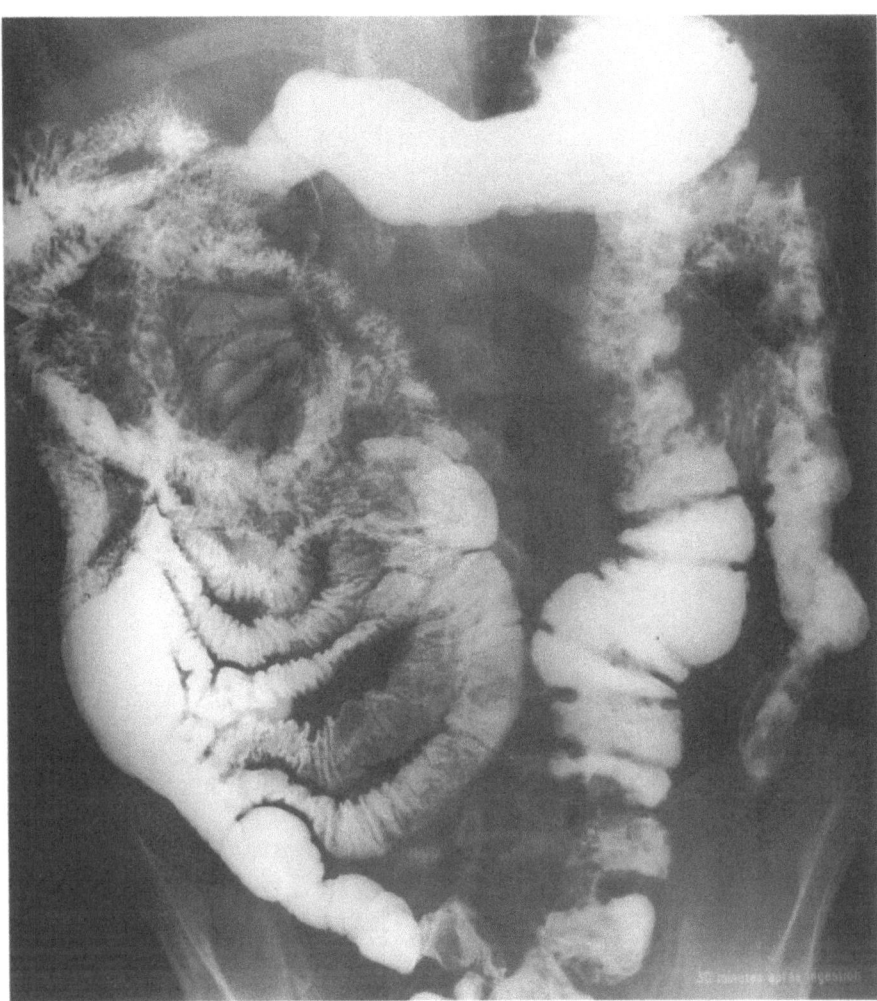

Fig. 7. Common mesentery. This 40-year-old man complained of abdominal plain. The SBFT demonstrated abnormal positioning of the small intestine which lied completely to the right of the midline

cases the vascular supply is from branches of the superior mesenteric artery, which anastomose with vessels from neighbouring loops. In 20%, a specific artery, the vitelline artery, originates in the upper mesenteric artery and courses through a relatively long mesentery to supply the diverticulum.

The wall of the diverticulum is histologically identical to that of the ileum, with fewer lymphoid structures in the absence of infection. It contains areas of tissue heterotopia in 25 to 60% of cases. Gastric heterotopia is more frequent than pancreatic heterotopia and they are found together in 5% of all cases. Gastric mucosa is present in 90% of bleeding diverticula because peptic ulcers, which sometimes perforate, appear either along the supporting loop or in the diverticular pouch. Colonic, duodenojejunal or biliary mucosa have rarely been noted to be present.

Clinical findings

Meckel's diverticula very often exhibit no clinical signs. The most frequent symptom is intestinal hemorrhage in the form of intermittent melena, sometimes haematochezia or anemia. Pain, when it exists, may resemble that of an ulcer and be associated with occlusive phenomena due to adhesions, volvulus or intussusception (inverted diverticulum). Inflammation of the diverticulum may simulate appendicitis and produce the same complications.

Radiological findings

The diagnosis of Meckel's diverticulum can and must be made with an upper barium study in most cases. Plain abdominal radiographs are usually un-

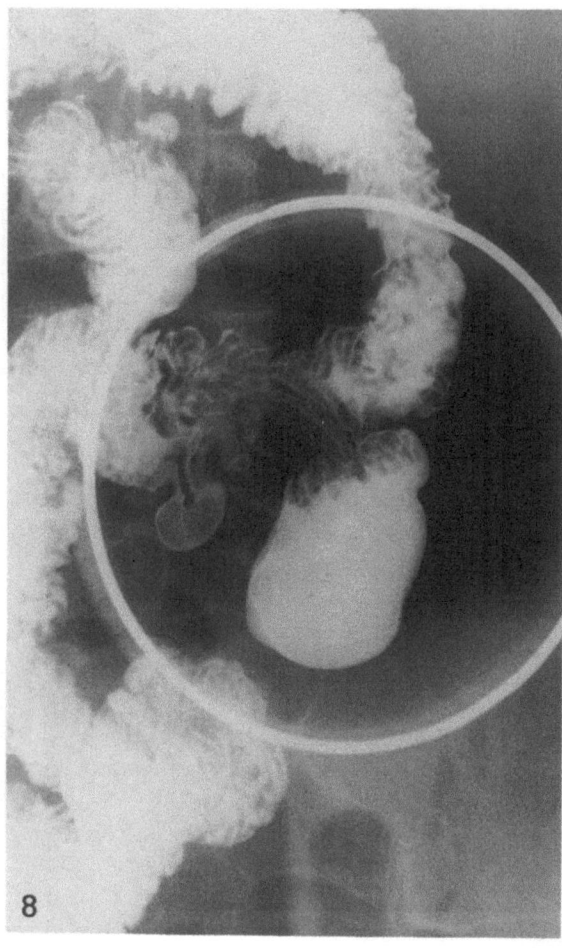

8

Fig. 8. Congenital jejunal diverticula. 62-year-old man with ileocolic Crohn's disease. The SBFT showed pedunculated diverticula of varying sizes along the antimesenteric aspect of the jejunal loops

contributory except in unusual cases of occlusion or of a giant diverticulum. Diagnosis based on barium enema with ileal backwash is only of anecdotal importance.

With barium contrast, a Meckel's diverticulum appears as a long, finger-shaped, rarely bulging, addition image. It is 8 cm long in average, but diverticula smaller than one centimeter may be observed as well as giant ones exceeding 15 cm. The end of the pouch is usually smooth and convex, although it can extend into one or several small secondary diverticula. Located on the antimesenteric aspect of an ileal loop, the diverticulum is perpendicular to the loop. Its wall is smooth or with folds similar to ileal folds, either longitudinal or transverse.

The radiologist must study carefully the opening of the diverticulum, which may be narrowed or widened, but most often is of the same diameter as the pouch. Diagnosis is confirmed when palpation evidences the T-shaped appearance described by

Bodart and formed by the insertion of the diverticulum onto the supporting loop. At the mouth of the diverticulum, compression sometimes isolates a triangular space surrounded by folds of the supporting loop at its insertion and by folds coursing into the diverticulum along its sides (Sellink). Demonstrating the opening of the diverticulum is essential for diagnosis as it rules out superposition of two branches of a loop. The diverticulum is less readily demonstrated when lying parallel to the supporting loop. A number of false-negative findings with barium studies are caused by the insufficient penetration of barium into the diverticulum due to an inflammatory narrowing of its neck, to an intradiverticular foreign body, to volvulus or simply to contraction of the diverticulum.

Once the diverticulum has been detected, it is necessary to search for complications, primarily ulceration, which often appears on the supporting loop opposite the neck of the diverticulum, although it so-

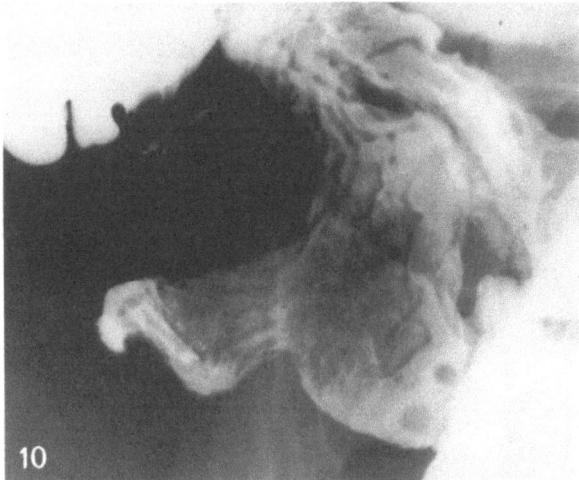

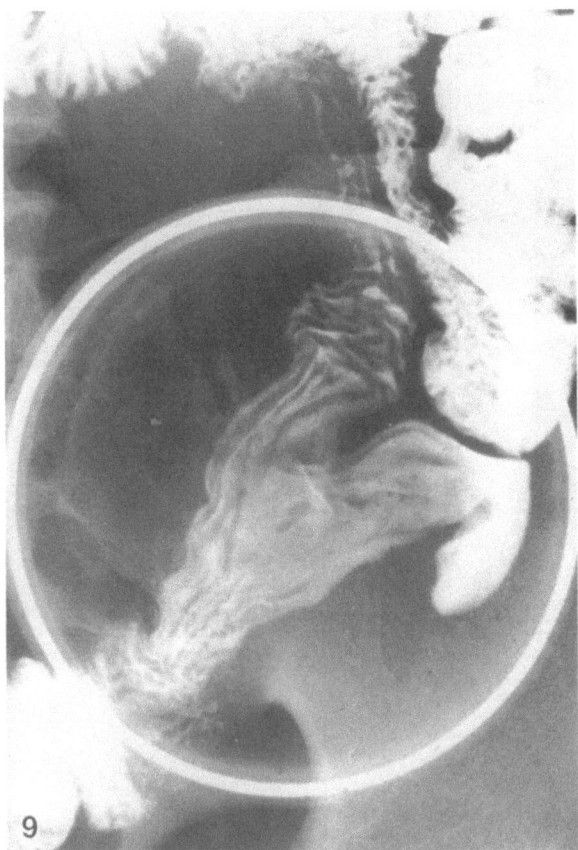

Fig. 9. Meckel's diverticulum. This 46-year-old man complained of pain and constipation. The SBFT detected a 80 x 20 mm diverticulum. Notice the triangular position of the folds at the base of the diverticulum

Fig. 10. Meckel's diverticulum. This 23-year-old man presented with right iliac pain. The SBFT showed a 40 x 20 mm diverticulum

metimes is found at the base and less often in the pouch of the diverticulum. The presence of gastric mucosa in the diverticulum can sometimes be demonstrated as images of nodules or sinuous folds similar to those of the fundus of the stomach. The heterogeneous appearance of a diverticulum may be linked to the presence of debris or of blood clots. Lymphoid hyperplasia, enterolithiasis or tumors (leiomyoma, carcinoid tumor) may be observed as well. Inflammation can occur in the diverticulum or the neighbouring loops, leading to abnormal fixation, angulation, or alterations of the folds, sometimes even to fistula formation. An inverted diverticulum is found after it has intussuscepted into the intestinal lumen. The diagnosis should be questioned if there is intussusception without the presence of a terminal nodule.

Complementary imaging

Arteriography plays only a secondary role in the diagnosis of a Meckel's diverticulum. In the case of considerable bleeding, it can localize the leakage as an opaque pool indicates extravasation of contrast medium. It may visualize a vitelline artery ending in a small vascular bundle, but this is present in only 20% of Meckel's diverticula.

On the other hand, technetium radionuclide scanning as an alternative to the radiological diagnosis of Meckel's diverticulum is especially helpful for children because of its low dose of ionizing radiation. The injection of sodium pertechnetate labelled with technetium 99 is reported to demonstrate 80% of cases of gastric mucosal heterotopia, which selectively takes up this product. False-positive results may be due to ectopia of other causes (e.g. duplication), to local vascular congestion (ulcer, abscess, vascular malformation) or to a malformation of the urinary tract (because of the normal renal excretion of the product). Some pediatricians use technetium scanning rather than barium studies. Our personal experience has led us to first perform a barium examination and to reserve radionuclide scanning for failures of the former technique because of the frequent false-negative results we have observed.

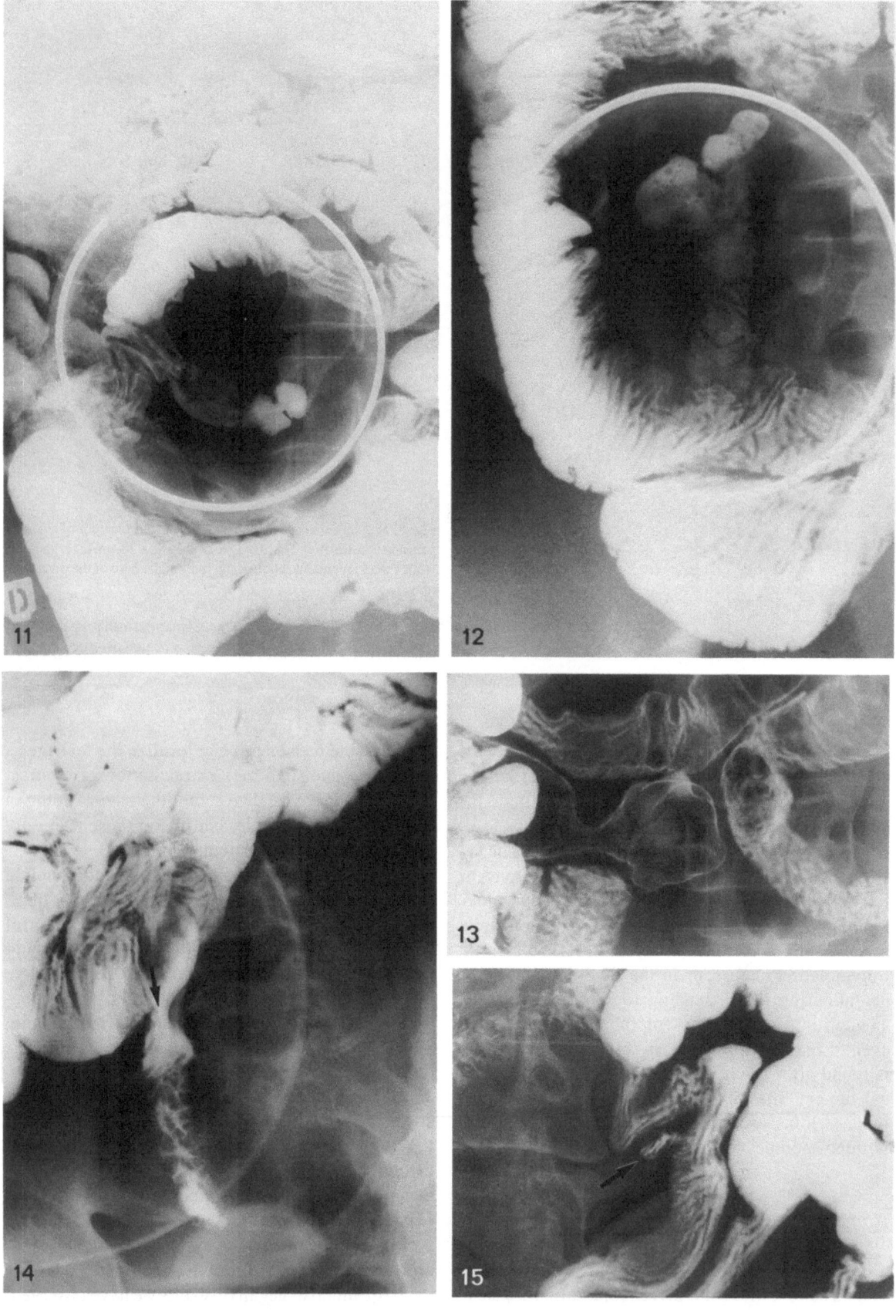

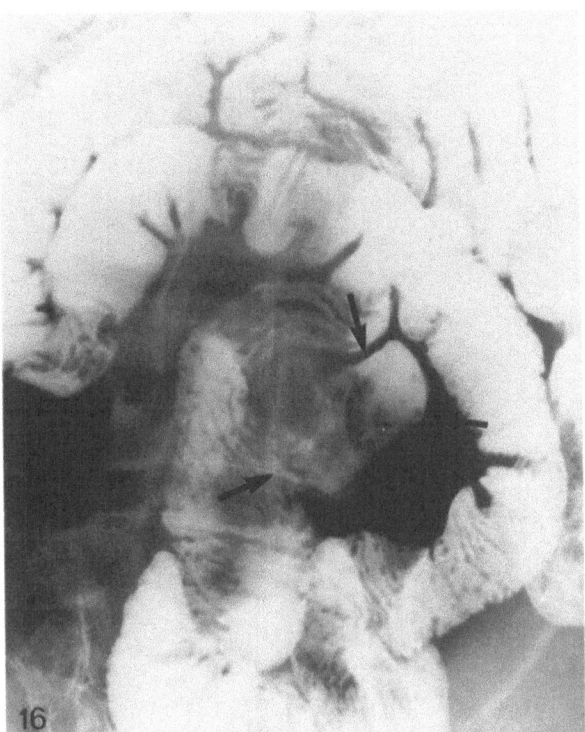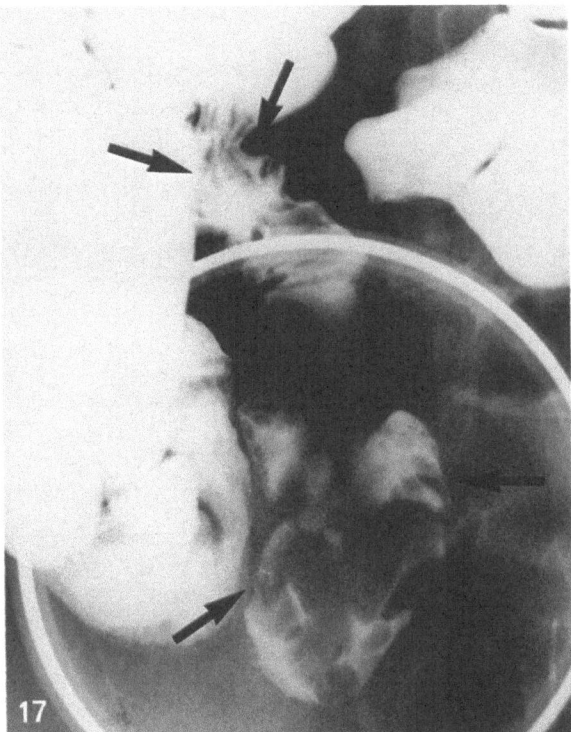

Fig. 16. Meckel's diverticulum. This 18-year-old man had his Meckel's diverticulum diagnosed during appendicectomy. The SBFT demonstrated a 30 x 15 mm diverticulum. Benign lymphoid nodulation of the diverticulum and the neighbouring loops can also be seen

Fig. 17. Meckel's diverticulum. This 22-year-old man developed profuse melena and underwent a negative mesenteric arteriography. The SBFT showed a 100 x 20 mm diverticulum with terminal saccular dilatation containing blood clots

◀ **Fig. 11.** Meckel's diverticulum. A 34-year-old man developed hematochezia. The SBFT found a 60 x 15 mm diverticulum with a fundal recess

Fig. 12. Meckel's diverticulum. A 24-year-old man complained of pain and constipation. The SBFT demonstrated a 60 x 15 mm diverticulum with three resess in its fundus

Fig. 13. Meckel's diverticulum. A 42-year-old man was admitted for abdominal pain. The SBFT visualised a 40 x 30 mm diverticulum with double contrast

Fig. 14. Meckel's diverticulum. A 19-year-old man experienced a bout of melena. The SBFT demonstrated a 90 x15 mm diverticulum with an abnormal pattern of folds due to associated gastric heterotopia

Fig. 15. Meckel's diverticulum. This 50-year-old woman complained of diarrhea. The SBFT showed a 15 x 5 mm diverticulum

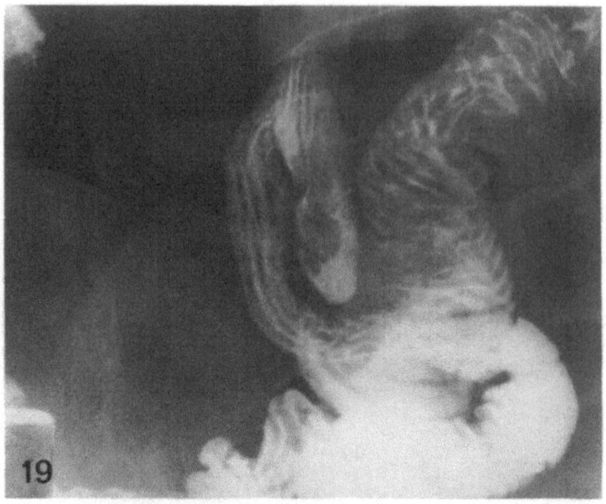

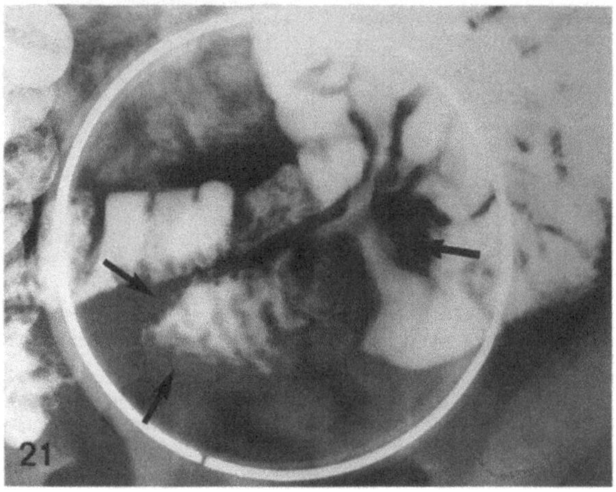

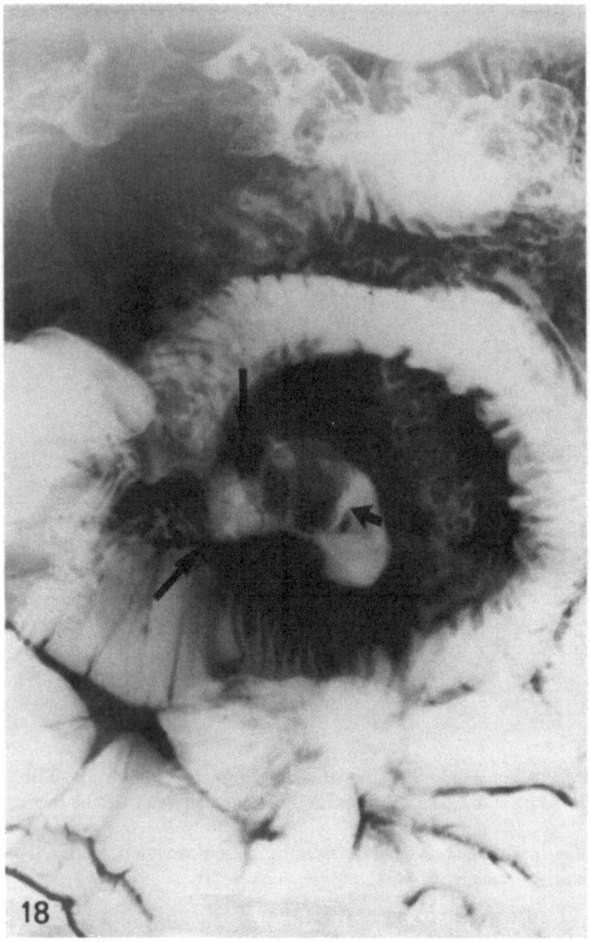

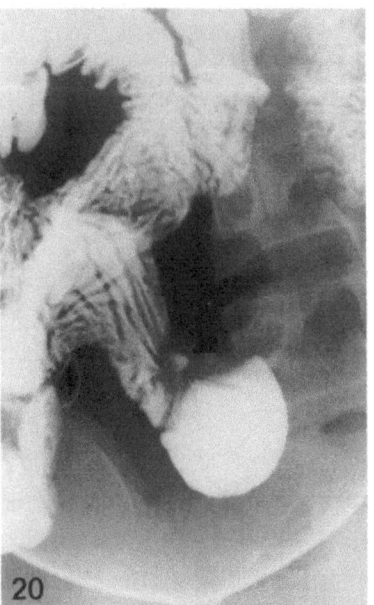

Fig. 18. Meckel's diverticulum. This 55-year-old man presented with an obstructive syndrome. The SBFT detected an enterolithiasis in 20 x 30 mm diverticulum

Fig. 19. Diverticulitis. This 52-year-old woman had suffered repeated bouts of melena for 25 years. The SBFT visualised this 15-cm long diverticulum (the polypoid image of the fundus corresponds to fundal heteropia), which was horseshoe-shaped, and fixed to a pelvic loop

Fig. 20. Ulcerated Meckel's diverticulum. This 31-year-old woman was investigated for hypochromic anemia. The SBFT demonstrated this 5 mm ulceration on the neck of an 80 x 30 mm diverticulum

Fig. 21. Ulcerated Meckel's diverticulum. A 7-year-old boy presented with melena. The SBFT showed a 5 mm ulceration at the base of a 40 x 20 mm diverticulum. The nodular folds in the pouch correspond to a focus of gastric heteropia

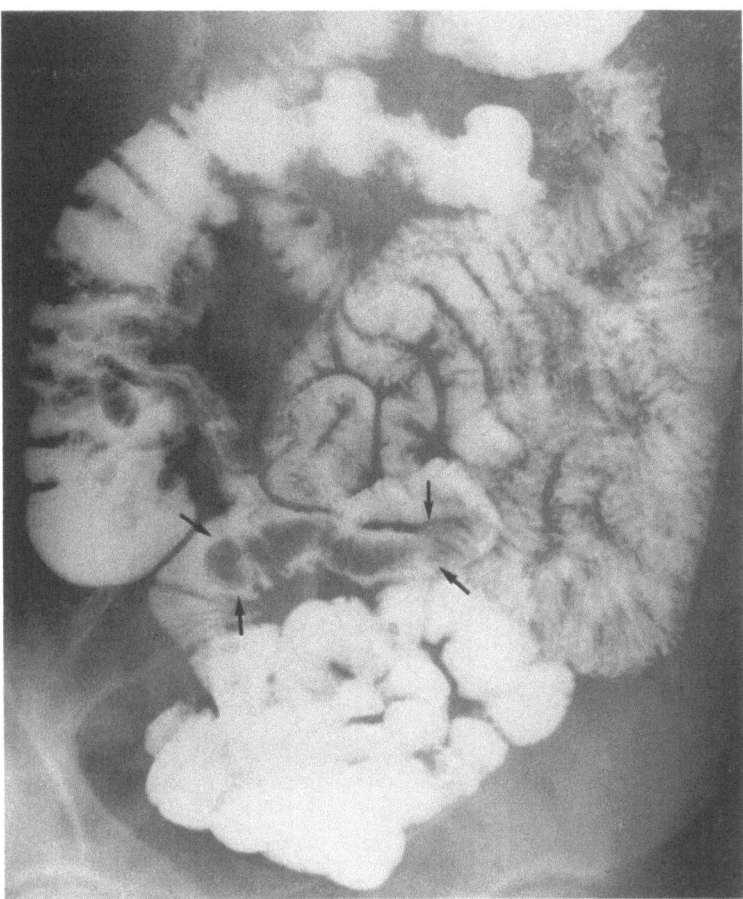

Fig. 22. Inverted Meckel's diverticulum (Courtesy of J P Barbut). This 40-year-old man presented with bouts of melena. The SBFT found this 100 x 15 mm polypoid image on an ileal loop

Duplication (fig. 24)

The duplication of a segment of small intestine leads to the formation of an enterogenous cyst when the additional segment is excluded from the intestinal tract and to a diverticulum when it is connected with the intestine (20% of all cases) or, exceptionally, to a double lumen when the pouch is connected at both ends. A duplication is less frequent than a Meckel's diverticulum and is more readily observed in children.

From an anatomical point of view, the two contiguous segments are included in the same mesentery, the additional segment being located on the mesenteric aspect of the normal loop, thus differenciating it from a Meckel's diverticulum. The location is nearly always on an ileal loop. Its wall is that of the normal small intestine, but it may contain ectopic tissue, mainly gastric or pancreatic. Associated vertebral abnormalities are observed in 20 to 33% of cases.

Clinically, duplication is discovered due to occlusion, hemorrhage, or sometimes because of a palpable mass.

Radiologically, duplication may appear as a round, homogeneous opaque area on plain abdominal radiographs if the enterogenous cyst is large enough. Ultrasound demonstrates the fluid content of the duplication. The image is that of a liquid-filled loop without peristalsis among the mobile images of the neighbouring loops. Computed tomography also demonstrates an oval image of liquid density. Opacification of a duplication connected with the intestine produces an image similar to that of a Meckel's diverticulum ; however, it is located on the mesenteric aspect of the ileum. The contribution of technetium scanning to the diagnosis is similar to that for a Meckel's.

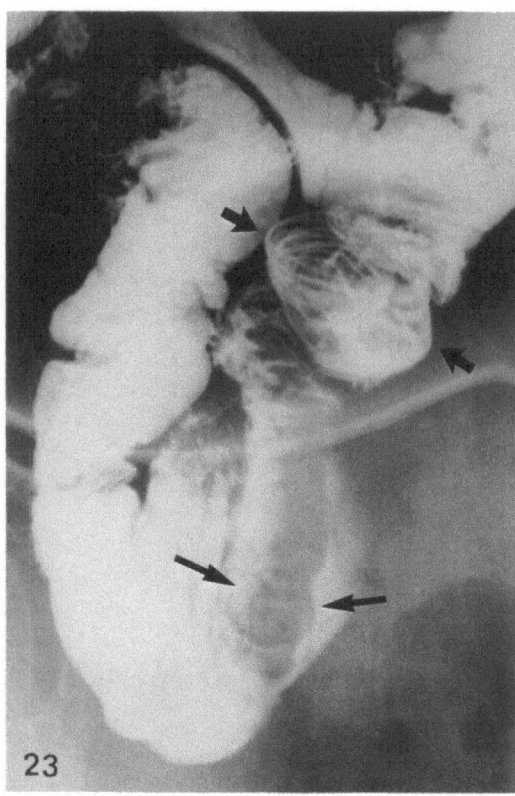

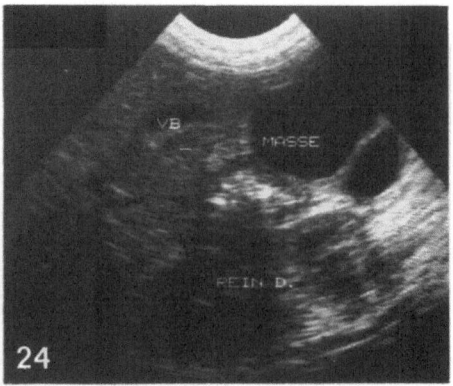

Fig. 23. Inverted Meckel's diverticulum. A 60-year-old woman was seen for anemia, melena and hematochezia. The SBFT visualised a polypoid image in a pelvic (retrovesical) loop with beginning proximal intussusception

Fig. 24. Ileal duplication (Courtesy of J M Pouillaude). A mass was discovered in the right iliac fossa of this 8-day-old infant. Ultrasound revealed a rounded transsonic image of the right flank, which was 3 cm diameter and fixed during several studies while remaining distinct from the gallblader and right kidney. Surgery showed an intramural terminal ileal duplication

Heterotopia

Besides the heterotopia observed in Meckel's diverticula or duplication, isolated heterotopia may be observed, such as an aberrant pancreas located in the jejunum in 7% of all cases and in the ileum in 0.9%, according to surgical series.

Vascular abnormalities

Most vascular abnormalities can be regarded as congenital abnormalities. They will be discussed in the following chapter, since these lesions have the appearance of tumors.

Practical conclusions

Apart from the neonatal period, Meckel's diverticu-lum is the most frequent of all congenital abnormalities.

It is most frequently found in the search for the source of intestinal hemorrhages that are often self-limited and recurrent, when the findings of gastroscopy and colorectal examination are negative.

Barium studies will detect most Meckel's diverticula even in children, thus it is the first examination to perform, with complementary radionuclide scanning as a second-line test in doubtful cases.

Arteriography is indicated only if the other methods have failed in the presence of abundant bleeding.

As no clinical symptoms may be observed, Meckel's diverticulum may be discovered incidentally when assessing intestinal hemorrhage of another origin.

Previous appendectomy does not rule out the diagnosis of a Meckel's diverticulum if uncertainty exists as to whether the small intestine was thoroughly palpated during surgery.

References

Stenosis and atresia

Agha F, Jenkins J (1983) Ileal mucosal diaphragm causing small bowel obstruction, Gastrointest Radiol 8 : 57-59

Pombo F, Arnal-Monreal F, Soler-Fernandez R, Alvarez-Fernandez JC, Carames J (1982) Multiple gastrointestinal atresias with intraluminal calcification. Br J Radiol 55 : 307-309

Segmental dilatation

Brown A, Carty H (1984) Segmental dilatation of the ileum. Br J Radiol 57 : 371-374

Morewod D, Cunningham (1985) Case report : segmental dilatation of the ileum presenting with anemia. Clin Radiol 36 : 267-268

Orenstein S, Magill M, Whitington P (1984) Ileal dysgenesis presenting with anemia and growth failure. Pediatr Radiol 14 : 59-61

Usselman J, Ghahremani G, Bordin G, Miller W, Safdi M, Warmath M, Conroy R (1981) Idiopathic localized dilatation of the ileum in adults. Gastrointest Radiol 6 : 313-317

Visceral myopathy and neuropathy

Berdon WE, Baker DH, Blanc WA, Gay B, Santulli TV, Donovan C (1976) Megacystis-microcolon-intestinal hypo-peristalsis syndrome : a new cause of intestinal obstruction in the newborn, report of radiologic findings in five newborn girls. AJR 126 : 957-964

Byrne WJ, Cipel L, Ament MF, Gyepes MT (1981) Chronic idiopathic intestinal pseudo-obstruction syndrome, Radiologic signs in children with emphasis on differentiation from mechanical obstruction. Diagn Imag 50 : 294-304

Ducastelle T, Tranvouez JL, Lerebourg E, Hemet J, Muller JM, Hecketsweiler P, Colin R (1986) Myopathie viscérale héréditaire : une entité au sein des pseudo obstructions intestinales chroniques. Gastroenterol Clin Biol 10 : 355-363

Dyer NH, Dawson AM, Smith BF, Todd JP (1969) Obstruction of bowel due to lesion in the myenteric plexus. Br Med J 1 : 686-689

Faulk DL, Anuras S, Gardner GD, Mitros FA, Summers RW, Christensen J (1978) A familial visceral myopathy. Ann Int Med 89 : 600-606

Moss AA, Goldberg HI, Brotman M (1972) Idiopathic intestinal pseudo-obstruction. AJR 115 : 312-317

Schuffler M, Lowe M, Bill A (1977) Studies holow visceral myopathy intestinal pseudoobstruction. Gastroenterology 73 : 327-338

Schuffler MD, Pagon RA, Schwartz R, Bill AH (1988) Visceral myopathy of the gastrointestinal tract in infants. Gastroenterology 94 : 892-898

Tanner MS, Smith B, Lloyd JK (1976) Functionnal intestinal obstruction due to deficiency of argyrophil neurones in the myenteric plexus, familial syndrome presenting with short small bowel, malrotation, and pyloric hypertrophy. Arch Dis Child 51 : 837-841

Teixidor HS, Heneghan Ma (1978) Idiopathic intestinal pseudo-obstruction in a family. Gastrointest Radiol 3 : 91-95

Hirschprung's disease

Berdon WE, Koontz P, Baker DH (1964) The diagnosis of colonic and terminal ileal aganglionosis. AJR 91 : 680-689

Vanhoutte JJ, Katzman D (1973) Roentgenographic manifestations of immaturity of the intestinal neural plexus in premature infants. Radiology 106 : 363-367

Malrotations

Balthazar E (1976) Intestinal malrotation in adults, roentgenographic assessment with emphasis on isolated complete and partial malrotations. AJR 126 : 358-367

Deprima S, Hardy D, Brant W (1985) Reversed intestinal rotation. Radiology 157 : 603-604

Griska LB, Popky GL (1980) Angiography in midgut malrotation with volvulus. AJR 134 : 1055-1056

Park RW, Watkins JB (1979) Mesenteric vascular occlusion and varices complicating midgut malrotations. Gastroenterology 77 : 565-568

Verma TR, Bankole MA (1973) Lymphovenous obstruction in anomalous midgut rotation. Arch Dis Child 48 : 154-157

Diverticula

Athey GN (1980) Unusual demonstration of a Meckel's diverticulum containing enteroliths. Br J Radiol 53 : 365-368

Bartam CI, Amess JA (1980) The diagnosis of Meckel's diverticulum by small bowell enema in the investigation of obscure intestinal bleeding. Br J Surg 67 : 417-418

Blumhardt R, Growcock GW, Hartshorne MF, Lasher JC, Benedetto AR, Bunker SR (1984) Patterns of intestinal activity with Meckel's scintigraphy. Gastrointest Radiol 9 : 353-356

Bogren HG, Billing L (1977) Multiple calculi in a Meckel's diverticulum. Report of a case. Acta Radiol Diagnosis 18 : 669-672

Bouyala JM, Derlon S, Aubrespy P (1966) Diverticule de Meckel chez l'enfant, à propos de 25 cas. Ann Chir Infant 7 : 11-16

Bree RL, Reuter SR (1973) Angiographic demonstration of a bleeding Meckel's diverticulum. Radiology 108 : 287-288

Bret P, Tran Minh V, Boisson M, Saint-Cyr M, Deliot JF, Burelle H (1974) Radiologie du diverticule de Meckel. Ann Radiol 17 : 479-485

Bretagne JF, Carré L, Ledu Y, Duvauferrier R, Gastatd J (1980) Léiomyome du diverticule de Meckel révélé par une hémorragie digestive. Diagnostic préopératoire par artériographie sélective. Sem Hôp Paris 56 : 1536-1539

Conway JJ (1980) Radionuclide diagnosis of Meckel's diverticulum. Gastrointest Radiol 5 : 209-213

Cornet A, Abelanet R, Chaumont P, Debesse P, Terris G, Dadoune JP, Epois A, Reboul P (1967) Diverticule de Meckel à forme hémorragique, dépistage artériographique. Sem Hôp Paris 53 : 3341-3450

Craig O, Murfitt J (1980) Radiological demonstration of Meckel's diverticulum. Br J Surg 67 : 881-883

Cross VF, Wendth AJ, Phelan JJ, Goussous HG, Moriarty DJ (1970) Giant Meckel's diverticulum in a premature infant. AJR 108 : 591-597

Cross VF, Wendth AJ, Phelan JJ, Goussous HG, Moriarty DJ (1970) Giant Meckel's diverticulum in a premature infant. AJR 108 : 591-597

Dalinka MK, Wunder MJ (1973) Meckel's diverticulum and its complications with emphasis of roentgenologic demonstration. Radiology 106 : 295-298

Danis R, Grauiss E (1982) Jejunal intraluminal diverticular duplication with recurrent intussusception. Pediatr Surg 17 : 84-85

Daumerie G, Descamps-Wallef G (1966) Hemorragie intestinale et diverticule de Meckel. Acta Gastroenterol Belg 29 : 879-910

Diamond T, Russel CF (1985) Meckel's diverticulum in the adult. Br J Surg 72 : 480-492

Dufour Y (1987) Diagnostic radiologique du diverticule de Meckel. Thèse Lyon

Faris JC, Whitley JE (1973) Angiographic demonstration of Meckel's diverticulum. Radiology 108 : 285-286

Fetterman LE (1968) Meckel's diverticulum radiographically appearing as a polyp (inverted). Br J Radiol 41 : 940-941

Fontaine R, Warter P, Wahl R, Weill F (1961) Apport de la radiologie dans la pathologie du diverticule de Meckel. J Radiol 42 : 327-333

Fresnel PL, Foucher G, Sibilly A (1973) A propos d'une statistique de 105 diverticules de Meckel. Ann Chir 27 : 943-952

Fries M, Mortensson W, Robertson B (1984) Technetium pertechnetate scintigraphy to detect ectopic gastric mucosa in Meckel's diverticulum. Acta Radiol Diagn 25 : 417-422

Gershater R (1976) Enterolith causing bleeding in a patient with Meckel's diverticulum. Angiographic demonstration. Radiology 120 : 327-328

Glick SN, Maglinte DDT, Herlinger H (1988) Association of Meckel's diverticulum and Crohn's disease. Gastrointest Radiol 13 : 67-71

Greenstein S, Bronwyn J, Fischmane E, Cameron J, Siegelmans (1986) Small bowel diverticulitis : CT findings. AJR 147 : 271-274

Hall TJ (1975) Meckel's bleeding diverticulum diagnosed by mesenteric arteriography. Br J Surg 62 : 882-884

Hemingway AP, Allison DJ (1982) Angiodysplasia and Meckel's diverticulum : a congenital association. Br J Surg 69 : 493-496

Jewett TC, Duszynsky DO, Allen Je (1970) The visualization of Meckel's diverticulum with 99 m Tc pertechnetate. Surgery 68 : 567-570

Johnson HR, Path MR (1973) Carcinoma of Meckel's diverticulum. Cancer 31 : 742-745

Kiprov DD, Griffel B (1975) Inversion of Meckel's diverticulum. Arch Surg 110 : 1154

Kleinclaus D (1980) Diagnostic radiologique et scintigraphique du diverticule de Meckel. Thèse Strasbourg

Maglinte DT, Elmore MF, Isengerg M, Dolan PA (1980) Meckel's diverticulum : radiologic demonstration by enteroclysis. AJR 134 : 925-932

Marion J, Chapuis JP, Daudet M, Bernex J (1969) Les accidents mécaniques du diverticule de Meckel, à propos de 5 observations. Pédiatrie 24 : 169-179

Meguid MM, Wilkinson RH, Canty T, Eraklis AJ, Treve S (1974) Utility of barium sulfate in diagnosis of bleeding Meckel's diverticulum. Arch Surg 108 : 361-362

Miller DL, Becker MH, Eng K (1981) Giant Meckel's diverticulum, a cause of intestinal obstruction. Radiology 140 : 93-94

Mosimann F, Bugnion M (1981) Intraluminal jejunal diverticulum. Gastrointest Radiol 6 : 309-311

Ohba S, Fukuda A, Kohno, Takeuchi S (1981) Ileal duplication and multiple intraluminal diverticula : scintigraphy and barium meal. AJR 5 : 992-994

Payne-James JJ, Law NW, Watkins RM (1985) Carcinoïd tumour arising in a Meckel's diverticulum. Postgrad Med J 61 : 1009-1011

Pellerin D, Harouchi A, Delmas P (1976) Le diverticule de Meckel, revue de 250 cas chez l'enfant. Ann Chir Inf 17 : 157-171

Rambaud P, Varloteaux C, Bessard G (1974) Le diverticule de Meckel chez l'enfant. Med Infant 81 : 445-451

Rosenthall L, Henry JN, Murphy DA, Freeman LM (1972) Radiotechnetate imaging ot the Meckel's diverticulum. Radiology 105 : 371-373

Rutherford RB, Akers DR (1966) Meckel's diverticulum : a review of 148 pediatric patients, with special reference to the pattern of bleeding and to mesodiverticular vascular bands. Surgery 59 : 618-626

Salomonowitz E, Wittich G, Hajek P, Jantsch H, Czembirek H (1983) Detection of intestinal diverticula by double-contrast small bowel enema : differentiation from other intestinal diverticula. Gastrointest Radiol 8 : 271-278

Schmutz G, Zeller C, Pauline D, Mugel JL, Kempf F (1982) Le diverticule de Meckel de l'adulte, étude en double contraste de 7 observations. J Radiol 63 : 543-548

Schoenbach SF (1978) Meckel's diverticulitis, oldest reported case. NY State J Med 78 : 1942-1943

Seagram CGF, Louch RE, Stephens CA, Wentworth P (1968) Meckel's diverticulum : a 10 year review of 218 cas. Can J Surg 11 : 369-373

Sfakianakis GN, Conway JJ (1981) Detection of ectopic gastric mucosa in Meckel's diverticulum and in other aberrations by scintigraphy : I. Pathophysiology and 10 year clinical experience. J Nucl Med 22 : 647-654

Sfakianakis GN, Haaseg M (1982) Abdominal scintigraphy for ectopic gastric mucosae, a retrospective analysis of 143 studies. AJR 138 : 7-12

Silver B, Desmos T (1983) Symptomatic inverted Meckel's diverticulum, case report. J Can Assoc Radiol 34 : 314-315

Simms MM, Corkery JJ (1980) Meckel's diverticulum : its association with congenital malformation and the significance of atypical morphology. Br J Surg 67 : 216-219

Sottero MJ, Bill AH (1976) The natural history of Meckel's diverticulum and its relation incidental removal, a study of 202 cases of diseased Meckel's diverticulum found in kind country : Washington. Am J Surg 132 : 168-173

Tabry IF, Nassar VH, Balikian JP (1973) Leiomyoma of Meckel's diverticulum, preoperatoire radiologic demonstration. Ann Surg 178 : 31-33

Tubiana JM, Dana A, Régent D, Dang Trang Son, Chermet J (1978) Etude critique de la valeur de l'artériographie mésentérique supérieure dans le diagnostic des diverticules de Meckel. J Radiol 59 : 689-696

Valle M, Hekali P, Kallio H, Keto P, Korhola O, Lehtinen E, Suoranta H (1978) Radiologic demonstration of Meckel's diverticulum. Gastointest Radiol 3 : 101-103

Weinstein EC, Dockerty MM, Waugh JM (1976) Neoplasms of Meckel's diverticulum, collective review. Int Abstr Surg 116 : 103

White AF, Kook Sank OH, Weber AL, James AE (1973) Radiologic manifestations of Meckel's diverticulum. AJR 118 : 86-94

Yamagushi M, Takeuchi S, Awazu S (1978) Meckel's diverticulum, investigation of 600 patients in Japonese. A J Surg 136 : 247-249

Duplication

Barkley R, Munoz O, Parkey R (1977) Intestinal duplication detected with technetium 99 m sodium pertechnetate imaging of the abdomen. Am J Digest 22 : 1121-1126

Bower R, Sieber W, Kiesewetter W (1978) Alimentary tract duplications in children. Ann Surg 188 : 669-674

Garcez J, Rosa M (1978) A propos d'un cas de duplication intestinale chez l'adulte. Acta Chir Belg 5 : 343-346

Grosfeld J (1970) Enteric duplications in infancy and childhood : 18 year review. Ann Surg 172 : 83

Gross P, Khadouri M (1981) Image hydroaérique d'une duplication iléale non communicante. Chir Pediatr 22 : 51-54

Kangarloo H, Sample W, Hansen G, Robinson JS, Sarti D (1979) Ultrasonic evaluation of abdominal gastro intestinal tract duplication in children. Radiology 131 : 191-194

Lamont A, Starinsky R, Cremin B (1984) Ultrasonic diagnosis of duplication cysts in children. Br J Radiol 57 : 463-467

Mabille JP, Montagnon J (1980) Duplication iléale avec entérolithe. Ann Radiol 23 : 445-447

Marliave M (de), Chouraqui JP, Bacle B, Muller P, Dyon JF (1985) A propos d'un cas d'hétérotopie gastrique diverticulaire de l'intestin grêle. Pédiatrie 40 : 115-122

Newmark H, Ching G, Halls J, Levy I (1981) Bleeding peptic ulcer caused by ectopic gastric mucosa in a duplicated segment of jejunum. Am J Gastroenterol 75 : 158-162

Rose J, Gribetz D, Krasna I (1978) Ileal duplication cyst : the importance of sodium pertechnetate TC 99 m scanning. Pediatr Radiol 6 : 244-246

Satoru O, Fukuda A, Khono S, Takeuchi S (1981) Ileal duplication and multiple intraluminal diverticula : scintigraphy and barium meal. AJR 136 : 992-994

Staudt F, Kuehle N, Maier W, Helwig H (1981) Ultraschalldiagnostic bei einem Neugeborenem mit einer Duplikatur des Ileums. Klin Pediatr 193 : 461-463

Symposium consacré aux duplications intestinales (1967) Ann Chir Infant 8 : 1

Tschappeler , Smith W (1977) Duplications of the intestinal tract : clinical and radiological features. Ann Radiol 20 : 133-139

Waterson T, Lyall MH, Longrigg N (1980) Diagnosis of intestinal duplication by 99 Tc. m pertechnetate scanning. Br J Surg 67 : 419-420

Neoplasms

Introduction

Tumors of the small intestine make up about 5% of all neoplasms of the gastrointestinal tract. They therefore represent a fairly uncommon occurrence. Radiologists must know these well since barium studies play an important part in their diagnosis. The relative frequency of the various neoplasms varies according to statistical sources and to whether or not duodenal tumors are taken into account (they are not considered in our discussion). Malignant tumors seem to be more frequent than benign tumors, but the latter often have no clinical symptoms. Mesenchymal tumors make up more than 2/3 of the benign, and carcinoid tumors and lymphoma about 2/3 of the malignant tumors.

The tumors of the small intestine appear at any age but most often are seen in adults. The clinical signs are often late manifestations and are not typical. They include abdominal pain that is more specific when periumbilical, occurring long after meals, accompagnied by changes in bowel habits (diarrhea, subocclusion), anemia and a palpable mass. Deterioration in the patient's general condition and signs of malabsorption herald a malignant tumor, usually widespread. The first sign is often an acute event: intestinal hemorrhage, occlusion and, less often, perforation.

Plain radiographs of the abdomen sometimes demonstrate the opacity of a large tumor; less often one can detect a localised pool of gas secondary to tumour necrosis or a cluster of calcifications.

A small bowel follow through (SBFT) leads to diagnosis of the tumor provided the technique is very rigorous. The histological type can sometimes be suggested. However, malignant and benign tumors cannot always be differentiated: some cancers have the appearance of intraluminal nodules with smooth contours and some necrosed benign tumors appear as a localised pool of gas with creviced contours. The radiological appearance reflects the anatomical structure of the tumor in the intestinal wall with its extension. The lesion is usually local or segmental:

- Appearing sessile or pedunculated, rarely ulcerated or intussuscepted, as an isolated intraluminal nodule; this corresponds to a benign or a carcinoid tumor. There may appear a stenosis, a segmental ectasia, or thickened walls and increased interloop gap; alteration of the folds may show them to be enlarged, nodular or disappearing. These appearances usually correspond to a malignant tumor.
- A marginal notch, flattened or displaced loops due to the exoenteric development of the tumour may be seen. When the tumor is large, central necrosis sometimes produces the image of a pool or a fistula, which is more frequent in malignant but is also observed with some benign tumors.

Ultrasound and computed tomography may detect a large tumor or suggest a little one if distension or intussusception of a loop of small intestine is observed.

Arteriography is useful for the diagnosis of vascular exoenteric tumors which may not be seen with small bowel follow-through. It is useful during hemorrhage as it can demonstrate extravasation of the dye into the bowel lumen.

Radionuclide scanning sometimes permits the localization of the source of such intestinal hemorrhages.

Benign tumors

Benign tumors of the various histological types have many points in common from a clinical and radiological point of view. The histology is sometimes suggested by a particular appearance of the lesion but most often by statistical frequency. We have included hamartomas and inflammatory pseudotumors in this chapter.

Pathology

Mesenchymal tumors most frequently appear in the submucosa (more than 2/3 of all cases): leiomyomas predominate in the jejunum, lipomas and fibromas in the ileum. The epithelial tumours are mostly adenomas, and exceptionally villous tumors. All these may be single or multiple. Some syndromes are characterized by the presence of multiple benign tumors, such as hamartomas in the Peutz-Jeghers syndrome, adenomas in Gardner's syndrome, or polyps in the Crohnkite-Canada syndrome.

All benign tumors may intussuscept or ulcerate. Some may also degenerate, such as leiomyomas, schwannomas, neuromas in von Recklinghausen's disease, adenomas or villous tumors. The benign character of a tumor may be difficult to demonstrate even at pathology.

Clinical findings

Benign tumors are equally frequent in both sexes. They appear at any age but are most often diagnosed in adults. They cause anemia, melena, subocclusion or complete obstruction, but may also exhibit no clinical signs and be discovered incidentally.

Radiological findings

The typical appearance during SBFT is a pedunculated polyp or a sessile nodule, either round or lobulated. A sessile nodule at right or obtuse angles to the intestinal wall and which preserves the mucosal folds, suggests a tumor originating in the submucosa or in the muscularis. This type of tumor also appears as a nodule at acute angles to the wall and may even intussuscept. When the tumor develops mainly outside the intestinal lumen, as it frequently occurs with a leiomyoma or a fibroma, a single notch on the bowel edge in association with displacement of the neighbouring loops or a barium pool image between loops due to central necrosis may be observed. The ulceration of a benign tumor is often difficult to demonstrate because of its superficial and localised character. On the other hand, intussusception often reveals the tumor. Multiple benign tumors produce the image of nodulation made up of juxtaposed or scattered elements.

Analysis of the lesions according to histological type

Leiomyomas (figs. 1 to 4)

The leiomyoma is the most frequent benign tumor of the small intestinal (about 30%), most often located in the jejunum. It has a highly variable diameter (1 to 20 cm) and a regular contour. A leiomyoma appears in the muscularis and tends to develop outside the intestinal lumen. It is overlooked if not displaced into the lumen of the neighbouring loop by the radiologist during palpation. The radiological image is that of a variably large marginal nodule producing a notch or displacing the involved loop while preserving its peristalsis or fold pattern.

Superficial ulceration is frequent ; necrosis may occur in large leiomyomas. This necrosis may appear as small calcifications, or more often as an extraluminal pool image that sometimes hig-hlights the tumor.

Arteriography can detect leiomyomas because of their dense vascularity. The appearance is that of a very vascular mass with sharp margins. The arterial vessels are enlarged and venous return occurs prematurely and is abundant. Leiomyomas are rarely hypovascular. Arteriography cannot always distinguish whether the tumor is benign or malignant.

Neurogenic tumors (figs. 5 to 8)

Neuromas, schwannomas and neurofibromas make up about 10% of the benign tumors of the small intestine. They have no site of predilection. Multiple neurofibromas can be observed in 10 to 25% of patients with von Recklinghausen's disease. These lesions carry a risk of sarcomatous degeneration. Gangliocytic paragangliomas are rare tumors, which are usually confined to the duodenum and only very rarely observed in the jejunum.

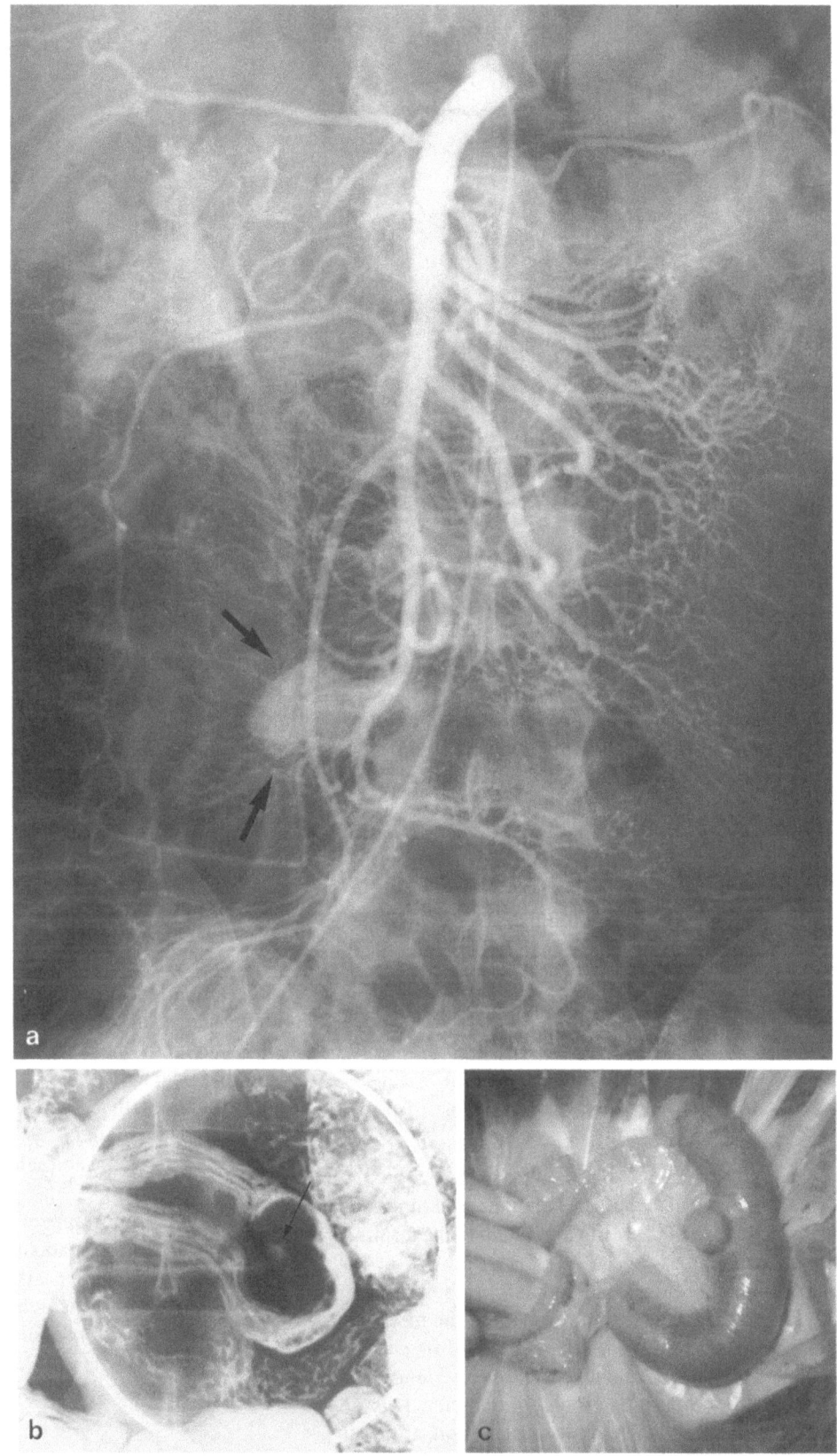

Fig. 1 a-c. Leiomyoma. 29-year-old man. Melena and acute anemia. **a** Arteriography : round tumor blush of 2 cm in diameter is supplied by an ileal artery, **b** SBFT : a 25 x 30 mm submucosal nodule with an ulcerated centre is seen developing outside the intestine, **c** surgical specimen: densely vascularized exointestinal tumor

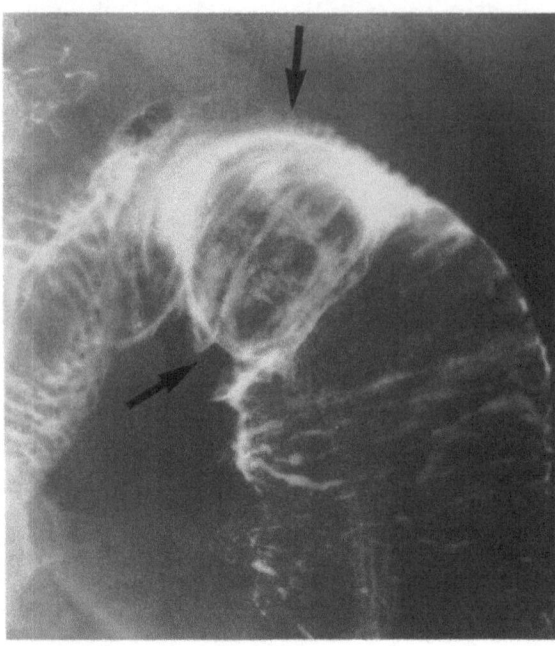

Fig. 2. Leiomyoma. 55-year-old woman. Epigastric pain relieved by bilious vomiting. SBFT : a round endoluminal nodule, 30 mm in diameter, is found distal to a jejunoileal intussusception. There was also an associated ovarian leiomyoma

The radiological signs of neurogenic tumors are similar to those of leiomyomas both on barium studies and arteriography.

Fibromas (figs. 9 to 12)

Fibromas represent 10% of all benign tumors of the small intestine. They appear mainly in the ileum and tend to intussuscept or protrude outside the intestinal wall as do leiomyomas. The appearance of a fibroma on SBFT is similar to that of a leiomyoma, but arteriography shows a less dense vascularity.

Lipomas (figs. 9 to 12)

Lipomas make up about 20% of all benign tumors of the small bowel and are most frequent in the terminal ileum near the ileocecal valve. The growth of the soft, malleable lipoma is hindered by the muscular layers, so that it tends to protrude into the intestinal lumen and even intussuscept, in spite of its submucosal origin. The lesion usually forms a round, oval or lobulated nodule 2 to 4 cm in diameter. It is relatively malleable and mobile on palpation, although it carries no pedicle. The peristalsis and folds of the involved loop are normal. Ulceration, if it occurs, is rarely demonstrated. Intussusception is frequent. Multiple lipomas may sometimes be observed. If the

tumor is large, computed tomography suggests the tissue diagnosis because of its hypodense image.

Epithelial tumors (figs. 13 to 15)

Epithelial tumors make up about 15% of all benign tumors of the small intestine. They are not found in a specific location, except for villous tumors which are more often located in the jejunum (the first most common site is the duodenum). These tumors are usually adenomas, and exceptionally can be villous. The radiological appearance is that of a small, round or ovoid nodule with a smooth or lobulated contour, sometimes pedunculated; they may be multiple. The ulceration is superficial and seldom visible; intussusception is frequent.

A villous tumor appears as a nodular, sometimes extensive, lesion made up of small conglomerated elements which are easily deformed on palpation. Unlike adenomas, which rarely degenerate in the small intestine, villous tumors become malignant in 30% of cases.

Vascular tumors (figs. 16 and 17)

Vascular tumors make up 10% of all benign tumors of the small intestine. Their histological classifica-

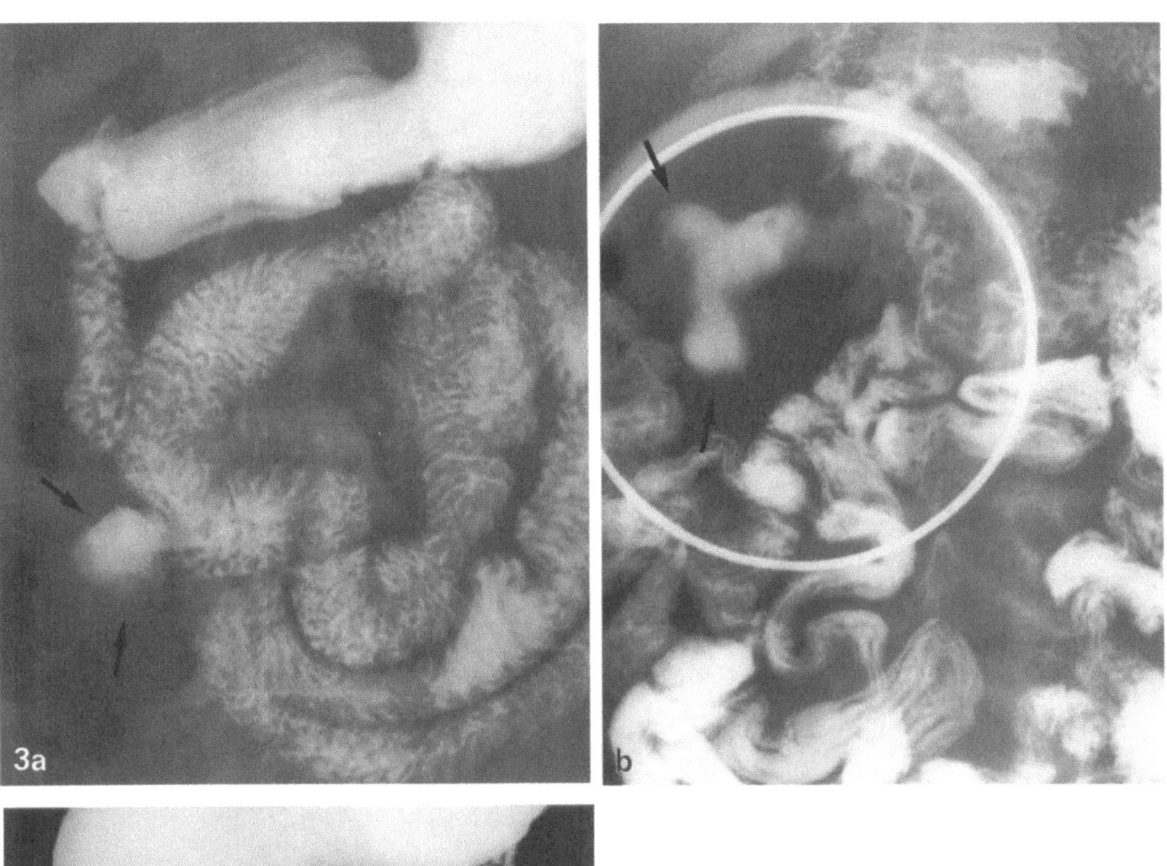

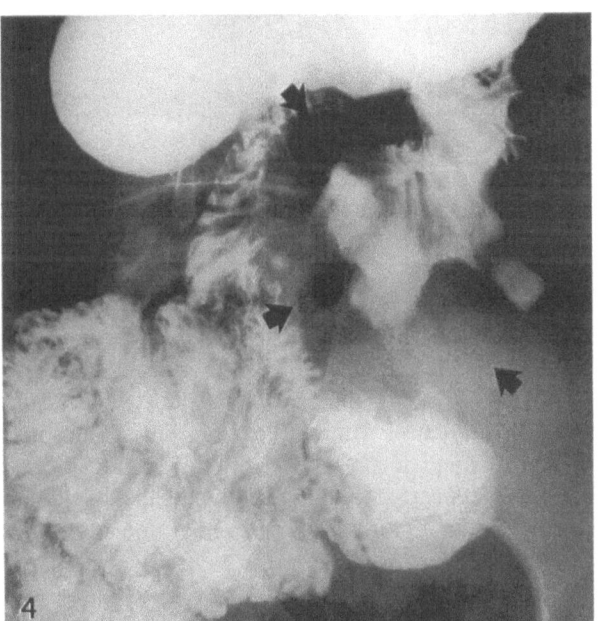

Fig. 3 a, b. Leiomyoma. 40 year-old man. 2 bouts of melena in 7 years. **a** SBFT : a 2 cm opaque pool image is shown contiguous to a jejunal loop. 7 years later a subhepatic mass is noted as a pseudokidney image on ultrasound. **b** SBFT : a trifoliated 5 cm pool of barium with a filiform connection to a slightly displaced jejunal loop is seen. Surgery found an exointestinal tumor with a necrotic centre.

Fig. 4. Leiomyoma. 41-year-old woman with known Recklinghausen's disease. Pain, vomiting, melena, and a palpable mass. SBFT : an opaque pool image with creviced contours is centered on a jejunal loop with a lucent area surrounding the lesion

tion is confusing. The main types of tumors are the hemangiomas which predominate in the jejunum, and the lymphangiomas mostly found in the ileum. They cause hemorrhage, which may be massive, obstruction, and intussusception due to intramural bleeding. The diffuse forms may cause a malabsorption syndrome. These tumors are often scattered throughout the bowel and appear as small, slightly protruding nodular elements, flattened by compression. Phleboliths sometimes appear in their vicinity. These tumors, especially small ones (angiodysplasia), are often not seen on SBFT.

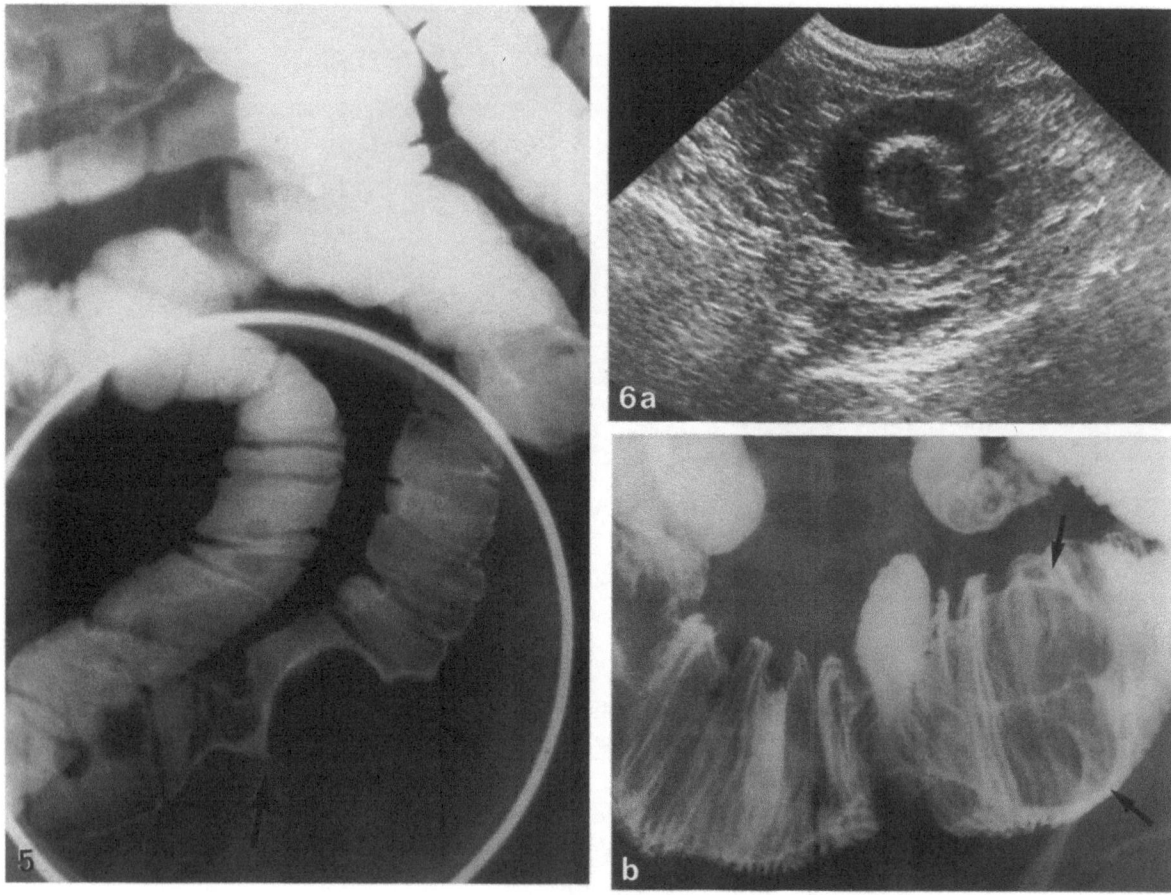

Fig. 5. Neurofibroma a, b. (Courtesy of J M Bruel). SBFT : a 2 cm marginal nodule is located on an ileal loop

Fig. 6 a, b. Neurofibroma a, b. 35-year-old man. Diabetes. Iron deficiency anemia. **a** Ultrasound shows an ileal intussusception. **b** SBFT : a bilobulated nodule is seen distal to an ileoileal intussusception

Some vascular tumors are part of a more diffuse vascular disease: the Osler-Weber-Rendu syndrome is a dominantly inherited disease, which includes multiple mucocutaneous telangectasiae. The blue rubber bleb nevus, the cutaneointestinal hemangiomas and the multiple jejunal phlebectasia syndromes are all rare diseases which involve both the integumentary and digestive tracts. Such lesions may also be observed in Turner's syndrome, the Sturge-Weber syndrome and tuberous sclerosis.

Angiography can demonstrate hypervascularity with vascular dilatation and early, massive venous filling. Preoperative arteriography is useful to locate these lesions.

Inflammatory tumors and pseudotumors

Some reports of inflammatory fibrous polyps, of isolated eosinophilic granulomas not part of eosinophilic gastroenteritis, and of talcomas and other types of postoperative granulomas (discussed in Chapter XIII) have been published. These present according to the literature as intramural or intraluminal, sometimes large, nodules with a smooth contour. They are more frequently found in the ileum than the jejunum, often in an area of stasis (proximal to a stenosis or in a blind loop). Endometriosis is described in Chapter XII.

Lymphoid nodular hyperplasia (LNH) presents as scattered nodulations made up of sessile and round elements, 2 to 3 mm in diameter. It is most often seen in the terminal ileum. In children it is a part of a nonspecific inflammatory reaction. In adults, LNH of the terminal ileum is observed in typhoid fever, yersiniosis, viral infections, etc. Diffuse involvement should lead to a search for hypogammaglobulinemia, giardiasis or a malignant non-Hodgkin's lymphoma.

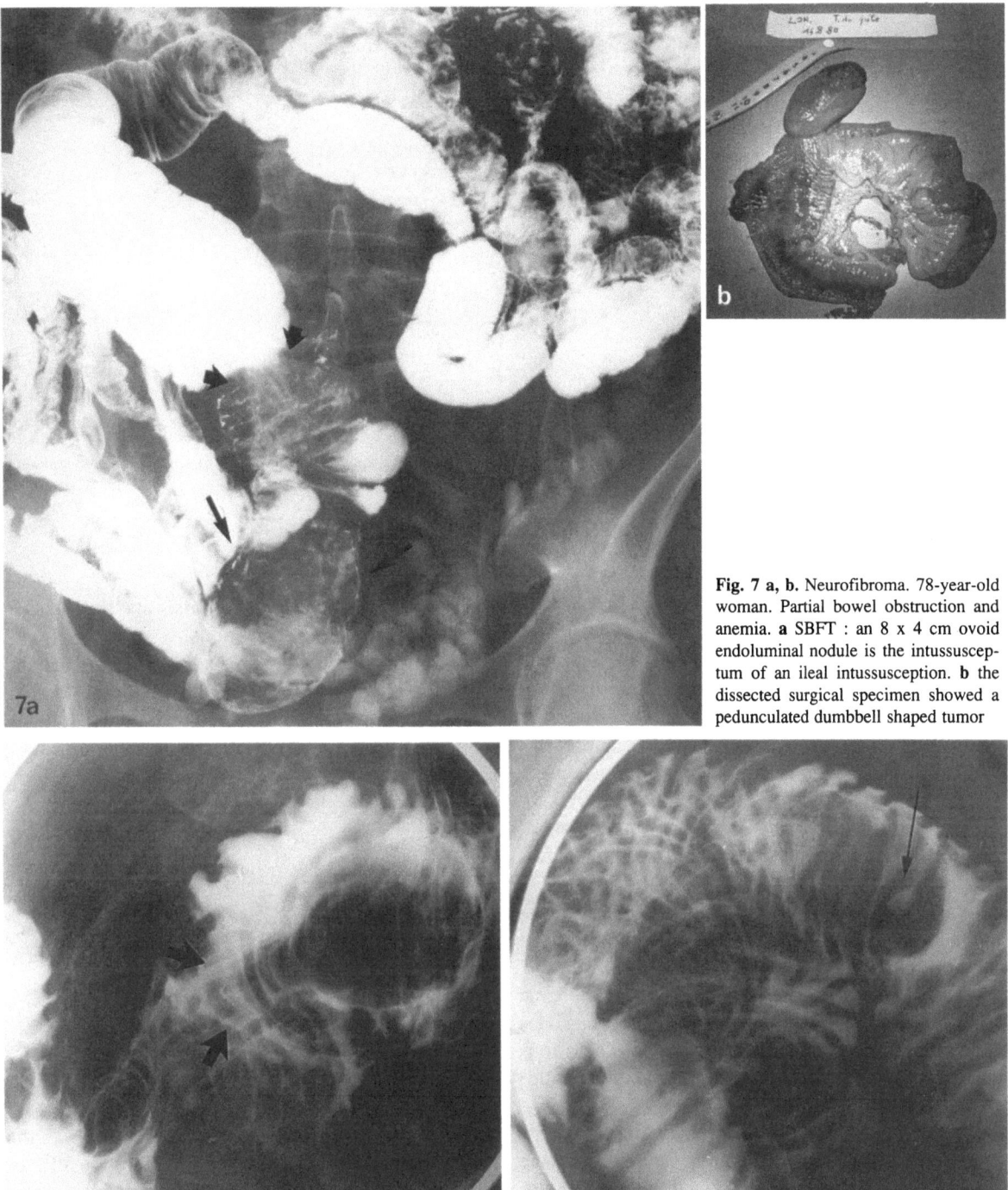

Fig. 7 a, b. Neurofibroma. 78-year-old woman. Partial bowel obstruction and anemia. **a** SBFT : an 8 x 4 cm ovoid endoluminal nodule is the intussusceptum of an ileal intussusception. **b** the dissected surgical specimen showed a pedunculated dumbbell shaped tumor

Fig. 8 a, b. Gangliocytic paraganglioma. 54-year-old woman. Melena and anemia. SBFT 4 x 3 cm polyp with an ovoid head and an ulcerated centre b at the level of ligament of Treitz

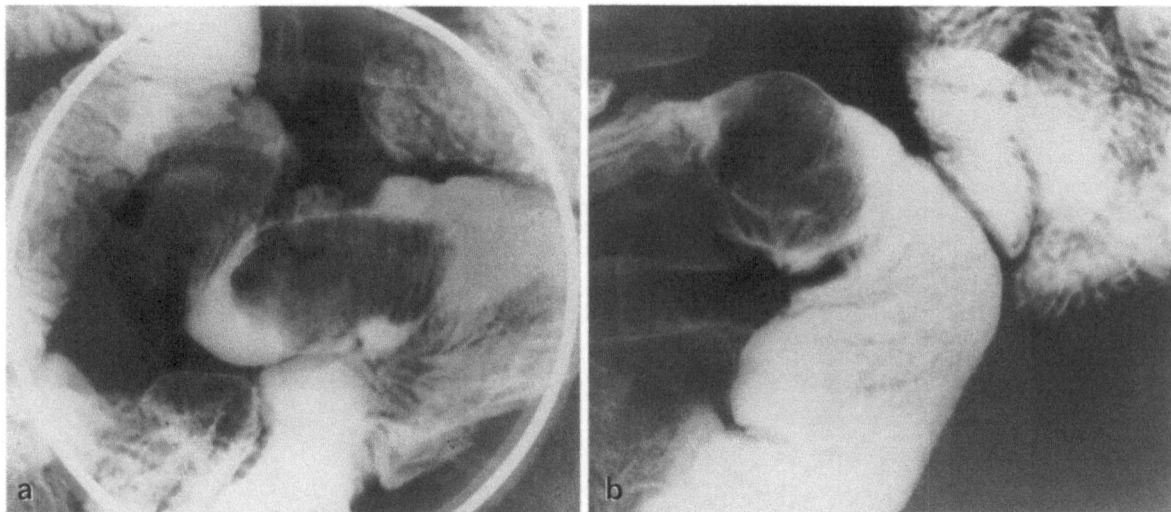

Fig. 9. ab Lipoma. 59-year-old woman. Anemia. SBFT : 25 x 35 mm ovoid, endoluminal jejunal nodule with sharp, slightly indented contours, which is mobile and malleable on palpation

The polyposis syndromes (figs. 18 and 19)

This term encompasses several syndromes, which all have in common a radiological appearance of diffuse nodulation:
- The Peutz-Jeghers syndrome is most frequent; this is an autosomal dominantly inherited disease, associating periorificial lentiginosis and digestive or, less frequently, non digestive hamartomas. The hamartomas frequently are present in the small intestine and sometimes in the colon and stomach. These lesions are made up of a fibrous connective and muscular axis covered with epithelium. They produce jejunoileal nodulations. These present as multiple, sometimes innumerable, sessile or pedunculated and sometimes lobulated elements of various sizes. Intussuceptions and hemorrhage due to ulcerations are frequent. Malignant transformation is exceptional on the small intestine.
- Gardner's syndrome, an autosomal dominantly inherited disease, includes the presence of soft-tissue tumors, rectocolic polyposis extending rarely into the terminal ileum, osteomas and various malignant tumors. Digestive involvement consists of adenomas that degenerate in 50% of cases.
- The unusual Crohnkite-Canada syndrome is not hereditary and associates skin hyperpigmentation, alopecia, nail dystrophy, malabsorption and the presence of gastric, ileal and colonic inflammatory polyps. The prognosis of this disease is not favorable.

-Juvenile, non-hereditary polyposis may be associated with various malformations.
- Multiple hamartomas of the small intestine may be observed in Cowden's disease, the Ruvalcaba-Myhre-Smith syndrome or tuberous sclerosis, and polyps are seen in Turcot's syndrome.

Malignant tumors

Malignant tumors are detected more often than benign tumours on radiographs. Carcinoid tumors and non-Hodgkin's lymphomas dominate in the ileum, adenocarcinomas in the jejunum.

Carcinoid tumors (figs. 20 to 43)

Carcinoid tumors are the most frequent tumors of the small intestine after lymphomas, making up 20% of all cases. Their frequency is underestimated, as confirmed by autopsy studies. Carcinoid tumors of the small intestine make up 25 to 30% of all carcinoid tumors. These belong to the apudomas and appear in many organs, especially the appendix (40 to 50% of the cases), the colon, the ovaries and the bronchi. Only the rectal and appendiceal tumors generally behave indolently. The other carcinoid tumors are malignant and may metastasize, especially to the liver.

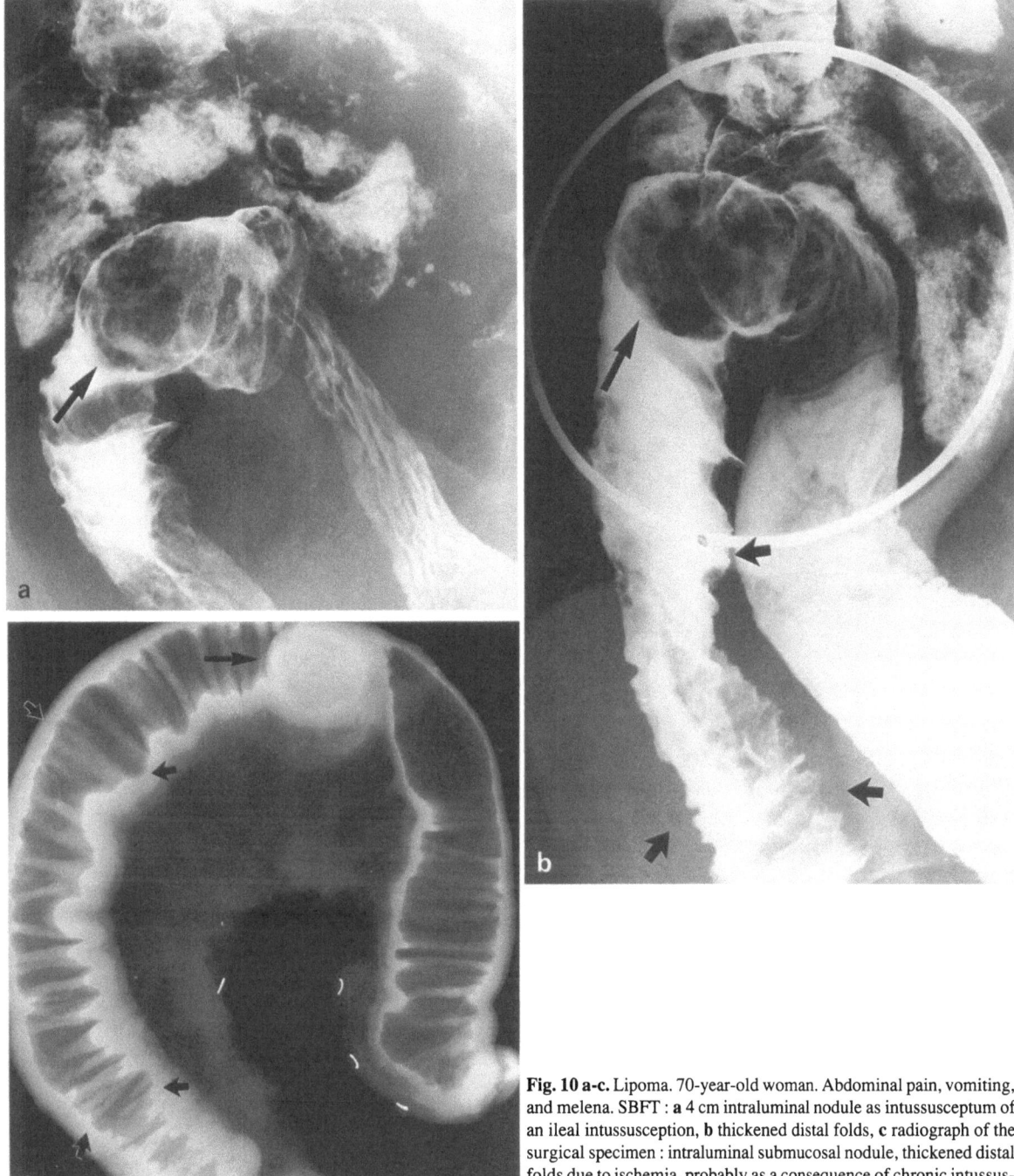

Fig. 10 a-c. Lipoma. 70-year-old woman. Abdominal pain, vomiting, and melena. SBFT : **a** 4 cm intraluminal nodule as intussusceptum of an ileal intussusception, **b** thickened distal folds, **c** radiograph of the surgical specimen : intraluminal submucosal nodule, thickened distal folds due to ischemia, probably as a consequence of chronic intussusception

Carcinoid tumors develop in Kultschistzky's cells, which are argentaffin cells ensuring the secretion of several hormones, including serotonin and bradykinin. The tumors and their metastases secrete great quantities of these hormones, which are too abundant to be inactivated by the liver and cause distal vascular lesions such as perivascular elastic tissue deposition and cardiac involvement (fibrous thickening of the tricuspid and pulmonary valves causing right ventricular failure).

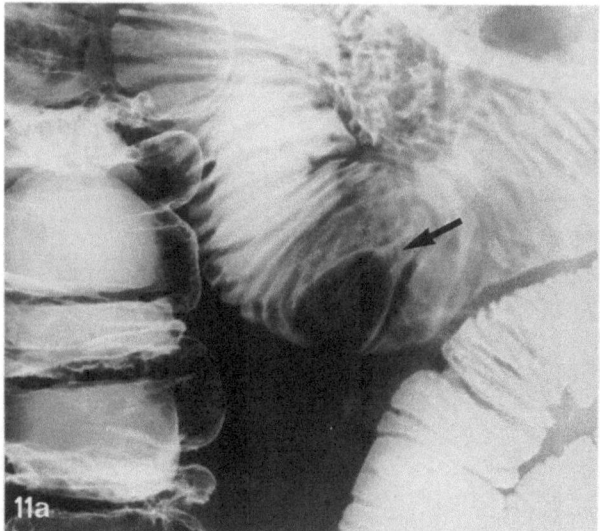
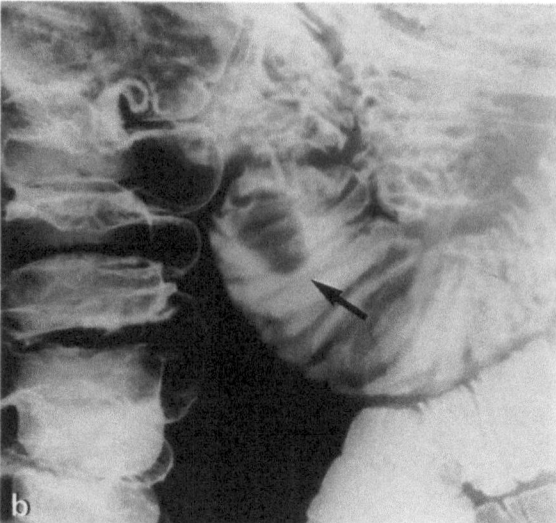

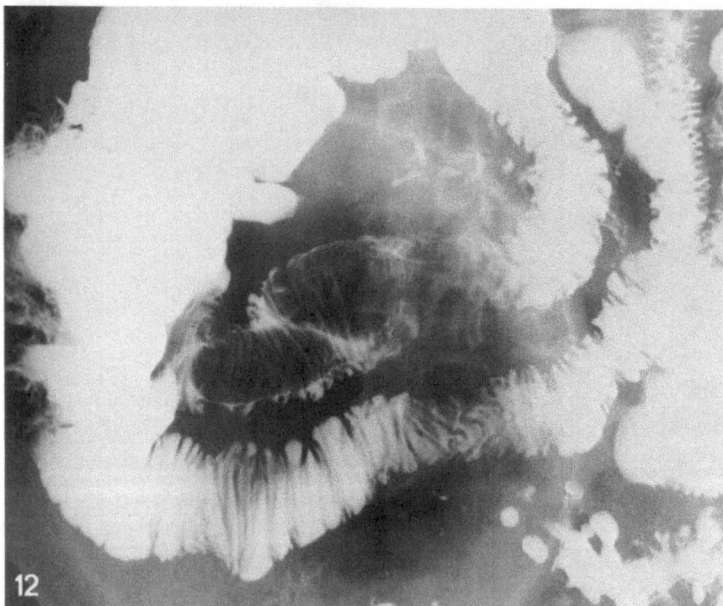

Fig. 11 a, b. Lipoma. 50-year-old woman. Delayed postprandial pains. SBFT : 25 x 15 mm intraluminal nodule with sharp contours, slightly deformed on palpation

Fig. 12. Lipoma. SBFT : two ovoid nodules with distinct margins, juxtaposed in the jejunal lumen

Pathology

Carcinoid tumors are 8 times more frequent in the ileum as in the jejunum; they predominate in the terminal ileum. Multiple tumors in the small intestine are observed in 10 to 30% of all cases. Some authors have even reported carcinoid tumors in Meckel's diverticula.

From a macroscopic point of view, these tumors are yellow, firm, sharply delineated and encased in the intestinal wall. They rarely ulcerate and are smaller than 3 cm in diameter. Invasion of the intestinal wall and mesenteric retraction are nearly constant when the tumor exceeds 2 cm.

Microscopically, the tumor originates in the crypts of Lieberkühn and invades the muscularis and serosa early on. Peritumoral calcifications are sometimes observed, and signs of contiguous ischemia are frequent.

Extension to the lymph nodes occurs quickly, and the risks of metastatic involvement is proportional to the size of the tumor: 5% when it is smaller than 1 cm, 95% when it is larger than 2 cm. Carcinoids are often associated with other tumors of

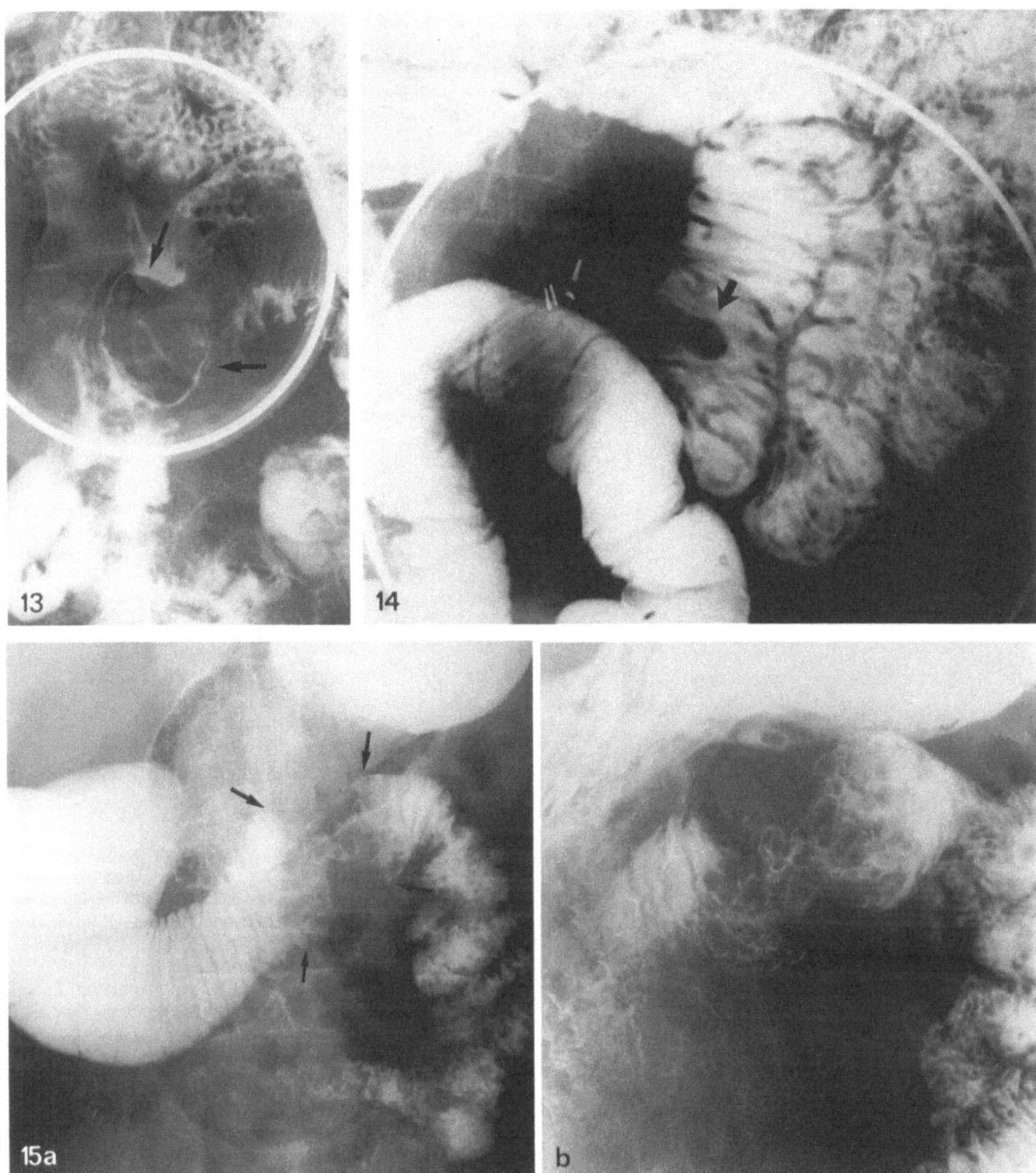

Fig. 13. Adenoma. 31-year-old woman. Anemia. SBFT : 35 mm intraluminal nodule as the intussusceptum of a jejunal intussusception

Fig. 14. Adenoma. 50-year-old man. Iron deficiency anemia. SBFT : a jejunal polyp

Fig. 15 a,b. Villous tumour. 76-year-old man. Bilious vomiting. SBFT : 5 cm long stenosing lesion at the level of the ligament of Treitz, formed by an area of nodulation with small conglomerated elements

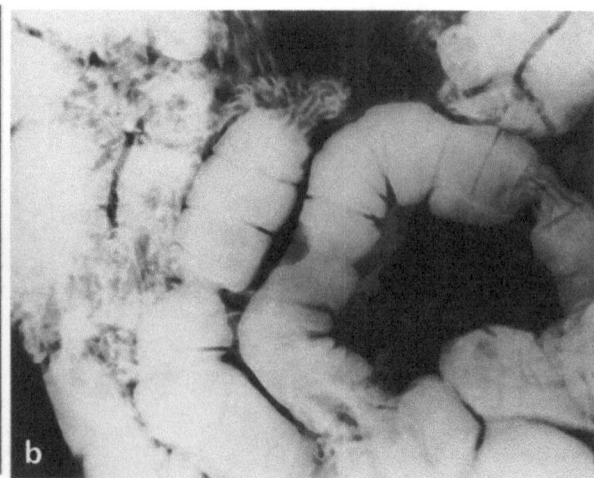

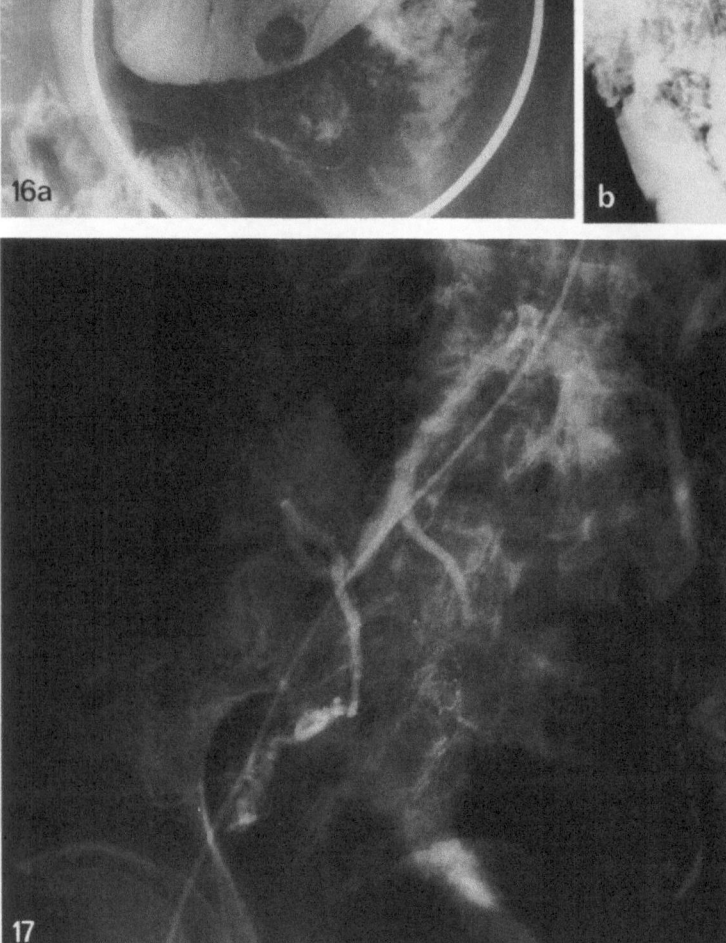

Fig. 16 a, b. Cystic lymphangioma. 67-year-old man. Abdominal pain. SBFT : 12 mm intramural nodule visible on frontal (a) and side (b) views in an ileal loop

Fig. 17. Angioma. 62-year-old patient. Known Rendu-Osler-Weber disease. Iron deficiency anemia. Superior mesenteric arteriography : an arteriolar ectasia is seen in the ileocecal region with an early venous return

different histological types in the digestive tract and in other sites.

Clinical findings

Men are affected twice as often as women, and the tumors are discovered around age 60. In 15 to 30% of all cases, the patient will typically report a sudden flush of the face and neck, a feeling of warmth and swelling; the subject will notice hypersialosis, hy-persalivation, tears, tachycardia and may develop low blood pressure and bronchospasm followed by a period of, first, cyanosis, then pallor. These symptoms are due to the secretion of bradykinin derivatives. These crises are triggered by emotions or certain foods and may last up to 30 min. The flush almost always indicates the presence of hepatic metastases. At more advanced stages, telangectasiae and hyperpigmentation become apparent.

Symptoms most often are nonspecific, and the patients will report pain and bowel habit changes, in-

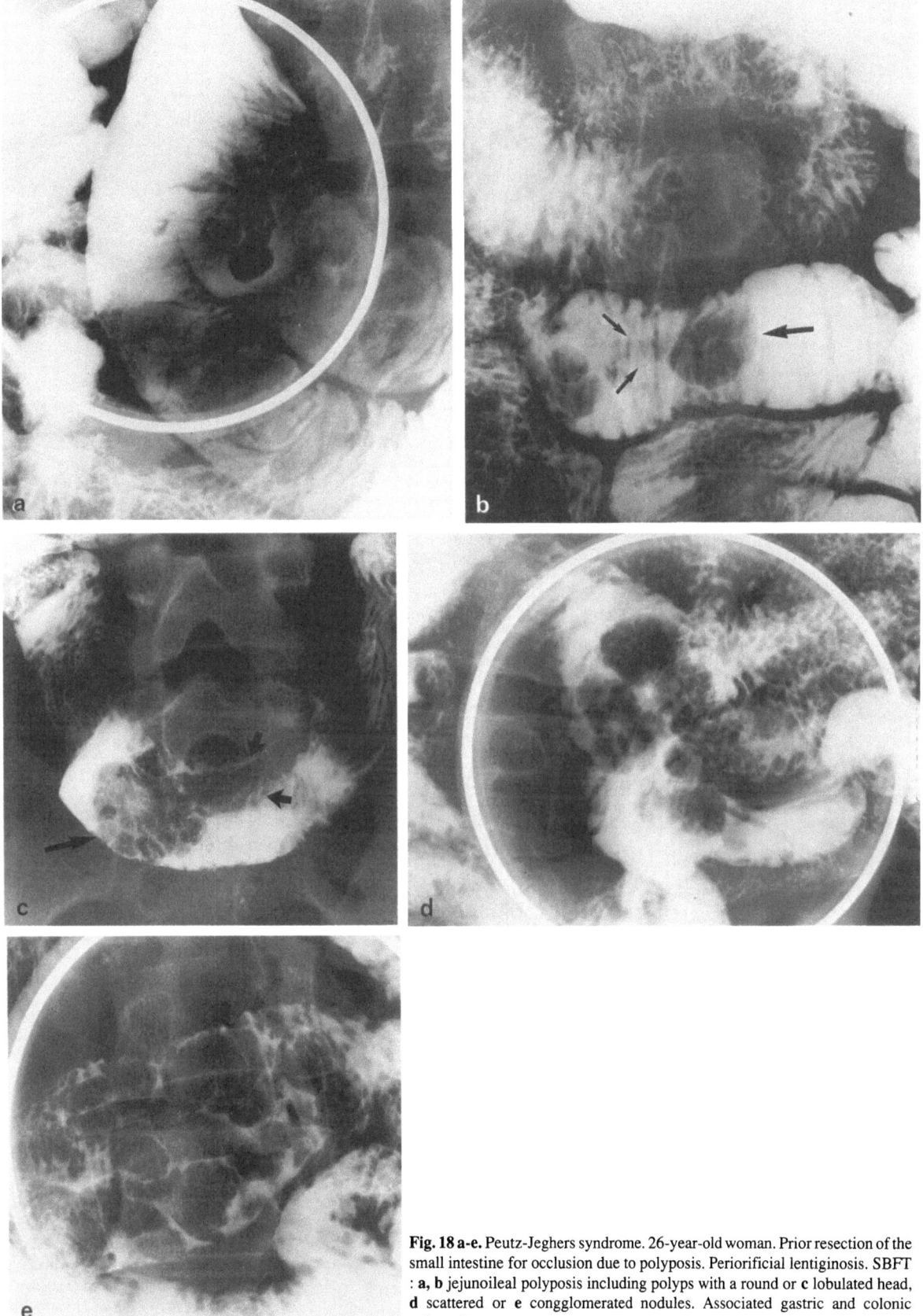

Fig. 18 a-e. Peutz-Jeghers syndrome. 26-year-old woman. Prior resection of the small intestine for occlusion due to polyposis. Periorificial lentiginosis. SBFT : **a, b** jejunoileal polyposis including polyps with a round or **c** lobulated head, **d** scattered or **e** congglomerated nodules. Associated gastric and colonic polyposis

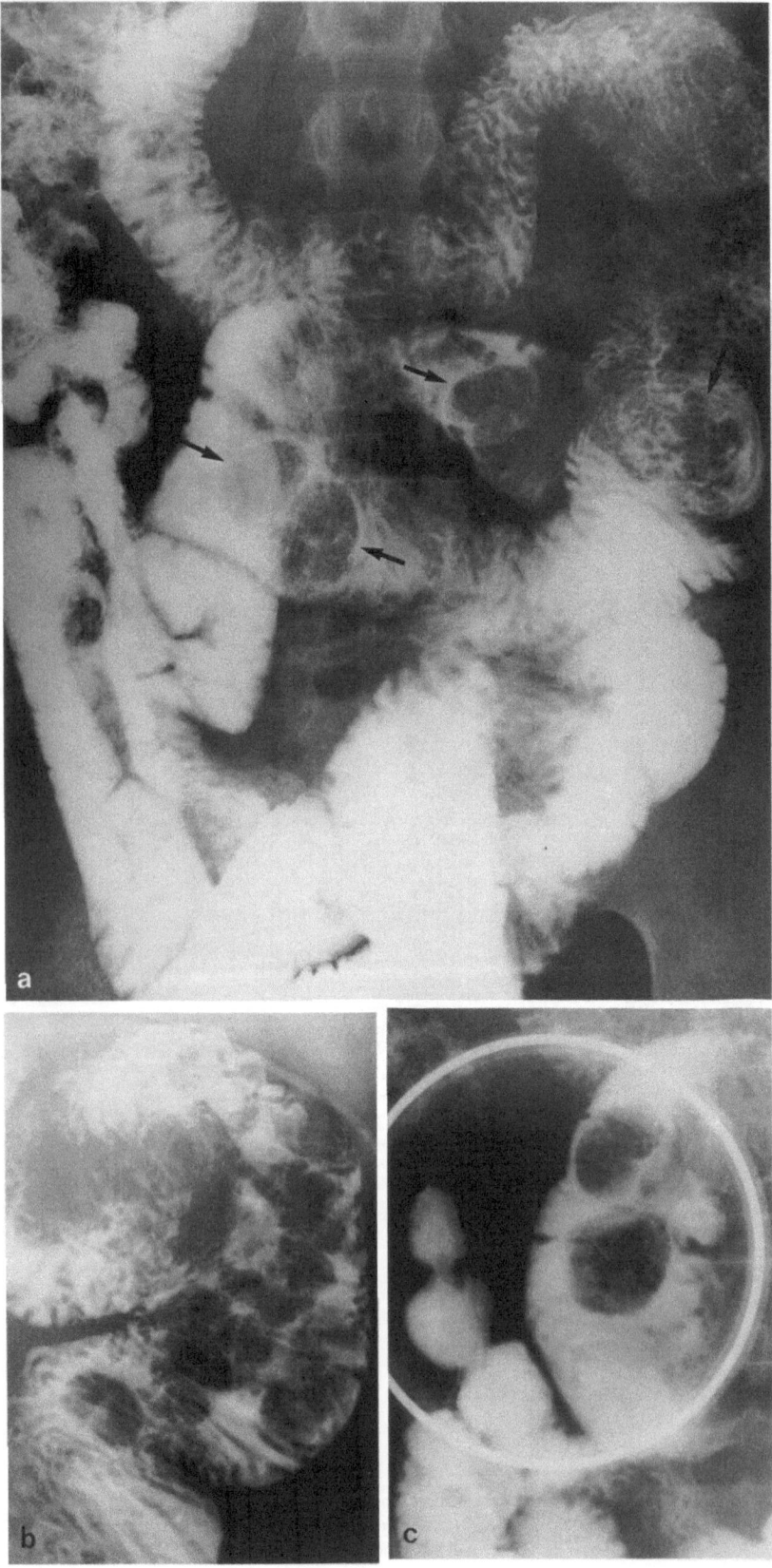

Fig. 19 a-c. Peutz-Jeghers syndrome. 32-year-old woman. Two anterior resections of small intestine for occlusion due to polyposis. Melena. Periorificial lentiginosis. SBFT : nodulation made up of scattered and juxtaposed elements

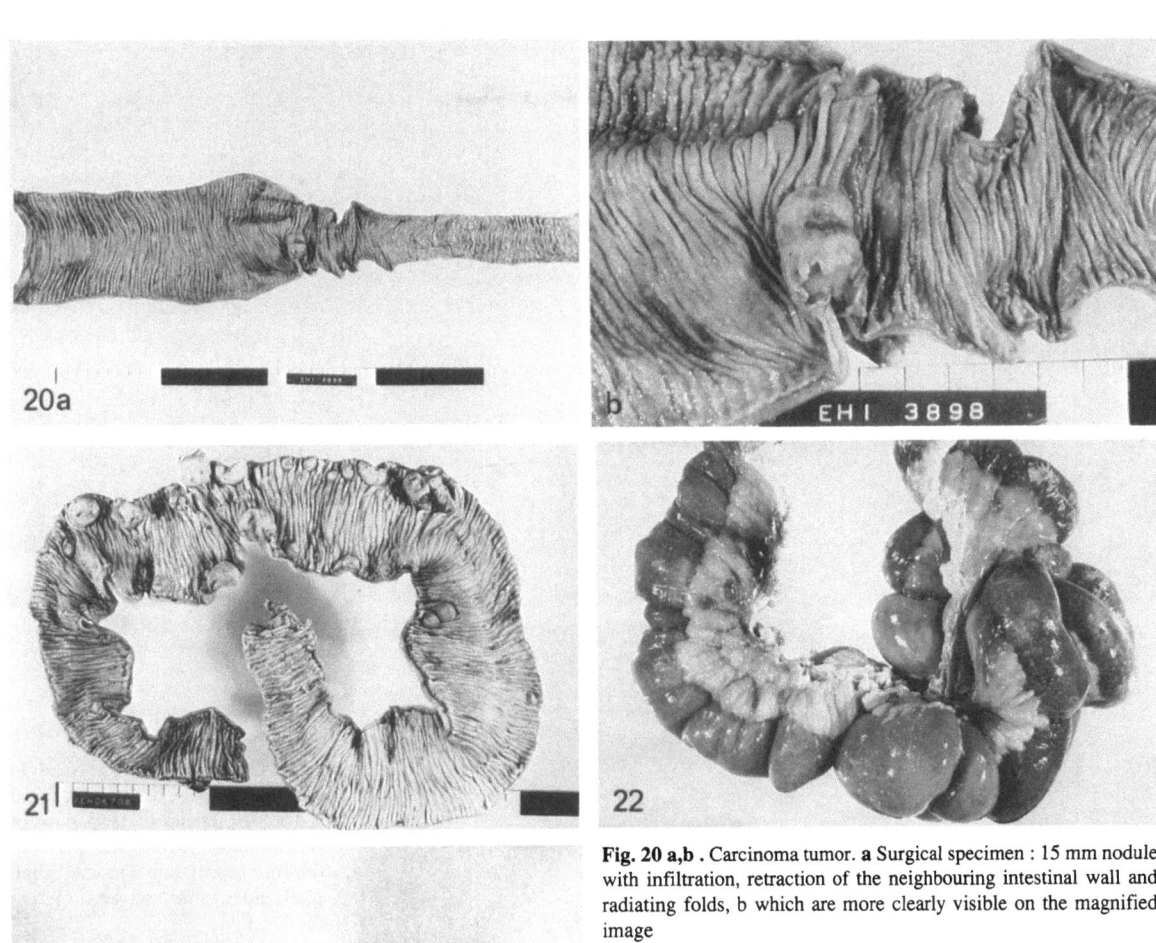

Fig. 20 a,b . Carcinoma tumor. **a** Surgical specimen : 15 mm nodule with infiltration, retraction of the neighbouring intestinal wall and radiating folds, **b** which are more clearly visible on the magnified image

Fig. 21. Multiple carcinoid tumors. Surgical specimen

Fig. 22. Carcinoid tumor. Surgical specimen : retractile infiltration of the mesentery

Fig. 23. Carcinoid tumor. Surgical specimen. Sagittal section demonstrating infiltration in the area of implantation

cluding diarrhea and melena. These patients have often been followed over several years for atypical abdominal pain or diarrhea, diagnosed as irritable bowel syndrome. An increasingly frequent mode of presentation is by incidental ultrasonographic detection of nodules in the liver. The puncture of these nodules reveals their endocrine nature.

The progression of disease is usually slow, death occurring as a consequence of cardiac failure. The 10-year survival is under 10%.

The measurement of blood and urine serotonin and urinary 5-hydroxy-indolacetic acid levels indicate the presence of the disease and metastases.

Radiological findings

Contrary to common belief, the diagnosis of a carcinoid tumor can most often be made or at least suspected on SBFT. Its appearance is often that of a round or oval, rarely ulcerated, marginal nodule with sharp contours, 1 to 3 cm in diameter. Its terminal ileal location is so characteristic that it is possible to consider carcinoid at the top of the differential diagnostic list. Despite such a benign appearance, the lesion may already have metastasized to the liver or lymph nodes.

The nodule may be associated with signs of

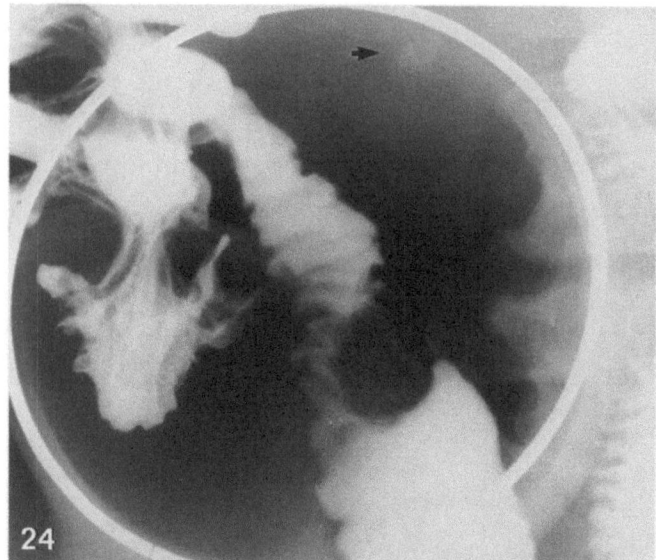

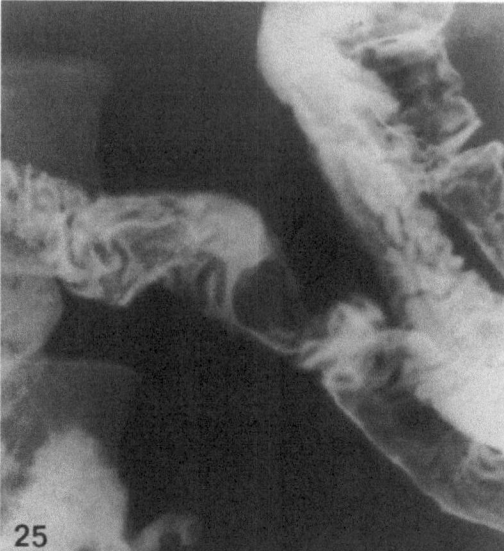

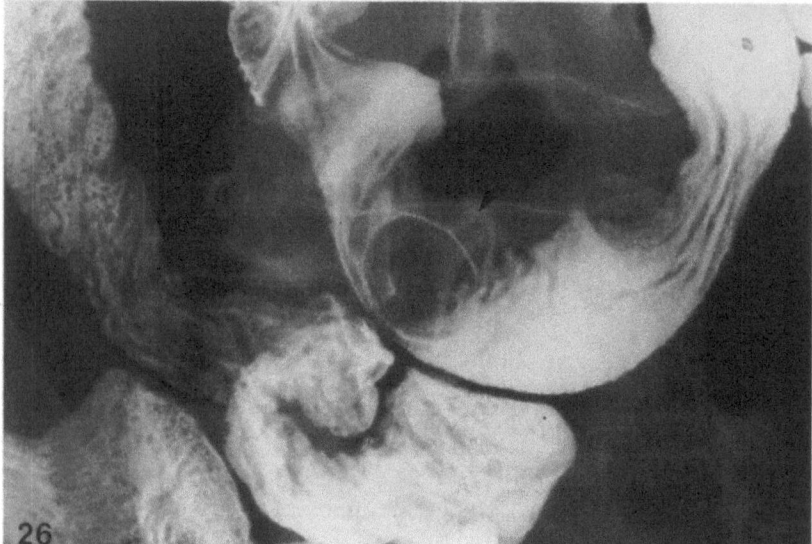

Fig. 24. Carcinoid tumour. 55-year-old man. Hepatomegaly. Hepatic ultrasound and cytological puncture : metastasis of endocrine tumour. SBFT : round nodule, 15 mm in diameter, in the terminal ileum. Calcifications in the soft tissues in the right iliac fossa

Fig. 25. Carcinoid tumour. A 41-year-old man. Episodes of diarrhea in a neurotonic patient. SBFT : 10 mm round nodule in the terminal ileum

Fig. 26. Carcinoid tumour. 37-year-old man. Two episodes of melena. SBFT : round nodule, 15 mm in diameter, perhaps ulcerated, on a pelvic loop

mesenteric infiltration producing a void image around the lesion. The involved loop is fixed and angulated and the neighbouring loops are arranged in circular or star-shaped patterns, the mesenteric edge is retracted and the antimesenteric margin sacculated.

Segmental crowding of the folds contiguous to the nodule or a short stenosis are signs of wall infiltration. Small calcifications may be seen in the soft tissues near the nodule and indicate calcified lymph node metastases.

The palisade arrangement of the folds of neighbouring loops reflects ischemia. Several jux-taposed or scattered nodules are sometimes observed in the ileum, with scattered micronodules.

The differential diagnosis of carcinoid tumors varies according to the lesion. If signs of mesenteric infiltration are present, only the appearance of the solitary marginal nodule may help differentiate a carcinoid tumor from peritoneal carcinomatosis. Endometriosis of the small intestine may give a similar picture where accompanying involvement of the sigmoid loop is most often the clue to the diagnosis. When the solitary ileal nodule is not located in the terminal portion, differentiation from

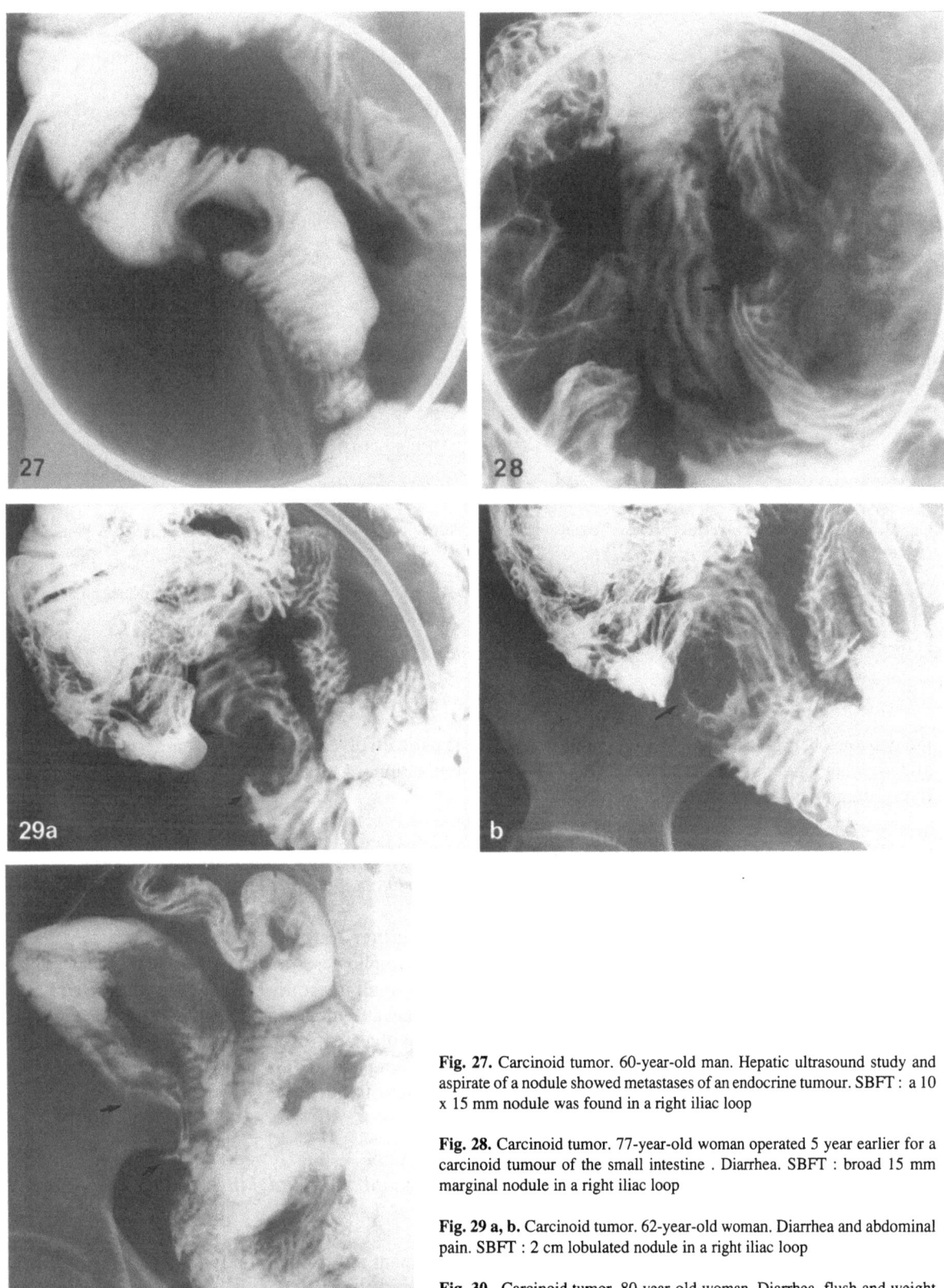

Fig. 27. Carcinoid tumor. 60-year-old man. Hepatic ultrasound study and aspirate of a nodule showed metastases of an endocrine tumour. SBFT : a 10 x 15 mm nodule was found in a right iliac loop

Fig. 28. Carcinoid tumor. 77-year-old woman operated 5 year earlier for a carcinoid tumour of the small intestine . Diarrhea. SBFT : broad 15 mm marginal nodule in a right iliac loop

Fig. 29 a, b. Carcinoid tumor. 62-year-old woman. Diarrhea and abdominal pain. SBFT : 2 cm lobulated nodule in a right iliac loop

Fig. 30 . Carcinoid tumor. 80-year-old woman. Diarrhea, flush and weight loss,. Hepatic ultrasound and cytological aspirate of a nodule : metastasis of carcinoid tumour. SBFT : broad 15 mm marginal nodule in a right iliac loop

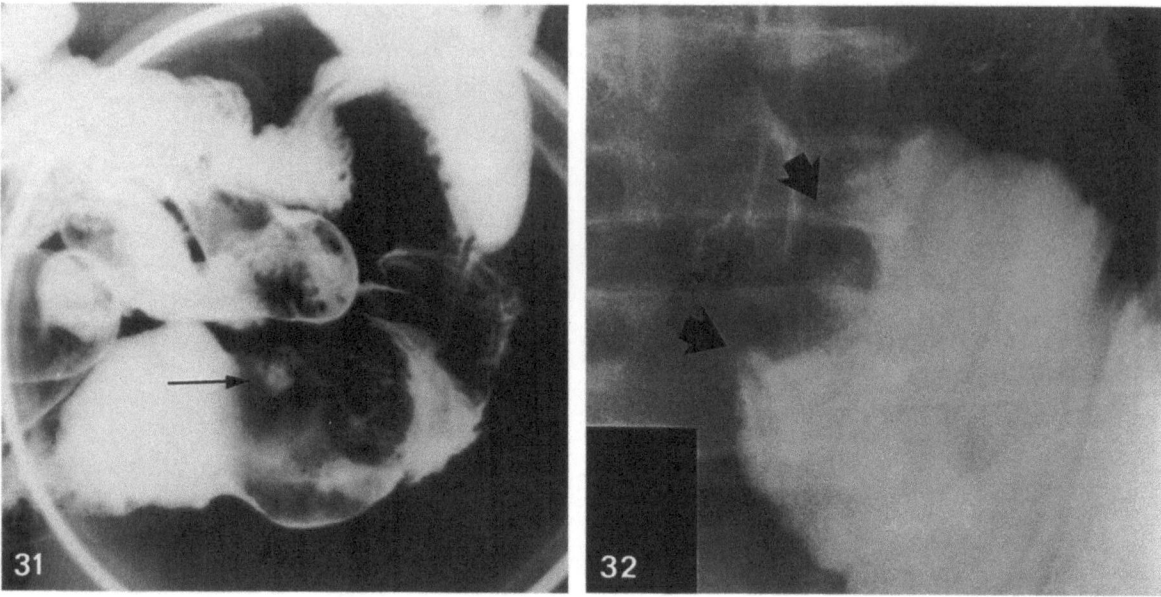

Fig. 31. Carcinoid tumor. 54 -year-old woman. Anemia and melena. SBFT : round ulcerated nodule, 3 cm in diameter, with moderate invagination, in a pelvic loop

Fig. 32. Carcinoid tumor. 54-year-old man with an obstructive syndrome. SBFT : 2 cm ileal nodule with stasis and proximal distention.

the various benign tumours is not readily made although statistically, a carcinoid remains the most likely diagnosis.

Complementary imaging

Ultrasound and computed tomography play a role in the assessment of the extension of carcinoid tumors into the mesentery, the lymph nodes and the liver. Ultrasound is increasingly used to diagnose these neoplasms as guided fine needle aspiration of the hepatic metastases in detects establishes the nature of the tumor.

Some authors consider arteriography necessary for the diagnosis of a carcinoid tumor: although the typical arteriographic appearance of the tumor itself is seen in only 20% of cases, mesenteric invasion, with the star-shaped radiating appearance of the vasa recta and terminal arterioles, as well as the winding, angulated, irregular arrangement of its associated distal arteries, is almost pathognomonic. In fact, arteriography is rarely essential for the diagnosis of a carcinoid tumor, but it is nevertheless useful for the study of mesenteric, nodal and, more importantly,

hepatic involvement in view to surgery or chemoembolization.

Lymphomas and immunoproliferative syndromes (Hematosarcoma)

This chapter deals mainly with malignant non-Hodgkin's lymphomas, which are the most frequent tumors of the small intestine. Alpha-chain disease and Mediterranean lymphoma are much less frequent, and the involvement of the small intestine with Hodgkin's lymphomas, plasmacytomas or leukemias is even less frequent.

Malignant non-Hodgkin's lymphoma (figs. 44 to 66)

Malignant non-Hodgkin's lymphoma (MNHL) is a lymphoid tissue tumor. It is considered a primary neoplasm of the digestive tract if there is absence of nodal, hepatosplenic or medullary involvement. Primary digestive MNHL make up 5% of all MNHL as

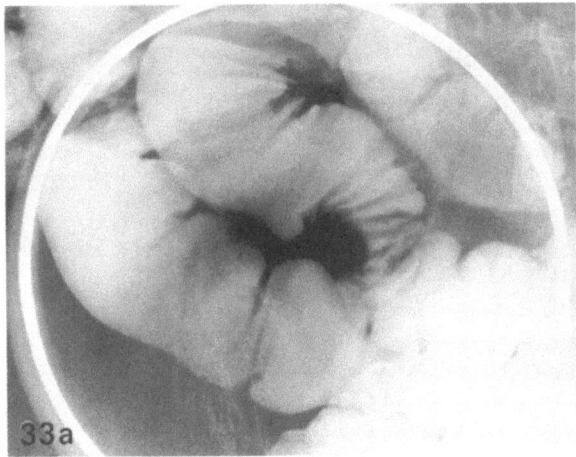

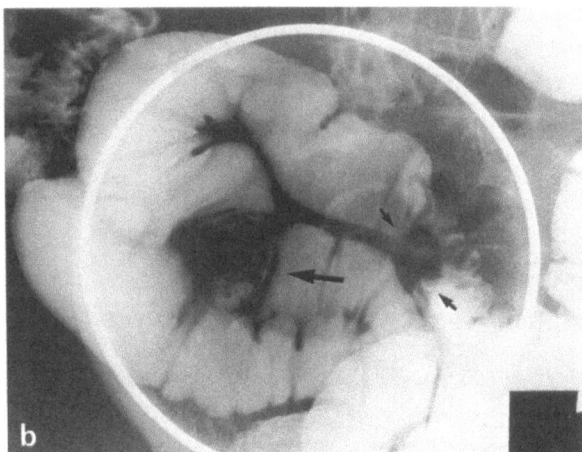

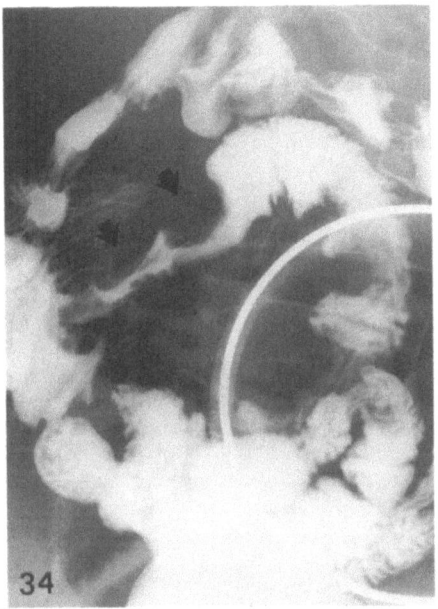

Fig. 33 a, b. Carcinoid tumors. 82-year-old man. Diarrhea. Arterial hypertension. Hepatic ultrasound and cytological aspirate of a nodule : metastasis of carcinoid tumour. SBFT : **a** 15 mm marginal nodule with crowded folds in a right iliac loop, **b** near the first nodule, one of the other three nodules detected during the examination is seen

Fig. 34. Carcinoid tumors. 61-year-old man. Weight loss. Hepatic ultrasound study and cytological aspirate of a nodule : metastasis of carcinoid tumour. SBFT : two 20 mm marginal nodules juxtaposed in the terminal ileum

metastatic lesions are much more frequent. More than 50% of patients with MNHL at its terminal stages present with an intestinal lesion, often silent. MNHL represent one third of all small intestinal malignant tumors. Other portions of the digestive tract are involved at the same time in one-third of cases.

Pathology

Lymphomas are more frequently found in the ileum owing to the distribution of lymphoid tissue. Particularly severe forms may be associated with cecal involvement. In half of the patients, the small intestinal lesions are multiple. The tumors are often large as one third exceed 10 cm in diameter.

Lymphomas originate in the intestinal wall and may grow into the lumen, remain confined to the wall or extend into the serosa and mesentery. When infiltrating the wall, these tend to destroy muscle and nerve fibres, resulting in characteristic ectasiae. They may also cause necrosis or a fistula. The MNHL produce little fibrosis, thus accounting for the relative malleability of the lesions and for the absence of proximal dilatation.

Several anatomicopathological classifications have been proposed. The international one takes the degree of malignancy and the histological features (diffuse or nodular, cell morphology, cell size, mitosis, etc.) into account. No correlation can be found between the histological characters and the macroscopic appearance of a lymphoma.

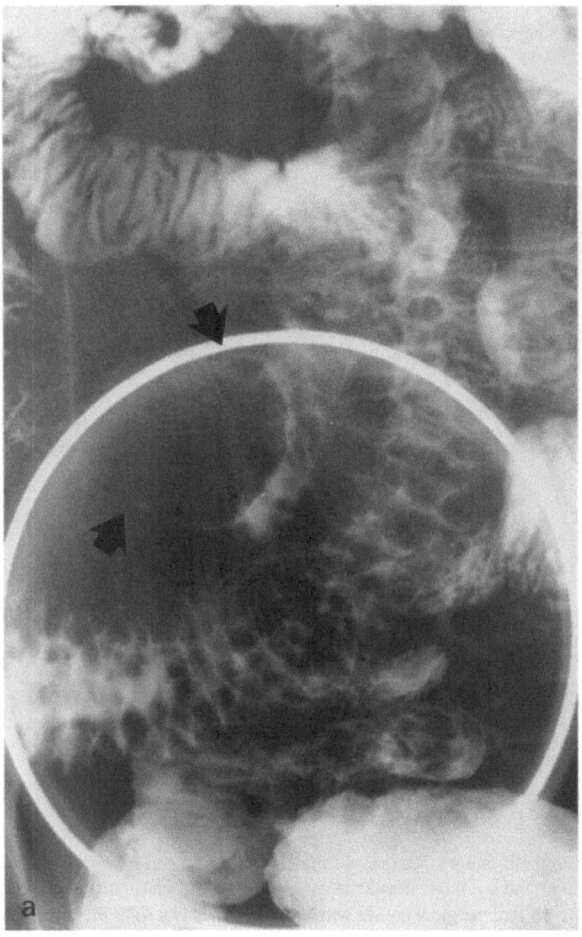

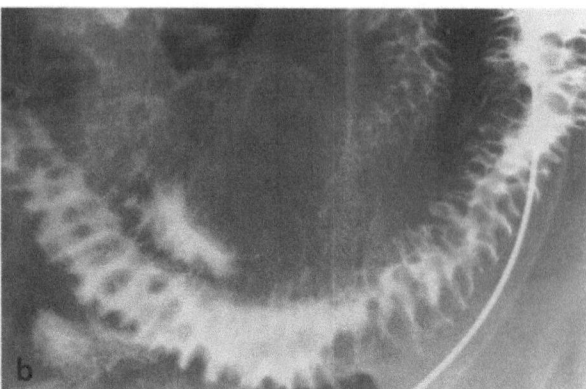

Fig. 35 a, b. Carcinoid tumors (Courtesy of A Fond). 61-year-old woman. Diarrhea and flushing. Hepatic ultrasound study and cytological aspirate of a nodule : metastasis of endocrine tumor. SBFT : **a** 3 cm marginal nodule in a right iliac loop and **b** proximal nodulation made up of multiple juxtaposed elements, several millimeters in diameter, proved to be small carcinoid tumours after histological analysis

Clinical findings

This disease most often affects men around age 50 but it is observed at any age even in children, where ileocecal forms with a fulminant course are frequent.

Lymphoma causes no specific symptoms. The patients present with pain, diarrhea, vomiting and an alteration of their general condition. A palpable mass is found in one-third of patients. In half, the disease is discovered during emergency surgery for obstruction or perforation. Clinical and biological malabsorption is observed in 10% of patients with MNHL, especially in the diffuse forms involving mesenteric lymph nodes, and sometimes because of associated infectious jejunitis. In these cases, partial villous atrophy is found and a gluten-free diet is not effective. Inversely, celiac disease may degenerate after a long time into a small bowel lymphoma.

The 5-year survival of patients with primary small intestine MNHL is 40%. The prognosis de-

pends on the extent of the tumour rather than on its histological type.

Duodenojejunoscopy and terminal ileoscopy may play an important role in the diagnosis. However, biopsies are often negative in the absence of mucosal involvement.

Radiological findings

Plain abdominal radiographs sometimes demonstrate a gas pool with irregular contours, which suggests the disease, a homogeneous opacity displacing the neighbouring intestinal loops may also be seen, or the combination of both signs.

Barium images vary according to the anatomic form.

The *nodular forms* make up 20% of cases. Isolated nodules are rare. They are round or oval,

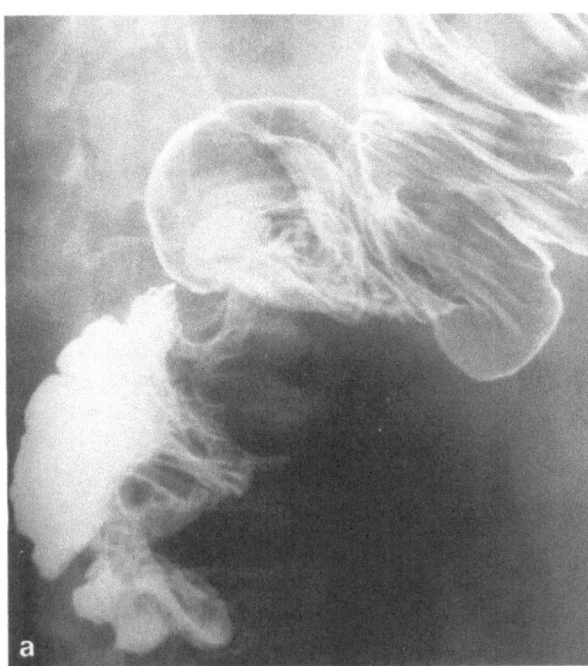

Fig. 36 a, b. Carcinoid tumor. 58-year-old man. Diarrhea and poor general condition. **a** Barium enema : extrinsec compression by tumour in the right colon. **b** SBFT : mitabdominal void. 20 mm nodule on a right iliac loop

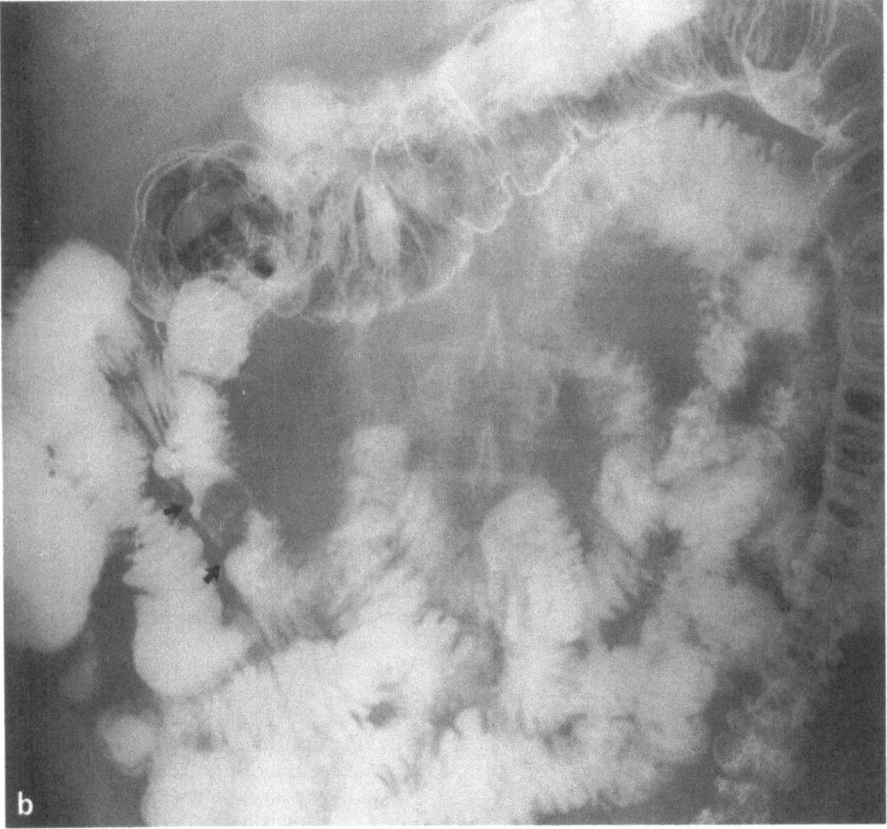

sometimes several centimeters in diameter. They develop in a loop, which retains its flexibility and peristalsis, and sometimes intussuscept. They may be slightly deformed on palpation. The nodules are most often multiple, with variable sizes and shapes, and are irregularly scattered in contiguous or distant

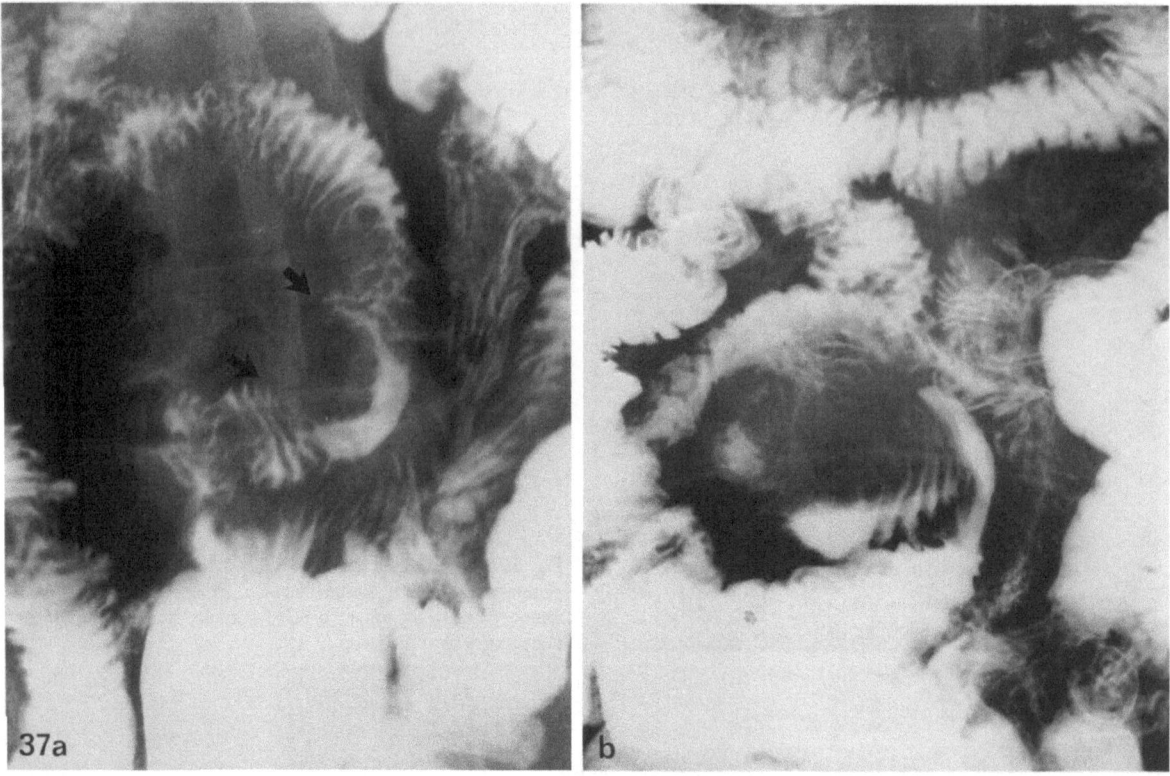

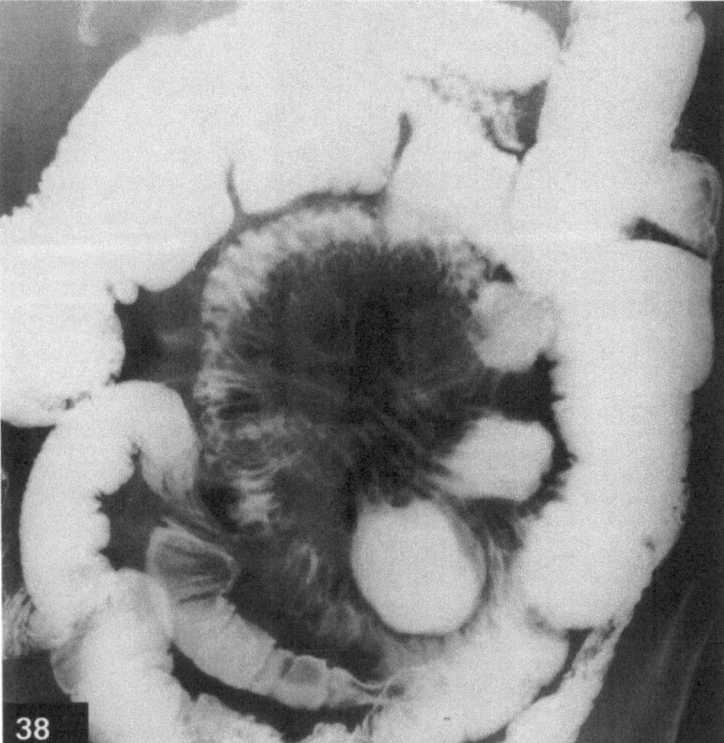

Fig. 37 a, b. Carcinoid tumor. 75-year-old woman. Abdominal pain. Diarrhea. Poor general condition SBFT : **a** 25 mm marginal nodule in an ileal loop, **b** underlying angulation, clearly demonstrated by palpation

Fig. 38. Carcinoid tumor. 69-year-old man. Periumbilical pain. SBFT : characteristic appearance of a mesenteric infiltration : a void image and a circular arrangement of an intestinal loop with spiculation of the mesenteric aspect coupled to sacculation of the opposite wall

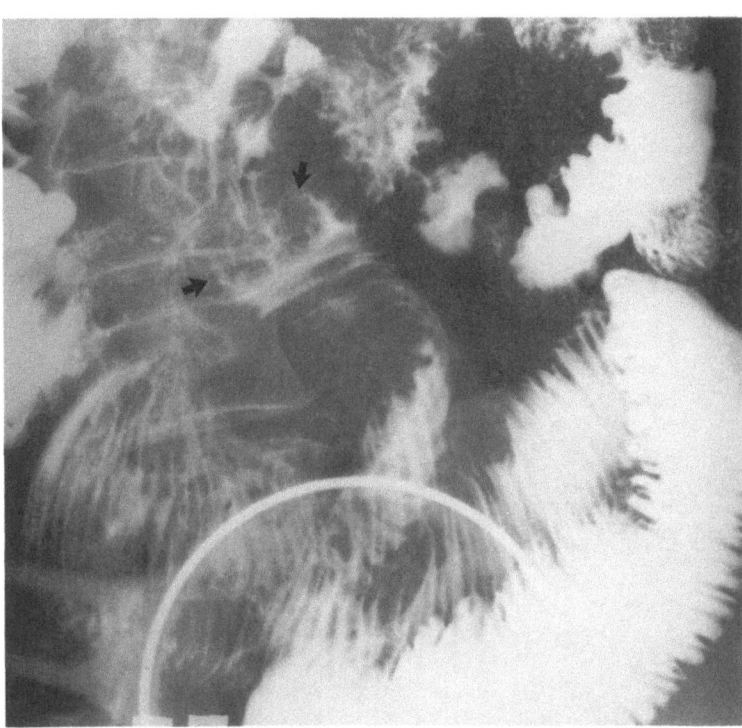

Fig. 39. Carcinoid tumor. 63-year-old woman. Abdominal pain. Diarrhea, and weight loss. SBFT: 2 x 3 cm lobulated nodule. Dilated and compressed proximal loops

loops. The nodules are sometimes juxtaposed or conglomerated and are enmeshed in large nodular folds, thus producing a convoluted appearance.

Digestive lymphoma in adults is sometimes associated with the image of diffuse nodulation made up of round elements of regular shape and size (smaller than 3 mm in diameter), similar to the image of benign lymphoid hyperplasia that is often observed in the terminal ileum of children.

The nodules are often ulcerated, with a large, round depression producing a concentric pattern covering a great part of the nodule. Ulceration may be the major sign, having the appearance of a ridge or meniscus. The image of a long fissure within the nodule sometimes mimicks the rhagade of Crohn's disease. However, the rhagade in the latter does not appear within a nodule but on the mesenteric edge of a loop, in an internodular recess.

The *infiltrating forms* are observed in over 50% of cases. They appear as alterations in the fold pattern with thickened intestinal walls. The folds are flattened and disappear or, on the contrary, are irregularly thickened. The most characteristic image is that of segmental marginal infiltration, usually on the convex edge of a loop, which is retracted by winding and nodular folds («scalloping»). The involved

segment is stiffened but still relatively malleable on palpation. The interloop gap is widened. The caliber of the intestinal lumen is rarely narrowed. In the stenosing forms, the involved segment may be short, with an image similar to that of other forms of tumoral stenosis, or long as is the case in ischemia. Several segments, often close to each other, may be involved. The disease may be diffuse and associated with a malabsorption syndrome manifested as early dilution and flocculation of the contrast medium with blurred contours.

The *ectasiating form*, described in 1954 by Hillemand and Chérigié as the aneurysmal form, produces a pool image on an intestinal loop, to which it is connected without any abnormal transition. The excavated contour of the image and its heterogeneous opacity indicate alternating nodules and depressions. Such images are characteristic of MNHL, but may also be observed with leiomyosarcomas, and some metastases as well.

Some MNHL develop mainly outside the intestinal wall. They displace the intestinal loop or, less frequently, cause retractile mesenteric infiltration («transverse stretch»). Such forms are not readily differentiated from those with exclusively nodal or mesenteric involvement. Cavities opacified by

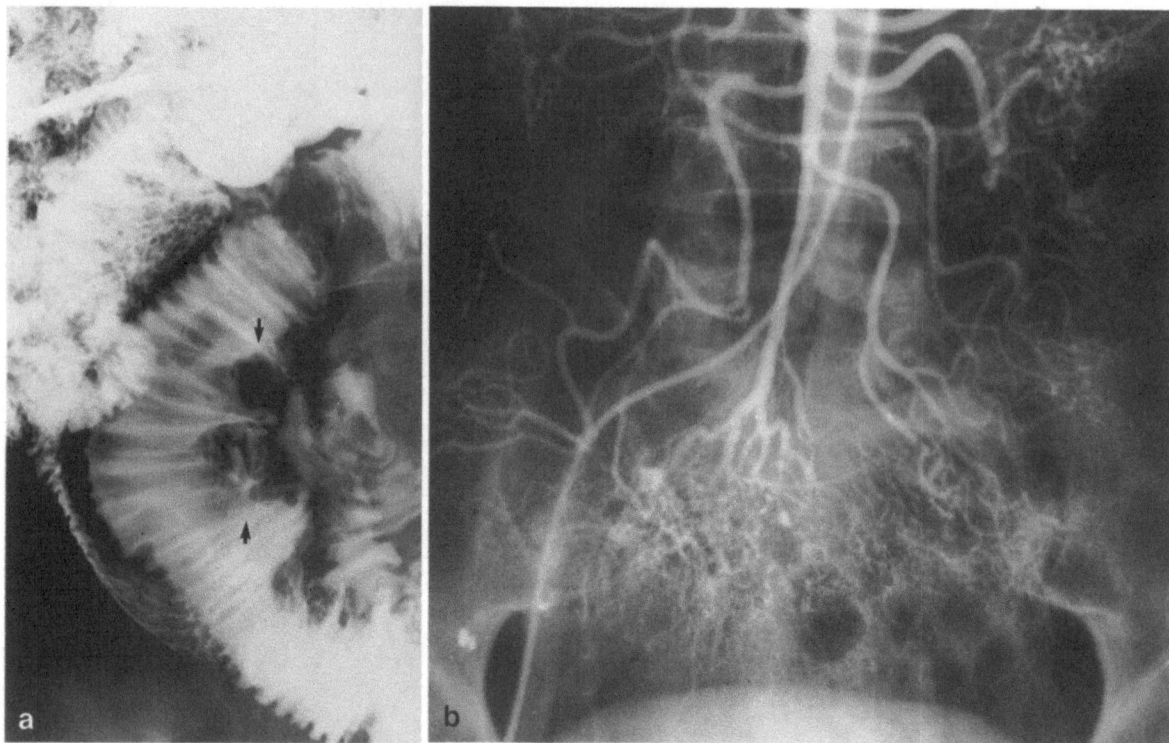

Fig. 40 a, b. Carcinoid tumors. 50-year-old man. Subocclusive crisis. **a** SBFT : two juxtaposed 10 mm mucosal nodules. thickened folds in the loop, suggestive of ischemia, **b** mesenteric arteriography : angulation and irregular caliber in the neighbouring blood vessels

barium, or fistulae producing pool images between, or connecting several loops, may be observed within these masses.

The diagnosis of MNHL is based on a number of elements:

- frequency of multiple lesions,
- size and extent of the pathological images,
- relative flexibility of the lesions,
- some specific images such as segmental marginal infiltration or the appearance of the ectasiating form.

Complementary imaging

Ultrasound sometimes makes it possible to think of the diagnosis of MNHL and guide percutaneous aspiration. The appearance observed is that of a «pseudokidney» with a large echogenic area surrounded by an asymmetric, irregular, hypoechogenic ring or a «sandwich» image, which is anechogenic or hypoechogenic and borders the echogenic intestinal lumen. The proximity of anechogenic nodules may indicate a subserosal lesion or the invasion of neighbouring lymph nodes (70% of all cases). Hepatosplenic invasion is well demonstrated. Hepatic metastases appear as poorly delineated, hypo- or anechogenic nodules, sometimes with increased echogenicity posteriorly. Focal lesions are less frequent in the spleen, although splenic involvement is likely in the case of splenomegaly.

Computed tomography is helpful for the assessment of the extra-intestinal spread of lymphoma, which is often more extensive than that indicated by barium studies. The density of the MNHL is that of soft tissue (40 to 60 HU), and its differentiation from invasion of the small intestine by a neighbouring tumour is not always easy to make. Computed tomography can demonstrate sites of retroperitoneal adenopathy as small as 1 cm and mesenteric lymph node masses as small as 3 cm. Nodal metastases are as dense as the primary tumour. Their evolution during treatment can be followed with computed tomography, which, like ultrasound, may guide percutaneous aspiration in lesions larger than 2 cm.

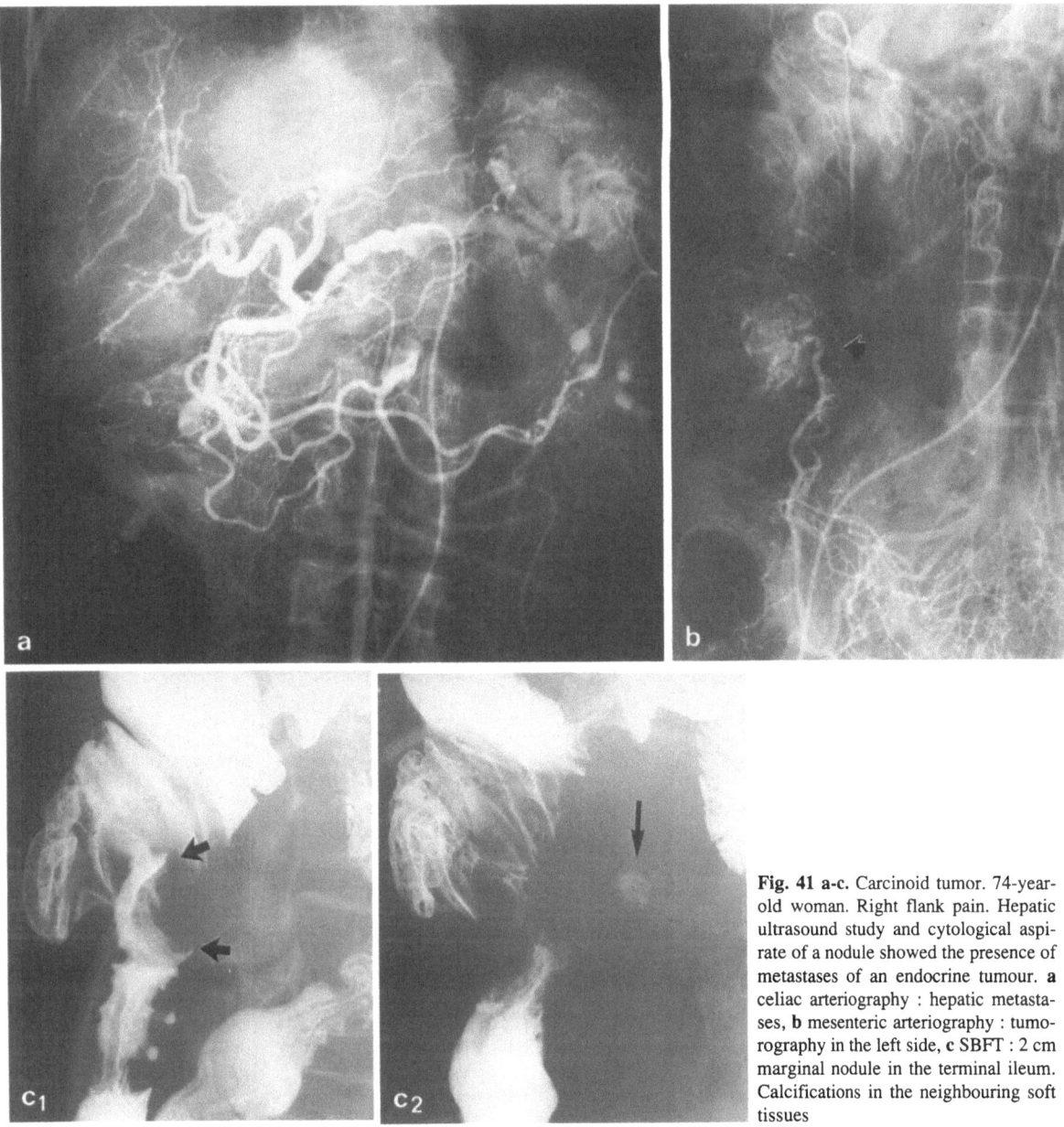

Fig. 41 a-c. Carcinoid tumor. 74-year-old woman. Right flank pain. Hepatic ultrasound study and cytological aspirate of a nodule showed the presence of metastases of an endocrine tumour. **a** celiac arteriography : hepatic metastases, **b** mesenteric arteriography : tumorography in the left side, **c** SBFT : 2 cm marginal nodule in the terminal ileum. Calcifications in the neighbouring soft tissues

Arteriography plays only an accessory role in the assessment of MNHL as most are hypovascular tumours.

In 10% of cases, lymphangiography may demonstrate nodal infiltration not seen on ultrasound or computed tomography. It permits the detection of 70% of recurrence during the first year; later in the course of disease, lymph node opacification is insufficient to allow for definite conclusions. It cannot assess hypogastric and subhepatic mesenteric adenopathy.

Hodgkin's disease (figs. 67 and 68)

Primary Hodgkin's disease rarely involves the small intestine: about one hundred cases have been reported in the literature. It is most often metastatic . The lesion probably develops in Peyer's patches.

Pathology
The intestinal wall is infiltrated by Reed-Sternberg cells, lymphocytes, eosinophils and plasma cells. Metastatic lymph nodes are often observed.

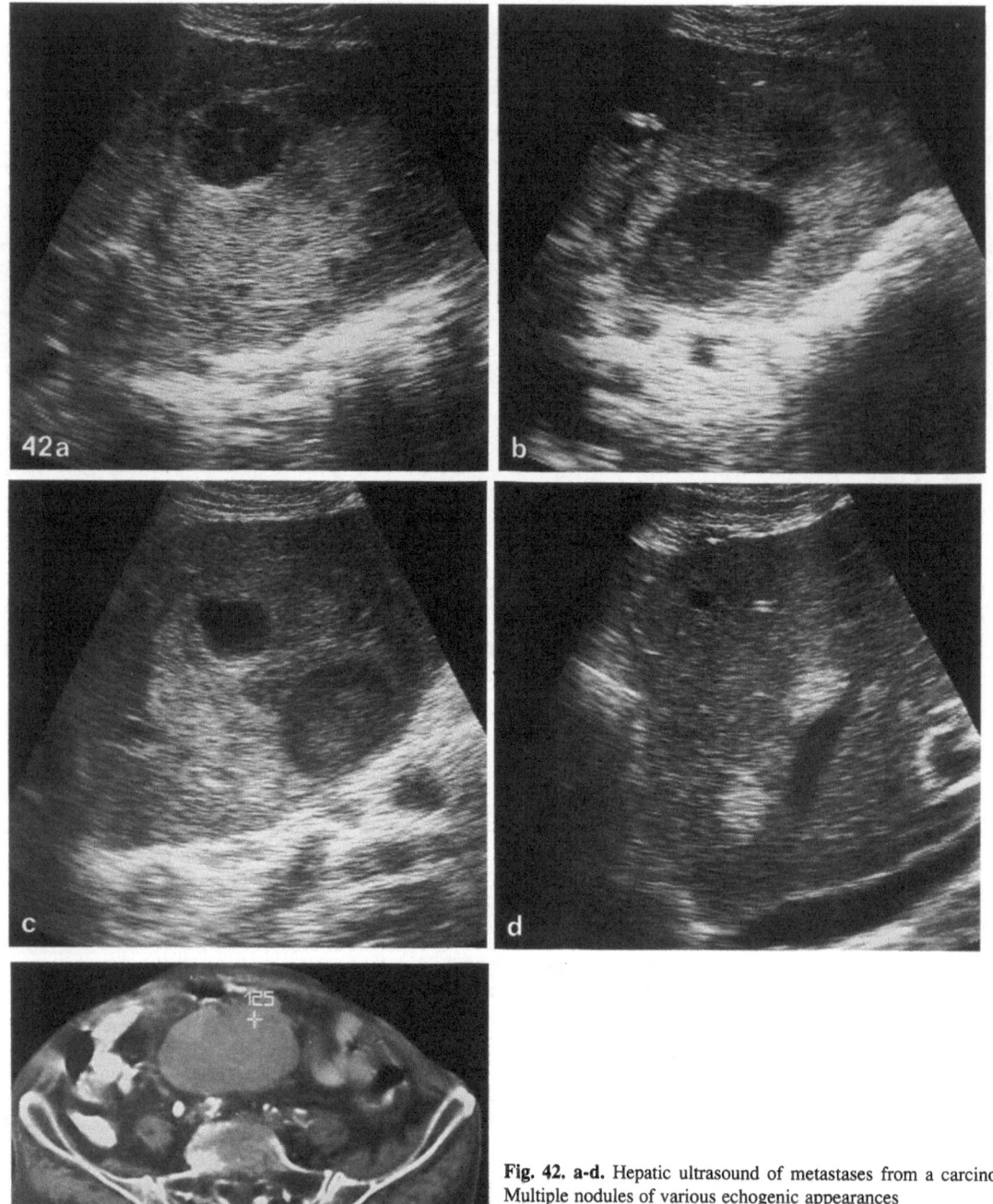

Fig. 42. a-d. Hepatic ultrasound of metastases from a carcinoid tumor. Multiple nodules of various echogenic appearances

Fig. 43. Abdominal computed tomography of a carcinoid tumor. Mesenteric nodal mass lying in front of the promontory

Clinical findings

The clinical signs are the same as with other malignant tumours of the small intestine and include pain, subocclusion, a palpable mass and an alteration in the patient's general condition. The diagnosis is usually not made before surgery in the primary forms. If it is, the preoperative workup must include the search for metastases. The prognosis of localized forms seems to be very favourable after surgery combined with radiation therapy (100% survival after 5 years). Survival is reduced to 50% after 5 years if metastatic lymph nodes are present near the primary lesion.

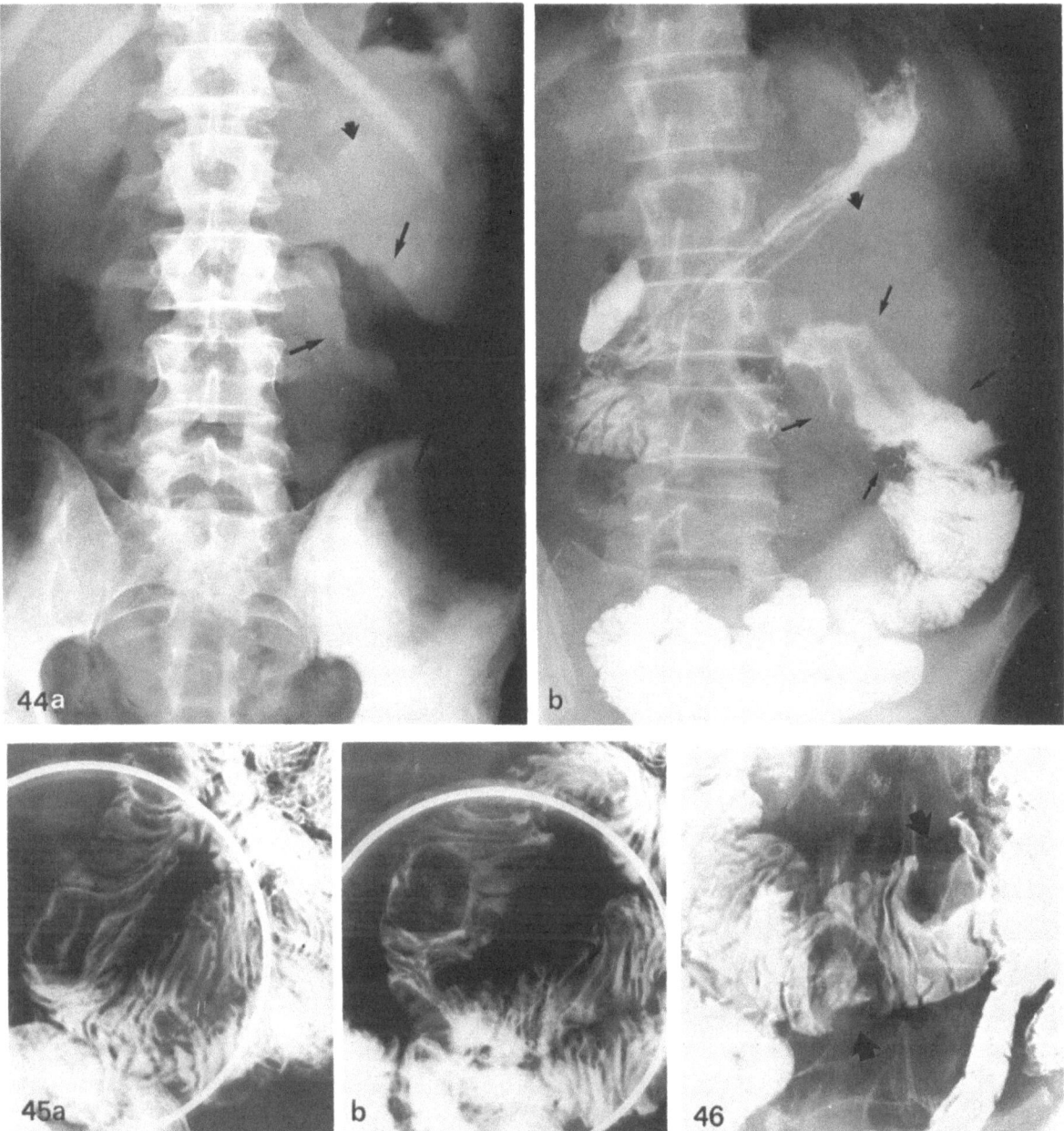

Fig. 44 a, b. Lymphoma. 25-year-old man with left-sided abdominal pain. **a** Plain radiography before urography : gas pool image within an opacity in the left hypochondrium, b SBFT : image confirming a lymphoma of the ectasiating form in the first jejunal loop

Fig. 45 a, b. Lymphoma. SBFT : isolated 30 x 15 mm nodule, slightly malleable on palpation, centered on a linear image which suggests an ulceration

Fig. 46. Lymphoma (Courtesy of P Moiroud). SBFT : two 20 mm nodules, one with extensive ulceration, juxtaposed in a jejunal loop

Radiological findings

On small bowel follow-through, the lesions most often appear as fixed stenoses extending over several centimeters, with disappearance of the folds and a tapered transition with the segments proximal and distal. A «mass effect» is usually observed, displacing and compressing the neighbouring loops. Nodular or ulcerated forms are very rare. No excavated forms

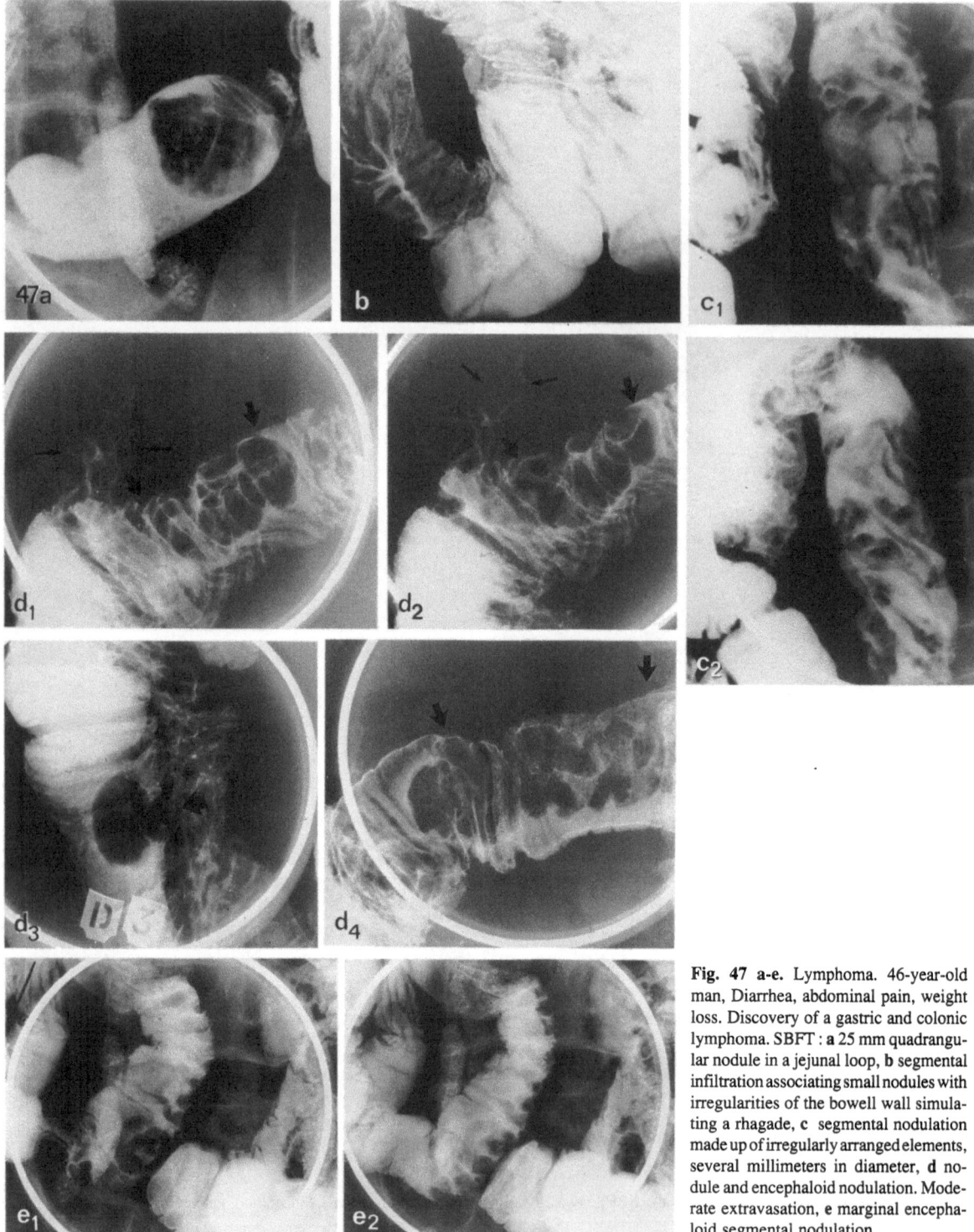

Fig. 47 a-e. Lymphoma. 46-year-old man, Diarrhea, abdominal pain, weight loss. Discovery of a gastric and colonic lymphoma. SBFT : **a** 25 mm quadrangular nodule in a jejunal loop, **b** segmental infiltration associating small nodules with irregularities of the bowell wall simulating a rhagade, **c** segmental nodulation made up of irregularly arranged elements, several millimeters in diameter, **d** nodule and encephaloid nodulation. Moderate extravasation, **e** marginal encephaloid segmental nodulation

or aneurysmal dilatation are observed in contrast to MNHL. The differential diagnosis includes adenocarcinoma and radiation-induced enteritis.

Complementary imaging
Ultrasound and computed tomography are very useful, as for MNHL. The ultrasound image is usually more

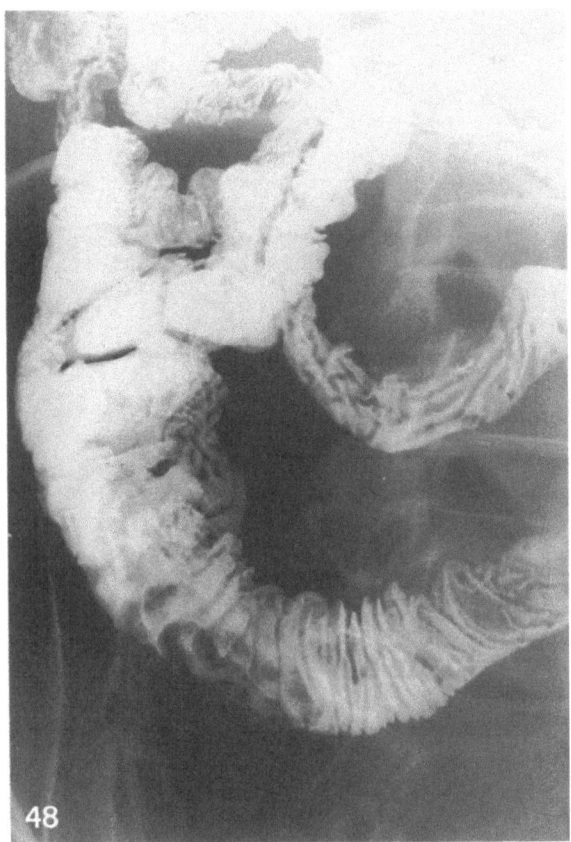

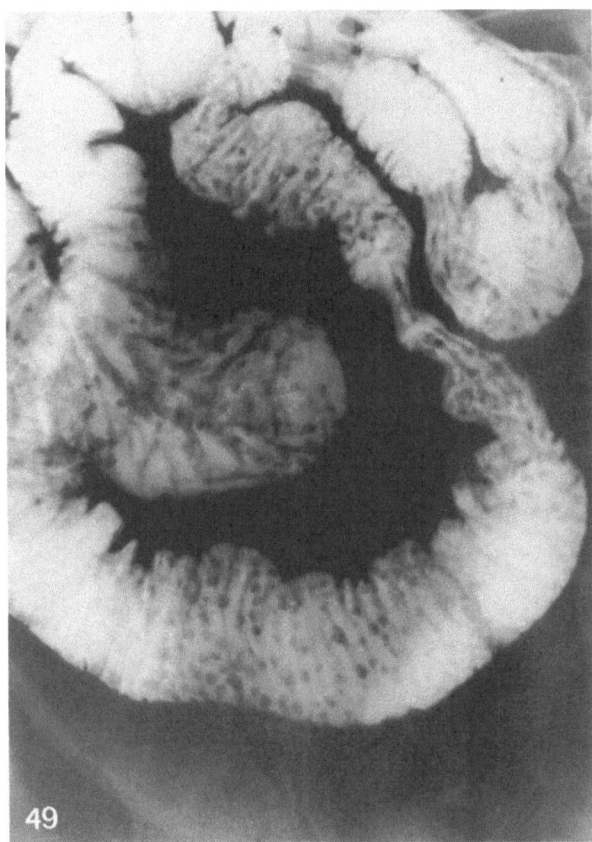

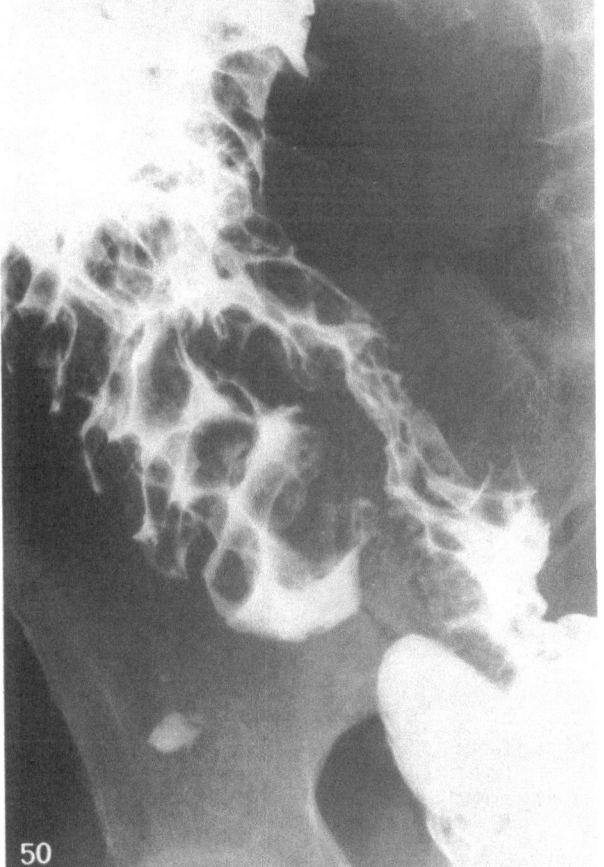

Fig. 48. Lymphoma. 63-year-old man. Gastric and colonic lymphoma. SBFT : encephaloid segmental nodulation

Fig. 49. Lymphoid nodular hyperplasia. 51-year-old man.
Malignant skin lymphoma. Assessment of tumor spread.
SBFT : nodulation of the ileal loops characteristic of
lymphoid nodular hyperplasia.

Fig. 50. Lymphoma. 40-year-old woman. Right iliac pain.
SBFT : ileocecal nodulation made up of juxtaposed elements of various sizes

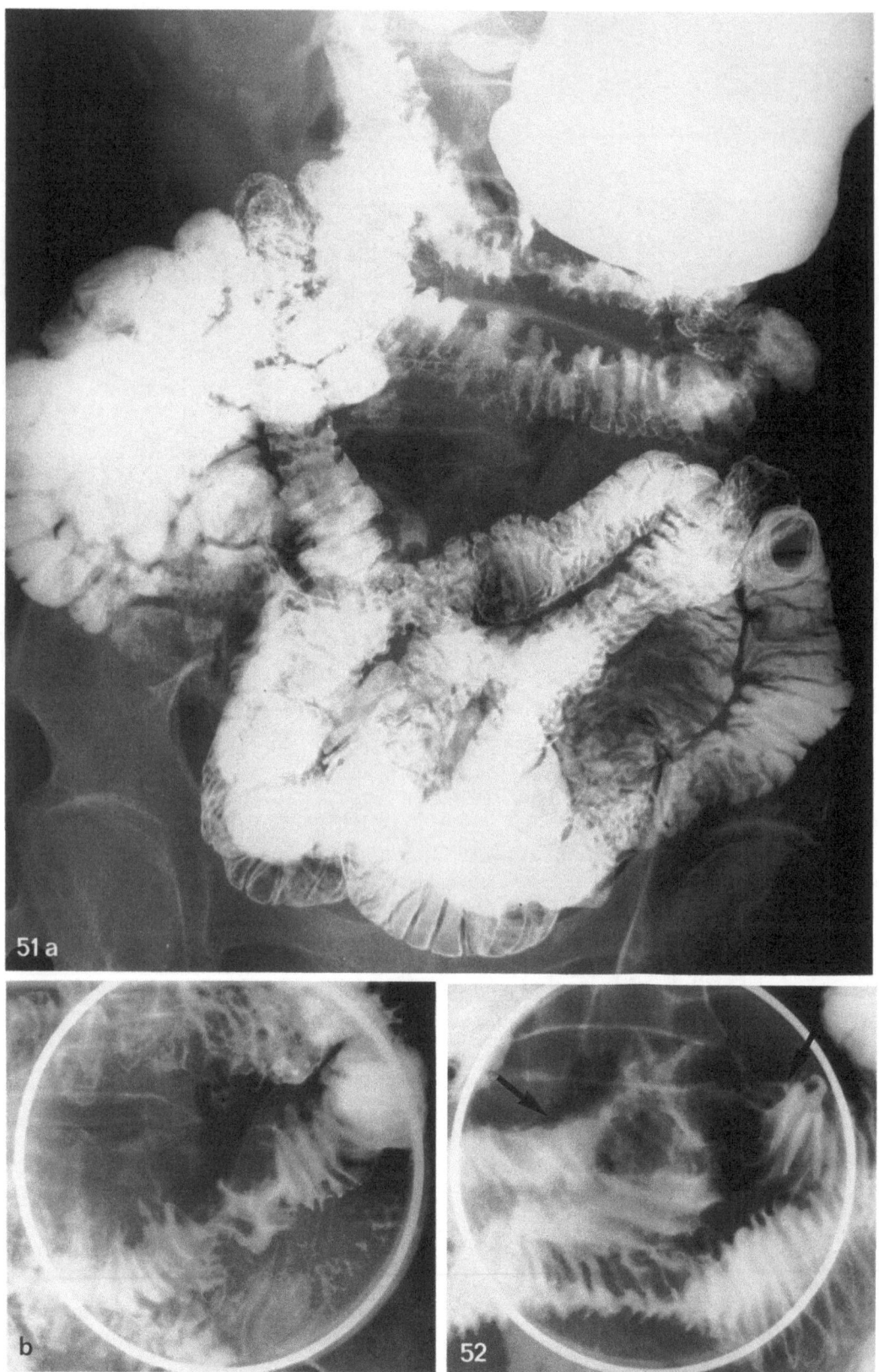

Fig. 51. Lymphoma. 75-year-old woman. Subocclusion. Deterioration in her general condition and melena. SBFT : nodulation and nodular folds in a jejunal loop

Fig. 52. Lymphoma. 44-year-old man. Abdominal pain and melena. SBFT : ileal ulceration with excavated contours, surrounded by a nodular ridge

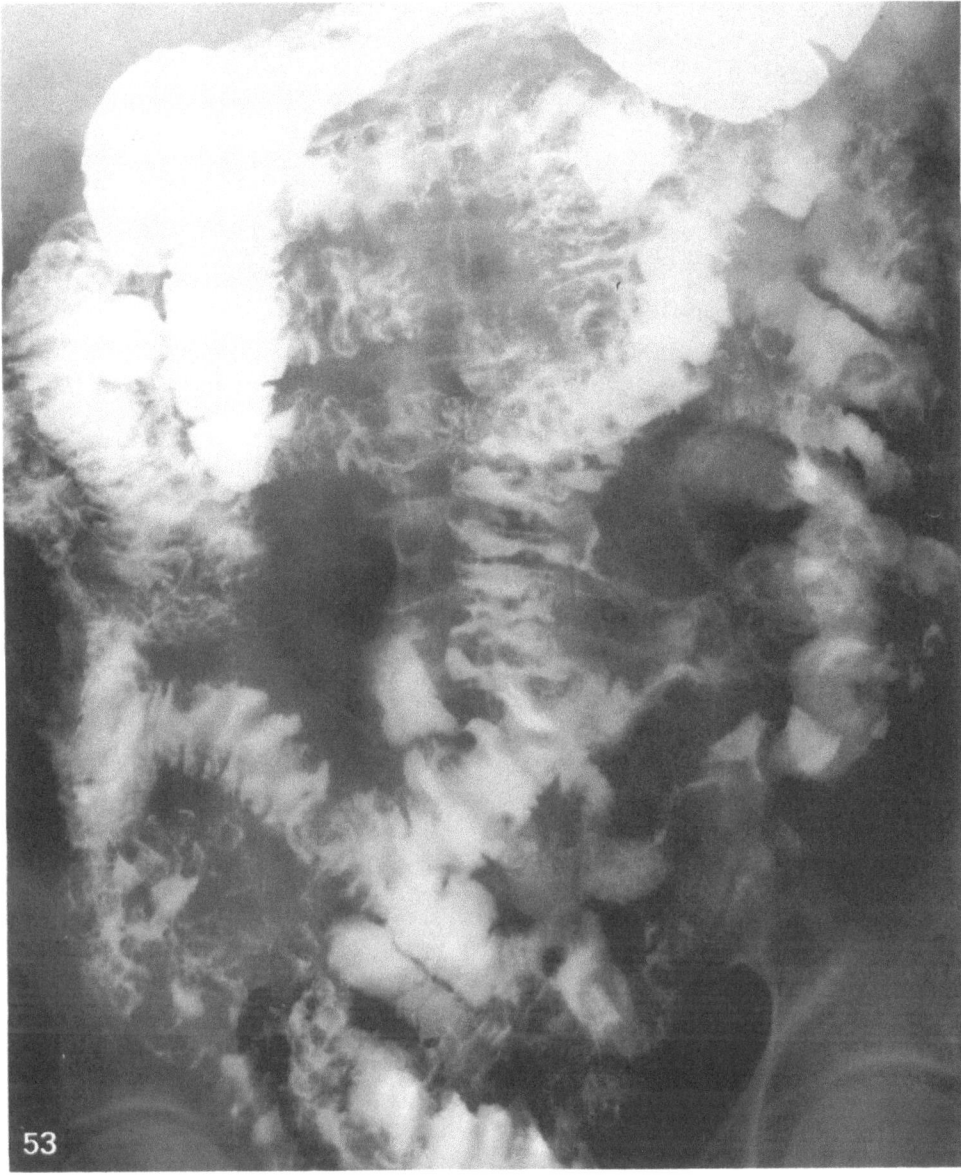

Fig. 53. Lymphoma. 64-year-old man. Abdominal pain. Deterioration of his general condition. SBFT : association of nodules and large nodular folds in the entire small bowel

echogenic than that of the MNHL because of more extensive fibrosis. Splenic lesions are much more frequent but 50% of normal-sized spleens may be histologically involved.

Alpha-chain disease and mediterranean lymphoma (figs. 67 to 73)

Alpha-chain disease is an immune disease caused by the proliferation of plasmacytes secreting an abnor-

mal immunoglobulin. In early stages, it can be cured by antibiotics; later it goes on to cause lymphomatous degeneration. The lesions mainly involve the small intestine and the mesenteric lymph nodes. Lung and bone involvement has also been described. Some authors consider that Mediterranean lymphoma, which is characterized by a malignant plasmocyte infiltration, could be regarded as independent from alpha-chain disease. This disease has been mainly described around the Mediterranean Basin and is associated with deficient nutrition, and poor hy-

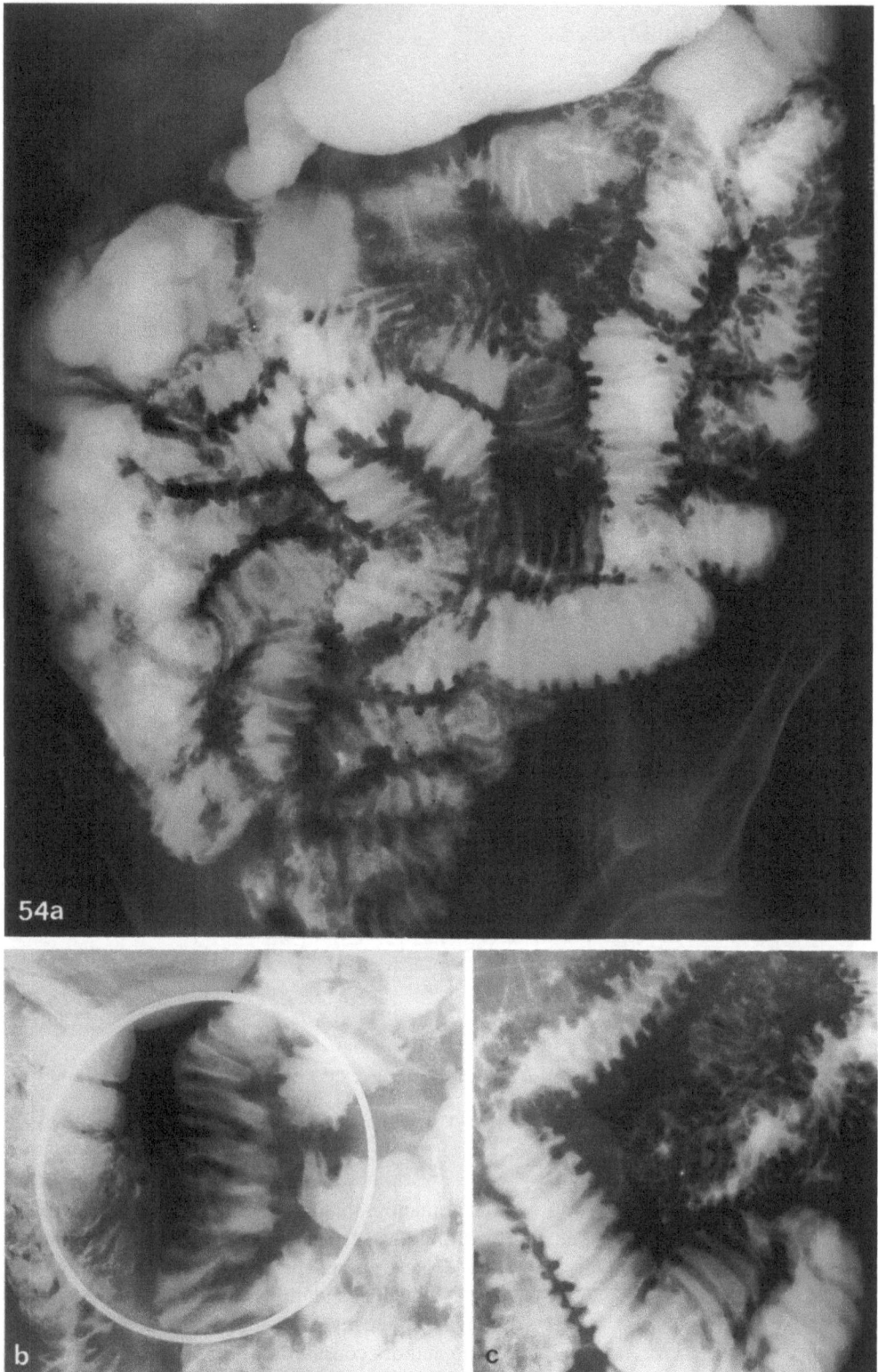

Fig. 54 a-c. Lymphoma. 57-year-old man. Diarrhea and weight loss. SBFT : diffuse, moderate thickening of the intestinal wall and nodular hypertrophy of the folds

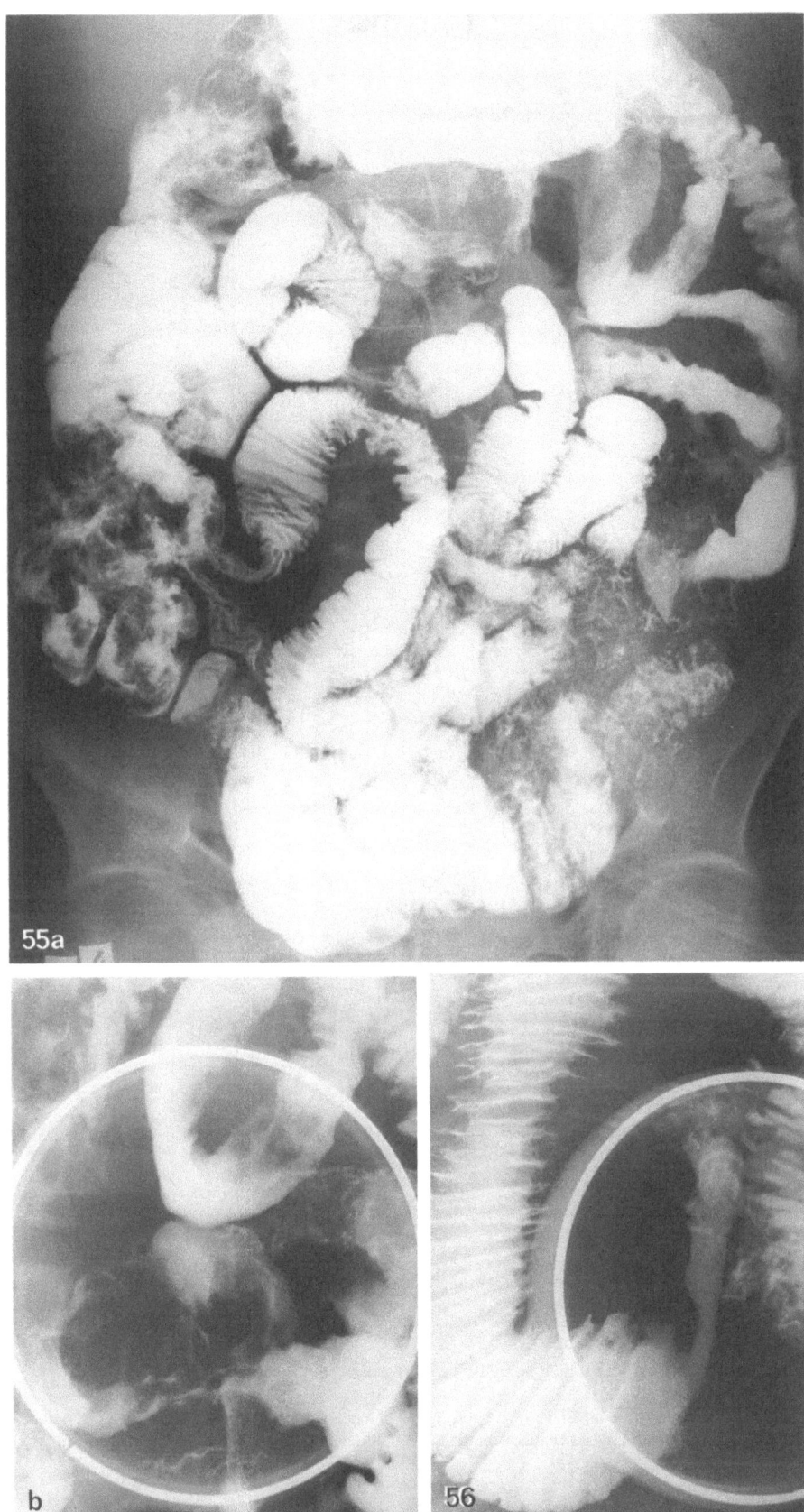

Fig. 55 a,b. Lymphoma. 37-year-old man. Postprandial pain. Weight loss. SBFT : fixed, stiff first jejunal loops, increased interloop gap, irregular narrowing and disappearance of the folds

Fig. 56. Lymphoma. 63-year-old man. Diarrhea and vomitting. SBFT : long jejunal stenosis. Dilatation of the proximal loop with broadened straight folds

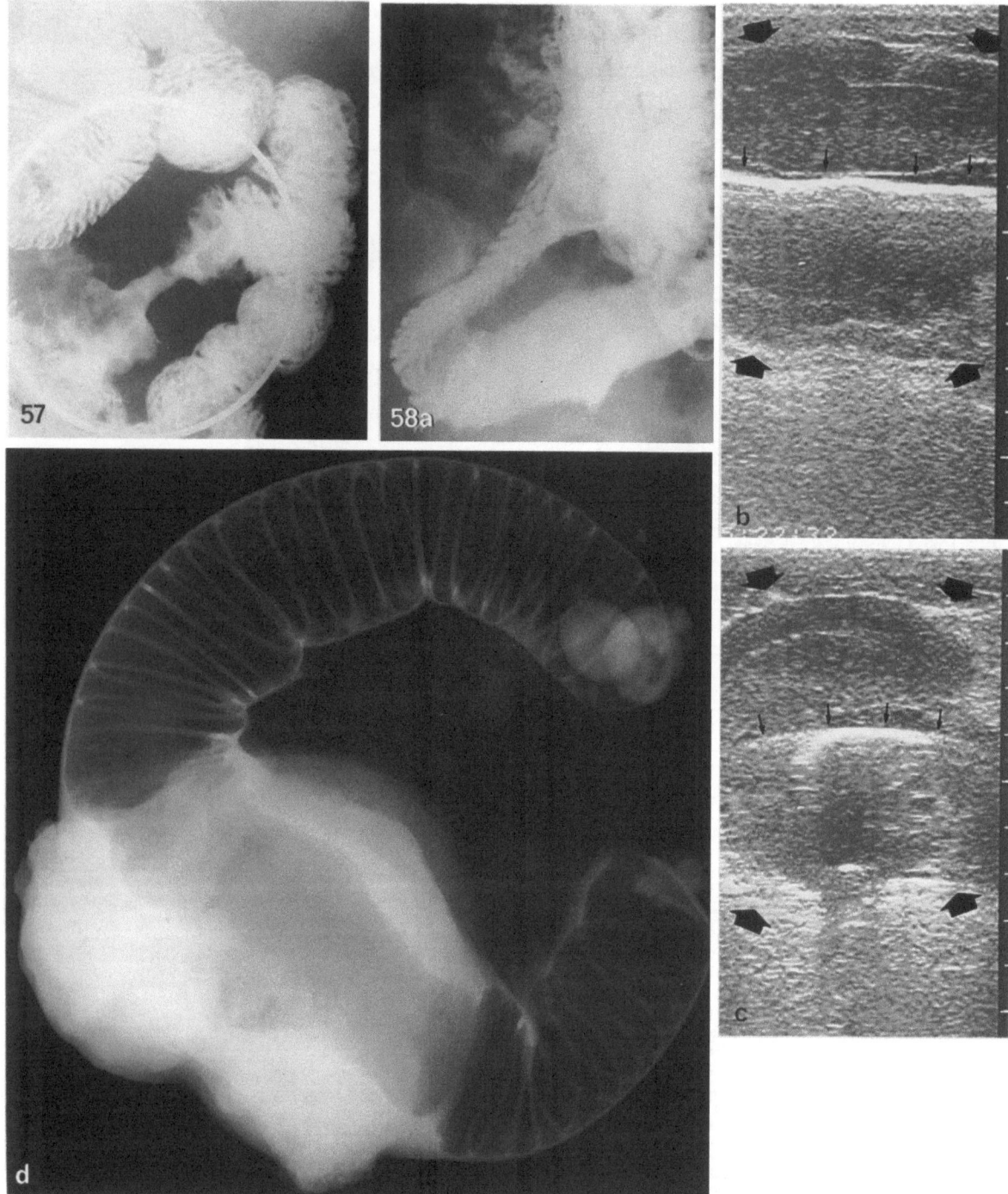

Fig. 57. Lymphoma. 55-year-old man. Postprandial pain and weight loss. SBFT : short stenosis of the second jejunal loop

Fig. 58 a-d. Lymphoma. 15-year-old boy. Abdominal pain. **a** SBFT : segmental ectasia of a pelvic loop with inferior marginal ulceration. **b** longitudinal and **c** transverse ultrasound sections : tumoral mass centered on the intestinal lumen, **d** radiograph of the surgical specimen

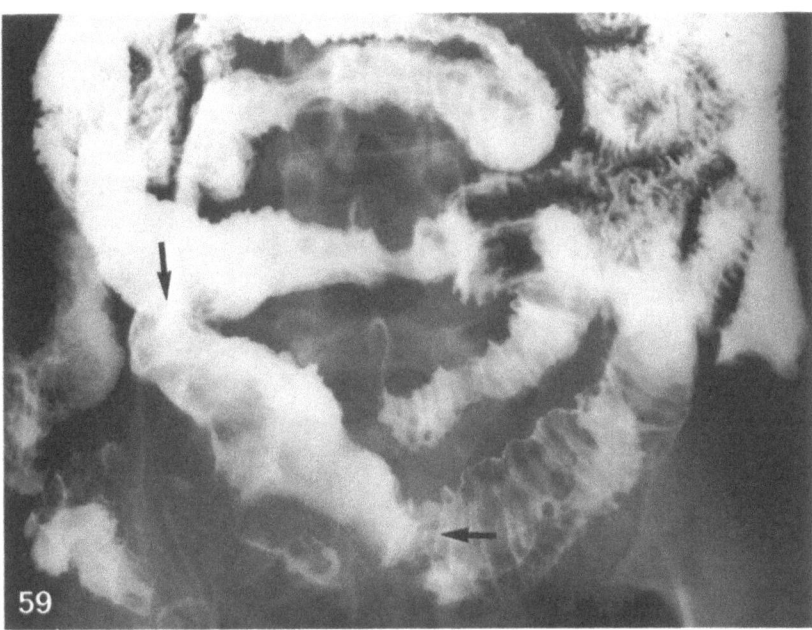

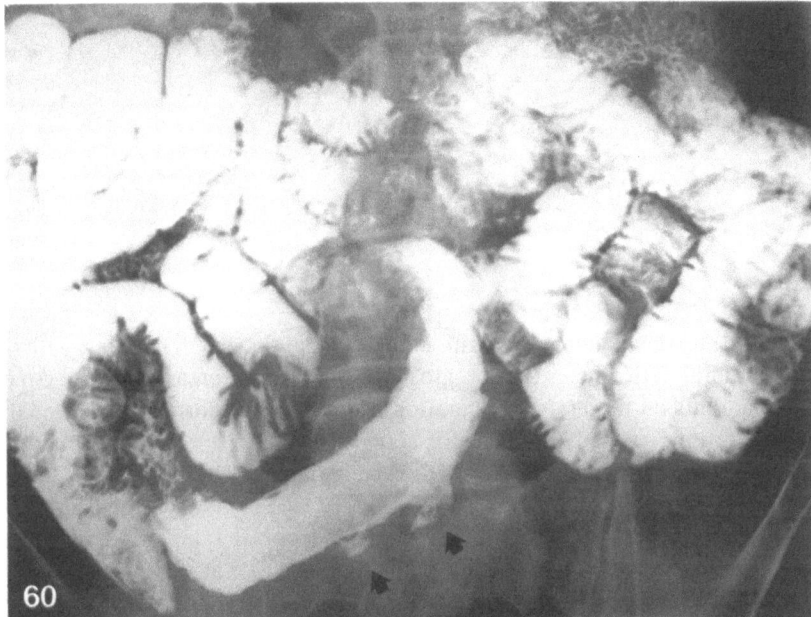

Fig. 59. Lymphoma. 32-year-old man. Abdominal pain. SBFT : segmental ectasia of an ileal loop with excavated margins

Fig. 60. Lymphoma. 66-year-old man with fever and diarrhea. SBFT : segmental ectasia of an ileal loop with excavated margins, with two inferior marginal ulcerations

giene. It may be triggered by repeated microbial and parasitic infections and is frequently associated with giardiasis.

Pathology

From a macroscopic point of view, the lesions dominate in the duodenum and the jejunum, which have thickened walls with nodular folds. There is usually no ulceration. The villi may be broadened, flattened or even atrophied. Adenopathy is usually observed regardless of the stage. Microscopic studies show massive lymphoplasmocytic infiltration of the intestinal wall. Edema caused by malabsorption with hypoalbuminemia contributes to thickening of the walls.

Clinical findings

Alpha-chain disease affects both sexes equally, at any age but mainly between ages 20 and 40. It manifests as signs of malabsorption including diar-

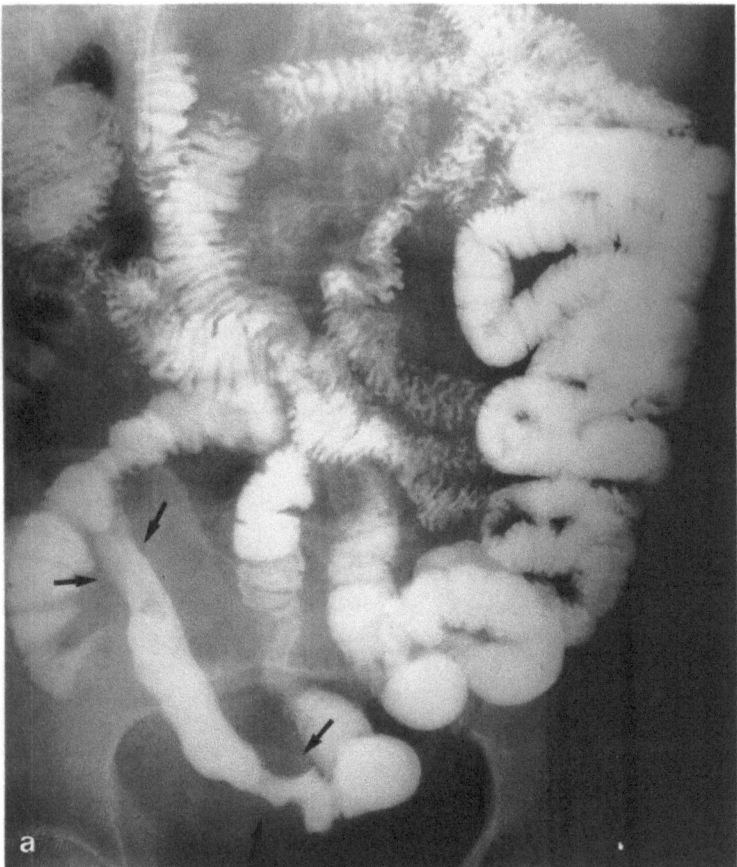

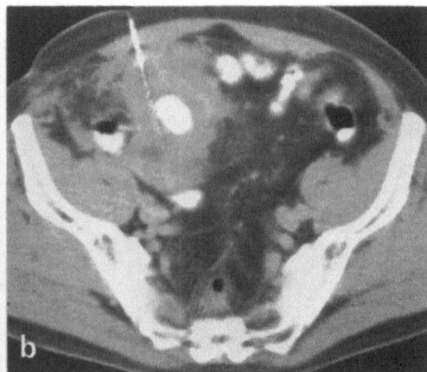

Fig. 61 a, b. Lymphoma (Courtesy of M Breta-golle). 50-year-old man with abdominal pain and low-grade fever. **a** SBFT : stiff, fixed terminal ileal loop with widened interloop gap and disappearance of the folds, **b** computed tomography : thickened intestinal walls. Cytologic aspirate : Burkitt's lymphoma

rhea, steatorrhea, abdominal pain, signs of vitamin and mineral deficiencies (pallor, glossitis, hair loss, edema, clubbed fingers) and alteration of the general condition. At the lymphomatous stage, an abdominal mass is sometimes palpated. Death occurs within 5 years.

The laboratory studies show anemia, leucocytosis and decreased serum calcium. Immunoelectrophoresis is the major means of diagnosis since it demonstrates a pathological protein made up of a heavy alpha chain without a light chain. This protein is found in blood, urine and digestive secretions.

Radiological findings

The barium study shows diffuse enteropathy principally in the duodenum and jejunum. Early on, it combines signs of malabsorption, and abnormalities of the wall and the mucosa. If present, signs of malabsorption are not specific, causing dilution, flocculation and segmentation of the contrast medium. An increase in the interloop gap and in the curvature of the loops can be observed. The folds are broade-

ned, nodular, with clear margins and a normal or decreased height. An evocative sign is the mucosal abnormality, caused by partial villous atrophy forming a very thin reticulation with micronodulation in the luminal space and microspiculation of the margins. Nodulations are sometimes larger and caused by lymphoid hyperplasia. Adenopathy is rarely visible at this stage.

The abnormalities observed initially are still present at the stage of lymphoid degeneration. Peristalsis decreases and signs of segmental infiltration of the walls with a decreased caliber and tapering folds are noted. The image of concentrically ulcerated nodules can be seen. Duodenal infiltration, a rare sign in MNHL, is observed in 30% of all cases and suggests the disease. Adenopathy is sometimes visible as an extrinsic compression, especially in the duodenum, simulating swelling of the pancreas.

Differential diagnosis mainly deals with severe intestinal infections and with Whipple's disease at the first stage and with the other forms of lymphoma at the second stage. The association of duodenal infiltration, of nodular jejunal folds and of an abnor-

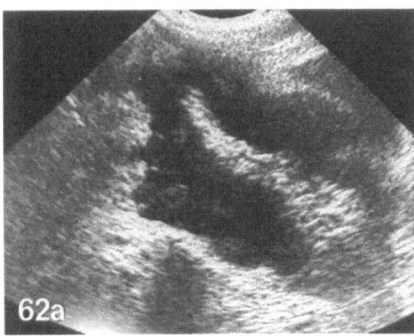

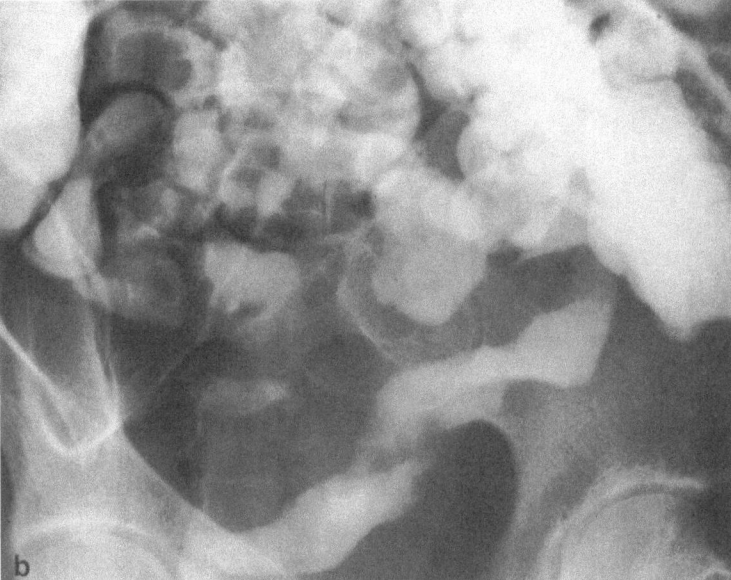

Fig. 62 a,b . Lymphoma. 28-year-old man. Pelvic mass. **a** ultrasound tumoral thickening of an ileal loop with ectasia of the lumen, **b** SBFT : ileal lymphoma of the aneurysmal form

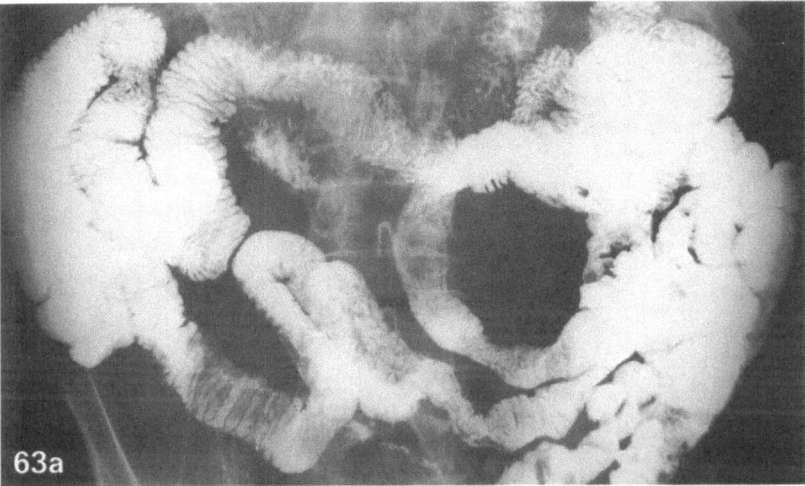

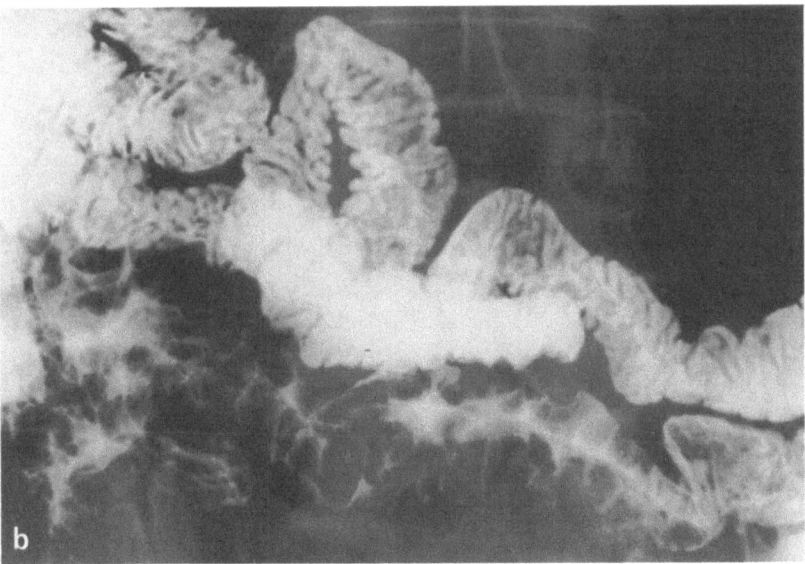

Fig. 63 a, b. Lymphoma. 74-year-old man. Diarrhea. Diffuse duodenal and colonic lymphoma. SBFT : **a** image of extrinsic compression of the jejunal loops, **b** nodulation in the terminal ileum made up of elements of various sizes

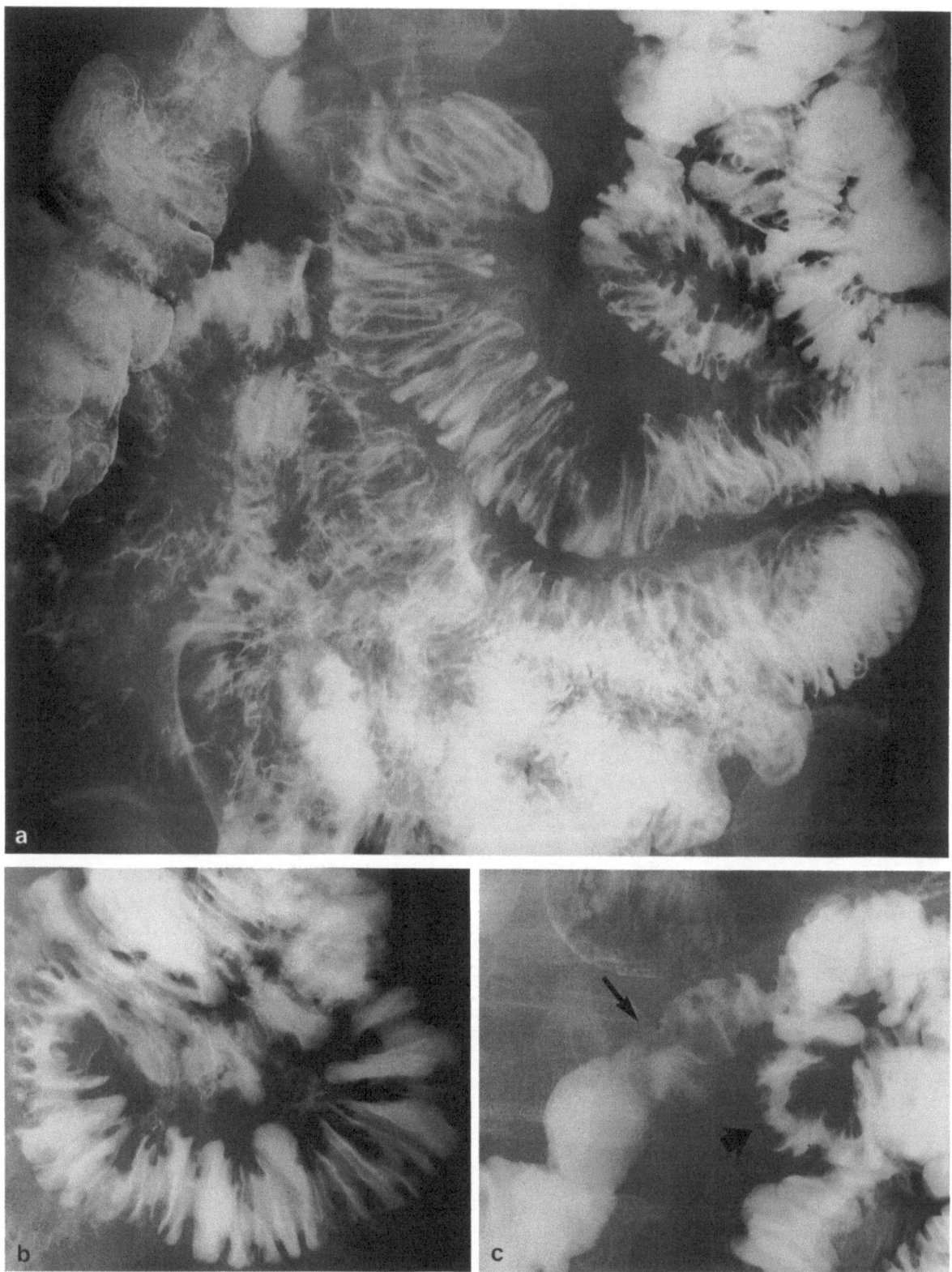

Fig. 64 a-c. Lymphoma. 59-year-old man. Diarrhea and and colicky pains. Fever and deterioration of general health. SBFT : **a** diffuse alterations of the small intestine with broadened, nodulated folds, **b** circular arrangement of a jejunal loop suggesting a mesentric infiltration, **c** ridge ulceration and stenosis suspicious of as an extrinsic lesion

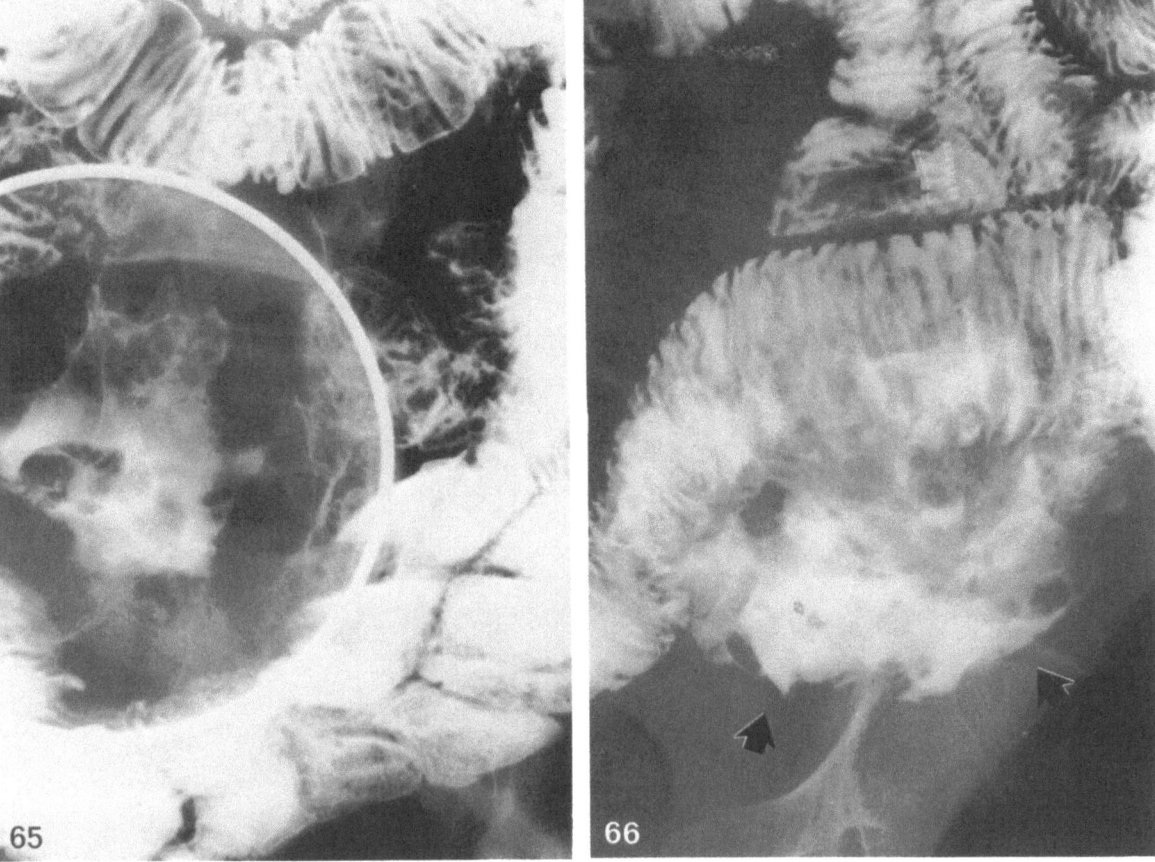

Fig. 65. Lymphoma. 24-year-old man. Hematochezia and abdominal pain. SBFT : pool image with irregular margins, apparently isolated, due to perforation of a jejunal lymphoma

Fig. 66. Lymphoma. 72-year-old woman with anemia, fever, and melena. SBFT : heterogeneous pool image with creviced contours due to central necrosis in a tumour originating in a jejunal loop

mal villous pattern should make the radiologist suspect the diagnosis of Mediterranean lymphoma.

Leukemia, Waldenström's disease, plasmacytoma (figs. 74 and 75)

These diseases are akin to each other and may cause extensive infiltration of the intestinal wall with neoplastic cells.

Intestinal infiltration is found at autopsy in 25 to 50% of the subjects with leukemia, according to the histological type. Acute intraabdominal events (hemorrhage, occlusion, perforation, abscess) are frequent, more so when there are several contributing factors. Besides tumoral infiltration, these may be accounted for by lymph node compression, ische-

mia, secondary infection, concomitant neoplasm or complications of treatment.

Richter's syndrome is the additional development of a malignant non-Hodgkin's lymphoma as observed in 5% of cases of chronic lymphocytic leukemia. Isolated involvement of the small intestine is extremely rare, since the lymphoma is generalized.

Waldenström's macroglobulinemia is characterized by a monoclonal IgM serum peak and causes hepatosplenomegaly, adenopathy and signs of blood hyperviscosity. It may lead to various complications, including lymphoplasmocytic infiltration of the digestive tract. Waldenström's disease affects mainly men over 40.

Multiple myeloma causes a plasmocytic neoplastic infiltration, mainly in bones but also in other tissues, including the digestive organs. An isolated

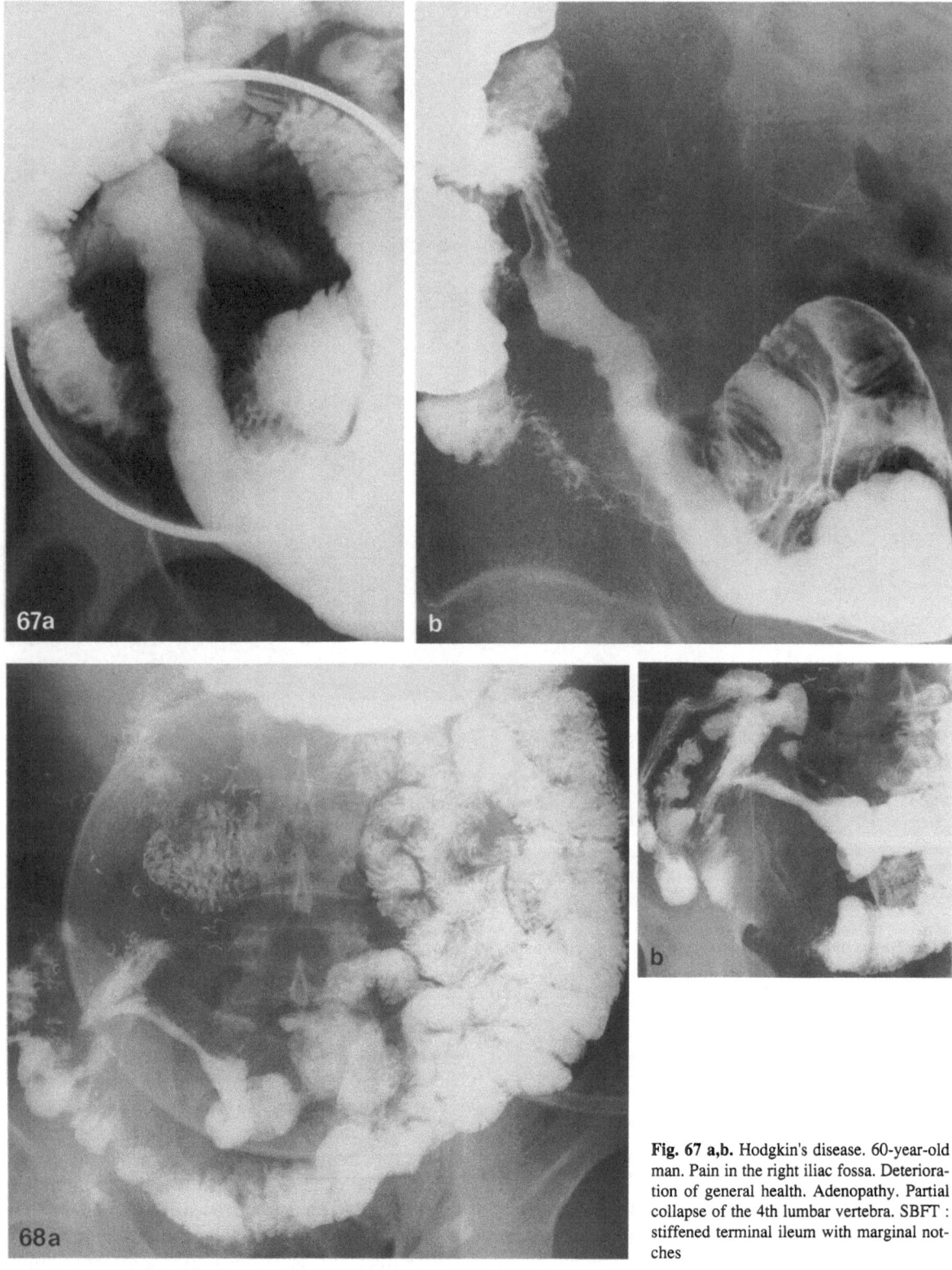

Fig. 67 a,b. Hodgkin's disease. 60-year-old man. Pain in the right iliac fossa. Deterioration of general health. Adenopathy. Partial collapse of the 4th lumbar vertebra. SBFT : stiffened terminal ileum with marginal notches

Fig. 68 a,b . Hodgkin's disease 20-year-old man treated for Hodgkin's disease by abdominal radiation therapy 20 years earlier. Right iliac mass. SBFT : fixed, stenosed ileal loop opposite an extrinsic compression

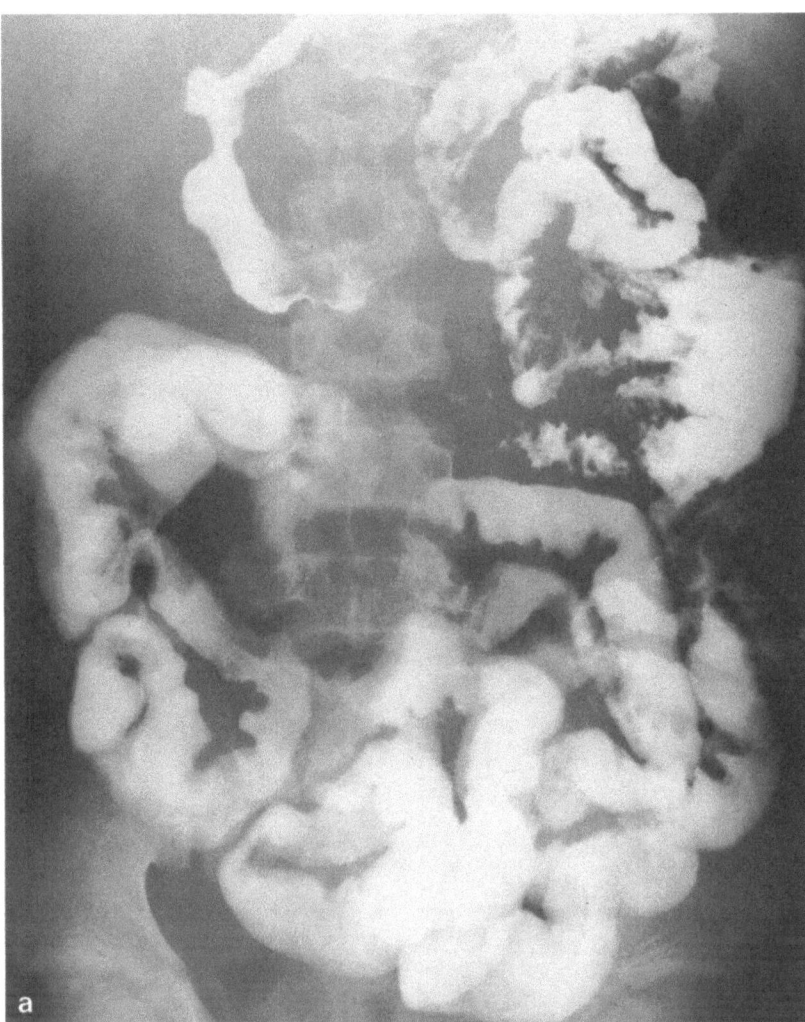

Fig. 69 a-c. Alpha chain disease. 20-year-old man. Steatorrhea not cured by a gluten-free diet. Poor general condition. Malabsorption. SBFT : **a, b** stifferring of the intestinal wall and disappearance of the duodenal folds, dilution of contrast medium and diffuse jejunoileal alteration with thickened walls and disappearing folds (total villous atrophy), **c** one year later. ulcerated nodule of the third stage of the duodenum

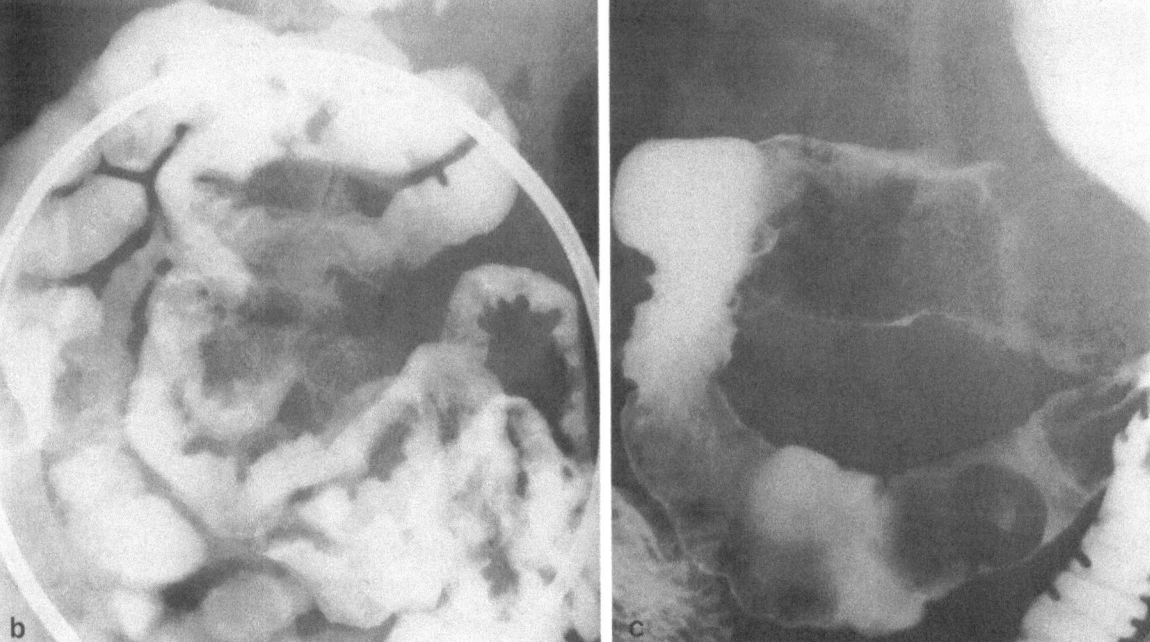

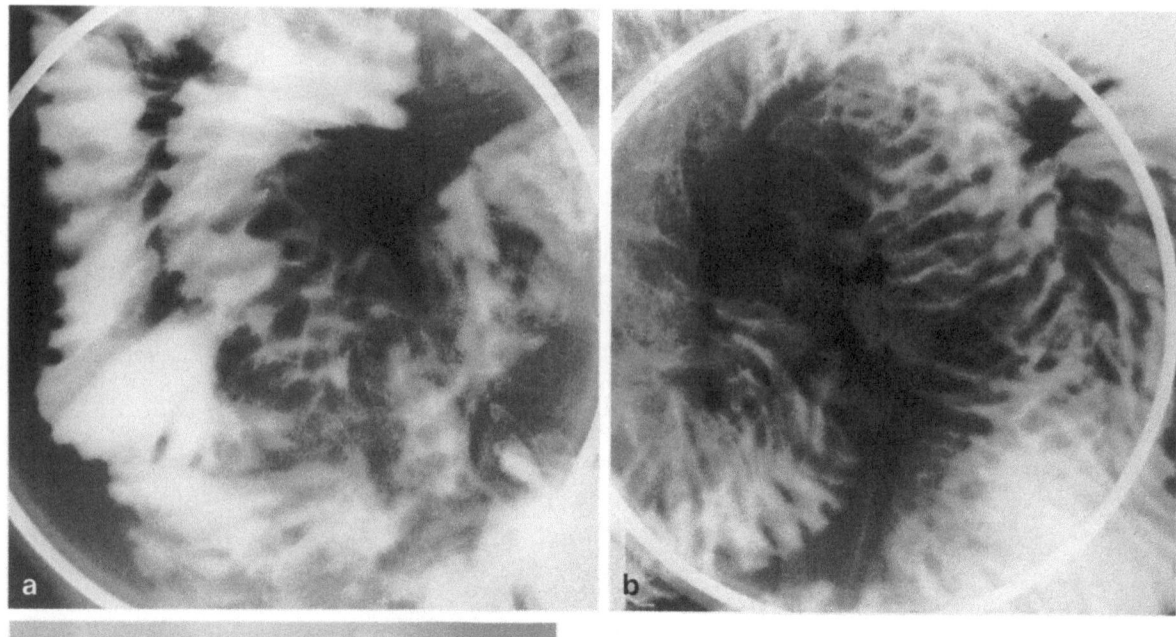

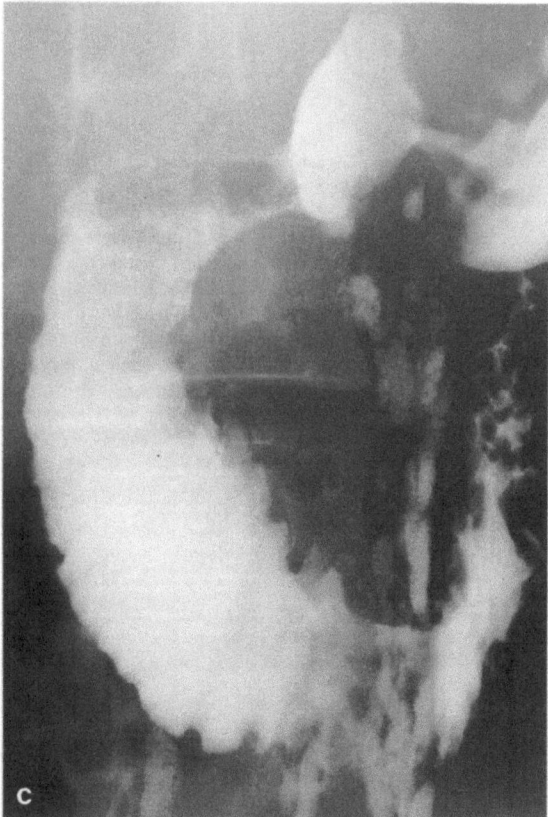

Fig. 70 a-c. Alpha chain disease. 26-year-old man. Chronic diarrhea. Poor general condition and abdominal pain. SBFT : a irregular, nodular folds in the jejunum and the ileum, b punctated appearance of the wall (partial villous atrophy), c broadened, flattened duodenal folds with microspiculation

digestive plasmacytoma is very rare. The characteristic findings which usually present in the peripheral smear are then absent. The prognosis depends on whether the tumor is localized or not.

In these diseases, the small bowel follow-through often shows extensive or multiple lesions.

Infiltration of the wall may be observed, resulting in rigid loops with thickened walls. Nodula-

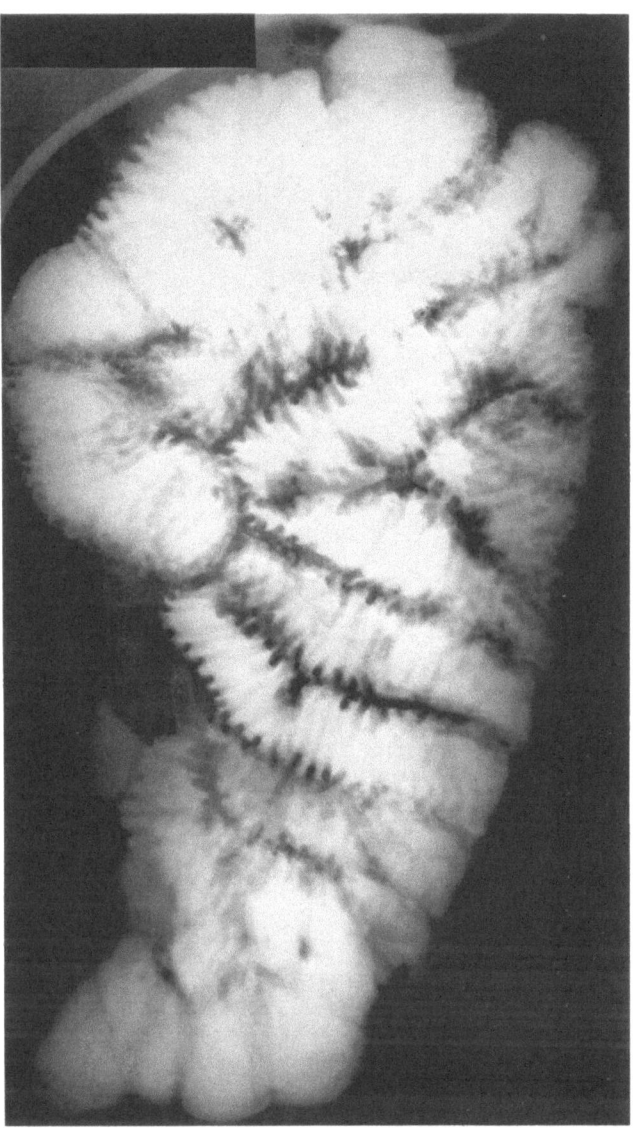

Fig. 71. Alpha chain disease. 40-year-old woman. Diarrhea and malabsoption. The abdominal ultrasound study showed mesenteric adenopathy. SBFT : Mild dilution, mild dilatation of the jejunal loops, widening of the interloop and interfold distances

tions are made up either of elements with a one to several centimeters diameter, or of micronodulation due to the broadened villi, or to the enlarged lymphatics. This appearance is particularly visible in Waldenström's macroglobulinemia.

The appearance may be that of a malignant tumor, the mass lesions may cause intussusception or occlusion. Ulceration is rare.

Signs of malabsorption, of compression by lymph nodes, or of segmental ischemia can be demonstrated, as can pneumatosis cystoides intestinalis.

Sarcoma (other than hematosarcoma) (figs. 76 to 79)

Primary sarcoma makes up 10% of the malignant tumors of the small intestine.

Pathology

Sarcomas can be found throughout the small bowel. The most frequent form is a densely vascularized, encapsulated, budding tumor with a necrotic center, sometimes developing in the lumen but most often

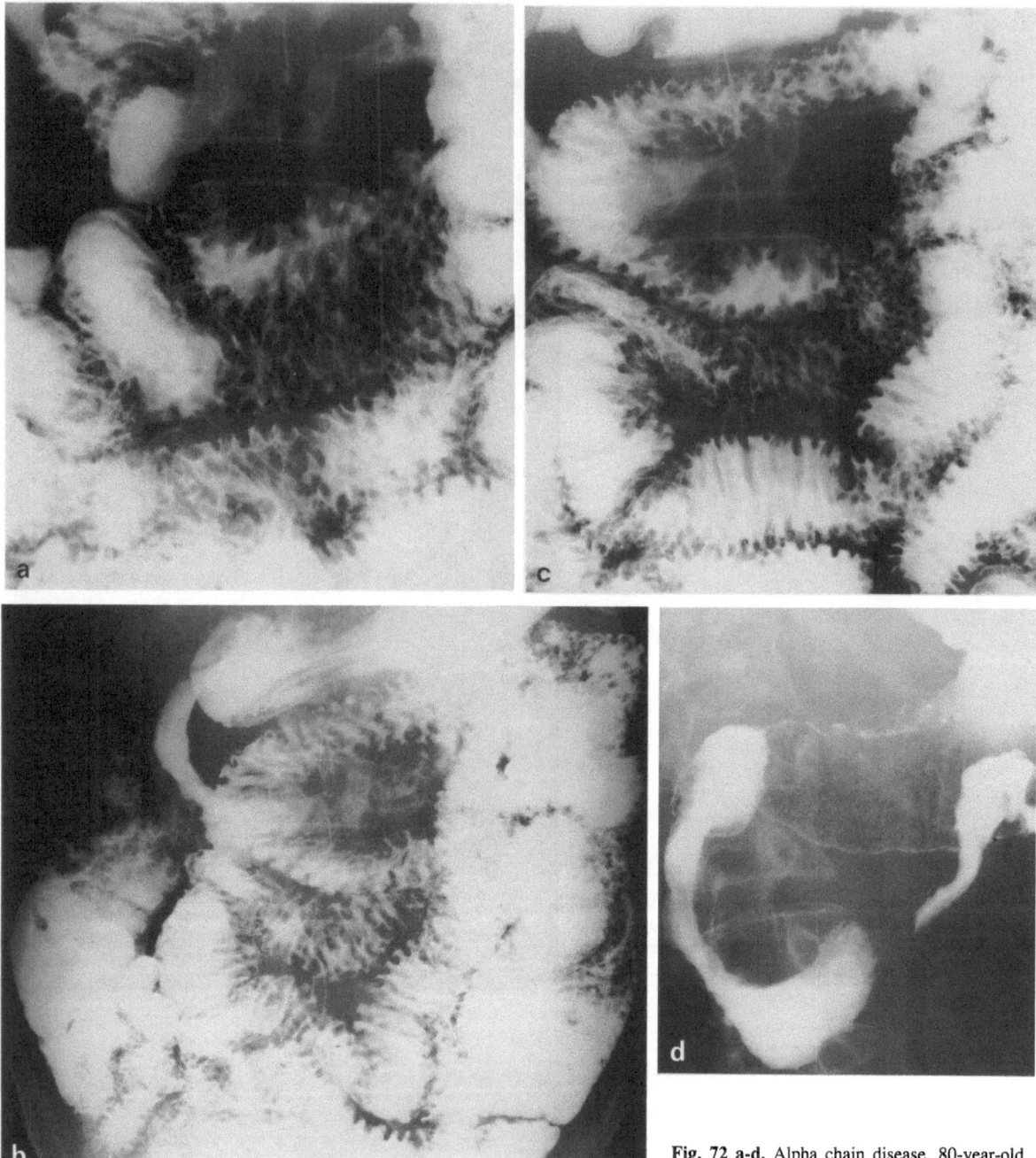

Fig. 72 a-d. Alpha chain disease. 80-year-old. Chronic diarrhea and poor general condition. SBFT: **a, b, c** nodulation and microspiculation of the jejunal folds (partial villous atrophy), **d** disappearance of the duodenal folds and reticulated image of the walls

extending outside the intestine. At diagnosis, the tumor is usually larger than 5 cm in diameter. Kaposi's sarcoma includes multiple, soft, reddish submucosal nodules of variable sizes, which are scattered in the stomach and the intestine and are sometimes ulcerated or umbilicated. This sarcoma seldom appears as an infiltrating and stenosing tumor.

The histological type of Kaposi's sarcoma is angiosarcomatous. The other sarcomas include leiomyosarcomas and sometimes fibrosarcomas, reticulosarcomas, schwannosarcomas or liposarcomas.

Clinical findings

Sarcoma equally affects men and women. It is cha-

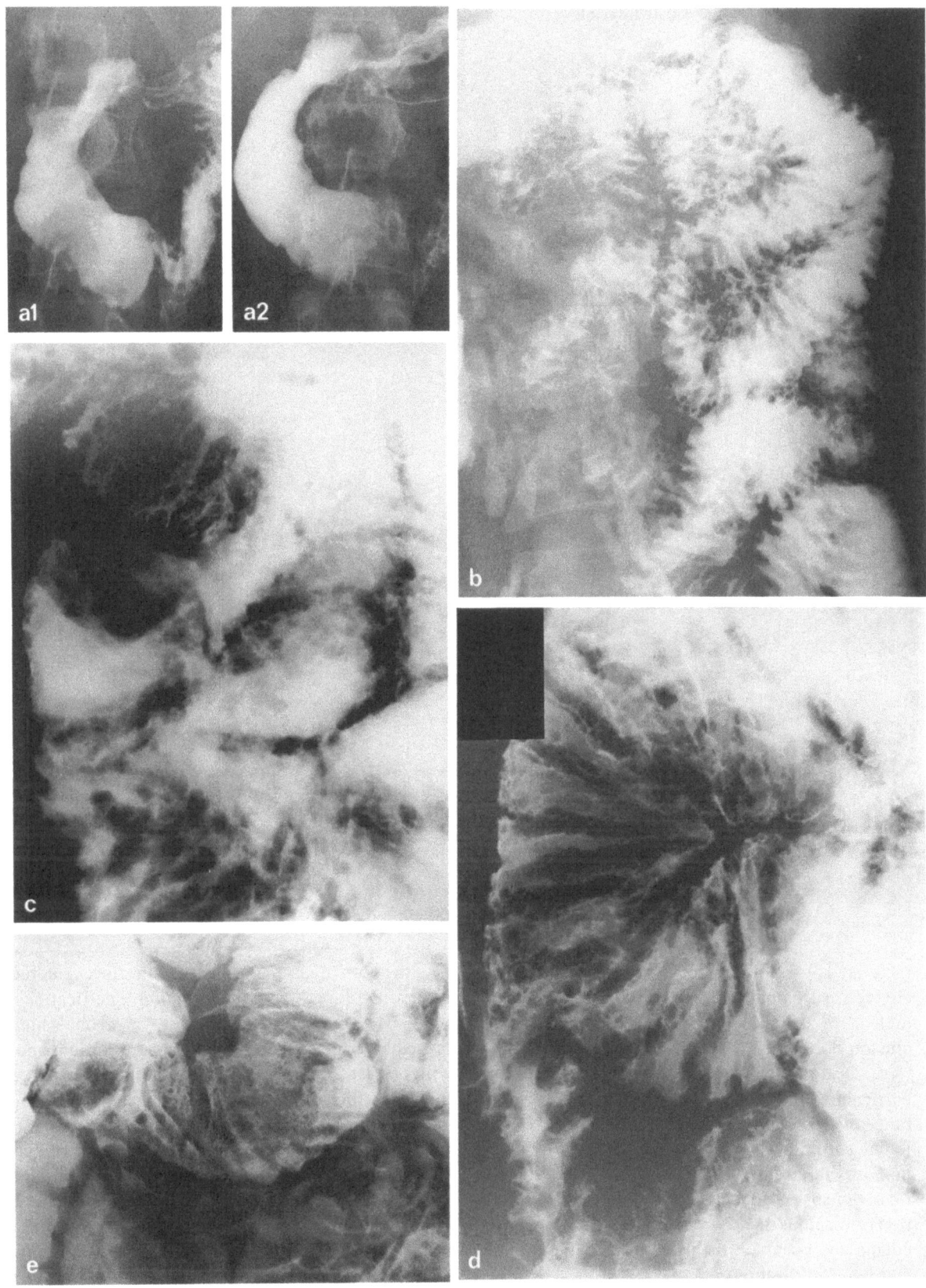

Fig. 73 a-f. Alpha chain disease. 19-year-old woman. Chronic diarrhea and abdominal pain. SBFT : **a** disappearance of the duodenal folds, **b, c, d, e,f** decreased height or nodular appearance of the jejunal folds with microspiculation of the margins and micronodulation in the luminal space (partial villous atrophy)

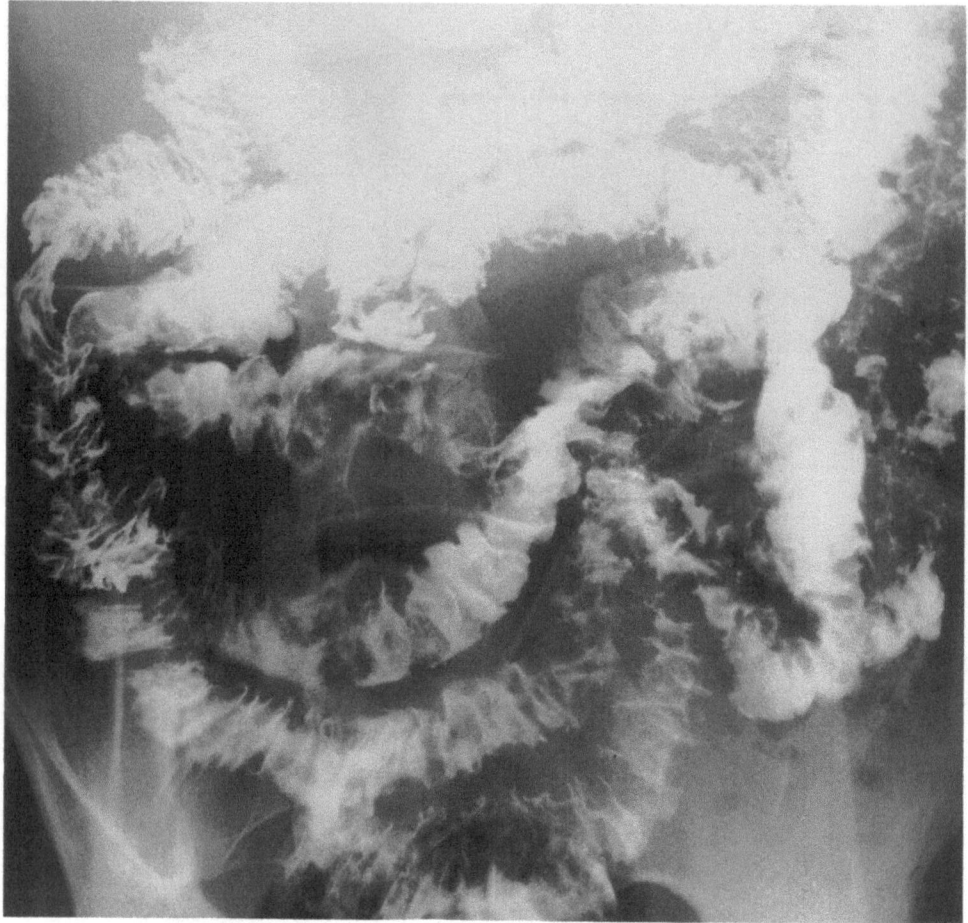

Fig. 74. Lymphoblastic leukemia. 47-year-old man with acute lymphoblastic leukemia. Abdominal pain and diarrhea. SBFT : association of nodules and enlarged nodular folds in the jejunum

racterized by its long clinical latency and is often discovered as a palpable mass during the assessment of melena, or abdominal pain. Signs of chronic subocclusion occur later. Survival at 5 years is 50%.

The clinical signs of Kaposi's sarcoma are particular. This sarcoma was rare before the appearance of AIDS and represents a frequent and rapidly lethal evolution of the disease, especially in the homosexual group (1/3 of all cases). The digestive involvement is often preceded by a cutaneous eruption (violacious macules or papules) associated with edema and occurs at the same time as lymph node and bone infiltration.

Radiological findings
Plain radiographs can demonstrate an opacity displa-

cing the normal gas pattern of the intestine, centered on an irregular gas pool or containing calcifications.

The ectatic form is the most typical one which presents as a heterogeneous, often large barium pool with creviced contours, either along the course of a loop to which it is abruptly connected or in the middle of an empty space, displacing the neighbouring loops suggesting a mass with a necrotic center. Usually, no intestinal dilatation is observed proximally. The diagnosis of malignancy is likely but it is not always possible to differentiate a sarcoma from the aneurysmal form of a lymphoma, from some metastases, from the invasion of the small intestine by neighbouring tumors or even from benign mesenchymal tumors.

In Kaposi's sarcoma, the most frequent findings are multiple submucosal nodules, sometimes

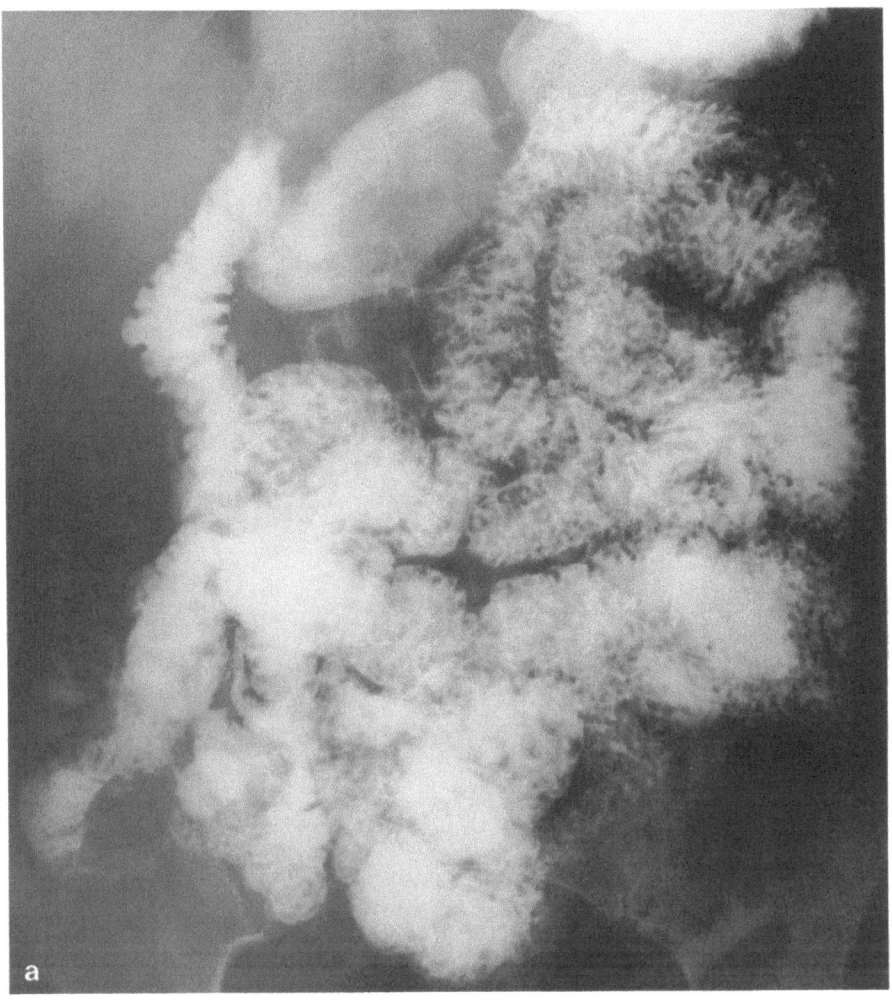

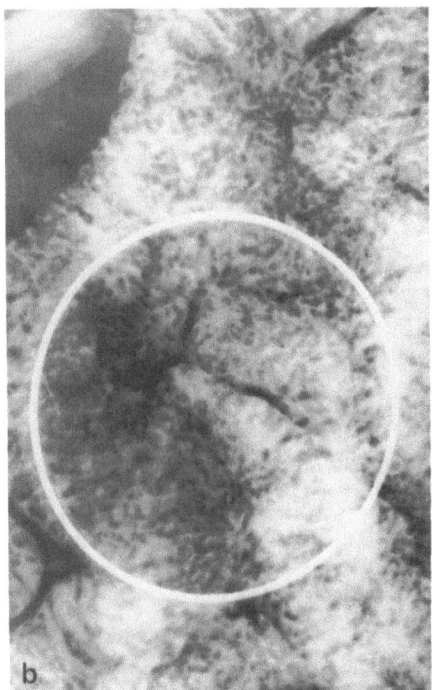

Fig. 75 a,b. Waldenström's disease. 50-year-old man. Pain, colic, meteorism, and diarrhea. SBFT : diffuse micronodulation predominantly in the jejunum

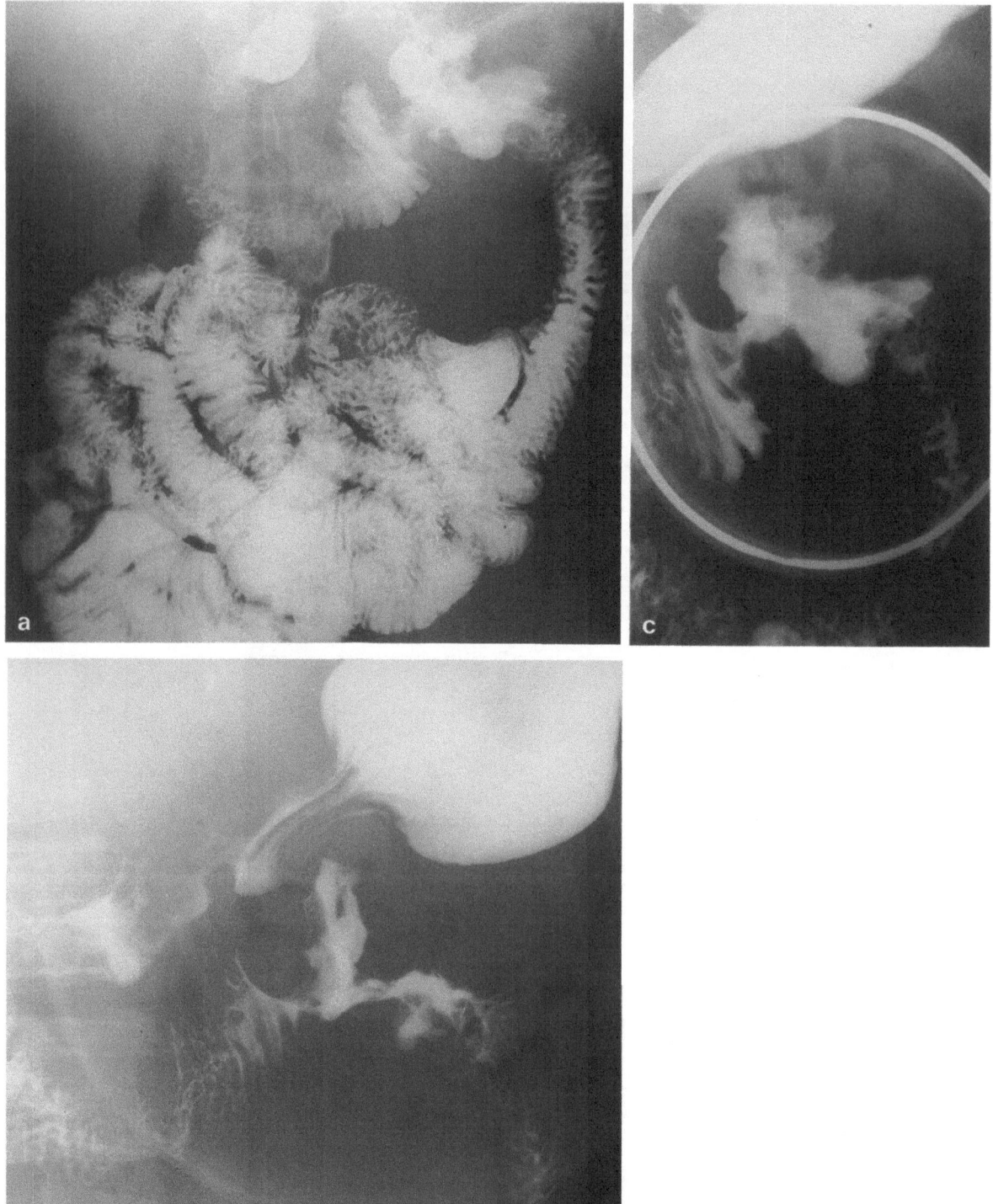

Fig. 76 a, c. Leiomyosarcoma. 33-year-old man. Melena and degradation of general condition. SBFT : 6 cm barium pool with irregular margins, located at the level of the ligament of Treitz and displacing jejunal loops markedly, thus demonstrating the size of the tumour

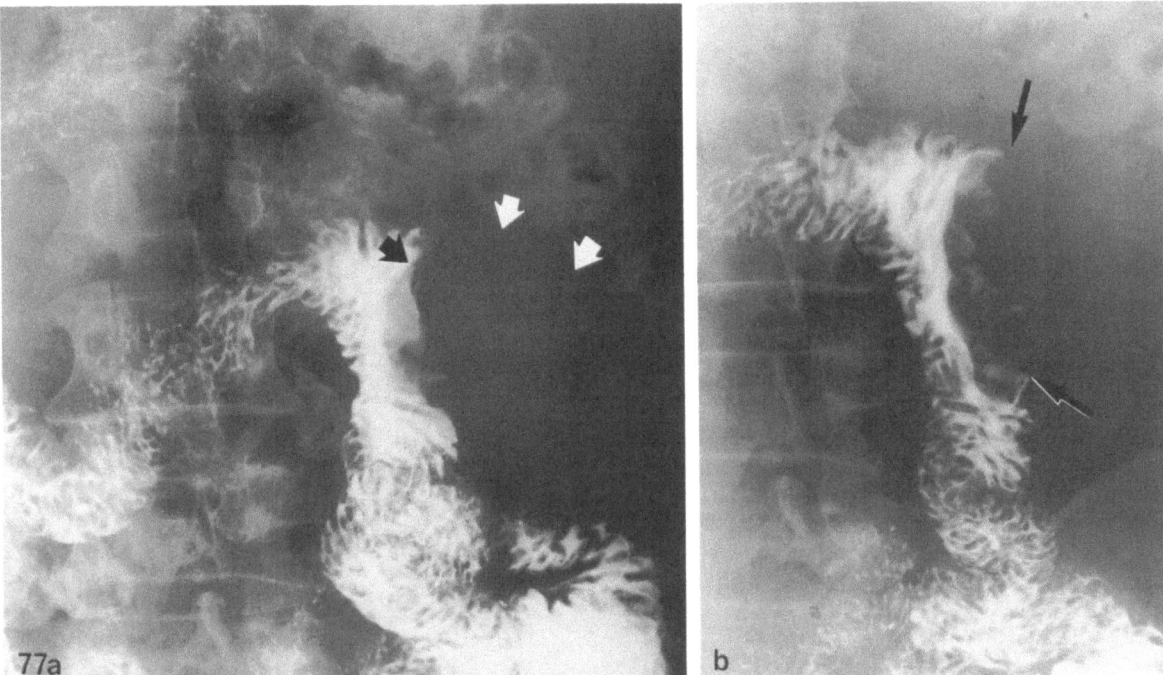

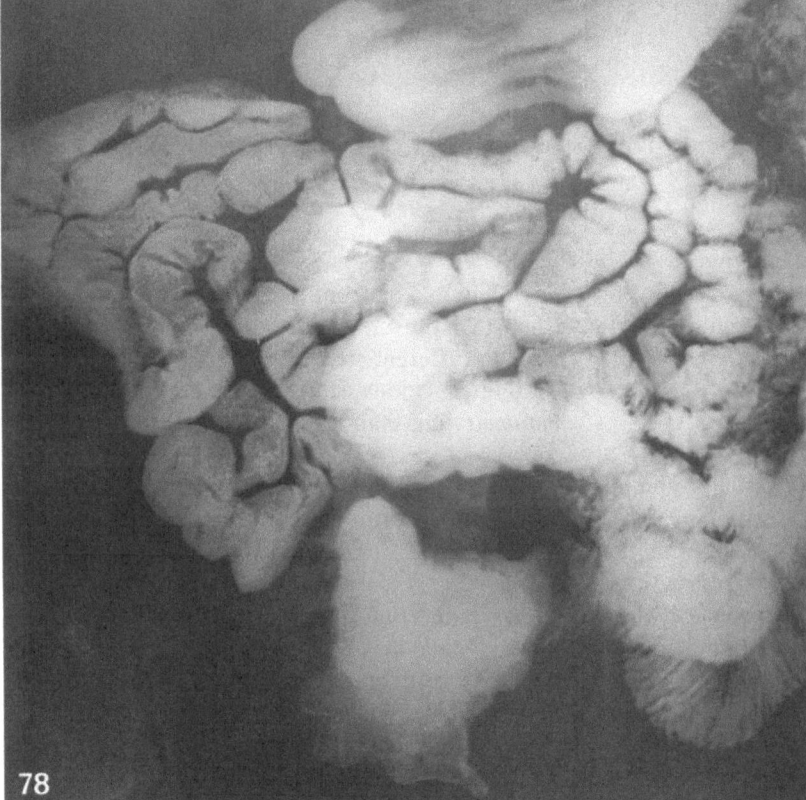

Fig. 77 a, b. Leimyosarcoma. 40-year-old man. Iron deficiency anemia. SBFT: **a, b** 6 cm marginal notch of the first jejunal loop with slightly lobulated contours, separated from the colon by an opacity representing the tumour mass

Fig. 78. Leimyosarcoma. 68-year-old man. Digestive symptoms, apparently of functional origin. SBFT : 6 cm, roughly triangular barium pool in the pelvis with irregular contours and without proximal distention

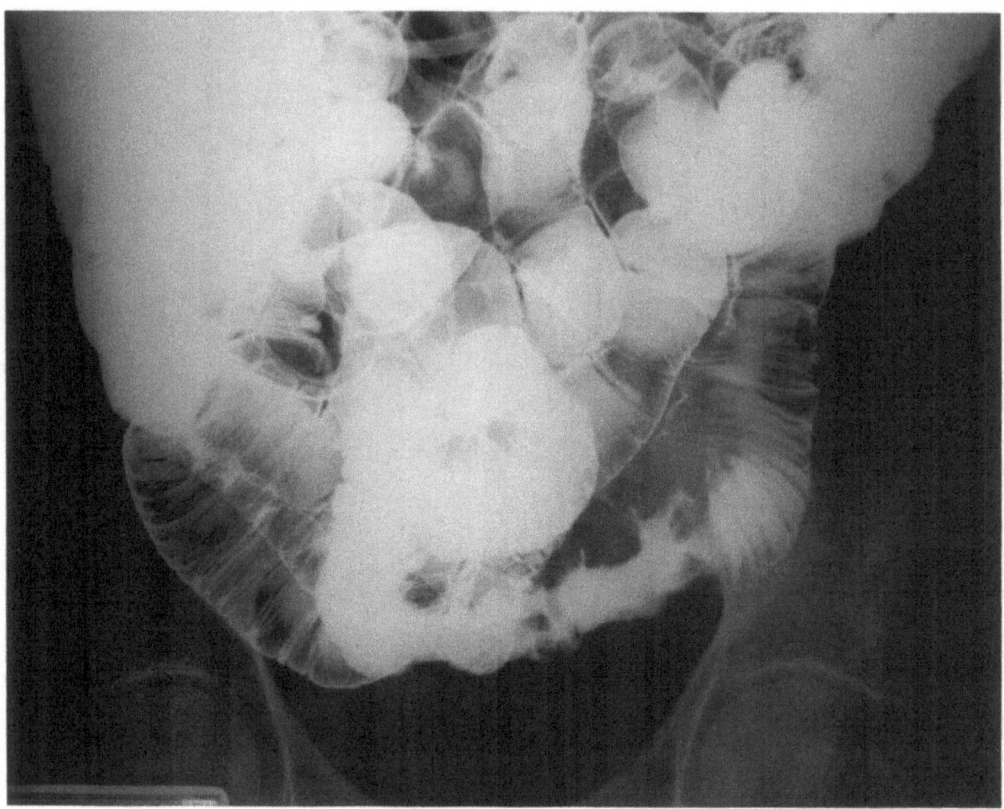

Fig. 79. Leiomyosarcoma (Courtesy of J M Bruel). 41-year-old man. Diarrhea and vomiting. Asthenia, and anemia. SBFT : moderate narrowing with irregular contours and a heterogeneous appearance (nodules and disappearance of the folds) in a pelvic ileal loop, extending over 15 cm with associated moderate proximal dilatation

ulcerated or pedunculated, varying in size from several millimeters to centimeters. Segmental rigidity is less frequent.

Complementary imaging

The complementary modalities (ultrasound, computed tomography, arteriography) are very useful to define the volume, extent and location of the tumours as well as to detect possible metastases. A large tumour may be detected by ultrasound, which demonstrates a hypoechogenic pseudoliquid, lobulated mass surrounded by a more echogenic ring of variable thickness amongst the intestinal loops. Its appearance may be similar to that of some pancreatic pseudocysts.

Arteriography shows a dense tumour blush with a hypovascular center (necrosis) supplied by normal or enlarged blood vessels in which the usual signs of malignancy must be searched for. In fact, malignancy can be demonstrated only if hepatic metastases are found, because it is difficult to distinguish leiomyoma from leiomyosarcoma by arteriography. On the other hand, arteriography sometimes helps to differentiate sarcoma from some forms of small intestinal invasion by neighbouring tumors by demonstrating their vascular pedicles.

Adenocarcinoma (figs. 80 to 84)

Primary small intestinal adenocarcinomas are rare tumours since they make up only 1% of cancers of the digestive tract and less than 25% of malignant tumours of the small intestine. From a macroscopic and histological point of view, it is impossible to differentiate the primary and metastatic forms.

Pathology

Adenocarcinomas are located in the jejunum in 80% of all cases and in half, they are found in the first

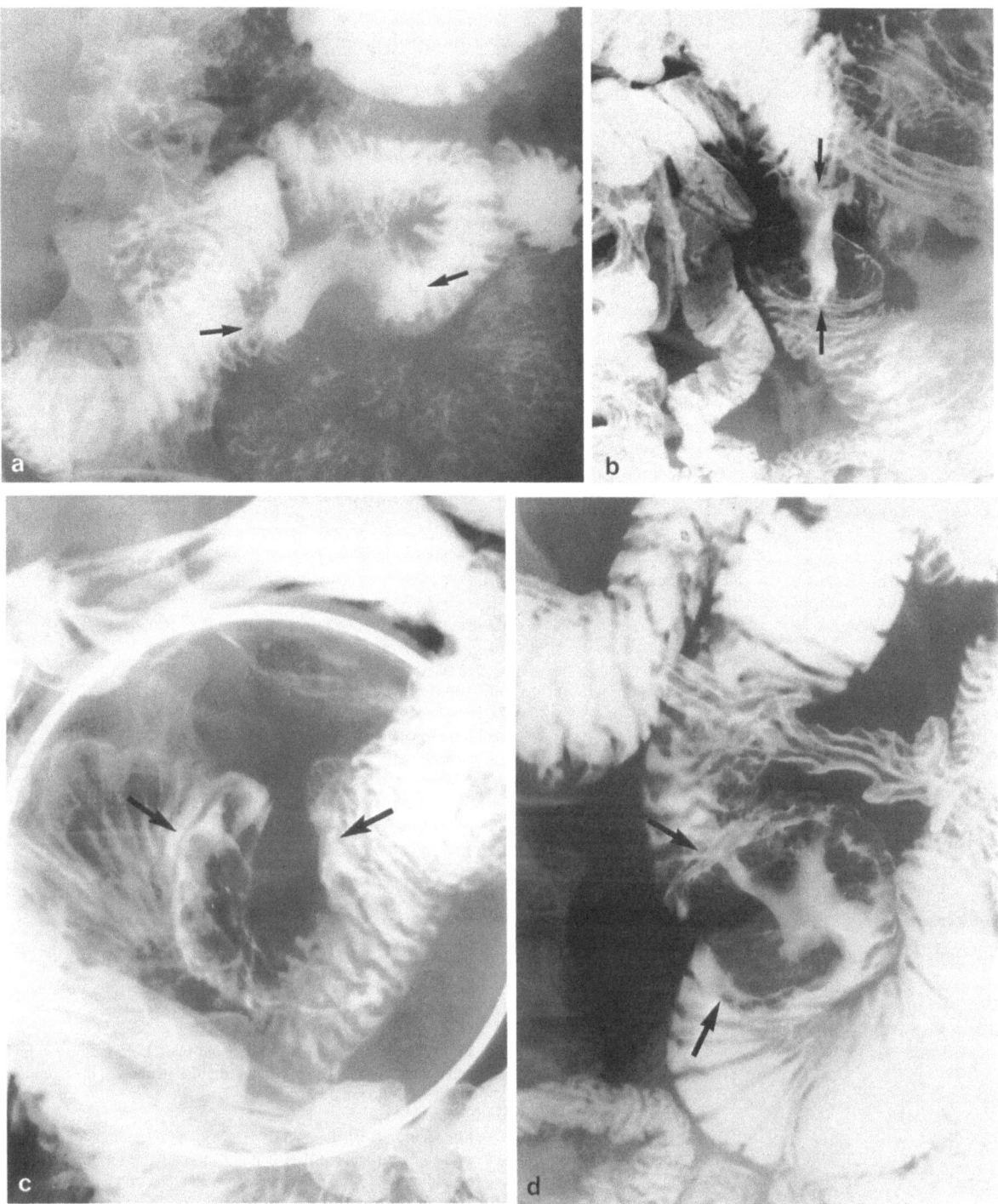

Fig. 80 a-d. Adenocarcinoma. 48-year-old man. Epigastric pain. Anemia and melena. SBFT : tumoral image with an appearance varying with compression : **a** segmental infiltration of the first jejunal loop, **b** stenosis with a short intussusception cuff, **c** nodule with a broad stalk or **d** 4 cm ulcerated nodule

jejunal loop near the ligament of Treitz. When located in the ileum, they often extend to the terminal ileum.

The appearance may be that of a stenosis, or an ulcerated nodule. The neoplasm is usually lieber-

kühnian in origin, sometimes undifferentiated or anaplastic, and exceptionally brünnerian or mucinous. Cancers caused by the degeneration of a villous tumor are exceptional because of its rarity in the

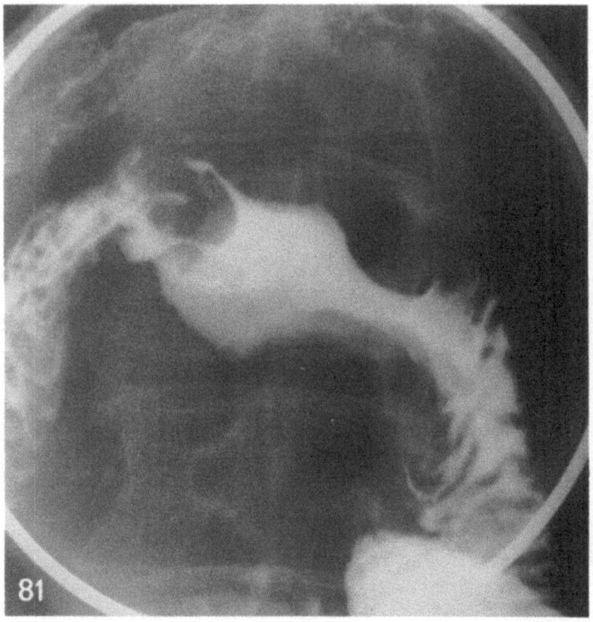

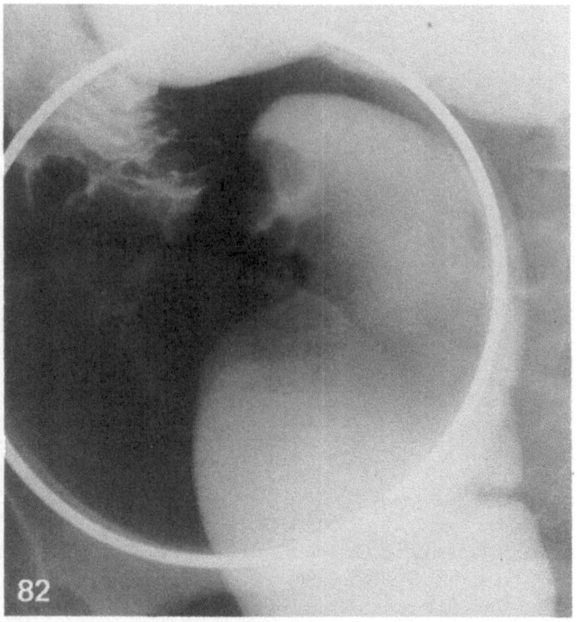

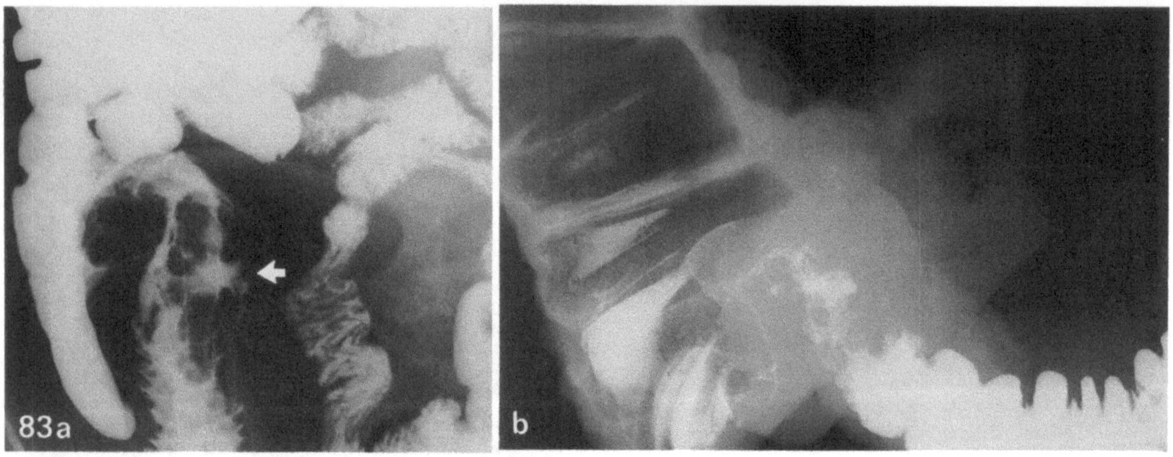

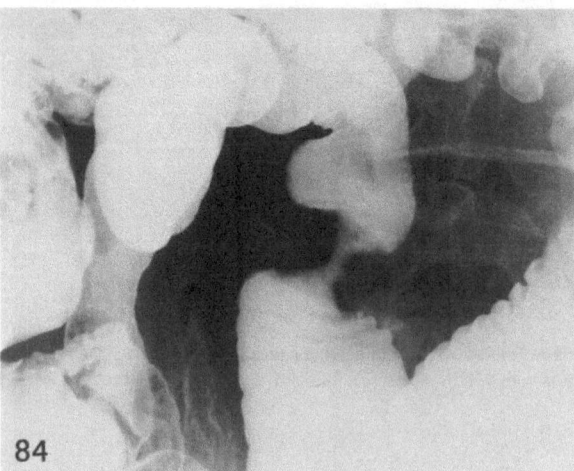

Fig. 81. Adenocarcinoma. 74-year-old man. Anemia. SBFT : stenosis of the first jejunal loop with stiff contours, distal to a nodule at the level of the ligament of Treitz

Fig. 82. Adenocarcinoma. 88-year-old man. Deterioration in his general health. SBFT : 3 cm long irregular stenosis of the terminal ileum with proximal dilatation

Fig. 83 a, b. Adenocarcinoma. 43-year-old man. Abdominal pain and constipation. **a** SBFT : nodulation in the terminal ileum, extending over 5 cm and centered on an ulceration with displacement of the medial margin of the cecum, **b** radiograph of the surgical specimen : ulcerated, budding tumor from the ileal aspect of the ileocecal valve

Fig. 84. Adenocarcinoma. 89-year-old woman. Subocclusion. SBFT: 20 mm long ileal stenosis demarcated at both ends by over hanging edges

small intestine. Celiac disease and Crohn's disease have already been mentioned as predisposing factors for the appearance of a carcinoma.

Clinical findings

Adenocarcinoma is most frequent in men over 50. The clinical signs are nonspecific and include abdominal pain, a poor general condition changes in bowel habits, and anemia. The lesion is often discovered when treating one of its complications (occlusion, hemorrhage, perforation). Survival at 5 years does not exceed 20%.

Radiological findings

Barium studies most often show short stenoses averaging 5 cm but sometimes as long as 10 to 15 cm, usually in the first jejunal loop. The stenotic segment may be centred or excentred, and is often fixed and featureless. Its contours are smooth, irregular or nodular and it is connected abruptly to the segments proximal and distal, sometimes with an incomplete intussusception. Suprastenotic dilatation occurs later on. Displacement of the neighbouring loops and fistulous formation are less frequent than with sarcoma. When located in the terminal ileum, the tumor may simulate Crohn's disease.

Malignant ulceration produces a pool image with excavated contours and a heterogeneous appearance, usually surrounded by a nodular ridge with sharp margins. The involved loop is sometimes fixed and angulated.

Adenocarcinoma rarely forms an isolated nodule which can be ulcerated or intussuscepted.

The diagnosis of malignancy is made on the basis of the barium images, but it is difficult to differentiate adenocarcinoma from lymphoma or metastases.

Complementary imaging

Ultrasound and computed tomography are useful to study the extent of the tumor and detect the presence of adenopathy and hepatic metastases.

Arteriography shows a hypovascular mass, thus permitting to differentiate it from Crohn's disease in doubtful cases. The intratumoral blood vessels are irregular, but no neovascularization is usually present.

Metastases (figs. 85 to 96)

Invasion of the small intestine by a neighbouring tumour and peritoneal carcinomatosis are discussed in the chapter dealing with exointestinal (extrinsic) pathology. The actual frequency of metastases is probably significantly higher that that observed by radiology, since many cases go undetected in the terminal stage of a cancer if no acute complications occur. Incidence figures vary between 16 and 39% of all malignant tumors of the small intestine.

Pathology

The most frequent primary tumor is colonic which with the other sites of origin for adenocarcinomas (stomach, rectum, pancreas, prostate, ovaries) makes up more than 40% of metastases located in the small intestine.

Malignant melanoma produces more than 30% of intestinal metastases, but any mesenchymal tumor (e.g. soft tissue sarcoma) can produce metastases.

Malpighian epitheliomas are rarely encountered, except with cancers of the cervix.

The presence of multiple metastases is a frequent occurrence.

Clinical findings

Patients are often female over 60.

The clinical signs (pain, vomiting, change in bowel habits, alteration of the general condition, anemia, etc.) are frequently followed by acute complications including occlusion and perforation.

The average period of survival is 1 year.

Radiological findings

The radiological appearance of metastases on small bowel follow-through includes all the patterns observed in the tumoral pathology of the small intestine such as those seen in lymphomas, sarcomas, adenocarcinomas, and sometimes even those of benign tumours.

Metastases most often present as a short stenosis without folds, with an abrupt transition proximally and distally, with or without an intussuscepting sleeve. The typical image is seen in metastases from colonic cancer. Tumoral infiltration may produce segmental marginal stiffening with preserved contralateral folds without a true stenosis.

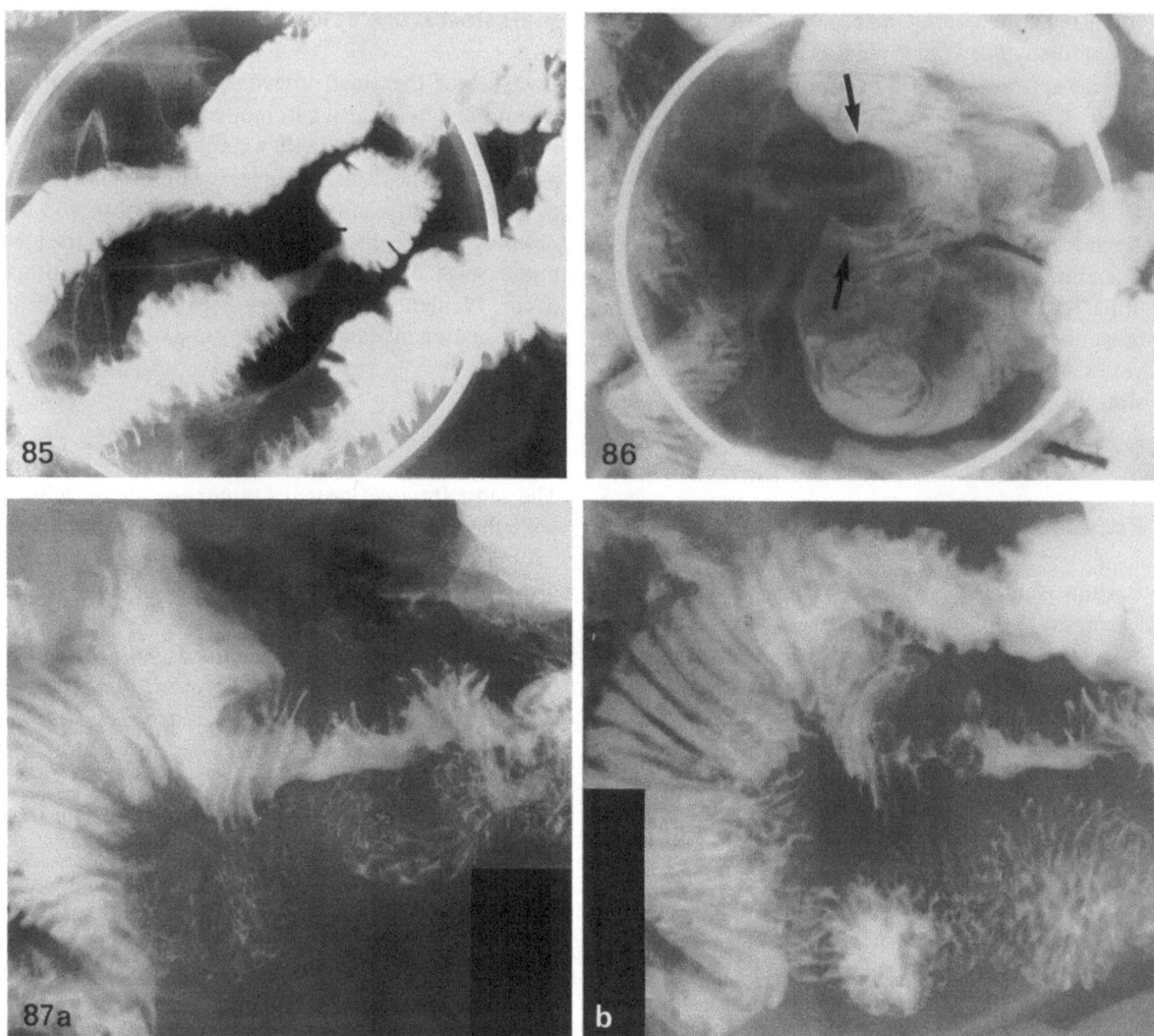

Fig. 85. Metastasis from a sigmoid colon cancer. 64-year-old man. Pain and weight loss. SBFT : 2 cm long tumoral stenosis.

Fig. 86. Metastasis from small bowell leiomyosarcoma. 66-year-old woman. Right ovariectomy and ileal resection for leiomyosarcoma one year earlier. SBFT : 2 cm marginal nodule in a jejunal loop

Fig. 87 a, b. Metastasis from colonic adenocarcinoma. 45-year-old woman. Resection of a cancer of the transverse colon 18 years earlier with complete colectomy for recurrence in the sigmoid colon 17 years later. SBFT : 4 cm long stenosis in the first jejunal loop with lower marginal stiffening partially preserving the folds of the upper margin

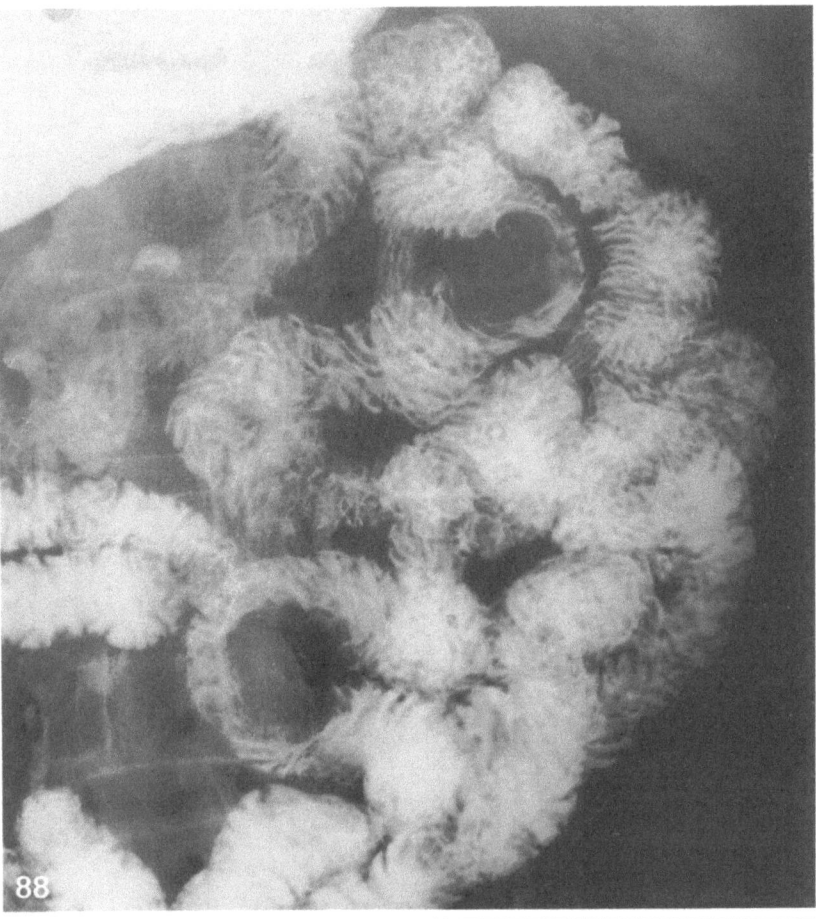

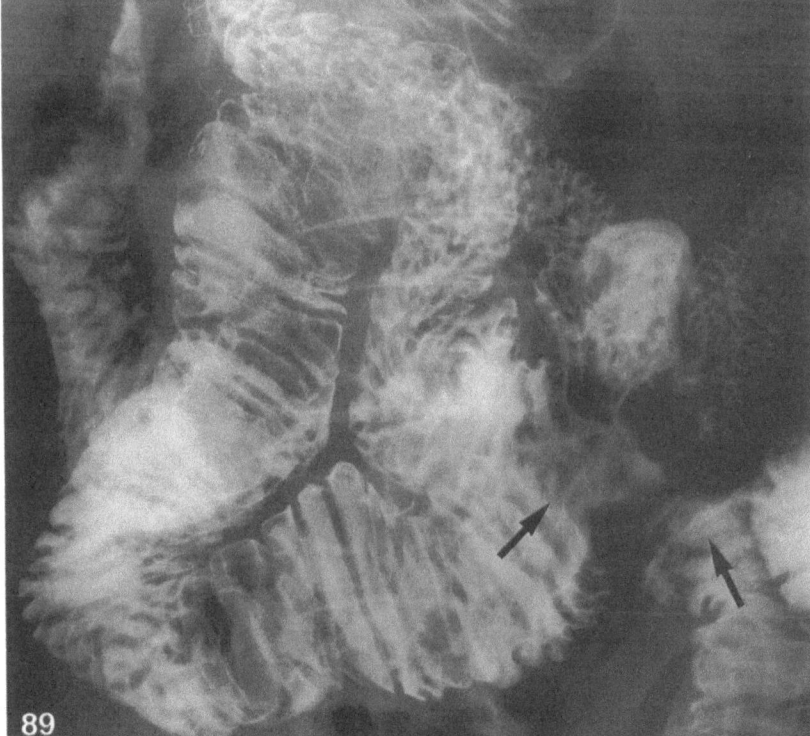

Fig. 88. Metastases from histiocytic sarcoma. 57-year-old man. Radiation therapy and chemotherapy for cervical histiocytic sarcoma two years earlier. Melena. SBFT : jejunal nodulation made up of multiple, round submucosal elements, ranging from a few to 35 mm in diameter (two are visible above)

Fig. 89. Metastasis from gastric adenocarcinoma. 50-year-old man having had a gastrectomy for cancer two years earlier. Subumbilical pain. SBFT : malignant ulceration in the jejunum

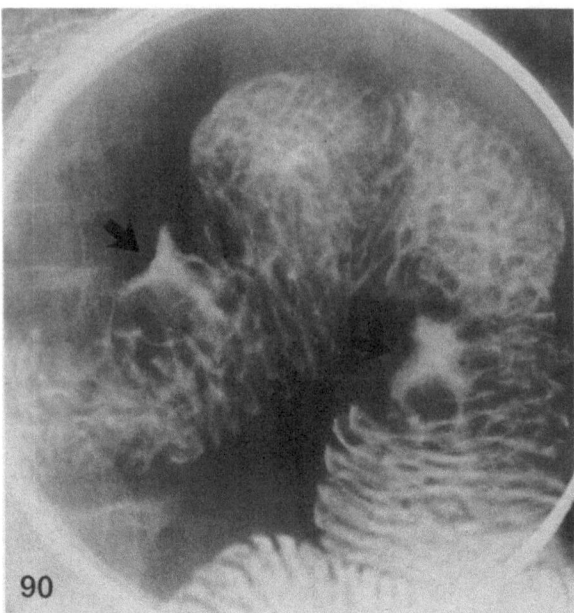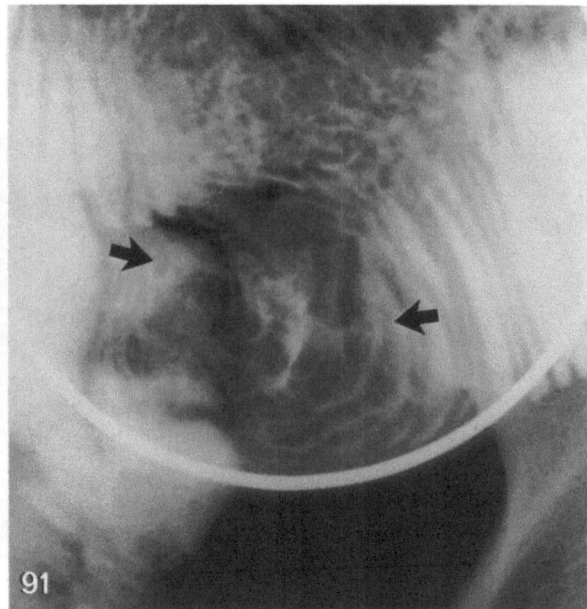

Fig. 90. Metastasis from a digestive adenocarcinoma (Courtesy of P Buffard). 58-year-old man. Subocclusion.SBFT : malignant jejunal ulcerations

Fig. 91. Metastasis from colonic adenocarcinoma. 65-year-old man. Sigmoidectomy for a cancer one year earlier. SBFT : malignant ulceration in the jejunum

Nodules are frequently seen in metastatic disease, especially with melanomas where single, endoluminal or marginal nodules, often multiple and ulcerated, sometimes simulate hereditary polyposis. The flexibility of the neighbouring loops favours intussusception. The round central ulceration produces a concentric image. The ulceration may also be quadrangular and often deep or with a ridge, and is sometimes multiple.

The ectasiating form produces pool images centered on the intestinal lumen or off center, similar to those observed in the aneurysmal form of lymphomas or sarcomas.

Complementary imaging

Ultrasound may show a hypoechogenic thickening of the intestinal wall with anechogenic areas, off center relative to the digestive lumen, as well as an invagination or the dilatation of one or several intestinal loops.

Computed tomography contributes in the assessment of the spread of the tumor.

The tumoral images obtained with arteriography do not show any specific features.

Practical conclusions

Any ileal nodule smaller than 3 mm in diameter must be suspected a priori of being a carcinoid tumour. Humoral assessment and hepatic ultrasound are needed to search for metastases, and surgery is required in the absence of contraindications.

The presence of mesenteric retraction should lead to a search in the neighbouring loops of small intestine for a marginal nodule, which may be a carcinoid tumor, before invoking the diagnosis of peritoneal carcinomatosis.

A segmental marginal infiltration is highly suggestive of the presence of lymphoma.

A segmental ectasia with creviced contours, although characteristic of lymphoma, can also be observed in leiomyosarcoma and metastases.

Diffuse alteration of the jejunal folds associated with duodenal infiltration must lead to a search for a Mediterranean lymphoma.

A stenosing tumor of the first jejunal loop is most often an adenocarcinoma. Stenosing tumours in other sites are most often metastases. Carcinomatous stenosis of the terminal ileum may mimick Crohn's disease.

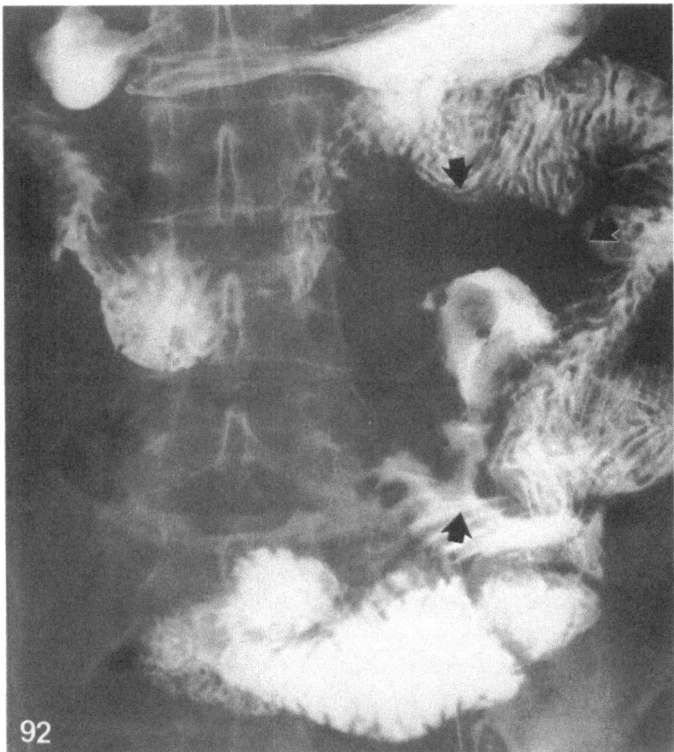

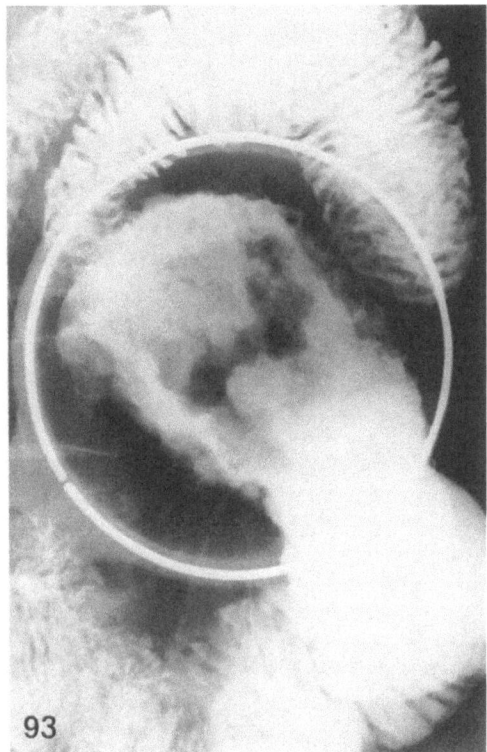

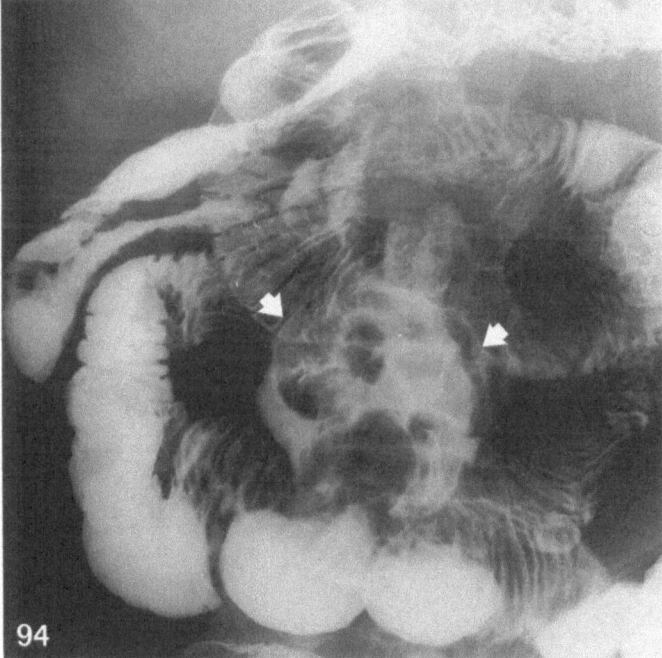

Fig. 92. Metastasis from cancer of the ovary. 70-year-old woman. Ovariectomy 19 years earlier for cancer of the ovary. Subocclusion and worsening of her general health. Anemia. Left abdominal mass. SBFT : Barium pool with irregular contours in the second jejunal loop within a tumor mass

Fig. 93. Metastasis from bronchial cancer. 76-year-old man. Left lung lobectomy for cancer 5 years earlier. Anemia. SBFT : 8 x 10 cm heterogeneous barium pool with irregular contours in a jejunal loop

Fig. 94. Metastasis from colonic adenocarcinoma. 79-year-old man. Right hemicolectomy for cancer 4 years earlier. Pain, diarrhea, deterioration in his general condition, palpable mass. SBFT : heterogeneous barium pool hanging from an ileal loop with lucent area around the lesion

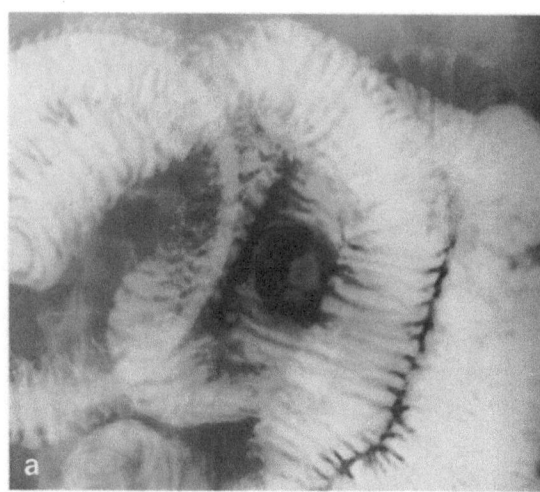

Fig. 95a, b. Metastases from melanoma (Courtesy of CL L'Hermine). 64-year-old woman. Melanoma of the right leg. Chemotherapy. Right inguinal adenopathy. SBFT : concentrically ulcerated nodules with an irregular stenosis of the first jejunal loop

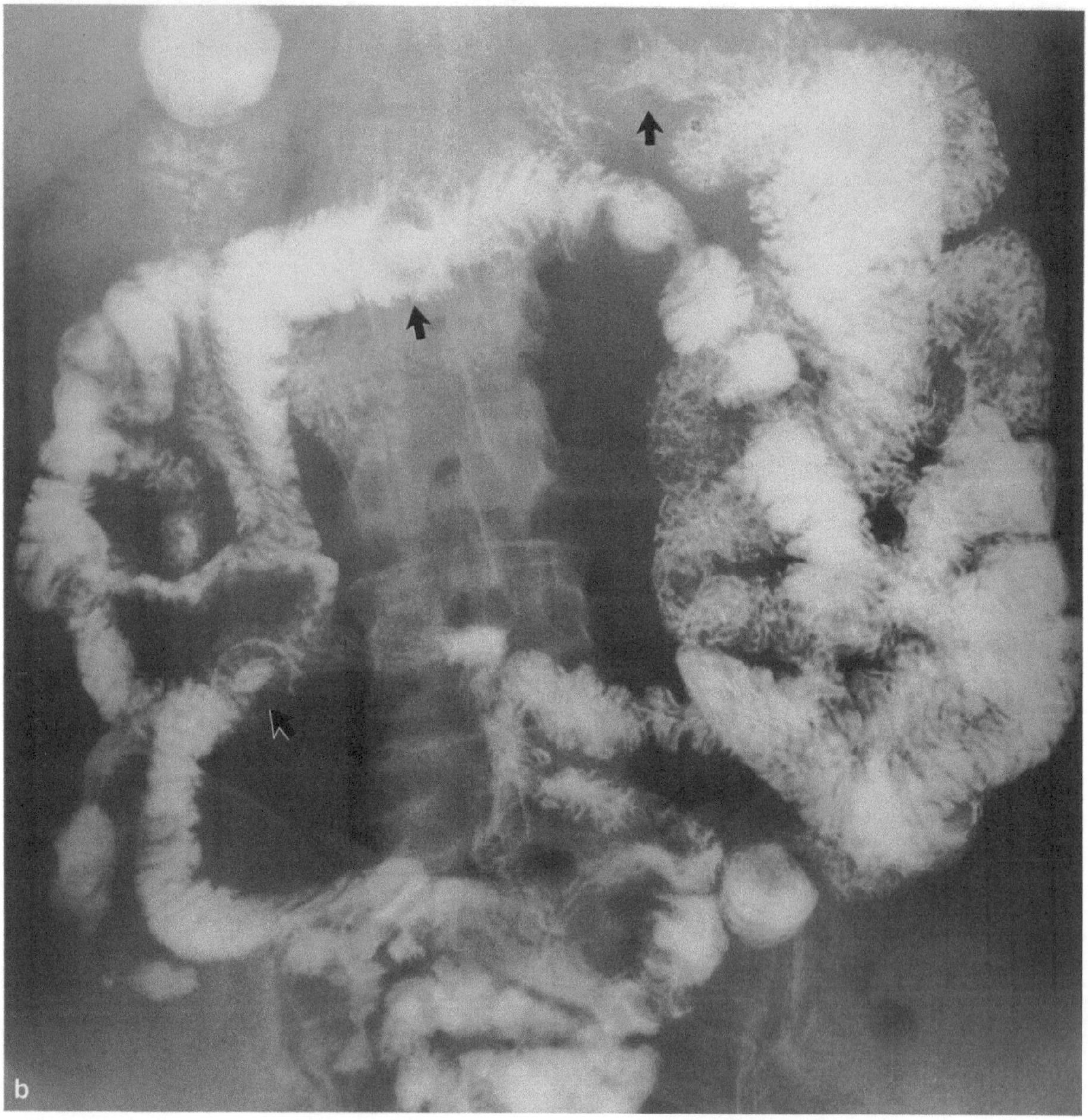

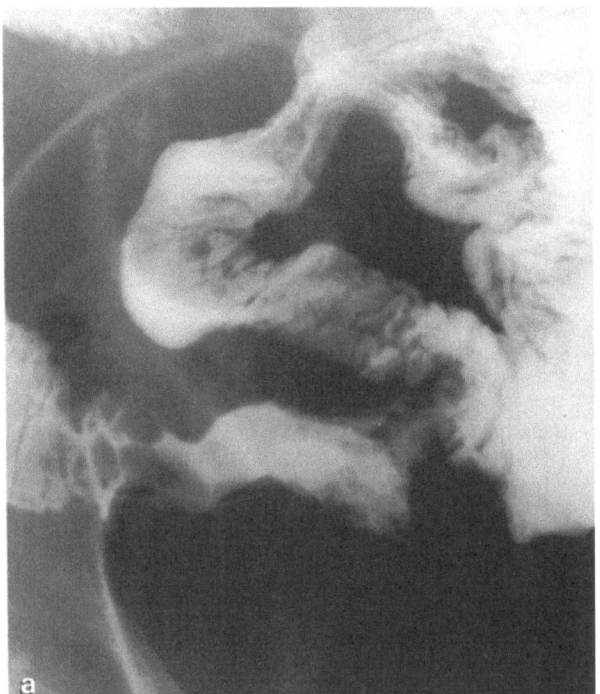

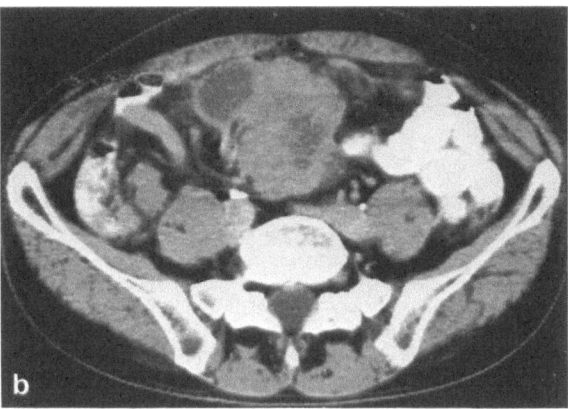

Fig. 96 a, b. Metastases from bronchial cancer. 65-year-old man with bronchial cancer ; digestive symptoms. **a** SBFT : segmental stiffness of a pelvic ileal loop, with excavated margins and decreased caliber, **b** computed tomography : lobulated, partially necrosed pelvic mass. A percutaneous cytological aspirate yielde the diagnosis of metastases from a bronchial cancer

References

Generalities

Beggs I, Freeman AH (1982) Excavated tumours of the gut. Clin Radiol 33 : 523-527

Benacerraf R (1974) Apport de l'artériographie digestive au diagnostic des tumeurs du grêle. Ann Radiol 17 : 751-764

Bernardino ME, Jing BS, Wallace S (1979) Computed tomography diagnosis of mesenteric masses. AJR 132 : 33-36

Bloch P, Eisenmann B (1972) Les tumeurs de l'intestin grêle. Vie Med 53 : 4725-4738

Bockus HL, Kelsey JR Jr (1976) Small bowel tumours. In : Gastroenterology. WB Saunders, Philaldelphie, 3rd ed, vol II, pp 459-468

Botsford TW, Crowe P, Crocker DW (1962) Tumors of the small intestine, a review of experience with 115 cases including a report of a rare case of malignant hemangioendothelioma. Am J Surg 103 : 358-365

Brookes VS, Waterhouse JA, Powell DJ (1968) Malignant lesions of the small intestine, a 10 year survey. Br J Surg 55 : 405-410

Carlson HC, Good CA (1973) Neoplasms of the small bowel in : Margulis AR, Burhenne HJ (eds) Alimentari tract Roentgenology. CV Mobsy Co, Saint-Louis, 2nd Ed, Vol II, pp 865-902

Collins SM, Hamilton JD, Lewis TD, Laufer I (1978) Small-bowel malabsorption and gastro-intestinal malignancy. Radiology 126 : 603-609

Coscina WF, Arger PH, Levine MS, Herlinger H, Cohen S, Coleman BG, Mintz MC (1986) Gastrointestinal tract focal mass lesions : role of CT and barium evaluations. Radiology 158 : 581-587

Debray C, Leymarios J, Hernandez CL (1968) L'artériographie sélective dans les tumeurs de l'estomac, du grêle et du colon. Ann Radiol 11 : 806-812

Delorme G, Tavernier J, Labat JP, Grelet Ph, Lafitte JJ, Fagola M, Diard F (1971) Apport de l'angiographie dans le diagnostic des tumeurs du grêle. J Radiol 52 : 673-680

De Schepper A, Hubens A, Van Vooren W (1974) Angiography in diagnosis of small bowel tumours. Radiology 14 : 425-430

Ebert PA, Zuidema GD (1965) Primary tumors of the small intestine. Arch Surg 91 : 452-455

Ekberg O, Ekholm S (1980) Radiography in primary tumors of the small bowel. Acta Radiol (Diagn) 21 : 79-84

Fakhry JR, Berk RN (1981) The « Target » pattern : characteristic sonographic feature of stomach and bowel abnormalities. AJR 137 : 969-972

Favriel JM, Cerf M, Benhamou G, Bocquet L, Debray CH (1979) Tumeurs jéjunales, révélation hémorragique, intérêt de la jéjunoscopie. Ann Gastroenterol Hépatol 15 : 475-480

Franken TH, Schirmer G, Sobbe A (1975) Roentgenologische Diagnose und differentiale Diagnose der Tumoren des Jejunum und Ileum. Roentgenbl 28 : 389-399

Garin CH, Lanitis G, Rousta B, Saegesser F (1976) Anatomo-clinical review of 104 cases of small intestine tumors. Int Surg 61 : 518-526

Ghahremani GG, Meyers MA, Port RB (1978) Calcified primary tumors of the gastrointestinal tract. Gastrointest Radiol 2 : 331-339

Greenstein JA, Sachar DB, Smith H, Janowitz HD, Aufses AH (1980) Pattern of neoplasia in Crohn's disease and ulcerative colitis. Cancer 46 : 403-407

Guinev B, Yanev S (1979) Signes clinico-radiologiques des tumeurs malignes de l'intestin grêle. Radiol Diagn (Berlin) 20 : 705-711

Hamzah, Ben Romdhane MH, Allegue M, Fodha M, Tlili-Graiess K, Kraiem C, Letaief R, Laarif M, Jeddi M (1987) Les lésions tumorales cavitaires du grêle. Diagnostic radio-échographique. A propos de 4 observations. J Radiol 68 : 537-544

Hancock RJ (1970) An 11-year review of primary tumours of the small bowel including the duodenum. Can Med Assoc J 103 : 1177-1179

Harris OD, Cooke WT, Thompson H (1967) Malignancy in adult : coeliac disease and idiopathic steatorrhea. Am J Med 42 : 899-912

Honoré H, Monsaingeon V, Escure MN (1981) Apport de l'échotomographie au diagnostic des tumeurs digestives. JEMU 2 : 137-145

Le Néel JC, Nomballais MF, Leborgne J, Mousseau M (1975) Les tumeurs malignes primitives de l'intestin grêle. Réflexions à propos de 25 observations. Gaz Méd Fr 82 : 2983-2993

Levine M, Drooze A, Herlinger H (1987) Annular malignancies of the small bowel. Gastrointest Radiol 12 : 53-58

Levitt RG, Sagel SS, Stanley RJ (1978) Detection of neoplasic involvement of the mesentery and omentum by computed tomography. AJR 131 : 835-838

Lowenfels AB (1973) Why are small-bowel tumours so rare ? Lancet I : 24-25

Maglinte D, Hill R, Miller RE, Chernish SM, Rosenak B, Elmore M, Burney B (1984) Detection of surgical lesions of the small bowel by enteroclysis. Am J Surg 147 : 225-229

Meriggi F, Cavallero M, Bonini C, Scotti Foglieni C (1978) Pathologia tumorale del diginuo, a proposito di 5 osservazioni. Est Minerva Chir 33 : 1243-1256

Miles RM, Crawford D, Duras S (1979) The small bowel tumor problem, an assessment based on 20 years experience with 116 cases. Ann Surg 189 : 732-740

Mittal VK, Bodzin JH (1980) Primary malignant tumors of the small bowel. Am J Surg 140 : 396-399

Olmsted WW, Ros PR, Hjermstad BM, McCarthy MJ, Dachman AH (1987) Tumors of the small intestine with little or no malignant predisposition : a review of the literature and report of 56 cases. Gastrointest Radiol 12 : 231-239

Peterson LR, Cooperberg PL (1978) Ultrasound demonstration of lesions of the gastrointestinal tract. Gastrointest Radiol 3 : 303-306

Peycelon R, Corréard RP (1970) Etude anatomoclinique d'une série de 29 tumeurs de l'intestin grêle. Ann Chir 24 : 1261-1272

Queloz J, Realini S, Candardjis G (1974) Le problème radiodiagnostique posé par les tumeurs de l'intestin grêle. Arch Fr Mal App Dig 63 : 269-278

Ribet M, Wurtz A, Latreille JP, Henriet PH (1972) Etude anatomoclinique de 24 tumeurs de l'intestin grêle. Lille Méd 17 : 101-103

River L, Silverstein J, Tope JW (1956) Benign neoplasms of small intestine, critical comprehensive review with reports of 20 new cases. Surg Gynecol Obstet 102 : 1-38

River L, Silverstein J (1956) Benign neoplasms of the small intestine. Surgery 102 : 11-21

Roux M, Delavierre PH, Vayre P, Hureau J, Hillemand P, Besançon F, Martignon CL (1973) Les tumeurs primitives du grêle, à propos de 30 observations. Sem Hôp Paris 49 : 2055-2061

Schey WL, Emanuel B, Raffensperger J (1979) Benign neoplasia and pseudoneoplasia of the small bowel in children. Gastrointest Radiol 4 : 47-55

Schier Y (1969) Diagnosis and therapeutic aspects of tumors of the small bowel. Arch Surg 98 : 659-662

Schnyder PA, Candardjis G (1983) CT detection of benign and malignant abnormalities of the small bowel. Eur J Radiol 3 : 33-38

Sethi G, Hardin CA (1969) Primary malignant tumors of the small bowel. Arch Surg 98 : 659-661

Silbermann H, Crichlow RW, Caplan HS (1974) Neoplasms of the small bowel. Ann Surg 180 : 157-160

Spelberg F, Schmidtler F (1980) Primary malignant tumors in the small bowel, a report about 43 of our own cases and 1134 cases from literature. Acta Chir Jugosl 27 : 39-46

Treadwell TA, White RR (1975) Primary tumors of the small bowel. Am J Surg 130 : 749-754

Vuori JVA, Vuori MK (1971) Radiological findings in primary malignant tumours of the small intestine. Ann Clin Res 3 : 16-21

Wytock DH, Bartholomew LG, Sheps SG (1983) Digital ischemia associated with small bowel malignancy. Gastroenterol 84 : 1025-1027

Leiomyomas

Baker HI, Good CA (1955) Smooth-muscle tumors of the alimentary tract, their roentgen manifestations. AJR 74 : 246-255

Bruneton JN, Drouillard J, Roux P, Lecomte P, Tavernier J (1981) Leiomyoma and leiomyosarcoma of the digestive tract, a report of 45 cases and review of the literature. Eur J Radiol 1 : 291-300

Calafat JF (1983) Place de la radiologie dans le diagnostic des tumeurs gastro-intestinales d'origine musculaire. Thèse Médecine, Nancy

Mabille JP, Cortet P, Gaudet M, Seigneuric C, Gambert B (1973) Les léiomyomes de l'intestin grêle. Ann Radiol 16 : 773-779

Miller RE, Lehman G (1978) Gastrointestinal hemorrhage from ileal leiomyoma, utility of the complete reflux small bowel examination. Gastrointest Radiol 2 : 367-369

Skandalakis JE, Gray SW, Shepard D (1964) Smooth muscle tumors of small intestine. Am J Gastroenterol 42 : 172-190

Tête R, De Montgolfier R, Piante M (1970) Léiomyome et léiomyosarcome de l'intestin grêle, intérêt de l'artériographie sélective. Arch Fr Mal App Dig 59 : 621

Uflacker R, Amaral NM, Lima S, Wholey M, Pereira EN, Nobrega M, Tavares T (1981) Angiography in primary myomas of the alimentary tract. Radiology 139 : 361-369

Neurogenic tumors

Capdeville R, Bennet J, Dubois F, Toulet J (1970) L'artériographie des tumeurs du grêle, à propos de 3 cas de schwannomes. Arch Fr Mal App Dig 59 : 453-462

Carney JA, Go VLW, Sizemore GW, Hayles AB (1976) Alimentary tract ganglioneuromatosis, a major component of the syndrome of multiple endocrine neoplasia, type 2b. N Engl J Med 295 : 1287-1291

Debray CH, Hardouin JP, Gouin B, Marche CL (1971) Les localisations digestives de la maladie de Recklinghausen. Gaz Med France 78 : 965-974

Demos TC, Blonder J, Schey WL, Braithwaite SS, Goldstein PL (1983) Multiple endocrine neoplasia (MEN) syndrome. Type IIB : Gastrointestinal manifestations. AJR 140 : 73-78

Keller D, Bringer JP, Veillon F (1981) Une étiologie rare d'invagination chez l'adulte : le neurofibrome intestinal. J Méd Strasbourg 12 : 334-336

Uflacker R, Alves MA, Diehl JC (1985) Gastrointestinal involvement in neurofibromatosis : angiographic presentation. Gastrointest Radiol 10 : 163-165

Fibromas

Chapuy A, Cognat M, Taillard G, Chavrier F (1969) Fibrome pur du grêle, à propos d'un cas. Arch Fr Mal App Dig 58 : 716-718

Lipomas

Dreze C, Cornil A, Lewalle L (1973) Lipomes multiples du jéjunum. J Belge Radiol 56 : 147-148

Heiken JP, Forde A, Gold P (1982) Computed tomography as a definitive method for diagnosing gastrointestinal lipomas. Radiology 142 : 409-414

Klepping C, Viard H, Ferry C, Villand J (1973) Les lipomes du tube digestif. Rev Fr Gastroentérol 87 : 19-32

Margolin FR, Lagios MD (1980) Polypoid lipomatosis of the small bowel. Gastrointest Radiol 5 : 59-60

Epithelial tumors

Delevett AF, Cuello R (1975) True villous adenoma of the jejunum. Gastroenterology 69 : 217-219

Keeley AF, Gottlieb LS (1969) Villous adenoma of the small bowel : an unusual lesion. Gastroenterology 57 : 185-190

Mir-Madjlessi SH, Farmer RG, Hawk WA (1973) Villous tumours of the duodenum and jéjunum, report of 4 cases and review of the literature. Am J Dig Dis 18 : 467-476

Perzin KH, Bridge MF (1981) Adenomas of the small intestine : a clinico-pathologic review of 51 cases and a study of their relationship to carcinoma. Cancer 48 : 799-819

Vascular tumors

Alfidi RJ, Esselstyn CD, Tarar R, Klein HJ, Hermann RE, Weakley LF, Turnbull RB (1971) Recognition and angiosurgical detection of arteriovenous malformations of the bowel. Ann Surg 174 : 573-582

Bambach CP, Coupland GAE, Sorby W, Roche J (1978) Angiodysplasia of the small bowel : a method of intraoperative identification. Aust NZ J Surg 48 : 317-321

Chevrel JP, Gouffier E, Boddaert A, Gueraud JP (1974) Deux cas d'angiomatose du grêle, intérêt de la jéjuno-iléoscopie per-opératoire. Chirurgie 100 : 412-421

Cooperman AM, Kelly KA, Bernatz PE, Huizenga KA (1972) Arteriovenous malformation of the intestine, an uncommon cause of gastrointestinal bleeding. Arch Surg 104 : 284-287

Hansen PS (1948) Hemangioma of the small intestine. Am J Clin Pathol Tech Bull 18 : 14-42

Hines R, Stryker SJ, Neiman HL, Royce Larsen L, Gottlieb J, Craig RM, Poticha SM (1981) Intraoperative angiography in intestinal angiodysplasia. Surg Gynecol Obstet 152 : 453-460

Nyman U, Boijsen E, Lindstrom C, Rosengren JE (1980) Angiography in angiomatous lesions of the gastrointestinal tract. Acta Radiol (Diagn) 21 : 21-31

Nys A, Buyssens N (1963) Diffuse cavernous hemangiomatosis of the small intestine, report of a case. Gastroenterology 45 : 663-666

Ochsner S, Penick RM (1957) Hemangioma of the small intestine. Radiology 68 : 845-848

Sandhu KS, Cohen H, Radin R, Buck FS (1987) Blue rubber bleb nevus syndrome presenting with recurrences. Dig Dis Sci 32 : 214-219

Inflammatory tumors

Chandrasoma P, Wheeler D, Randall-Radin D (1985) Traumatic neuroma of the intestine. Gastrointest Radiol 10 : 161-162

De Laguillaume B, Lagarde N, Delage J (1966) Les pseudo-tumeurs inflammatoires de l'intestin grêle. Arch Fr Mal App Dig 55 : 949

Eisenberg RL, Hedgcock MW, Brooke R, Montgomery CK (1977) Ulcerative pseudopolyposis mimicking neoplasm proximal to a jejunal obstruction. AJR 129 : 503-505

Gudjonsson H, Jones M, Krawitt FI, Kaye MD (1987) Pseudolymphoma of the jejunum. Dig Dis Sci 32 : 1314-1318

Matuchansky C, Duprey F, Briaud M, Babin P, Touchard G, Bloch P, Lenormand Y, Morichau-Beauchant M (1982) Hyperplasie nodulaire lymphoïde diffuse de l'intestin grêle, chez l'adulte sans déficit reconnu de l'immunité générale ni digestive. Gastroenterol Clin Biol 6 : 239-248

Matuchansky C, Touchard G, Babin P, Lemaire M, Cogne M, Preudhomme JL (1988) Diffuse small intestinal lymphoid infiltration in non immunodeficient adults from Western Europe. Gastroenterology 95 : 470-477

Molas G, Potet F, Nogig P (1985) Hyperplasie lymphoïde focale (pseudo-lymphome) de l'iléon terminal chez l'adulte. Gastroenterol Clin Biol 9 : 630-633

Rambaud J-C, De Saint-Louvent P, Marti R, Galian A, Mason DY, Wassef M, Licht H, Valleur P, Bernier J-J (1982) Diffuse follicular lymphoid hyperplasia of the small intestine without primary immunoglobulin defficiency. Am J Med 73 : 125-132

Robinson MJ, Padron S, Rywlin AM (1973) Enterocolitis lymphofollicularis, morphologic, pathologic, and serum immunoglobulin patterns. Arch Pathol 96 : 311-315

Weofel GF, Campbell DN, Penn I, Reichen J, Warren GH (1983) Inflammatory polyposis in an ileal blind loop. Gastroenterology 84 : 1020-1024

Polyposis syndromes

Dawson I (1969) Hamartomas in the alimentary tract. Gut 10 : 691-694

Dodds WJ (1976) Clinical and roentgen features of the intestinal polyposis syndromes. Gastrointest Radiol 1 : 127-143

Foster MA, Kilcoyne RF (1986) Ruvalcaba-Myhre-Smith syndrome : a new consideration in the differential diagnosis of intestinal polyposis. Gastrointest Radiol 11 : 349-350

Fritsch P, Pechlaner R, Czarnecki N, Hinter H (1981) The multiple hamartoma (Cowden) syndrome. Der Hautarzt 32 : 285-291

Linos DA, Dozois RR, Dahlin DC, Bartholomew LG (1981) Does Peutz-Jeghers syndrome predispose to gastrointestinal malignancy ? A later look. Arch Surg 116 : 1182-1184

Marshak RH, Lindner AE, Maklansky D (1977) Familial polyposis. Am J Gastroenterol 67 : 177-189

Naylor EW, Lebenthal E (1980) Gardner's syndrome : recent developments in research and management. Dig Dis Sci 25 : 945-959

Carcinoïd tumors

Anthony PP (1970) Gangrene of the small intestine, a complication of argentaffin carcinoma. Br J Surg 57 : 118-122

Balthazar EJ (1978) Carcinoïd tumors of the alimentary tract. I. Radiographic diagnosis. Gastrointest Radiol 3 : 47-56

Bancks NH, Goldstein HM, Dood GD (1975) The roentgenologic spectrum of small intestinal carcinoïd tumors. AJR 123 : 274-280

Besson A, Hofstetter JR, Saegesser F (1981) Tumeurs carcinoïdes, syndromes carcinoïdiens et tumeurs associées, à propos de 104 observations. Rev Fr Gastroenterol 172 : 53

Bjorn-Hansen R, Aakhus T (1973) Angiography in intestinal carcinoïd. Acta Radiol (Diagn) 14 : 721-727

Boijsen E, Kaude J, Tylen U (1974) Radiologic diagnosis of ileal carcinoïd tumours. Acta Radiol (Diagn) 15 : 65-82

Bruneton JN, Roux P, Drouillard J, Elie G, Tavernier J (1980) Etude radiologique des tumeurs carcinoïdes du tube digestif, revue de 150 cas de la littérature. Bordeaux Méd 13 : 881-888

Bruneton J-N, Sabatier J-C, Drouillard J, Elie G, Amouretti M, Tavernier J (1978) Apport de l'angiographie dans le diagnostic radiologique des carcinoïdes du grêle, à propos de 2 observations. Med Chir Dig 7 : 509-513

Clements JL, Hixson GL Jr, Berk RN, Dodds W, Goldstein H (1984) Gastrointestinal carcinoid tumors : an analysis of 104 cases. Mount Sinaï J Med 51 : 351

Gen C (1988) Les Tumeurs carcinoïdes du grêle, à propos de 2 observations. Thèse, Lyon

Goldstein HM, Miller M (1975) Angiographic evaluation of carcinoïd tumors of the small intestine : the value of epinephrine. Radiology 115 : 23-28

Hermanutz KD, Bucheler E, Biersack HJ (1974) Zur Röntgendiagnose des Karzinoïds. Fortschr Röntgenstr 121 : 186-196

Jeffree MA, Barter SJ, Hemingway AP, Nolan DJ (1984) Primary carcinoid tumours of the ileum : the radiological appearances. Clin Radiol 35 : 451-455

Jouanneau P, Malafosse M (1971) Les tumeurs carcinoïdes du tube digestif. Masson Expansion Sci Fr, Paris

Jouanneau P, Malafosse M, Bourreille J, Hemet J (1970) Entérite nécrosante segmentaire et carcinoïde. Les lésions artérielles. Chirurgie 96 : 756-761

Kinkhabwala M, Balthazar EJ (1978) Carcinoid tumors of the alimentary tract. II. Angiographic diagnosis of small intestinal and colonic lesions. Gastrointest Radiol 3 : 57-61

Li Song-Nian, Zou Wan-Zhong, Xie Jing X, Zhu Shao-Tong, Chen Jincheng (1982) Gastrointestinal tract carcinoid : radiologic and pathologic morphology. Chin Med J 95 : 136-144

Miller ER, Herrmann WW (1942) Argentaffin tumors of small bowel, a roentgen sign of malignant change. Radiology 39 : 214-220

Morin ME, Panella J, Baker DA, Engle J (1979) Ultrasound detection of a carcinoid tumor. Gastrointest Radiol 4 : 359-360

Mugel-Riwer B, Bersani D, Mugel JL (1983) Tumeurs carcinoïdes de l'iléon : intérêt du transit de l'intestin grêle. J Radiol 64 : 331-333

Noonan CD (1972) Calcified carcinoïd of small bowel, a case report. Radiol Clin Biol 41 : 115-120

Picus D, Glazer HS, Levitt RG, Husband JE (1984) Computed tomography of abdominal carcinoid tumors. AJR 143 : 581-584

Pistolesi GF, Caresano A, Del Favero C, Frasson F, Fugazzola C (1976) Aspects angiographiques du carcinoïde du grêle, à propos de 2 observations. J Radiol Electrol 57 : 725-731

Reichardt W, Ingemansson S, Lunderquist A, Nobin A (1979) Selective mesenteric phlebography in patients with carcinoïd tumors. Gastrointest Radiol 4 : 179-189

Reuter SR, Boijsen E (1966) Angiographic findings in 2 ileal carcinoïd tumors. Radiology 87 : 836-840

Seigel RS, Kuhns LR, Borlaza GS, McCormick TL, Simmons JL (1980) Computed tomography and angiography in ileal carcinoïd tumor and retractile mesenteritis. Radiology 134 : 437-440

Swobodnik W, Wechsler JG, Ditschuneit H (1983) Sonographic diagnosis of malignant carcinoid of the small intestine. Ultraschall 4 : 47-48

Thompson GB, Van Heerden JA, Martin JK, Schutt AJ, Ilstrup DM, Carney JA (1985) Carcinoid tumors of GI tract : presentation, management, and prognosis. Surgery 98 : 1054-1063

Tournier C, Viallet JF, Fermaud H (1974) Apport de la radiologie dans les tumeurs carcinoïdes du grêle. J Radiol 55 : 927-928

Tran-Minh V, Partensky C, Pouillaude JM, Boisson M, Barthélemy C, Bret P, Anjou A (1974) Aspects radiologiques des tumeurs carcinoïdes du grêle, à propos d'un cas personnel. J Radiol 55 : 923-924

Wallon J, Rahier J, Noël H, Haot J (1981) Les tumeurs carcinoïdes du tube digestif, pathologie tumorale du système endocrinien diffus du tube digestif. Rev Fr Gastroenterol 174 : 45

Weidner FA, Ziter FM (1981) Carcinoid tumors of the gastrointestinal tract. JAMA 245 : 1153-1155

Zeitels J, Naunheim K, Kaplan EL, Straus F (1982) Carcinoid tumors. Arch Surg 117 : 732-737

Malignant non-Hodgkin's lymphoma

Aguilar FP, Alfonso V, Riva S, Lopez Aldeguer J, Portilla J, Berenguer J (1987) Jejunal malignant lymphoma in a patient with adult-onset hypogammaglobulinemia and nodular lymphoid hyperplasia of the small bowel. Amer J Gastroent 82 : 472-475

Al-Saleem T, Zardawi IM (1979) Primary lymphomas of the small intestine in Iraq : a pathological study of 145 cases. Histopathology, 3 : 89-106

Aspestrand F, Melsom M (1984) Gastrointestinal lymphoma with total involvement of the gut. Radiologe 24 : 524-526

Balikian JP, Nassar NT, Shamma'a MH, Shahid MS (1969) Primary lymphomas of small intestine including the duodenum, a roentgen analysis of 29 cases. AJR 107 : 131-141

Belaiche J, Jian R, Galian A, Valleur P, Villet R, Wassef M, Modigliani R (1983) Enteropathie avec perte de protéine

et hyperplasie nodulaire lymphoïde de l'intestin grêle. Gastroenterol Clin Biol 7 : 59-65

Blackledge G, Bush H, Dodge OG, Crowther D (1979) A study of gastrointestinal lymphoma. Clin Oncol 5 : 209-219

Bret P (1979) Lymphome malin jéjunal diagnostiqué sur la radiographie d'abdomen sans préparation. J Belge Radiol 62 : 387-390

Camilleri JP, Diebold J (1972) Sarcomes Lymphoréticulaires de l'intestin grêle. Ann Gastroenterol Hepatol 8 (3) : 279-297

Capelle J, Leclère J, Kraiem A (1984) Faits cliniques : un cas d'invagination intestinale au cours d'un lymphome de Burkitt, aspects échographiques et tomodensitométriques. J Radiol 65 : 471-474

Carroll BA, Ta HN (1980) The ultrasonic appearence of extranodal abdominal lymphona. Radiology 136 : 419-425

Cooper BT, Holmes GK, Cooke WT (1982) Lymphoma risk in coeliac disease of later life. Digestion 23 : 89-92

Contreary K, Nance FC, Becker WF (1980) Primary lymphoma of the gastrointestinal tract. Ann Surg 191 : 593-598

Freeman HJ, Weinstein WM, Shnitka TK, Piercey JRA, Wensel RH (1977) Primary abdominal lymphoma — presenting manifestation of celiac sprue or complicating dermatitis herpetiformis. Am J Med 63 : 585-594

Glick SN, Teplick SK, Goodman LR, Clearfield HR, Shanser JD (1984) Development of lymphoma in patients with Crohn disease. Radiology 153 : 337-339

Greiner M (1984) Contribution du transit du grêle au diagnostic des lymphomes malins non hodgkiniens de l'intestin grêle chez l'adulte, à propos de 40 observations. Thèse, Lyon

Hamdouch M, Sbihi AH, Barahioui M, Outarahout O, Benjelloun H (1982) Apport de la pansonographie abdominale dans le lymphome non hodgkinien du grêle de l'enfant, à propos de 9 cas. J Radiol 63 : 647-651

Harousseau JL (1984) Le point rapide aujourd'hui sur la classification des lymphomes. Presse Méd 13 : 2353-2356

Issacson P, Wright DH (1978) Intestinal lymphoma associated with malabsorption. Lancet 8055 : 67-70

Kaude JV, Joyce PH (1980) Evaluation of abdominal lymphoma by ultrasound. Gastrointest Radiol 5 : 249-254

Krikorian TG, Burke JS, Rosenberg SA (1979) Occurence of non-Hodgkin's lymphoma after therapy for Hodgkin's disease. N Engl J Med 300 : 452-458

Lamers CB, Wagener T, Assmann K, Van Tongeren J (1980) Jéjunal lymphoma in a patient with primary adult-onset hypogammablobulinemia and nodular lymphoid hyperplasia of the small intestine. Dig Dis Sci 25 : 553-557

Lewin KJ, Ranchod M, Dorfman RF (1978) Lymphomas of the gastrointestinal tract, a study of 117 cases presenting with gastro-intestinal disease. Cancer 42 : 693-707

Marshak R, Wolf BS, Eliasoph J (1961) The roentgen findings in lymphosarcoma of the small intestine. AJR 86 : 682-692

Megibow AJ, Balthazar EJ, Naidich DP, Bosniak MA (1983) Computed tomography of gastrointestinal lymphoma. AJR 141 : 541-547

Mueller PR, Ferrucci JT, Harbin WP (1980) Appearance of lymphomatous involvement of the mesentery by ultrasonography and body computed tomography : the sandwich sign. Radiology 134 : 467-473

Naqui MS, Burrows L, Kark AE (1969) Lymphoma of the gastrointestinal tract : prognostic guides based on 162 cases. Am Surg, pp 221-231

Nisard A, Lecharpentier Y, Louvel A, Galian A, Bleichner G, Boisson J, Rambaud JC (1976) Etude anatomo-pathologique d'un lymphome malin compliquant une maladie cœliaque de l'adulte. Arch Fr Mal App Dig 65 : 295-305

Pagani JJ, Bernardino ME (1981) CT radiographic correlation of ulcerating small bowel lymphomas. AJR 136 : 998-1000

Paliard P, Riou JP, Lesbros F, Abdessemed H (1976) Maladie coeliaque de l'adulte et lymphome malin jéjunal, présentation d'un cas. Lyon Med 236 : 581-584

Paling MR (1983) Necrotic tumor simulating intraabdominal abscess : a case report. CT 7 : 395-397

Rosenberg SA, Diamon HD, Jaslowitz B, Craver LF (1961) Lymphosarcoma : review of 1269 cases. Médecine (Baltimore) 40 : 31-84

Sartoris DJ, Harell GS, Anderson MF, Zboralske FF (1984) Small-bowel lymphoma and regional enteritis : radiographic similarities. Radiology 152 : 291-296

Schaeffer PS, Friedman AC (1981) Nodular lymphoid hyperplasia of the small intestine with Burkitt's lymphoma and dysgammaglobulinemia. Gastrointest Radiol 6 : 325-328

Vessal K, Dutz W, Kohout E (1980) Röntgenlogische Bedunfe bei Lymphonen des Dünndarms. Fortschr Röntgenstr 3 : 243-248

Zornaza J, Dodd GD (1980) Lymphoma of the gastrointestinal tract. Semin Roentgenol 15 : 272-287

Hodgkin's disease

Ornstein DH, Ruoff M (1977) The radiology corner, Hodgkin's disease of the small intestine. Am J Gastroenterol 68 : 182-187

Shaw J, Mulvaney N (1982) Hodgkin's lymphoma : a complication of small bowel Crohn's disease. Aust NZ J Surg 52 : 34-36

Wood NL, Usaf MC, Coltman CA (1973) Localized primary extranodal Hodgkin's disease. Ann Int Med 78 : 113-118

Alpha-chain disease

Doe WF, Henry K, Doyle FH (1976) Radiological and histological findings in 6 patients with alpha chain disease. Br J Radiol 49 : 3-11

Gauthier D (1981) Le transit du grêle dans la maladie des chaînes alpha. Thèse, Lyon

Lejonc JL, Netter-Pinon G, Reyes F (1976) Les maladies des chaînes lourdes. Concours Med 38 : 1031-1045

Monges H, Aubert L, Chamlian A, Remacle JP, Mathieu B, Cougard A, Arroyo H (1975) Maladie des chaînes alpha à forme intestinale, présentation d'un cas traité par antibiothérapie avec rémission clinique, histologique et immunologique. Arch Fr Mal App Dig 64 : 223-231

Monges H, Aubert L, Remacle JP, Chamlian A, Mathieu B, Cougard A, Quilichini R, Chaffanjon P (1980) Survenue d'une maladie de Hodgkin après rémission complète d'une maladie des chaînes alpha. Gastroenterol Clin Biol 4 : 181-187

Mussche M, Thienpont L (1974) Adult coeliac disease complicated by intestinal reticulum cell sarcoma with high serum IgA level. Acta Clin Belg 29 : 389-393

Rambaud JC (1980) Secondes néoplasies et maladie des chaînes alpha. Gastroenterol Clin Biol 4 : 177-180

Rambaud JCL, Galian A (1981) La forme digestive de la maladie des chaînes alpha. Ann Gastroenterol Hepatol 17 : 37-43

Rambaud JC, Hautefeuille M, Galian A (1983) La forme digestive de la maladie des chaînes alpha. Ann Gastroenterol Hepatol 19 : 111-118

Ramos L, Marcos J, Illanas M, Hernandez-Mora M, Perez-Paya F, Picouto JL, Santana P, Chantar C (1978) Radiological characteristics of primary intestinal lymphoma of the « Mediterranean » type : observations on 12 cases. Radiology 126 : 379-385

Teulieres JP, Lambert R, Vachon A (1978) La maladie des chaînes lourdes alpha. Sem Hôp Paris, 54 : 546-553

Vessal K, Dutz W, Kohout E, Rezvani L (1980) Immunoproliferative small intestinal disease with duodenojejunal lymphoma : radiologic changes. AJR 135 : 491-497

Leukemia, Waldenström's disease, plasmocytoma

Desablens B, Gineston JL, Joly JP, Piprot-Choffat C, Svestre H, Capron JP (1987) Lymphome immunoblastique de la région iléo-coecale au cours d'une leucémie lymphoïde chronique, syndrome de Richter localisé à l'intestin et révélé par une ascite. Gastroenterol Clin Biol 11 : 901-903

Goeggel-Lamping C, Kahn SB (1978) Gastrointestinal polyposis in multiple myeloma. JAMA 239 : 1786-1787

Goldberg HI, Sheft DJ (1976) Abnormalities in small intestine contour and caliber, a working classification. Radiol Clin North Am 14 : 461-475

Hoang C, Halphen M, Galian A, Brouet JC, Marsan C, Leclerc JP, Rambaud JC (1985) Atteinte intestinale et entéropathie exsudative au cours de la macro globulinémie de Waldenstrom. Gastroent Clin Biol 9 : 444-448

Hunter TB, Bjelland JC (1984) Review : gastrointestinal complications of leukemia and its treatment. AJR 142 : 513-517

Kushner DC, Weinstein HJ, Kirkpatrick A (1980) The radiologic diagnosis of leukemia and lymphoma in children. Semin Roentgenol 15 : 316

Mendenhall CM, Thar TL, Million RR (1980) Solitary plasmocytoma of bone and soft tissue. Int J Radiat Oncol Biol Phys 6 : 1497-1501

Prolla JC, Kirsner JB (1964) The gastrointestinal lesions and complications of the leukemias. Ann Int Med 61 : 1084-1103

Rogé J, Marche C, Camilleri JP, Druet P, Silvereano-Rogé F, Vernier G (1978) Entéropathie exsudative et macroglobulinémie. Gastroent Clin Biol 2 : 897-906

Spagnoli I, Gattoni F, Mazzoni R, Uslenghi C (1983) Primary gastrointestinal plasmocytoma. Diagn Imag 52 : 23-27

Sarcoma

Bryk D, Farman J, Dallemand S, Meyers MA, Wecksell A (1978) Kaposi's sarcoma of the intestinal tract : roentgen manifestations. Gastrointest Radiol 3 : 425-430

Chiotasso P, Fazio VW (1982) Prognostic factors of 28 leiomyosarcomas of the small intestine. Surg Gynecol Obstet 155 : 197

Clark RA, Alexander ES (1982) Computed tomography of gastrointestinal leiomyosarcoma. Gastrointest Radiol 7 : 127-129

De Santos LA, Ginaldi S, Wallace S (1981) Computed tomography in liposarcoma. Cancer 47 : 46-54

Frager DH, Frager JD, Brandt LJ, Wolf EL, Rand LG, Klein RS, Beneventano TC (1986) Gastrointestinal complications of AIDS : radiologic features. Radiology 158 : 597-603

Friedman-Kien AE, Laubenstein LS, Rubinstein P, Buimovici-Klein E, Marmor M, Stahl R, Spigland I, Sookim K, Zolla-Pazner S (1982) Disseminated Kaposi's sarcoma in homosexual men. Ann Int Med 96 : 693-699

Kaftori JK, Aharon M, Kleinhaus U (1981) Sonographic features of gastrointestinal leiomyosarcoma. J Clin Ultrasound 9 : 11-15

Keller D, Piombini JL, Lévy M, Hernandez N, Foster E (1980) Manifestations digestives de la maladie de Kaposi. Rev Fr Gastroenterol 162 : 11-16

Lunderquist A, Holmdahl S, Clemens F (1971) Selective superior mesenteric arteriography in reticulum-cell sarcoma of the small bowel. Radiology 98 : 113-115

Megibow AJ, Balthazar EJ, Hulnick DH, Naidich DP, Bosniak MA (1985) CT evaluation of gastrointestinal leiomyomas and leiomyosarcomas. AJR 144 : 727-731

Neff R, Kremer S, Voutsinas I, Waxman M, Mitty W (1987) Primary Kaposi's sarcoma of the ileum presenting as massive rectal bleeding. Amer J Gastroent 82 : 276-277

Rose HS, Balthazar EJ, Megibow AJ, Horowitz L, Laubenstein LJ (1982) Alimentary tract involvement in Kaposi sarcoma : radiographic and endoscopic findings in 25 homosexual men. AJR 139 : 661-666

Rowley VA, Cooperberg PL (1982) The ultrasonographic appearance of abdominal leiomyosarcomas. J Can Assoc Radiol 33 : 94-97

Tête R, De Montgolfier R, Piante M (1970) Léiomyome et léiomyosarcome de l'intestin grêle, intérêt de l'artériographie sélective. Arch Fr Mal App Dig 59 : 621

Urmacher C, Myskowski P, Ochoa M, Kris M, Safai B (1982) Outbreak of Kaposi's sarcoma with cytomegalovirus infection in young homosexual men. Am J Med 72 : 569-575

Adenocarcinoma

Bernard C, Schmitt M, Guillemin F, Olive D, Hoeffel JC, Marchal AL, Bretagne MCM (1987) Localisations rares d'adénocarcinome digestif chez l'enfant. A propos de 2 cas. J Radiol 68 : 339-344

Bruneton JN, Drouillard J, Bourry J, Roux P, Lecomte P (1983) L'adénocarcinome de l'intestin grêle, état actuel du diagnostic et du traitement, étude de 27 cas et revue de la littérature. J Radiol 64 : 117-123

Darke SG, Parks AG, Grogono JL, Pollock DJ (1973) Adenocarcinoma and Crohn's disease, a report of 2 cases and analysis of the literature. Br J Surg 60 : 169-175

Ekberg O, Ekholm S (1980) Radiology in primary small bowel adenocarcinoma. Gastrointest Radiol 5 : 49-53

Fresko D, Lazarus SS, Dotan J, Reingold M (1982) Early presentation of carcinoma of the small bowel in Crohn's disease (« Crohn's carcinoma »). Gastroenterology 82 : 783-789

Gallego MS, Pulpeiro JR, Arenas A, Colina F (1986) Primary adenocarcinoma of the terminal ileum simulating Crohn's disease. Gastrointest Radiol 11 : 355-356

Ginzburg I, Schneider KM, Dreizin DH, Levinson C (1956) Carcinoma of the jejunum occurring in a case of regional enteritis. Surgery 39 : 347-351

Holmes GKT, Dunn GI, Cockel R, Brokes VS (1980) Adenocarcinoma of the upper small bowel complicating coeliac disease. Gut 21 : 1010-1016

Keller RJ, Hertz L, Zimmerman M, Geller S (1982) Carcinoma of the ileum simulating Crohn disease. AJR 138 : 151-153

Kerber GW, Frank PH (1984) Carcinoma of the small intestine and colon as a complication of Crohn disease : radiologic manifestations. Radiology 150 : 639-645

Meyers S, Feinman L (1974) Free perforation complicating primary adenocarcinoma of the jejunum. Am J Dig Dis 19 : 850-854

Milman PJ, Gold BM, Bagla S, Thorn R (1980) Primary ileal adenocarcinoma simulating Crohn's disease. Gastrointest Radiol 5 : 55-58

Morgan DF, Busuttil RW (1977) Primary adenocarcinoma of the small intestine. Am J Surg 134 : 331-333

Nesbit RR, Elbadawi NA, Morton JH, Cooper RA (1976) Carcinoma of the small bowel, a complication of regional enteritis. Cancer 37 : 2948-2959

Ouriel K, Adams JJ (1983) Adenocarcinoma of the small intestine. Am J Surg 147 : 66-70

Swift AC, Smith GT, Douglas DL (1980) Dual primary adenocarcinoma of the duodenum and jejunum in a patient with previous colonic cancer. Postgrad Med J 56 : 871-874

Tankel JW, Galasko C (1984) Adenocarcinoma of small bowel in a 12-year-old girl. J R Soc Med 77 : 693-694

Traube J, Simpson S, Riddell RH, Levin B, Kirsner JB (1980) Crohn's disease and adenocarcinoma of the bowel. Dig Dis Sci 25 : 939-944

Métastases

Antler AS, Ough Y, Pitchumoni CS, Davidian M, Thelmo W (1982) Gastrointestinal metastases from malignant tumors of the lung. Cancer 49 : 170-172

Beckly DE (1974) Alimentary tract metastases from malignant melanoma. Clin Radiol 25 : 385-389

Caramella E, Bruneton J-N, Roux P, Aubanel D, Lecomte P (1983) Metastases of digestive tract, report of 77 cases and review of literature. Eur J Radiol 3 : 331-338

Dalmas H, Anfossi G, Dor JF, Basbous D, Guidicelli C (1976) Invaginations jéjuno-et iléo-iléales révélatrices de multiples métastases mélaniques de l'intestin grêle, présentation d'une observation. J Chir (Paris) 111 : 341-346

De Castro CA, Dockerty MB, Mayo CW (1957) Metastatic tumors of the small intestines. Surg Gynecol Obstet 105 : 159-165

Du Brow RA, Rubin JM (1982) Intraabdominal metastatic carcinoma : unusual presentation and potential pitfall in CT evaluation. J Comput Assist Tomogr 6 : 966-968

Farmer RG, Hawk WA (1964) Metastatic tumors of the small bowel. Gastroenterol 47 : 496-504

Fawaz F, Hill GJ (1983) Adult intussusception due to metastatic tumors. South Med J 76 : 522-523

Goldstein HM, Beydoun MT, Dodd GD (1977) Radiologic spectrum of melanoma metastatic of the gastrointestinal tract. AJR 129 : 605-612

Koury HI, Kenady D (1988) Perforation of a metastatic lung adenocarcinoma of the jejunum. Amer J Gastroent 83 : 462

Listrom MB, Davis M, Lowry S, Williams WW, Monsein LH, Kleinman R, Kogel HK (1988) Intussuception secondary to squamous carcinoma of the lung. Gastrointest Radiol 13 : 224-226

Meyers MA, Sweeney J (1972) Secondary neoplasms of the bowel. Radiology 105 : 1-11

Meyers MA (1975) Metastatic seeding along the small bowel mesentery, roentgen features. AJR 123 : 67-73

Moffat RE, Gourley WK (1980) Ileal lymphatic metastases from cecal carcinoma. Radiology 135 : 55-58

Oddson TA, Rice RP, Seigler HF, Thompson WM, Kelvin FM, Clark WM (1978) The spectrum of small bowel melanoma. Gastrointest Radiol 3 : 419-423

Reboul J, Delorme G, Bouyssou P (1953) A propos d'un épithélioma secondaire du jéjunum. J Radiol 34 : 796-797

Smith SJ, Carlson HC, Gisvold JJ (1977) Secondary neoplasms of the small bowel. Radiology 125 : 29-33

Wittich G, Salomonowitz E, Szepesi T, Czembirek H, Fruehwald F (1984) Small bowel double-contrast enema in stage III ovarian cancer. AJR 142 : 299-304

Yang PM, Sheu JC, Yang TH, Chen DS, Yu JY, Lee SC, Hsu HC, Sung JL (1987) Metastasis of hepatocellular carcinoma to the proximal jejunum manifested by occult gastrointestinal bleeding. Amer J Gastroent 82 : 165-167

Yuhasz M, Laufer I, Sutton G, Herlinger H, Caroline DF (1985) Radiography of the small bowel in patients with gynecologic malignancies. AJR 144 : 303-307

Zornoza J, Goldstein HM (1977) Cavitating metastases of the small intestine. AJR 129 : 613-615

Inflammatory diseases

The major disease in the inflammatory pathology of the small intestine is Crohn's disease.

Crohn's disease

In 1932, Crohn, Ginzburg and Oppenheimer differentiated tuberculosis from regional ileitis, which has since been referred to as Crohn's disease. This term has been expanded to describe an idiopathic, chronic, ulcerating and stenosing inflammatory disease of the digestive tract, the histological characteristics of which include noncaseating giant-cell granulomas. The etiology of the disease is not known. Many authors regard it as a reaction to environmental agents (food, bacteria, viruses) in subjects with a genetic predisposition.

Crohn's disease was more frequent in Anglo-Saxon and Scandinavian populations some decades ago and has widely spread in France and around the Mediterranean Basin in the past twenty to thirty years. This disease of young adults, affecting both sexes equally, is not rare in children. Familial cases have been reported, as well as similar evolution in identical twins.

Pathology

The usual site of the disease is the terminal ileum, but other locations are not rare in the ileum or the jejunum. The disease can involve any segment of the digestive tract from the stomach to the anus. Colonic involvement seems increasingly frequent, and 80% of these are associated with ileal lesions. Esogastro-duodenal involvement is exceptional in the absence of intestinal lesions. Anal and perineal involvement, especially fistulae, is frequent.

The fundamental macroscopic lesions are edema, ulcerations with fibrosis of the intestinal wall. Edema, the earliest sign, broadens the villi. All types of ulceration can be observed, in particular aphtoid ulcerations signalling mucosal erosion amidst a hypertrophied lymphoid follicle, linear ulcerations, a cobblestone appearance due to a crisscrossing of longitudinal and transverse ulcerations, and transmural ulcerations. Fibrosis of the bowel wall is often off centre, contributes to thickening of the submucosa and leads to stenosis. The extent of the process is usually transmural when the disease becomes evident.

Progression of the inflammation leads to mesenteric sclerolipomatosis with adhesions to the neighbouring organs, to the presence of inflammatory adenopathy and to peritoneal exudation. The extension of the ulcers leads to the formation of abscesses and fistulae (especially ileoileal and ileosigmoid). Peritonitis is rare because of the subacute character of the evolution. The ureters and the bladder are sometimes involved.

The histological criterion of the disease is the presence of epithelioid and giant-cell granulomas without caseating necrosis, most often in the submucosa and sometimes lying beneath a perfectly normal mucosa, so that a biopsy is not deep enough to demonstrate the disease in all cases. The granulomas are found in only 30 to 60% of all cases, hence the need for the recognition of other associated pathological changes including transverse fissures, sometimes deeper than the muscularis, increased number and size of the lymphoid follicles in the submucosa, and lymphangiectasia.

Clinical findings

The major symptom of Crohn's disease is a chronic diarrhea associated with abdominal pain, which is often located in the right iliac fossa and may be mistaken for appendicitis. The findings of the surgeon during appendectomy sometimes make it possible to suspect the diagnosis. In other cases, the postoperative complications of appendectomy unveil the correct diagnosis. Crohn's disease may also be discovered because of a perineal fistula that fails to heal.

The physical examination may show an abdominal mass or a cutaneous fistula. Alteration of the patient's general condition, weight loss and fever, though sometimes considerable, do not always indicate the extent of the disease.

The most frequent associated extradigestive signs include buccal aphtosis, eye lesions such as iritis and conjunctivitis, erythema nodosum, skin ulceration and rheumatic diseases (rheumatoid spondylitis, periostitis). Associated conditions may also be hepatobiliary (lithiasis or sclerosing cholangitis, although the latter is less frequent than with ulcerative colitis), urinary (lithiasis, amyloidosis) or neurological.

The progression of disease is very unpredictable, most often occurring intermittently with episodes of remission which occur either spontaneously or are induced by anti-inflammatory, steroid therapy, parenteral feedings or surgery (resection, myotomy, etc.). Half of all patient will undergo surgery at some time, although the surgical indications are confined to stenosis and abscesses. In order to preserve the function of the small intestine, the surgeons currently tend to perform myotomies rather than limited resections in case of stenosis, where the slow evolution of the disease makes it possible. After an ileocolic anastomosis, the disease frequently recurs on the ileal side of the anastomosis.

After 15 years with Crohn's disease, 10% of the patients have died because of it, two-thirds are in good condition and the others are afflicted with symptoms due to recurrence or residual disease. In patients with Crohn's disease, the long-term risk of ileal or colonic carcinoma is twenty times that of the general population. The diagnosis must be conside-

red if a stenosis become more pronounced or a mass grows in spite of treatment.

The laboratory signs of a flare-up are usually an increase in the sedimentation rate, and sometimes a leucocytosis. The most reliable indices of activity currently seem to be the blood levels of albumin and acute-phase proteins (oromucoid, C-reactive protein). Radionuclide scanning with labelled leucocytes has been used to locate developing lesions and gallium isotope scanning to detect abscesses.

Radiological findings

Crohn's disease rarely presents as a single abnormality. It often combines several lesions with variable appearance and extent.

Elementary images (figs. 1 to 30)

Functional abnormalities
Like all inflammatory diseases, Crohn's disease is associated with functional abnormalities, the most specific of which is hypertonia of the terminal ileum, which is difficult to opacify, thus simulating stenosis, but which can be visualized with drug-induced hypotonia. Inversely, atonia is frequent in recurrence following resection.

Hypersecretion blurs the contours of the folds. It sometimes causes local barium flocculation, which must be differentiated from the punctated appearance of villous abnormalities described below. In diffuse forms, considerable secretory abnormalities may suggest malabsorption.

Abnormal curvature and position
Stiff, fixed or angulated loops as well as omega-shaped loops are observed within a lucent space in the advanced forms of Crohn's disease, including mesenteric sclerolipomatosis. A widened interloop gap indicates bowel wall and mesenteric thickening. A compression image is sometimes associated with an abscess or adenopathy.

Abnormal caliber and bowel wall expansion
The most specific appearance is that of a long stenosis, sometimes involving several loops that are stiff and angulated, and may be disrupted by the images of saccules. When stenosis occurs in the terminal ileum, it usually tapers off near the ileocecal valve. The stenoses may be circular, with spiculated

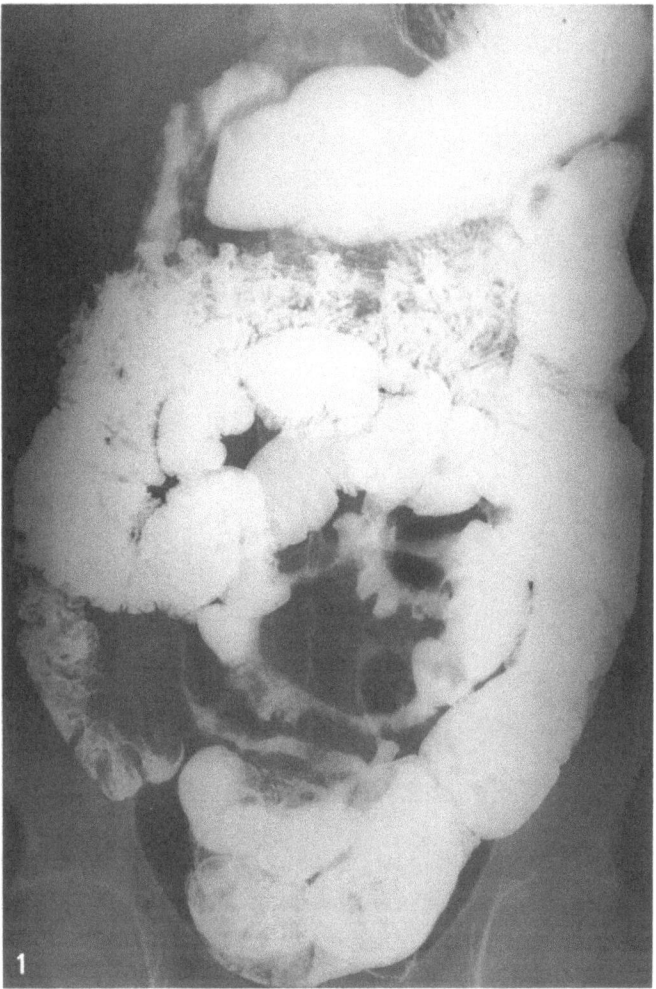

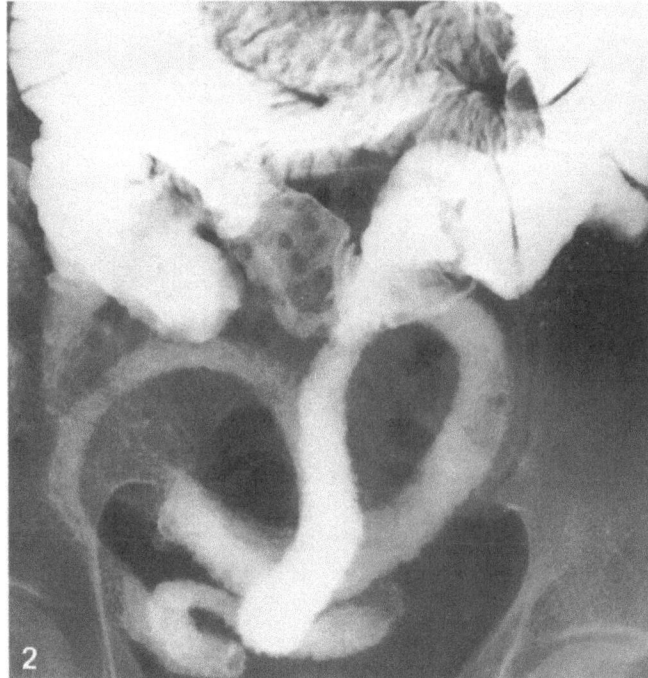

Fig. 1. Crohn's disease : abnormal position. Right infraumbilical void image drawing attention to the abnormal caliber and expansion of several ileal loops

Fig. 2. Crohn's disease : abnormal position. Unfolded and fixed pelvic loops drawing attention to the abnormal mucosal pattern

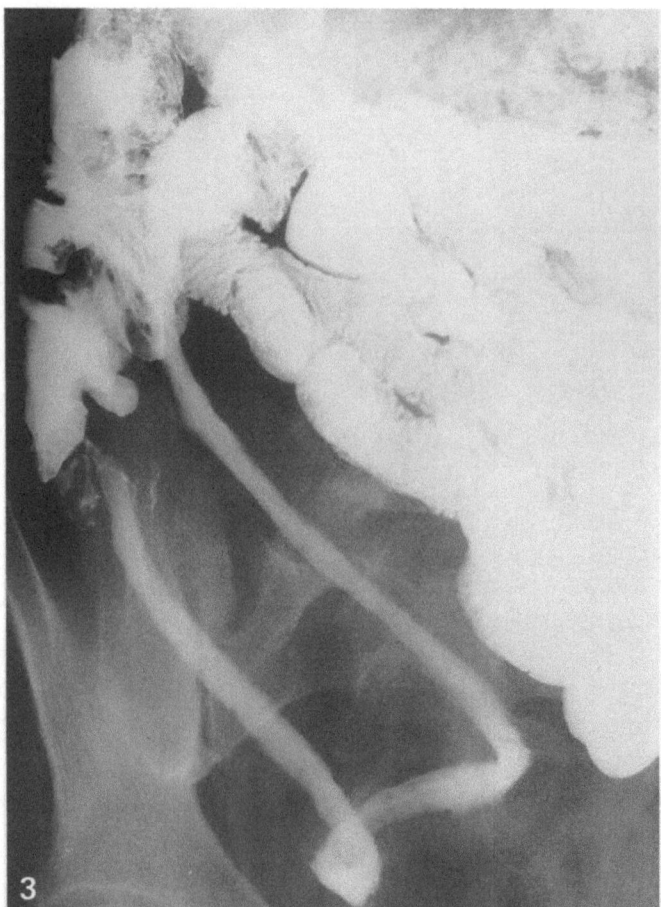

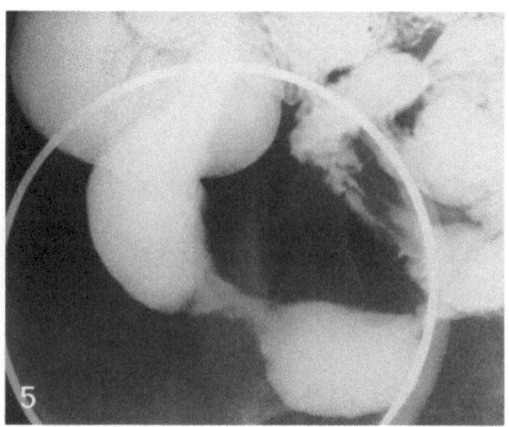

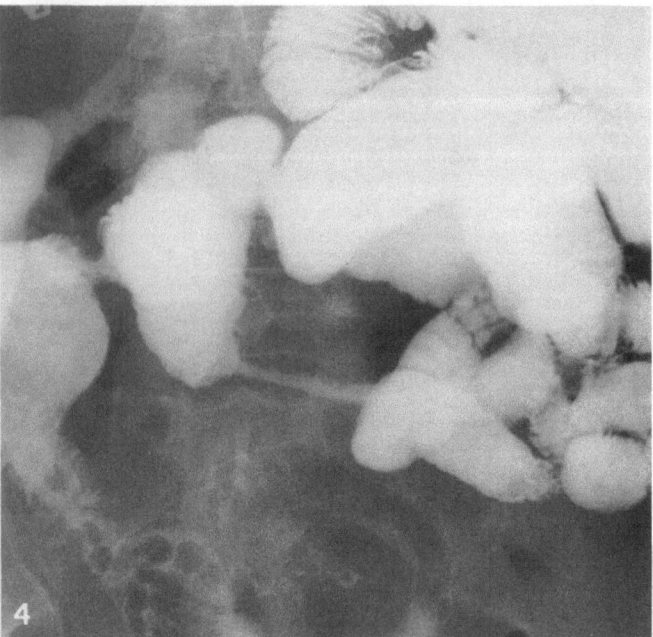

Fig. 3. Crohn's disease ; abnormal caliber. Angulated and fixed terminal ileum with a long stenosis and an abnormal mucosal pattern

Fig. 4. Crohn's disease : abnormal caliber. Ileal stenosis over 4 cm long with disappearance of the folds

Fig. 5. Crohn's disease : abnormal caliber. 2 cm long ileal stenosis with abnormal mucosal pattern

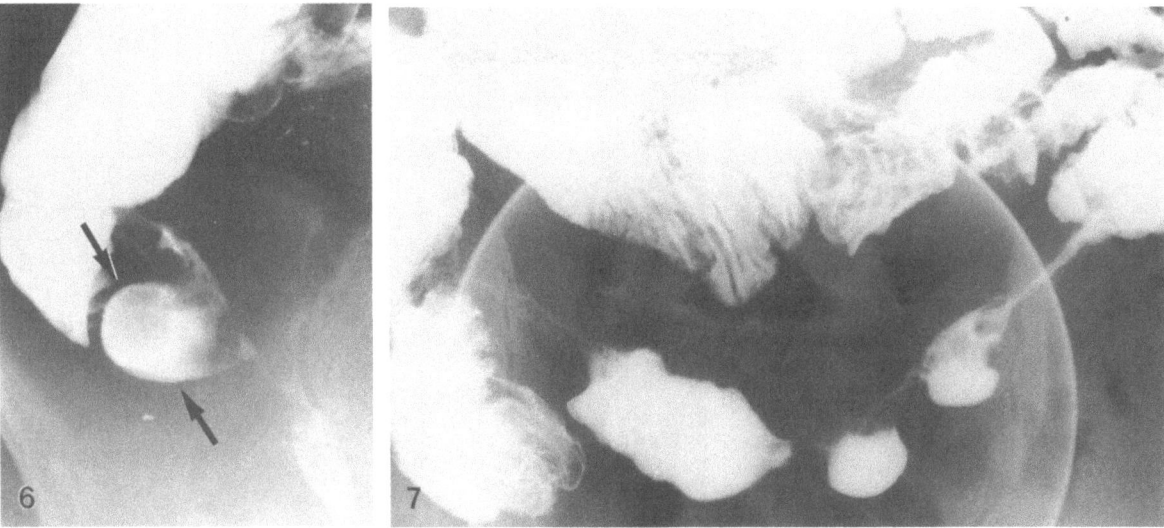

Fig. 6. Crohn's disease : abnormal expansion of the wall. Saccule in the stenosed terminal ileum

Fig. 7. Crohn's disease : abnormal expansion of the wall. Multiple saccules in the stenosed terminal ileum

contours more often than smooth ones. They are usually asymmetric, the mesenteric aspect being retracted while the opposite wall is sacculated. A short stenosis due to ulceration is sometimes observed. It is centered or asymmetric, often tiered and has a tapered transition area with the proximal and distal segments.

Nodulations

Nodulations in Crohn's disease often are flattened (cobblestone) reflecting protrusion of portions of the swollen mucosa indented by the intersection of multiple fissures. These produce a more or less regular network in the luminal space. On tangential views, the margin of the intestinal loop may have a slightly festooned or even straight appearance. This is often observed in narrowed and variably stiff loops, and indicates deep involvement of the intestinal wall.

At earlier stages, juxtaposed or distant nodules with blurred contours can be observed. They are due to hypertrophy of lymphoid follicles.

At the scarring stage, a cobblestone appearance due to crisscrossing fibrous tracts may be observed in a narrowed loop with smooth contours and may be difficult to distinguish from certain noduloulcerative images (which sometimes have a straight tangential appearance). Isolated, round or digitiform scarred polyps with sharply delineated margins are sometimes found on double contrast.

They are less frequent in the small intestine than in the colon.

Ulcerations

The *aphtoid* ulceration produces a concentric image on frontal views, consisting of a round, oval or polygonal opaque barium pool, one to several millimeters in diameter, surrounded by a lucent halo. On tangential views, the appearance is that of an addition image, not very deep and delineated by a ridge. An aphtoid ulceration is a sign of relatively superficial disease in the intestinal wall. It is seldom observed on severely diseased loops and must be searched for at the border of normal and injured areas, near the more advanced lesions. The right amount of compression must be applied since an ulceration does not appear if the compression is not sufficient and disappears if it is too strong. Aphtoid ulcerations are not specific for Crohn's disease, and are encountered in other diseases such as yersiniosis. However, it is a good indication of Crohn's disease and may be its earliest sign. It sometimes heals without scarring.

The linear ulcer or *rhagade* is the most specific sign of Crohn's disease. It appears on frontal views as a longitudinal opaque line, one to several centimeters long and surrounded by convergent folds. On tangential views, it produces a linear image, one to several millimeters thick, in the concavity of an

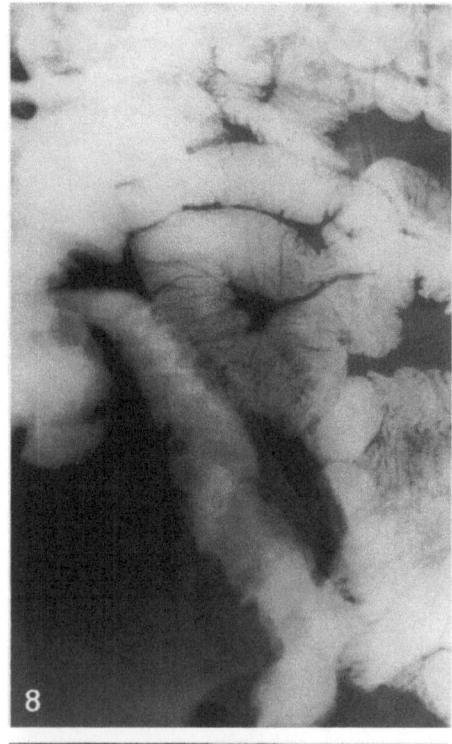

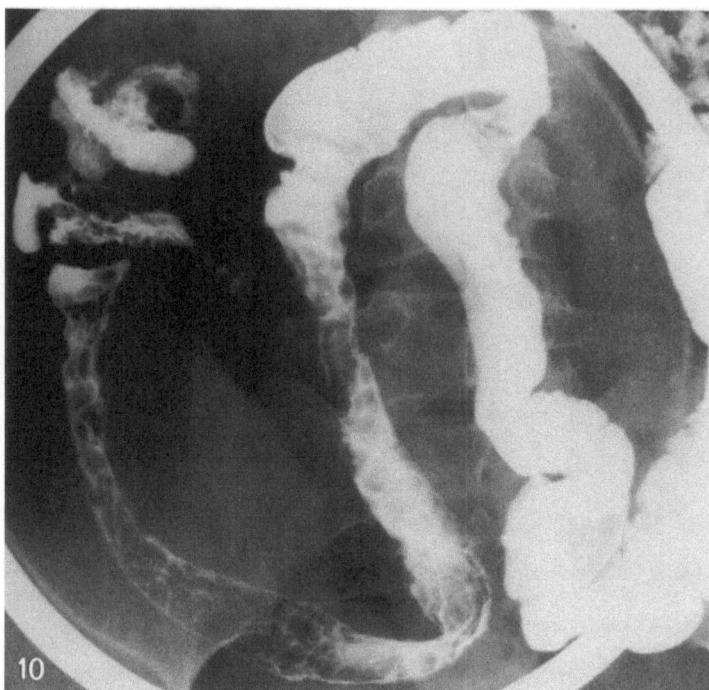

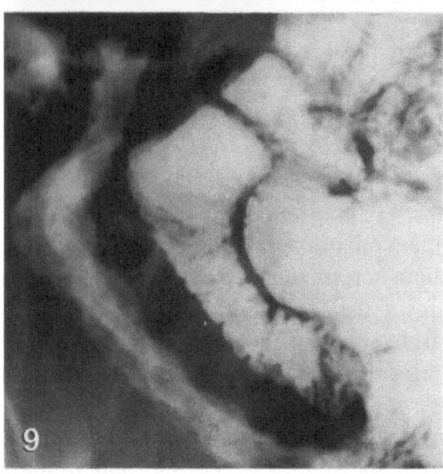

Fig. 8. Crohn's disease : nodulo ulcerated pattern of the terminal ileum

Fig. 9. Crohn's disease : nodulo ulcerated pattern and a mural expansion default in the terminal ileum

Fig. 10. Crohn's disease : flattened nodulation and narrowed terminal ileum

ileal loop from which it is separated by a lucent lining. The image is continuous or discontinuous and may be over twenty centimeters long. Like aphtoid ulcerations, it goes undetected with insufficient compression, and disappears with excessive compression. The lesion is often noticed because of large, transverse or slightly converging folds. The residual fissure left when a linear ulcer heals is difficult to distinguish from the evolving linear ulcer.

Triangular, diamond-shaped or polygonal ulcerations, either isolated or in continuity with a linear ulcer, can be observed. Connected aphtoid ulcerations may produce geographic ulcerations, but this is difficult to demonstrate unless double contrast is used.

Variably deep *transmural* ulcerations perpendicular to the wall are frequent in Crohn's disease but not specific, since they can also be observed in other diseases such as tuberculosis. They can heal or go on to produce peri-ileal abscesses.

Abnormal folds
Abnormal folds are observed at all stages of the

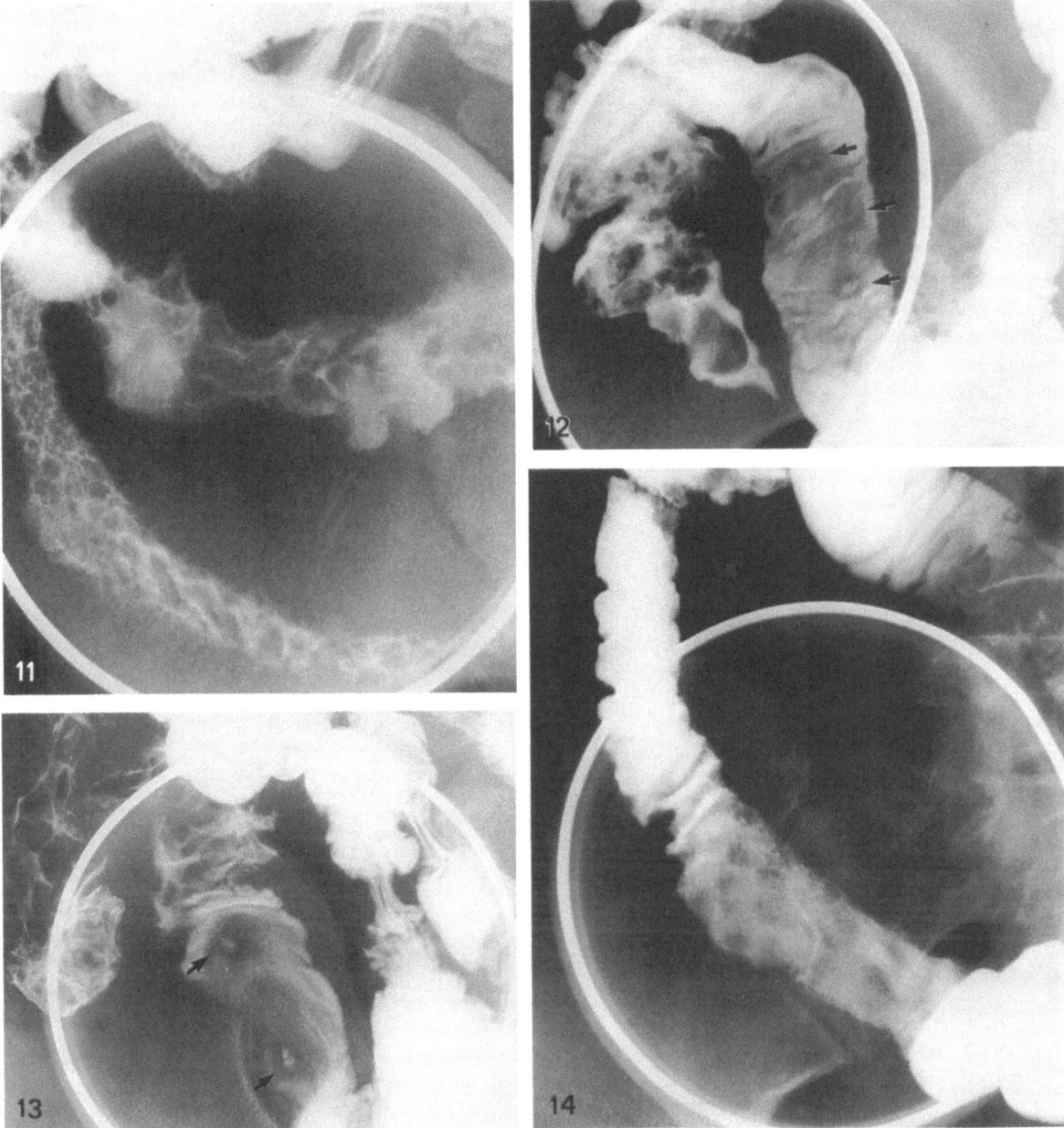

Fig. 11. Crohn's disease : reticulation and nodulo ulcerated pattern of a pelvic loop

Fig. 12. Crohn's disease. 3 aphtoid ulcerations in the terminal ileum

Fig. 13. Crohn's disease. 2 aphtoid ulcerations in the terminal ileum

Fig. 14. Crohn's disease. Scattered aphtoid ulcerations and punctated appearance of the terminal loop after ileocolic resection

disease and are sometimes its first sign when thickened or nodular transverse folds with degraded contours are observed. This is sometimes also the first sign of recurrence following intestinal resection. It may also be observed in the proximity of advanced lesions. Thickened transverse folds produce marginal spiculations, which may be difficult to distinguish from ulcerations, adhesions or internodular recesses. Fold abnormalities can disappear without residual signs.

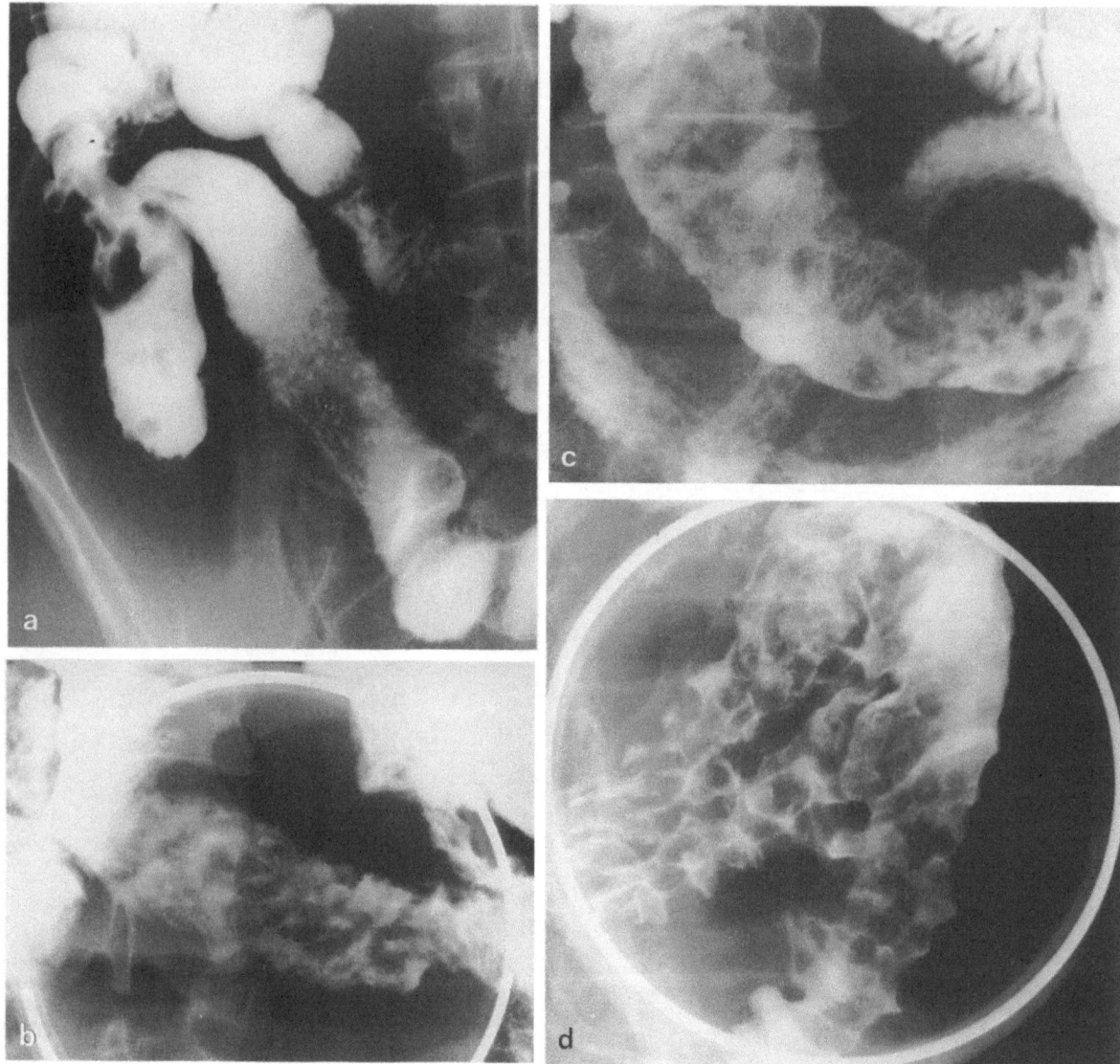

Fig. 15 a-d. Crohn's disease. Scattered aphtoid ulceration on a punctated background. The image are different according to whether the ulcerative or the nodular components dominate

Abnormal villous pattern

A fine punctated appearance of the mucosa, associated with a microspiculated image of its margins due to broadened villi, is frequently observed in Crohn's disease, either in areas without folds or on the thickened folds. Small aphtoid ulcerations or nodules are sometimes hardly visible when superimposed over this punctated background. This appearance may be the first sign of the disease or may be seen close to advanced lesions. It is not specific for Crohn's disease as it is observed in Whipple's disease, alpha-chain disease, radiation-induced enteritis, ischemia, hypoproteinemia, etc. After resection or in case of exten-

sive alteration of the small intestine, it indicates the functional adaptation of the villi in the remaining portion of the small intestine. Abnormalities of the villous pattern may disappear without residual signs.

Evolution of the radiologic appearance of the lesions in Crohn's disease

Grouping the basic lesions allows for the distinction of various stages in Crohn's disease. The disease does not automatically evolve from one stage to another and there is no absolute relation between the

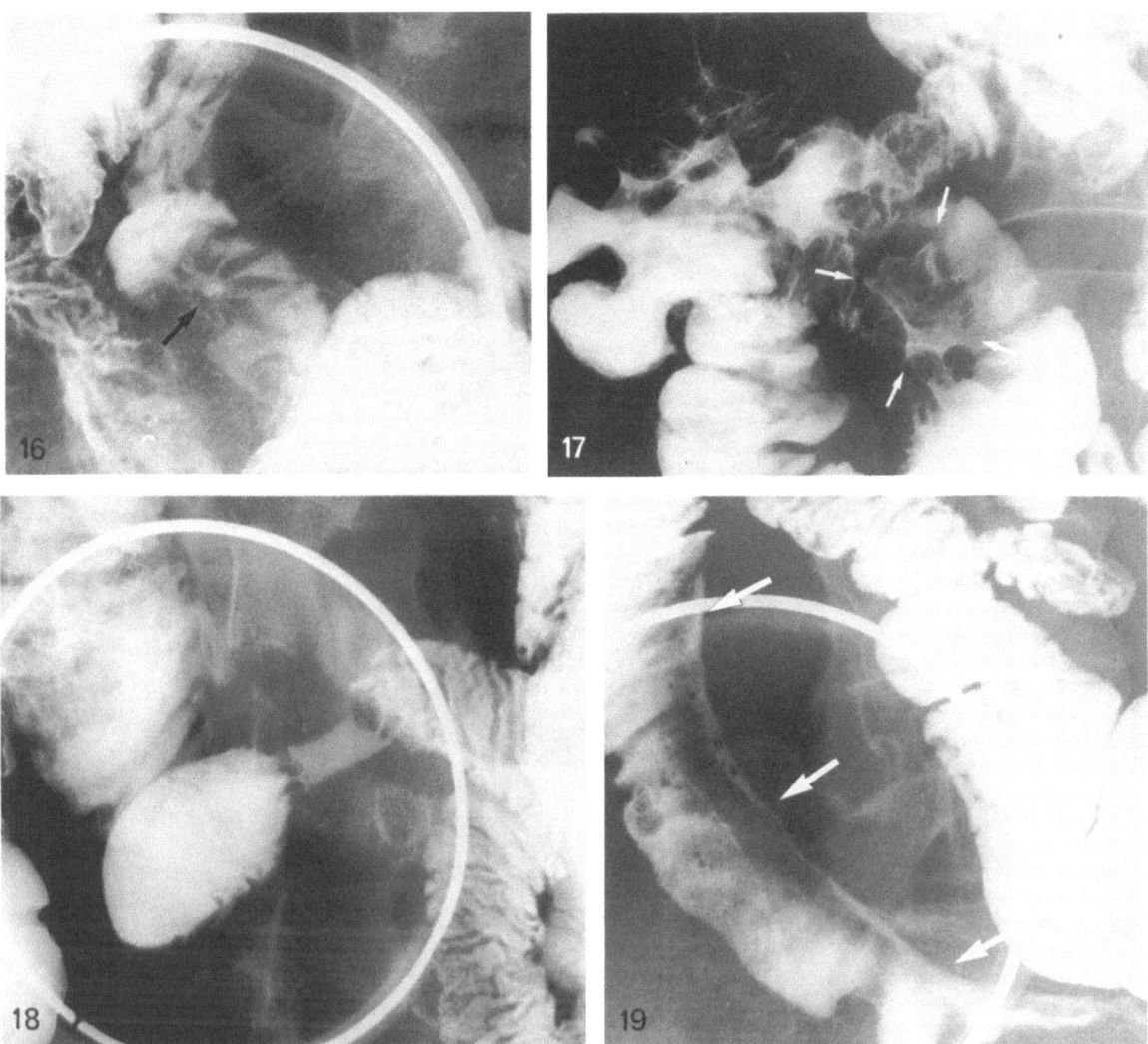

Fig. 16. Crohn's disease. Small star-shaped ulceration of the terminal ileum, outlined by converging folds

Fig. 17. Crohn's disease. Quadrangular ulceration of the terminal ileum, outlined by the convergence of large, nodular folds

Fig. 18. Crohn's disease. Quadrangular, stenosing ulceration

Fig. 19. Crohn's disease. Rhagade along the mesenteric aspect of an ileal loop, outlined by a ridge

age and stage of the disease, or between the clinical pattern and the radiological appearance. However, stenoses, occurence of fistulae and diffuse involvement usually correspond to an aggravation of the clinical signs.

Follow-up examinations permit the assessment of the progress of Crohn's disease: length of the affected intestinal segment, depth of the ulcers, caliber of stenosis, suprastenotic dilatation, extent of mesenteric involvement and of fistulae as well as the occurrence of distant lesions.

Terminal ileitis (figs. 31 to 43)
The most frequent site of Crohn's disease is the terminal ileum. The length of involvement usually exceeds 10 cm.

Stage 1 is characterized by superficial involvement of the intestinal wall, which may heal completely. Early disease is manifested as a punctated appearance, thickened and nodular folds, and aphtoid ulcerations. The three are often found together, with any one being more prominent according

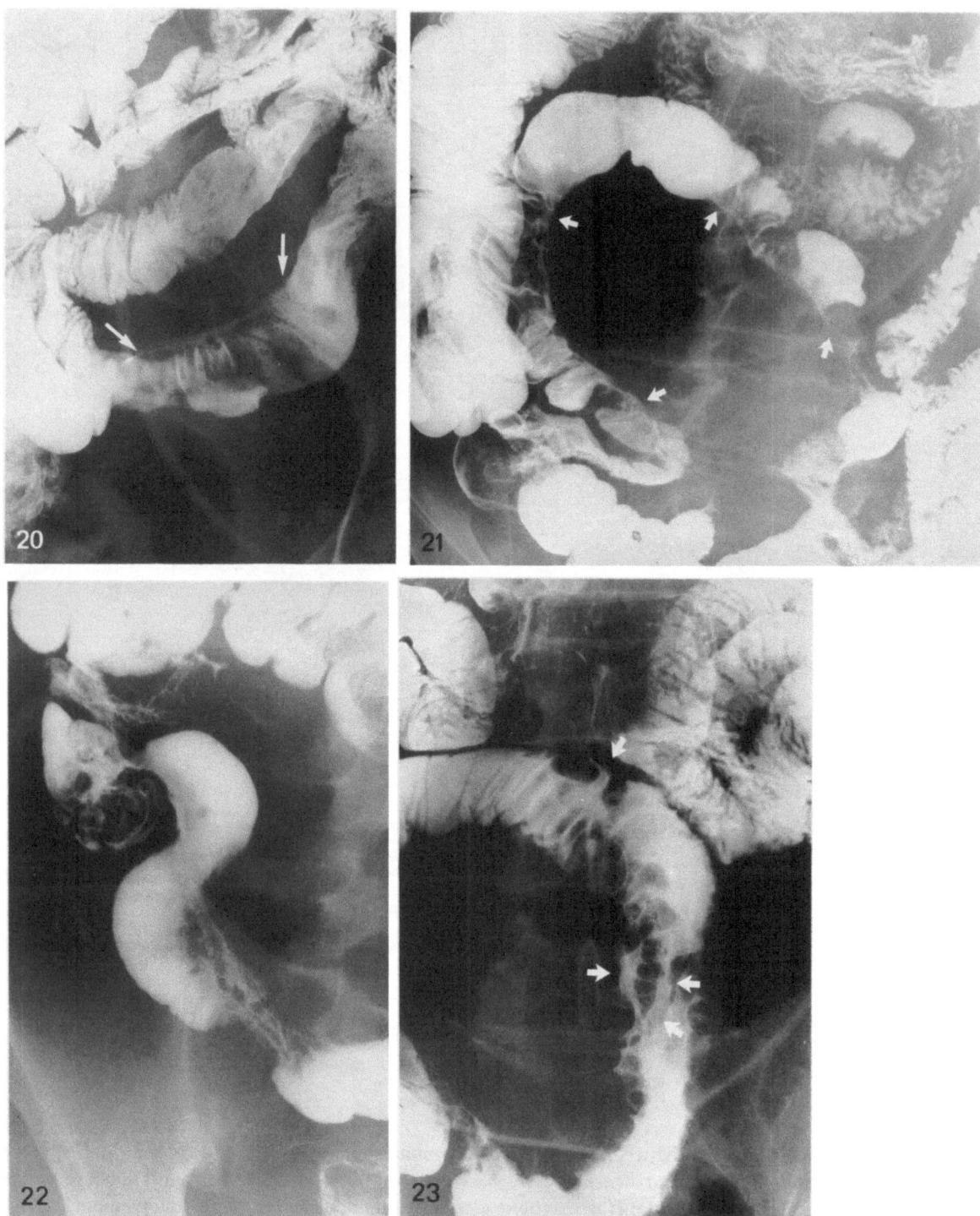

Fig. 20. Crohn's disease. Rhagade along the mesenteric aspect of an ileal loop, outlined by converging folds

Fig. 21. Crohn's disease. 25 cm rhagade, the course of which is interrupted in its upper part because of insufficient compression

Fig. 22. Crohn's disease. Rhagade in the terminal ileum on frontal view, outlined by a nodulation

Fig. 23. Crohn's disease. Ulceronodular appearance of an ileal loop

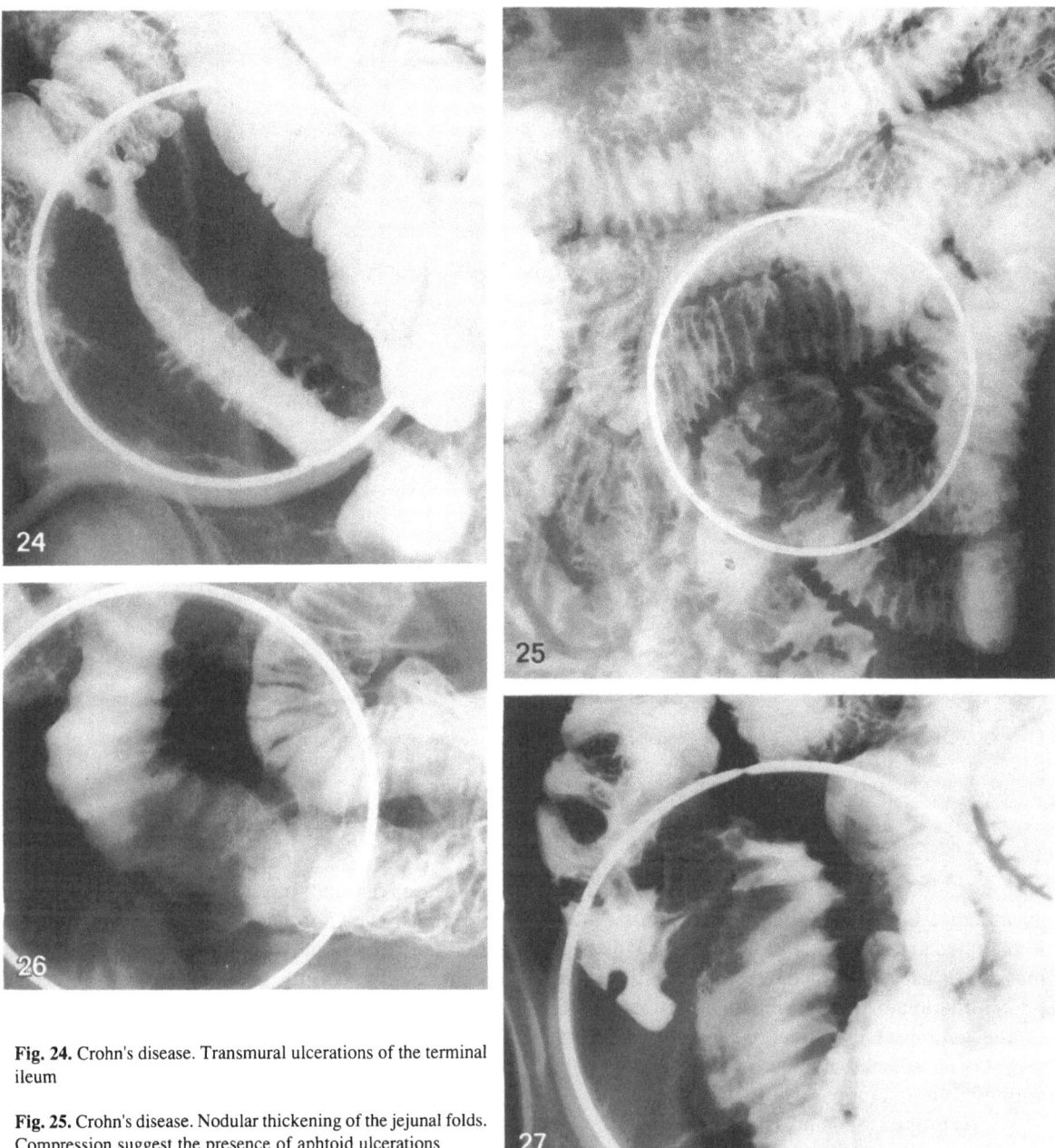

Fig. 24. Crohn's disease. Transmural ulcerations of the terminal ileum

Fig. 25. Crohn's disease. Nodular thickening of the jejunal folds. Compression suggest the presence of aphtoid ulcerations

Fig. 26. Crohn's disease. Large nodular folds with indistinct contours (contrast medium dilution) in the terminal ileum, with scattered aphtoid ulcerations

Fig. 27. Crohn's disease. Large, slightly nodular transverse folds in the terminal ileum

to how vigorously compression is applied. The attention of the radiologist is invariably drawn to the thickened folds of the terminal ileum. Appropriate compression demonstrates the punctated surface on which aphtoid ulcerations begin to appear. The association of these three signs evokes Crohn's disease but may be observed in other forms of ileitis.

Stage 2 is characterized by the occurrence of ulcerating lesions in the intestine and the mesentery, which will heal with scar formation.

The most typical appearance of Crohn's disease has been perfectly described by Bodart, who distinguished three segments in the terminal ileum: the more seriously affected terminal segment is

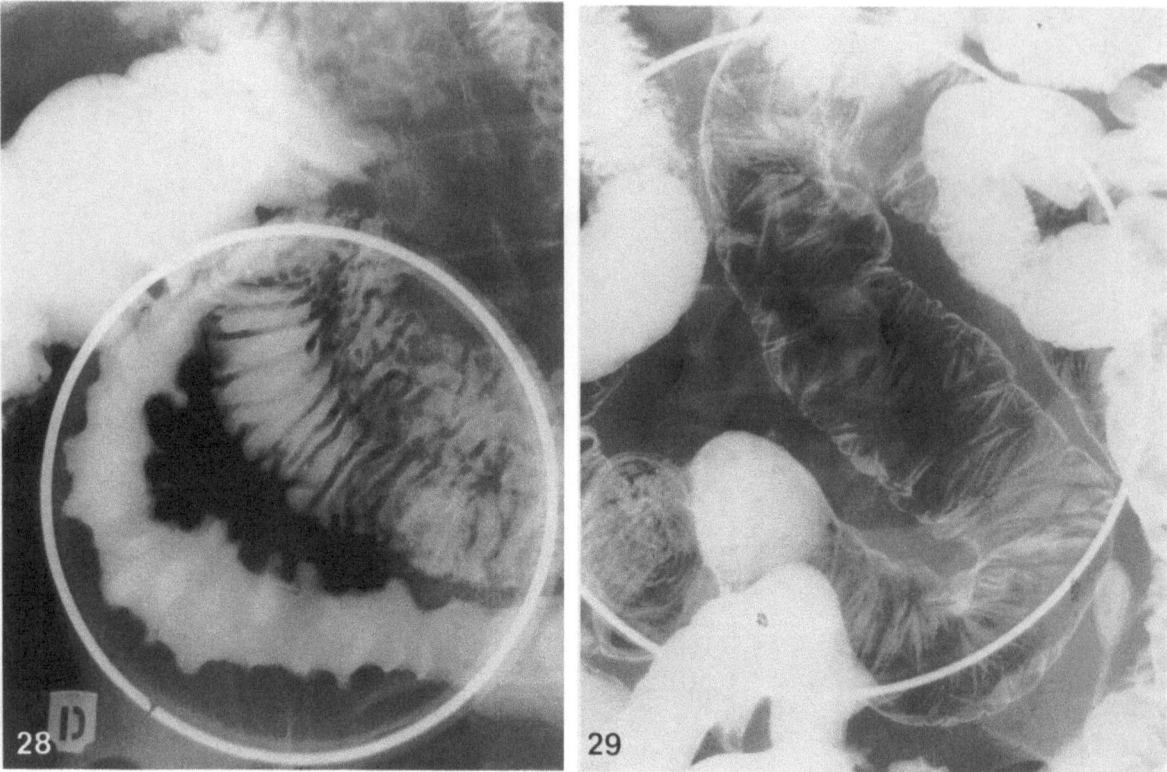

Fig. 28. Crohn's disease. Large, partially effaced nodular folds. the interfold recesses are not easily distinguished from the mucosal ulcerations

Fig. 29. Crohn's disease. Loss of orientation of the jejunal folds because of scarring

narrowed down to a «string»-like appearance ; the asymmetric intermediate segment exhibits a noduloulcerated pattern, sometimes with a rhagade on the mesenteric aspect outlined by large, slightly convergent, inflammatory transverse folds, and sacculation of the antimesenteric side; the proximal segment presents an edematous mucosa with nodular folds, and aphtoid ulcerations.

Appropriate compression and hypotonia often demonstrate the relative extent of the stenosed terminal segment in which a noduloulcerated pattern is detected. They also demonstrate the punctated appearance of the proximal segment.

A widened interloop gap and even a void image near the affected loops are signs of mesenteric extension in Crohn's disease.

The involvement of the ileum is more or less extensive, either continuous or presenting as «skip lesions» with preservation of apparently normal segments. Cecal involvement is often associated with terminal ileitis.

Stage 3 is that of complications of Crohn's disease. The most frequent complication is the ap-

pearance of fistulae, often secondary to transmural ulcerations. They produce opaque lines which course parallel or perpendicular to an intestinal loop where a stenosis is generally present. The variably long course may end abruptly or in a pool image, or the fistula may connect the affected loop to another ileal loop, or to the sigmoid colon, the bladder, neighbouring organs or the skin. The fixed or angulated loops may converge, or remain too distant from each other.

The appearance of an extrinsic compression suggests the presence of an abscess, especially if a neighbouring loop unaffected by the disease demonstrates an inflammatory pattern (hypersecretion, large folds).

In the long term, the extension of a stenosis or the appearance of excavated margins may indicate the presence of a cancer, the clinical and radiological diagnosis of which is difficult. The tumor may develop in a postoperative excluded segment.

Segmental jejunal or ileal involvement (fig. 44)
Some cases of ileal disease without terminal ileum

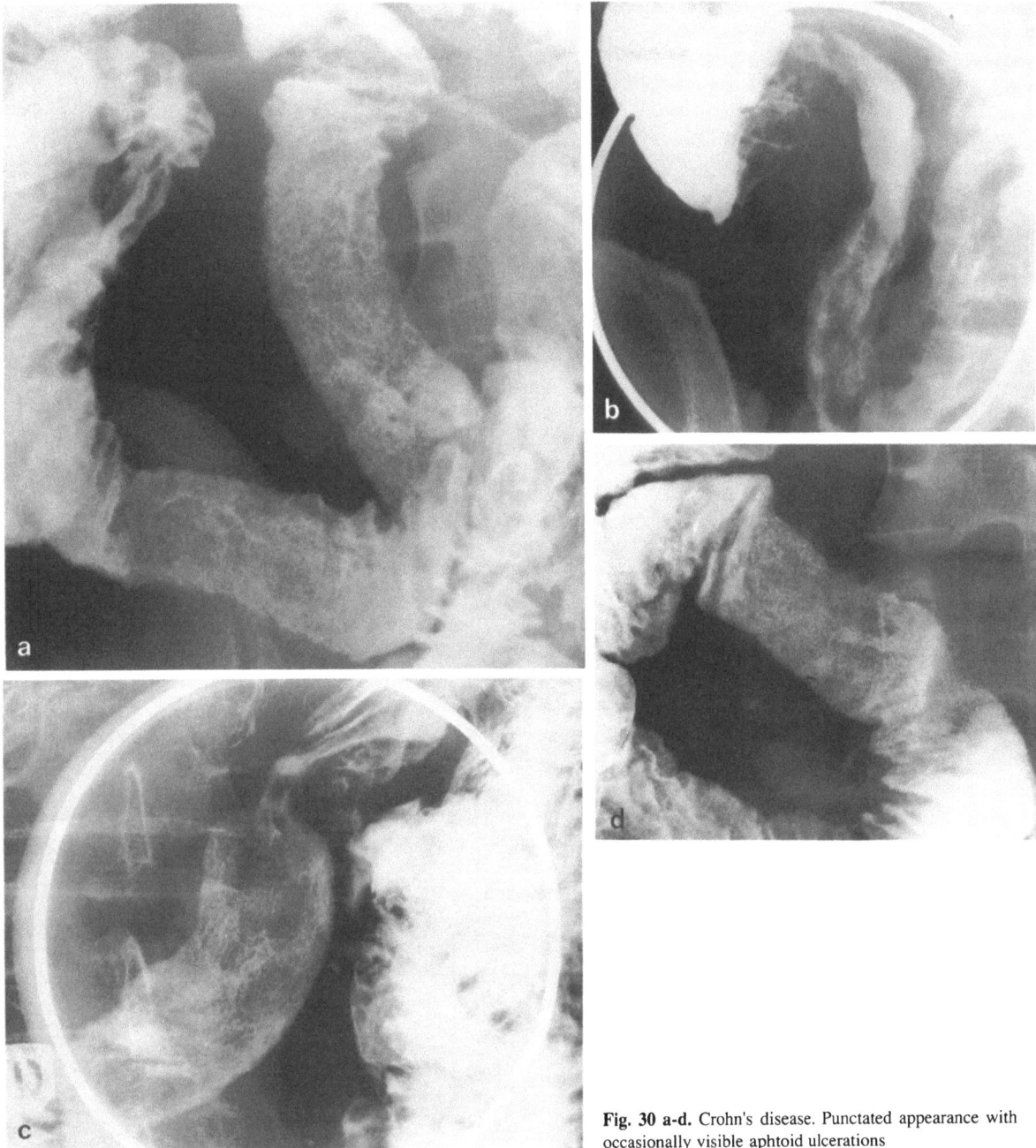

Fig. 30 a-d. Crohn's disease. Punctated appearance with occasionally visible aphtoid ulcerations

involvement have the same appearance as terminal ileitis.

Staggered stenosis may be seen and are often short, tapered either symmetric, sometimes centered on a star-shaped ulceration, or asymmetric with a rhagade on its mesenteric aspect. The junction with the proximal and distal segments is smooth. If the terminal ileum is not involved, the diagnosis of Crohn's disease may be difficult as small aphtoid ulcerations or a punctated appearance may not be visible near the narrowed portions.

Diffuse jejunoileal involvement (figs. 45 to 48)
Crohn's disease may appear as diffuse jejunoileitis with hypersecretion and large folds with indistinct contours. If careful compression of the loops shows micronodulation and little aphtoïd ulcers, there is a high probability of the existence of the disease.

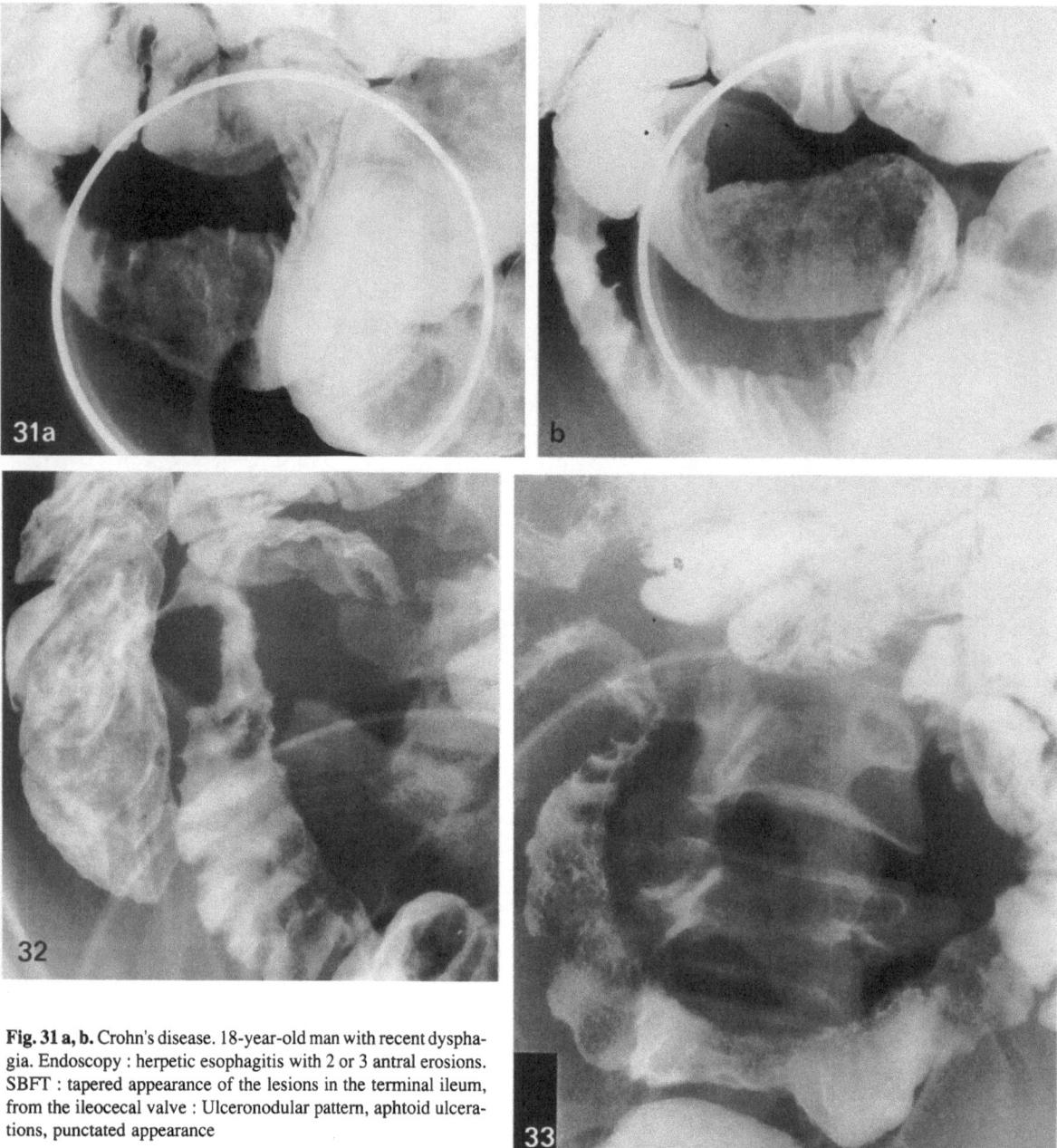

Fig. 31 a, b. Crohn's disease. 18-year-old man with recent dysphagia. Endoscopy : herpetic esophagitis with 2 or 3 antral erosions. SBFT : tapered appearance of the lesions in the terminal ileum, from the ileocecal valve : Ulceronodular pattern, aphtoid ulcerations, punctated appearance

Fig. 32. Crohn's disease. 36-year-old woman. Diarrhea, weight loss. SBFT : tapered appearance of the lesions in the terminal ileum, from the ileocecal valve. Microulcerated narrowing, asymmetric segment with large nodular folds, rare aphtoid ulcerations and punctated appearance

Fig. 33. Crohn's disease. SBFT : microulcerated narrowing, asymmetric segment with large nodular folds, rare aphtoid ulcerations and punctated appearance

Besides the mucosal disease, malabsorption may be a complication if Crohn's disease is very extensive or has required considerable intestinal resection. The degree of functional alterations, either motor or secretory, may partially hide the lesions produced by Crohn's disease.

Postoperative recurrence (figs. 42 and 43)
Postoperative recurrence often presents after resection of the terminal ileum and ileocolic anastomosis, whether associated or not with right hemicolectomy. It can be obvious and produce ulceronodular lesions like in terminal ileitis. If superficial, it presents as

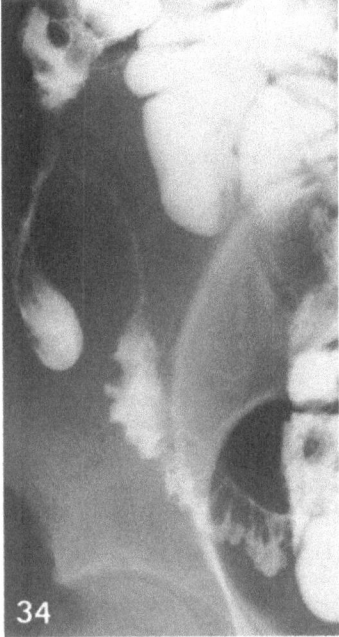

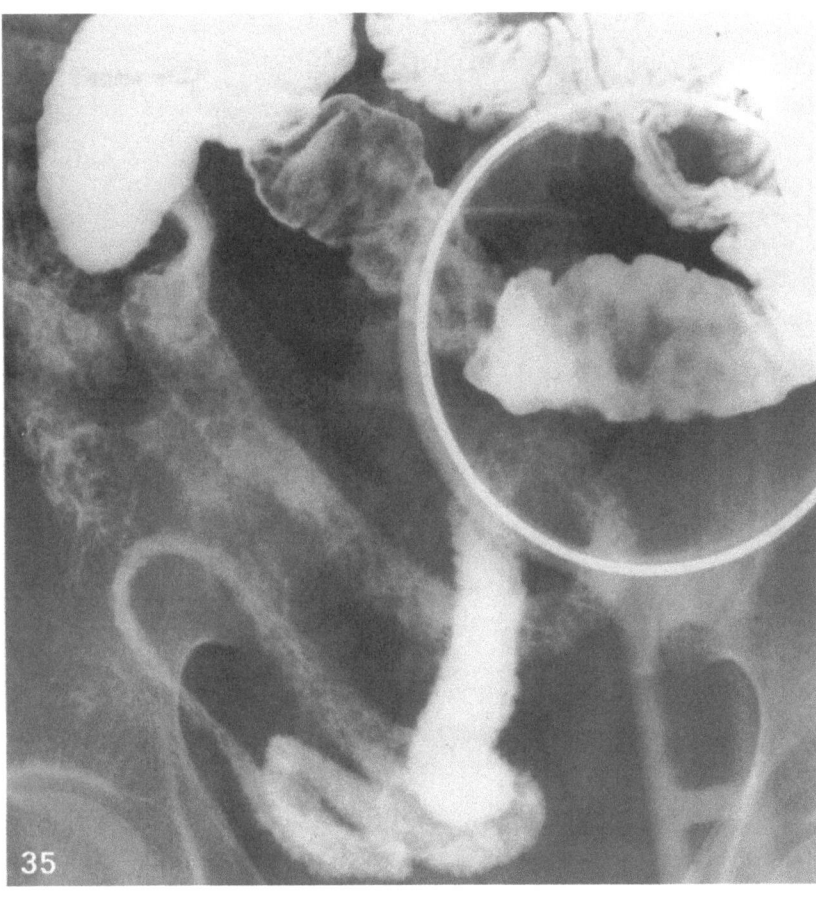

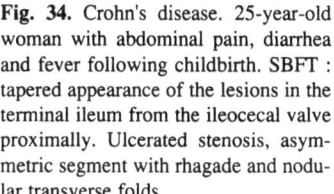

Fig. 34. Crohn's disease. 25-year-old woman with abdominal pain, diarrhea and fever following childbirth. SBFT : tapered appearance of the lesions in the terminal ileum from the ileocecal valve proximally. Ulcerated stenosis, asymmetric segment with rhagade and nodular transverse folds

Fig. 35. Crohn's disease. 38-year-old man. Pain, diarrhea and weight loss over several years. SBFT : tapered appearance of the lesions in the terminal ileum from the ileocecal valve proximally. Abnormal curvature, long stenosis with ulceronodular pattern in the distal loops, with proximal aphtoid ulcerations

an atonic terminal loop with large inflammatory folds, and a punctated appearance or small aphtoid ulcerations. In doubtful cases, a double-contrast barium enema can be helpful in demonstrating recurrence in the anastomosis.

Differential diagnosis

When Crohn's disease combines ulcerative and stenosing lesions at various stages of evolution, the differential diagnosis is inexistant. It becomes more difficult with isolated monomorphic or atypical lesions. Prominent nodulations may suggest lymphoma. One or several sites of stenosis, sometimes ulcerated, suggest ischemia, adenocarcinoma, tuberculosis or metastases. Predominant mesenteric involvement may be found in carcinoid tumors, endometriosis or contiguous inflammation. The careful search for aphtoid ulcerations proximally and distal-

ly, can confirm the diagnosis of Crohn's disease. This is also true in the case of diffuse jejunoileitis.

Disease of the terminal ileum can be caused by yersiniosis, tuberculosis, Behcet's disease or any inflammatory ileitis. The involvement is often less extensive than in Crohn's disease, and rhagades are exceptional. In difficult cases, terminal ileoscopy with biopsy can help in making the diagnosis. In some cases, diagnosis is only made based on the evolution of the disease.

Complementary imaging (figs. 37 to 39)

The radiological search for other sites of Crohn's disease, especially colonic, but gastroduodenal as well, is useful for diagnosis. A radiological assessment of the biliary ducts or of the urinary tract is sometimes necessary to study the extent of disease.

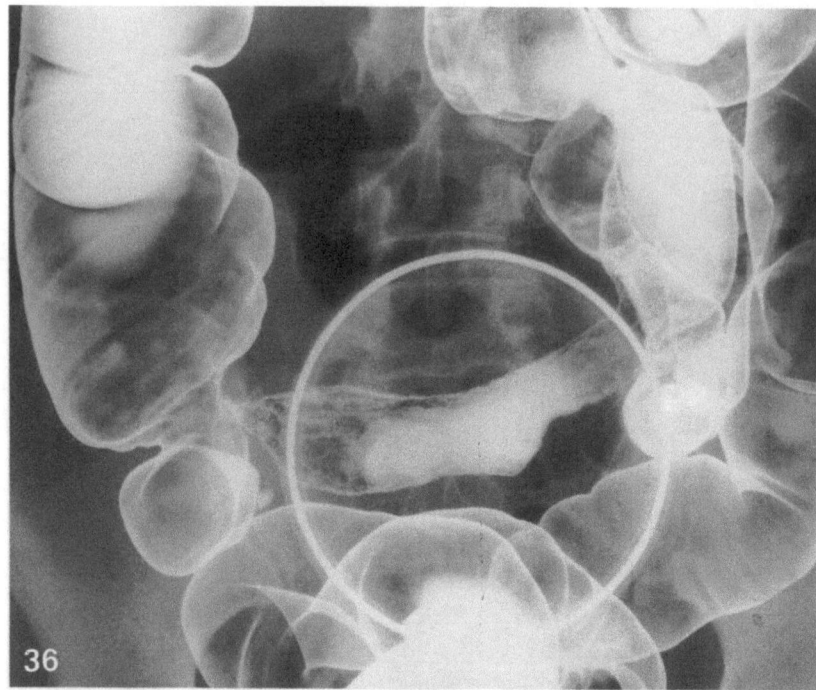

Fig. 36. Crohn's disease. 32-year-old woman,. Diarrhea and abdominal pain aggravated 6 months earlier, following appendicectomy. Double-contrast barium enema : retraction of the cecum and reticulonodulation of the terminal ileum

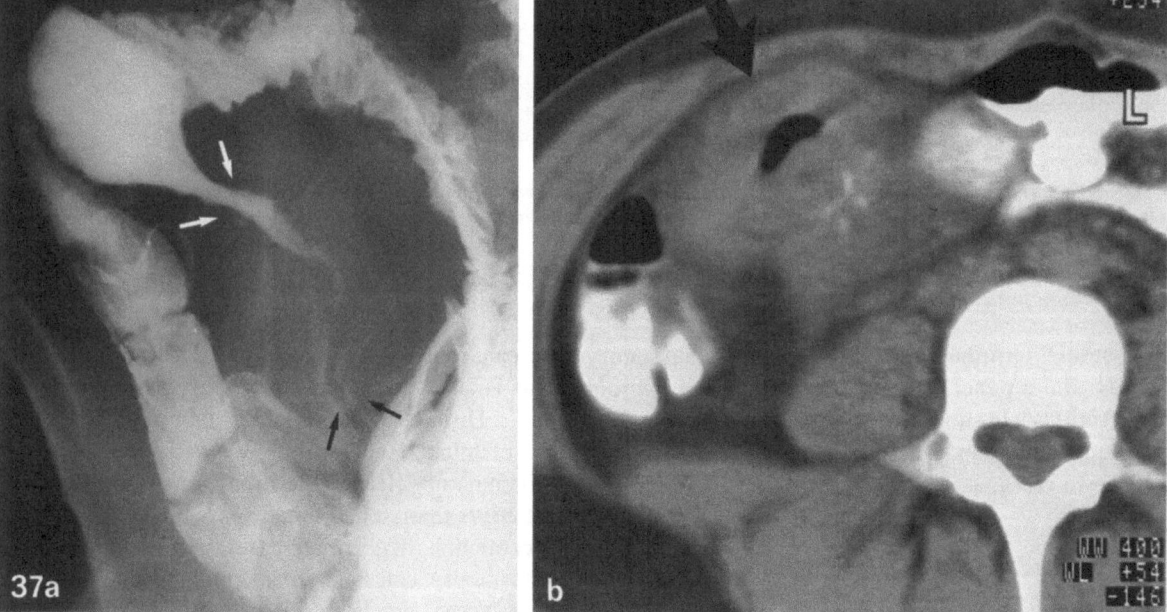

Fig. 37 a-c. Crohn's disease. 24-year-old woman followed up for 4 years, presenting with a febrile exacerbation after pregnancy, with a mass in the right iliac fossa. **a, b** SBFT : 6 cm long ulcerated stenosis of the terminal ileum 5 cm proximal to the ileocecal valve, **c** computed tomography : pseudotumoral thickening of the wall of the terminal ileum

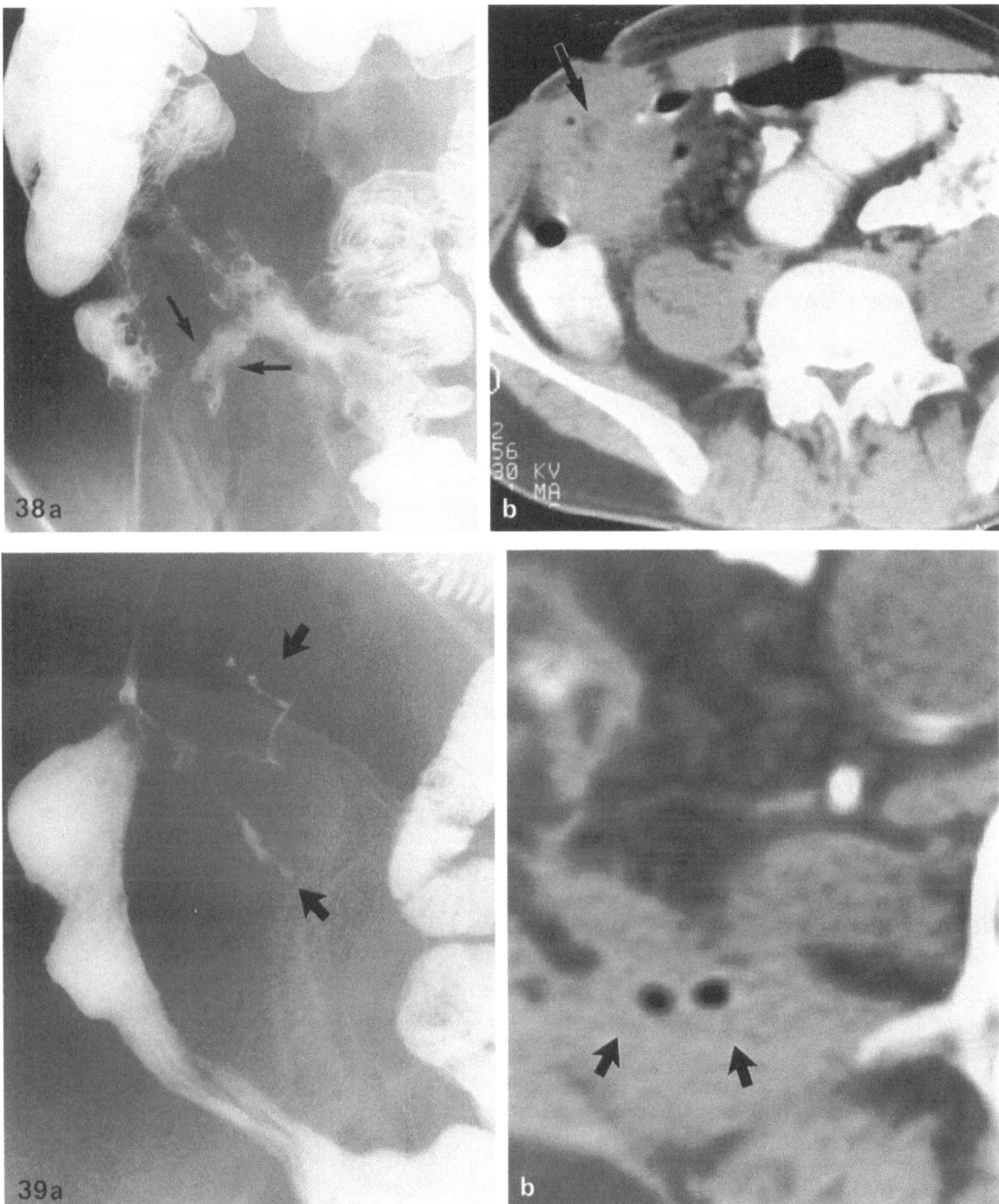

Fig. 38 a, b. Crohn's disease. 35-year-old man operated for a presumed acute perforated appendicitis. **a** SBFT : fistulous course perpendicular to the stenosed and ulceronodular terminal ileum. Cutaneous fistula, **b** computed tomography : abscess in the right iliac fossa

Fig. 39 a, b. Crohn's disease. 37-year-old woman. Abdominal pains, diarrhea, and weight loss. **a** SBFT : branching fistulous tract starting at the ileocecal junction **b** CT : right iliac fossa abscess anterior to the psoas muscle

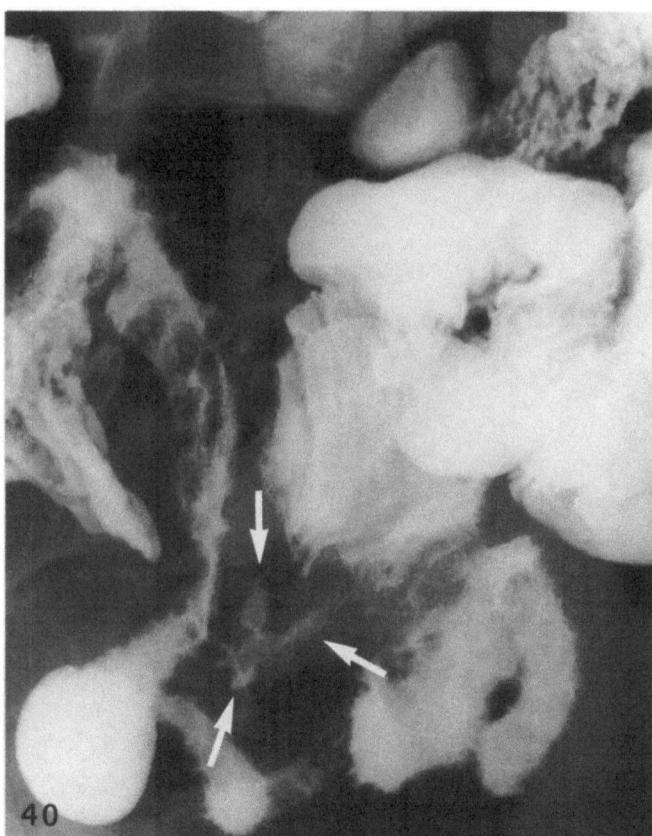

Fig. 40. Crohn's disease. 25-year-old man operated for suppurative appendicitis with a complicating cutaneous fistula. SBFT : convergence of several fixed, angulated and ulceronodulated ileal loops into a small opaque pool representing a peri-ileal abscess

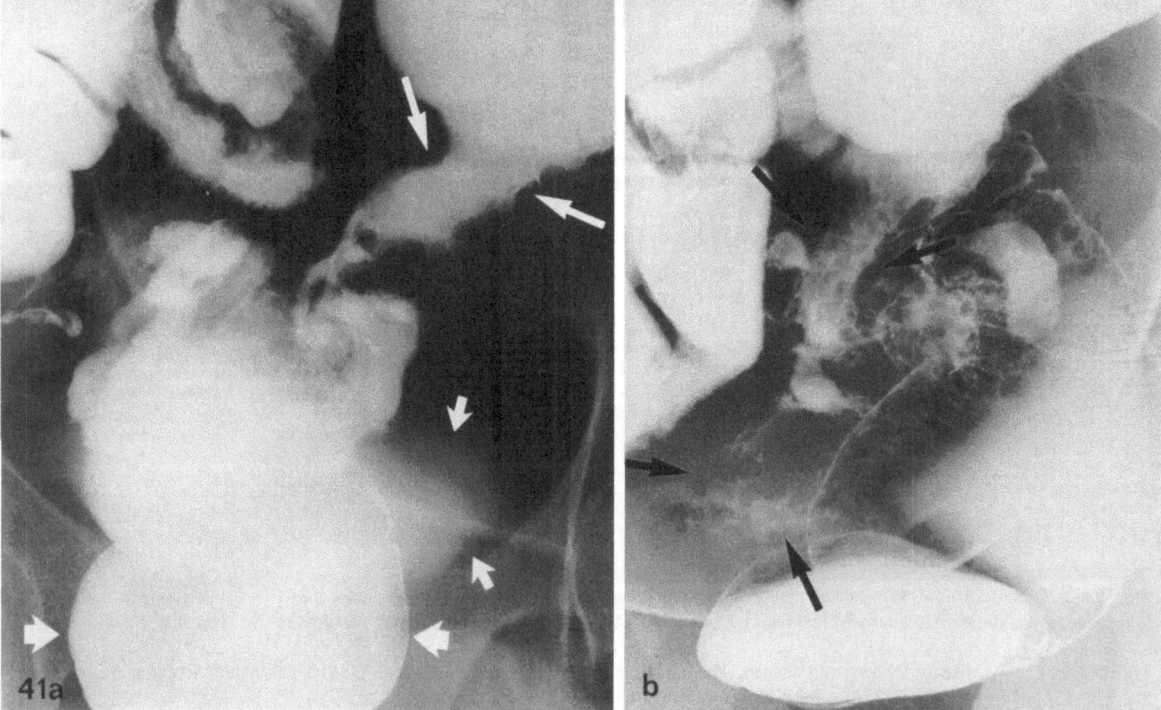

Fig. 41 a, b. Crohn's disease. 30-year-old man. Abdominal colics and weight loss. SBFT : distended ileal loop proximal to an ulcerated stenosis with an irregular fistula standing to both rectum and bladder

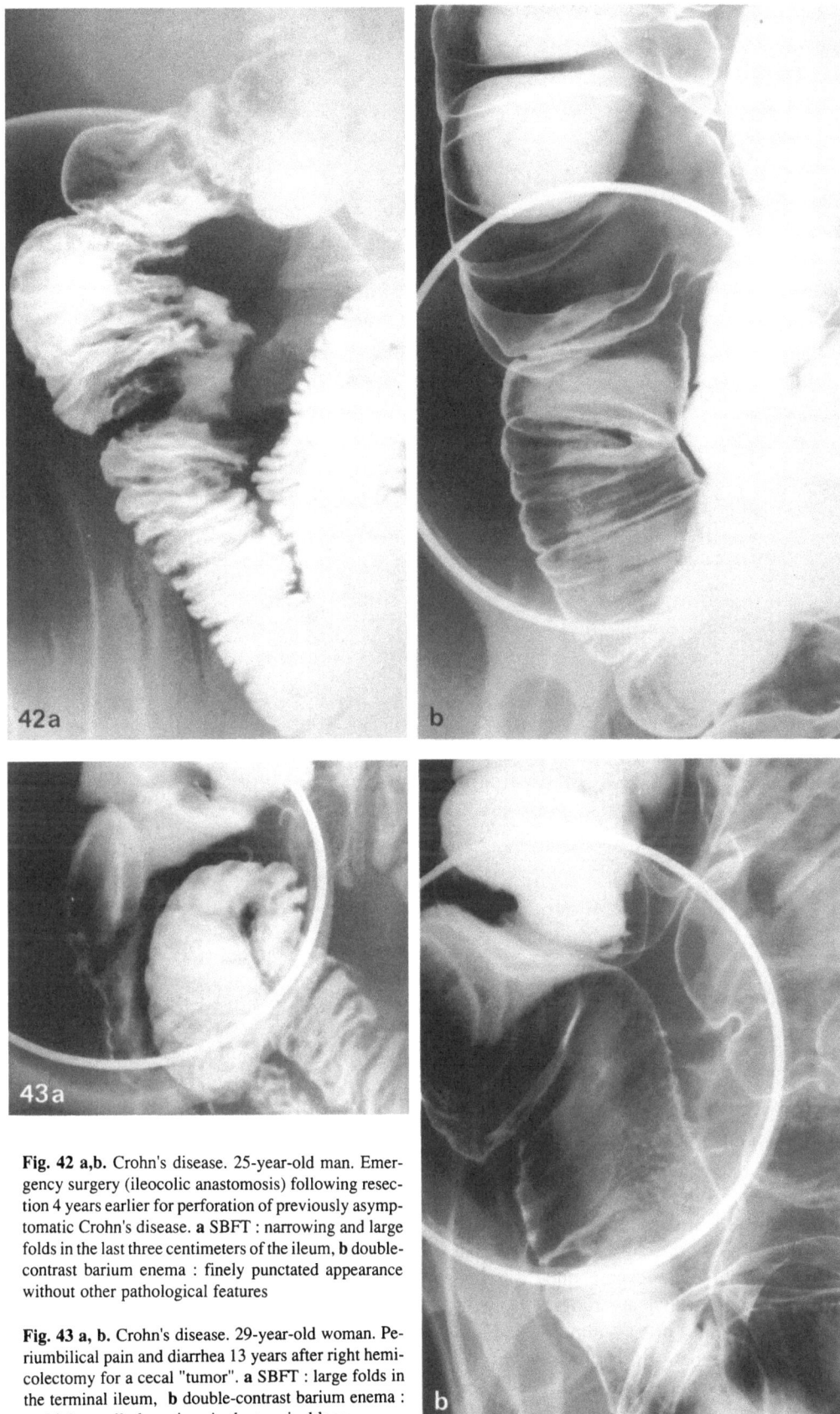

Fig. 42 a,b. Crohn's disease. 25-year-old man. Emergency surgery (ileocolic anastomosis) following resection 4 years earlier for perforation of previously asymptomatic Crohn's disease. **a** SBFT : narrowing and large folds in the last three centimeters of the ileum, **b** double-contrast barium enema : finely punctated appearance without other pathological features

Fig. 43 a, b. Crohn's disease. 29-year-old woman. Periumbilical pain and diarrhea 13 years after right hemicolectomy for a cecal "tumor". **a** SBFT : large folds in the terminal ileum, **b** double-contrast barium enema : multiple small ulcerations in the terminal loop

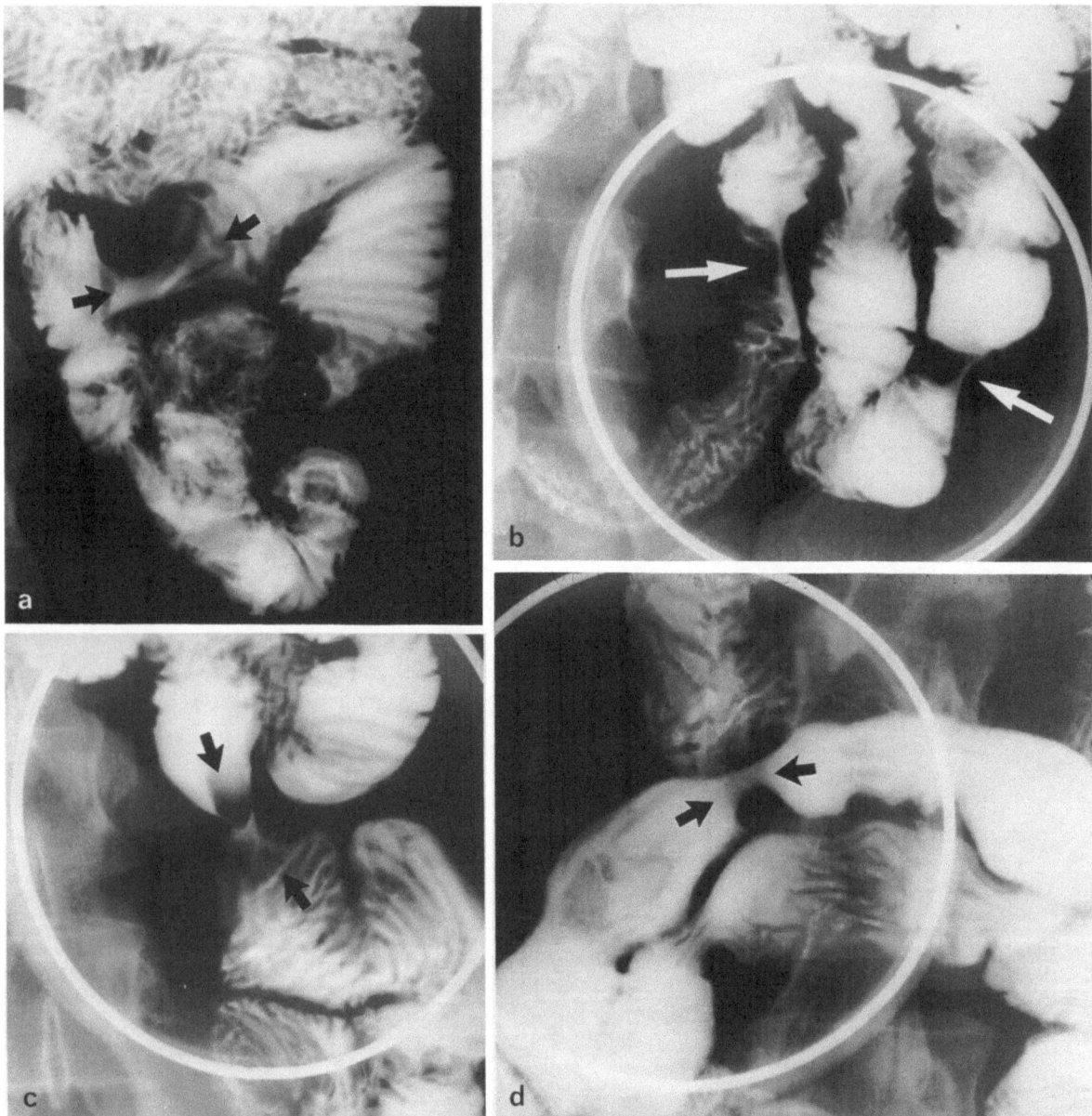

Fig. 44 a-d. Crohn's disease. 26-year-old woman with diarrhea and 8 kg weight loss. SBFT : tiered, short jejunal stenosis, with ulcerations of most of these

Initial *ultrasound* examination sometimes suggests the diagnosis of Crohn's disease if the walls of one or several loops are thickened, thus producing a «sandwich» image on longitudinal and oblique sections, and a concentric image on axial sections, with an echogenic center and a hypoechogenic periphery with a thickness ranging from 5 to 20 mm. The image is most often symmetric and is sometimes lined by a hyper- or hypoechogenic, sometimes heterogeneous, peripheral halo. The visibility of the parietal layers and the gradual, tapered transition

with normal areas differentiate this image from tumoral thickening. Ultrasound can demonstrate the presence of distended or, on the contrary, narrowed loops, either fixed or stiff, a mass lesion produced by a cluster of superimposed loops, a hypoechogenic abscess.

Computed tomography is usually preferred to ultrasound to study the extent of Crohn's disease. It can study the thickness of the intestinal wall, which is usually increased circumferentially, with a narro-

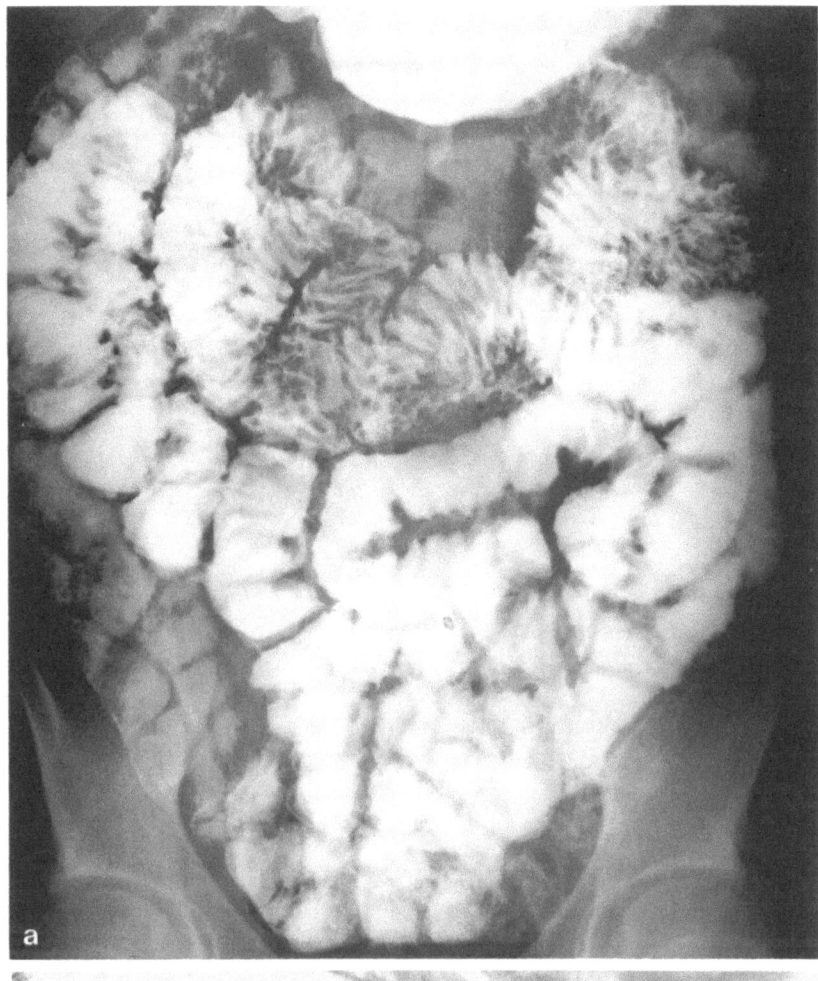

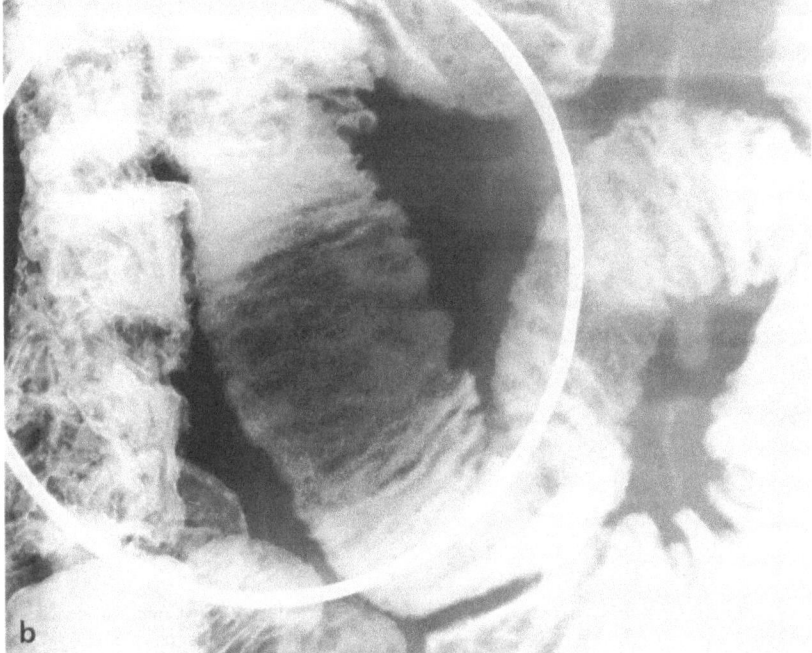

Fig. 45 a, b. Crohn's disease. 19-year-old woman. Febrile diarrhea fot 2 months. **a** SBFT : moderate, diffuse thickening of the wall and folds of the small intestine, suggesting the diagnosis of jejunoileitis. **b** SBFT : 5 months later, scattered aphtoid ulcerations on a punctated background

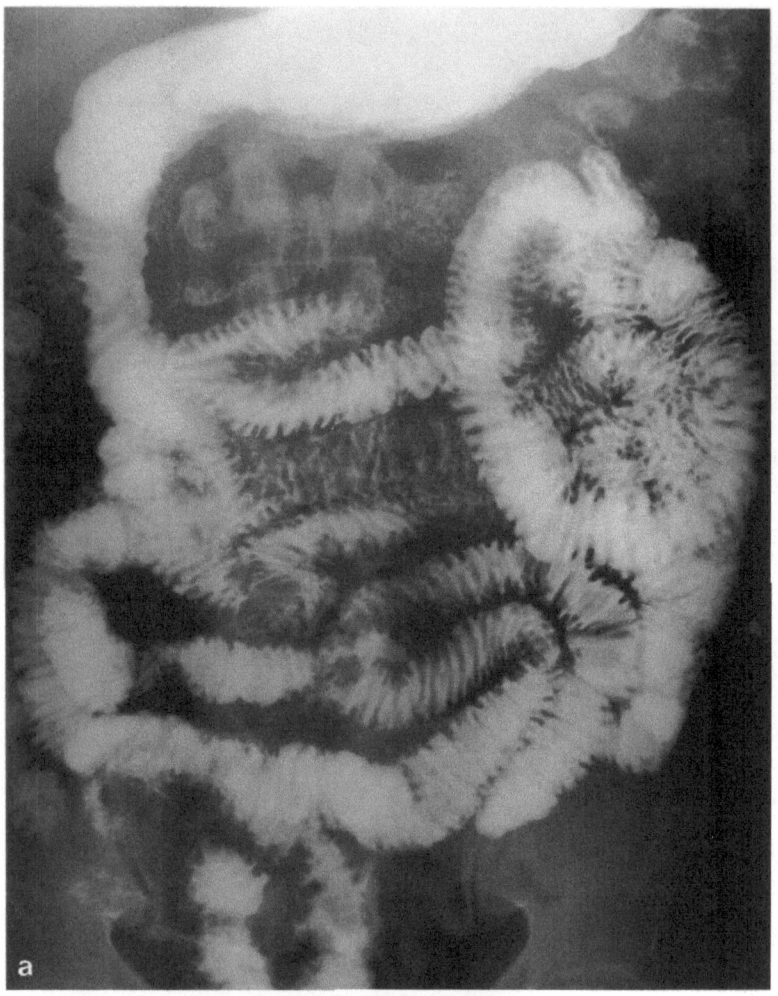

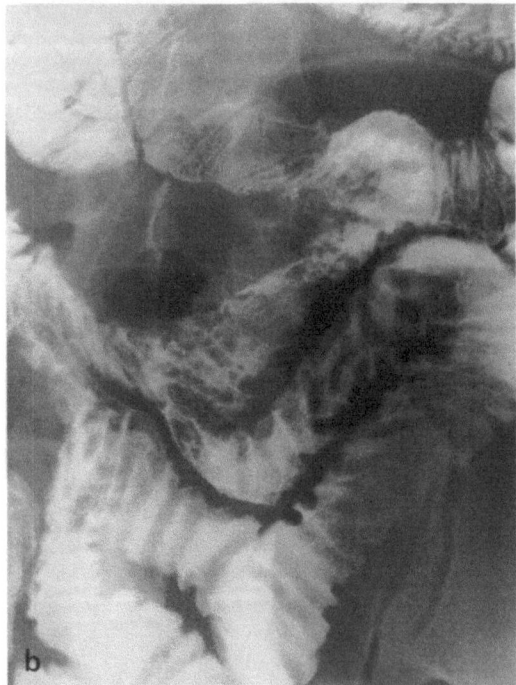

Fig. 46 a, b. Crohn's disease. 43-year-old man. Chronic diarrhea, eczema and polyarticular pains. SBFT : a hypertonia and moderate inflammatory thickening of the duodenojejunal and ileal folds , suggesting inflammatory changes. b compression demonstrates the thickened folds indistinct contours and rare aphtoid ulcerations over a punctated background

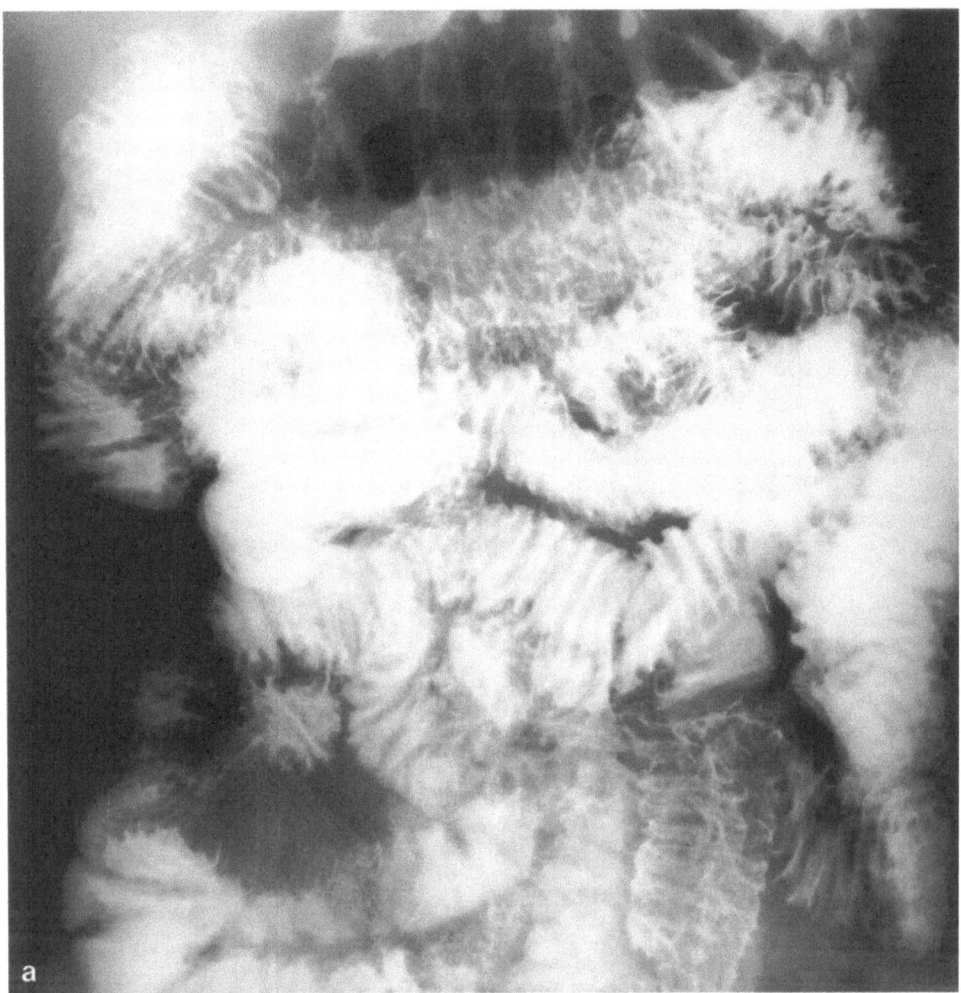

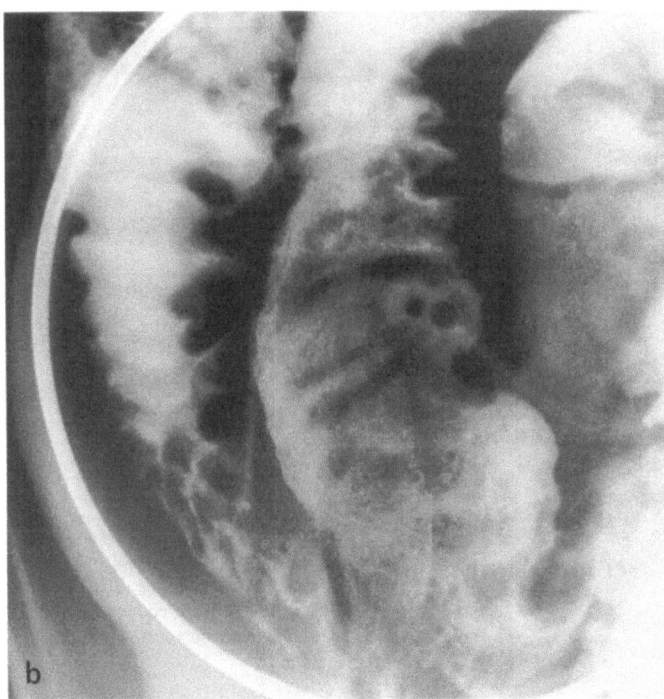

Fig. 47 a, b. Crohn's disease. 24-year-old. Diarrhea, weight loss and leukocytosis. SBFT : **a** appearance of intense jejunoileitis with moderate atonia and contrast medium dilution. **b** compression demonstrates a punctated background with occasional over lying aphtoid ulcerations

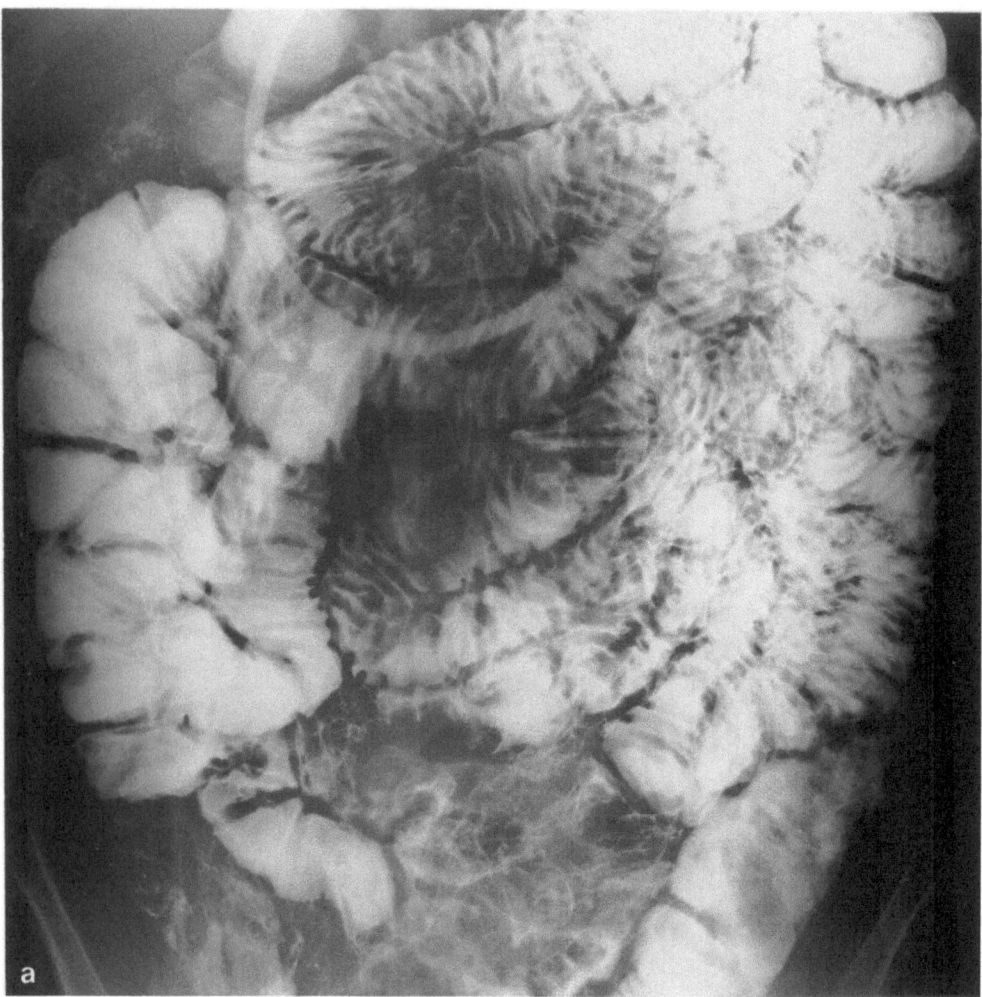

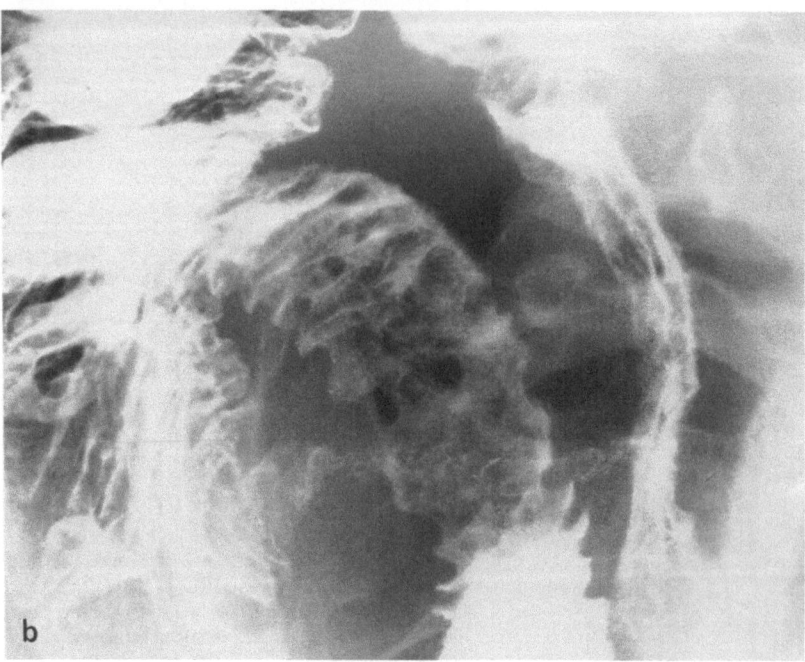

Fig. 48 a, b. Crohn's disease. 25-year-old man. Recent acute diarrhea with an inflammatory syndrome. SBFT : **a** diffuse jejunoileitis. **b** compression of the terminal ileum demonstrates aphtoid ulcerations

wed lumen, and irregular internal and external contours, and rarely visible ulcerations. The density of the thickened wall is the same as that of a normal wall. An annular image has been described after iodinated injection, representing hyperaemia in the mucosal and serosal layers.

Computed tomography is particularly useful to study the extent of the disease outside the intestine, particularly the presence and nature of mesenteric lesions. Focal hypertrophy of the mesenteric fat, without changes in its density, may be observed in early forms of Crohn's disease. Increased density indicates edematous infiltration of the mesentery. Fibrosis accounts for opaque lines or stripes converging towards the root of the mesentery. Mesenteric, and sometimes retroperitoneal adenopathy is frequent. Abscesses can be demonstrated only if all intestinal loops are well opacified, because a mass of loops stuck together may produce a misleading image. Abscesses appear as hypodense areas (sometimes isodense with muscle) with rim enhancement following contrast injection. They sometimes contain gas bubbles, or displace the neighbouring organs. They are sometimes located in the muscles of the anterior abdominal wall, in the extraperitoneal fat or the right psoas muscle, and may extend towards the kidney, the mesentery, the pelvis or the perivesical space. The fistulae causing these abscesses are not always demonstrated. Computed tomography shows the associated lesions of Crohn's disease in other organs such as the colon, the anus, the kidney, the bladder, the hip joints, etc.

In practice

A small bowel follow-through is necessary for the diagnosis and assessment of Crohn's disease.

The fact that lesions vary in severity inversely to their distance from the ileocecal valve is a main element in making the *diagnosis*. Other helpful findings include the presence of asymmetric lesions, their length a rhagade, aphtoid ulcerations, a punctated, appearance and a void surrounding the lesions. Evolutive ulcerated lesions of various ages and severity often coexist with fibrotic scars.

Assesment of the extent of Crohn's disease requires the radiological or endoscopic exploration of the colon and the upper digestive tract after the small bowel follow-through. Computed tomography must be used when the extent of the disease outside the intestine must be known and plays a pivotal role in the detection of abscesses.

Considering the period of evolution of Crohn's disease and the desire to avoid irradiation, radiological examinations must be carried out only when they are likely to alter therapeutic decisions. Comparison with previous examinations is necessary to assess the evolution of the disease. The radiological changes are not always related to the clinical course. However, radiology plays an important role in the assessment of «activity» of Crohn's disease along with the clinical and biological evaluations.

Tuberculosis (figs. 49 to 59)

Small intestinal tuberculosis is due to an infection by Mycobacterium tuberculosis of human or bovine origin. When caused by the human bacillus, the infection is often secondary to pulmonary tuberculosis. In Western countries, about 1% of cases of pulmonary tuberculosis will develop the intestinal form of the disease. This percentage increases with the severity of the disease and reaches 80% for lethal cases. If the bacillus is of bovine origin, the intestine is the primary focus of disease.

Tuberculosis has become rare in France, and one case of intestinal tuberculosis is diagnosed for every 30 cases of Crohn's disease. It is more frequent in poorer populations. It is often primary in these cases, with no associated pulmonary focus (90% of the cases in certain series). The disease appears in young adults between 20 and 40 but may be observed at any age. Women are more frequently affected.

In 85% of the cases, digestive tuberculosis is ileocecal, almost always involves the ileocecal valve. In other cases, multiple jejunoileal lesions are observed. Accompanying involvement of other digestive sites is not rare. Extradigestive involvement, either evolutive or cicatricial, is also frequent in the lungs (50% of all cases), lymph nodes, liver and spleen, kidneys, peritoneum (peritonitis encapsulans and ascites) or bones.

Pathology

Tuberculosis is characterized by inflammation and fibrosis of the intestinal wall and the neighbouring lymph nodes, with a variable appearance according to the stage of disease. At the early stage, the lymphoid follicles and Peyer's patches are swollen, and neighbouring tissue edematous and inflamed. Follicular necrosis and vascular thrombosis are associated with mucosal ulcerations. Subtotal villous atrophy some-

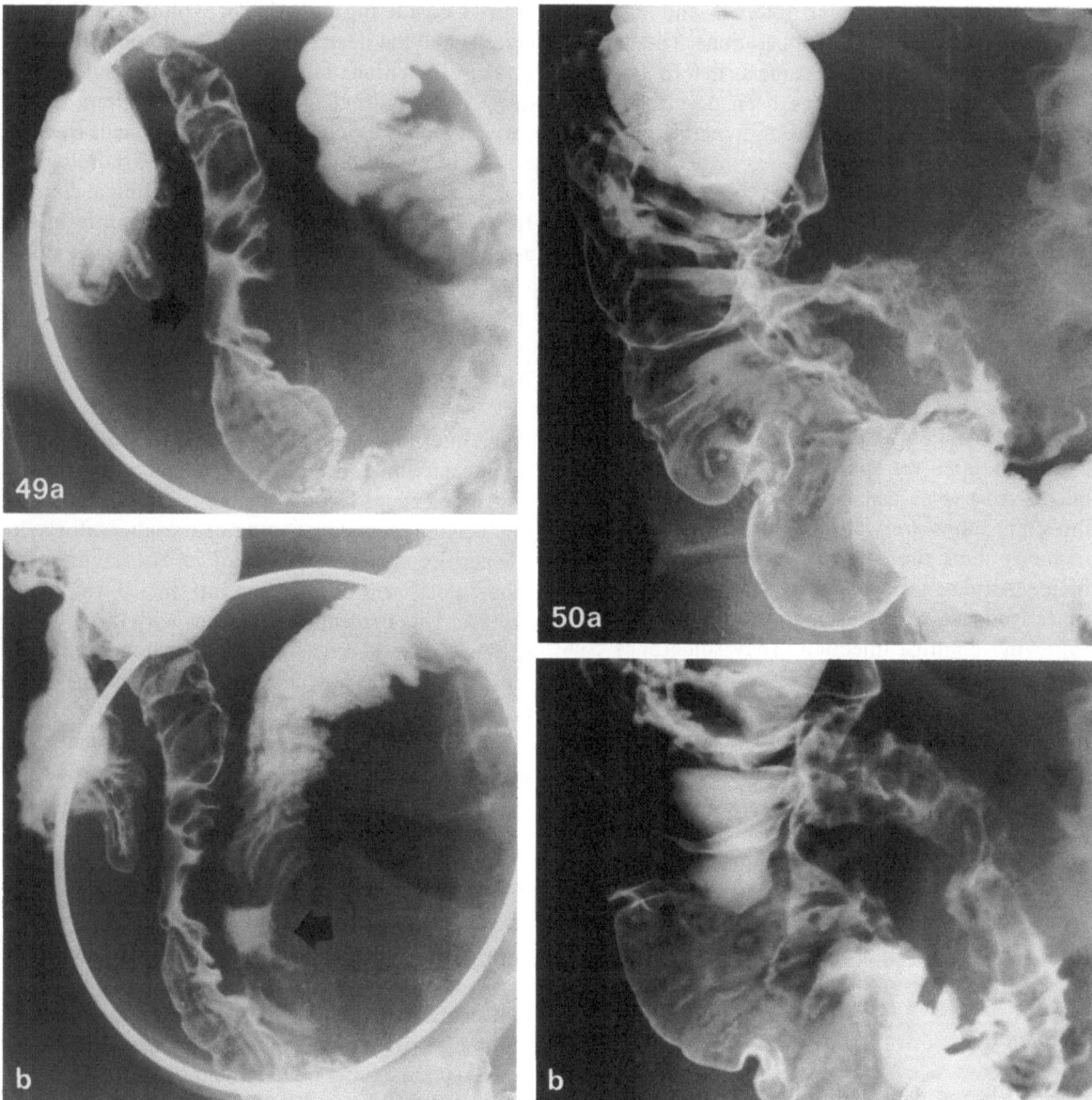

Fig. 49 a, b. Ileocecal tuberculosis. 72-year-old man. Active pulmonary tuberculosis. Recent diarrhea. SBFT : **a** asymetric narrowing, noduloulcerated appearance and quadrangular ulceration of the terminal ileum, **b** quadrangular ulceration of an ileal loop

Fig. 50 a,b . Ileocecal tuberculosis. 28-year-old man. Poor general status and abdominal pain. SBFT : noduloulcerated appearance of the terminal ileum. Abnormal expansion of the wall, aphtoid ulcerations and inflammed cecal folds

times occurs in the diffuse forms. At this stage, complete healing without scarring is possible, even without therapy. If the disease progresses, extensive fibrosis and the persistence of inflammation leads to bowel wall thickening with retraction, and to stenosis of short segments with smooth contours. Ulcers are superficial, multiple, several mm long, linear or star-shaped and surrounded by convergent folds or a ridge. Their course is usually transverse or circu-

lar. Fistulae may appear, burrowing into other intestinal loops, neighbouring organs or the skin. The transition with the normal segments is gradual. In the ileocecal forms, the ileocecal valve is enlarged, stiff and gaping. The walls are thickened, adhesions are prominent, and numerous sites of adenopathy appear. At this stage, treatment cannot prevent stenosis and retraction. The wall has a smooth appearance with some nodules or shows cobblestone nodulation

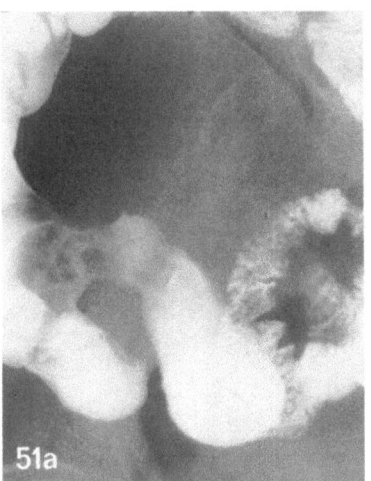
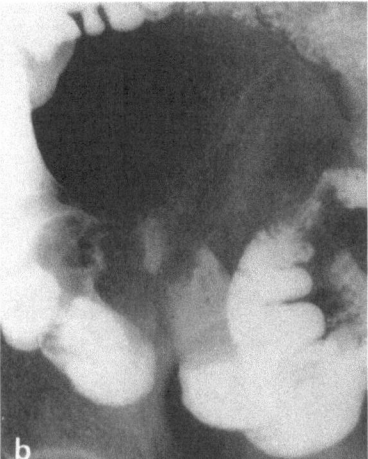
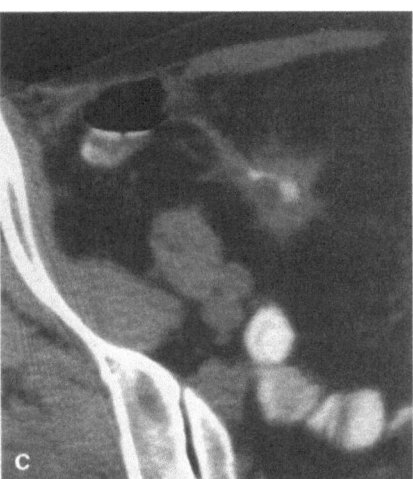

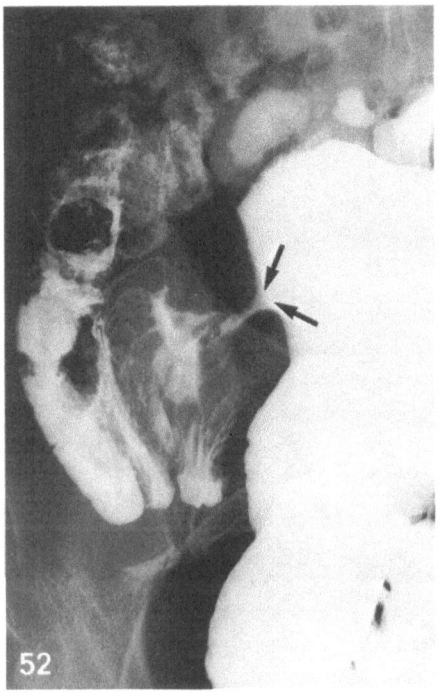

Fig. 51 a, b. Ileocecal tuberculosis. 50-year-old man. Ileocecal tuberculosis discovered 32 years earlier during appendicectomy. Medical treatment. Restant diarrhea and mass in the right iliac fossa. **a** SBFT : large ulceration ridge on the ileal aspect of the ileocecal valve and retraction of the medial edge of the cecum, **b** computed tomography : bowel wall thickening in the terminal ileum with retractile mesenteritis and neighbouring adenopathy

Fig. 52. Ileocecal tuberculosis. 29-year-old man. Subocclusive syndrome. Normal chest X-ray. SBFT : stenosis of the last centimeter of the ileum with considerable proximal distention

due to fibrosis and to the retractile healing of ulcers.

Microscopic study shows the characteristic lesion of tuberculous granulomas, particularly in the submucosa, the serosa and the lymph nodes. Each granuloma is made up of epithelioid cells and giant cells lying at the periphery of caseating necrosis (more frequently in lymphoid tissue). The granulomas are of various sizes, and are often contiguous to edematous and inflammed tissue. Ulcers are superficial and usually do not reach the muscularis. Considerable fibrosis forms septae in the muscularis, the serosa and the lymph nodes.

Clinical findings

Intestinal tuberculosis sometimes has no symptoms, as autopsies series have demonstrated. The clinical signs, if any, are nonspecific and sometimes occur years before the diagnosis is made. In order of decreasing frequency, the signs include abdominal, sometimes not unlike appendiceal pain, a deterioration in the patient's general condition, anorexia, fever, intermittent diarrhea, a palpable mass, nausea and symptoms of partial bowel occlusion. Hemorrhage, perforation, or the development of amyloido-

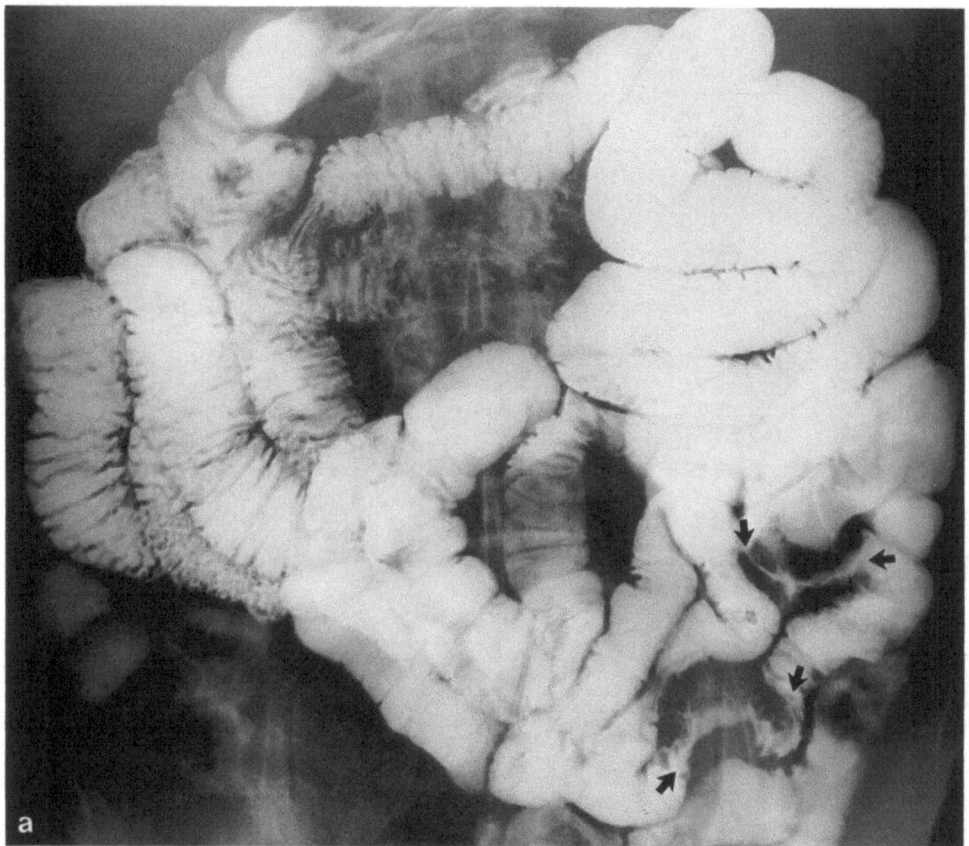

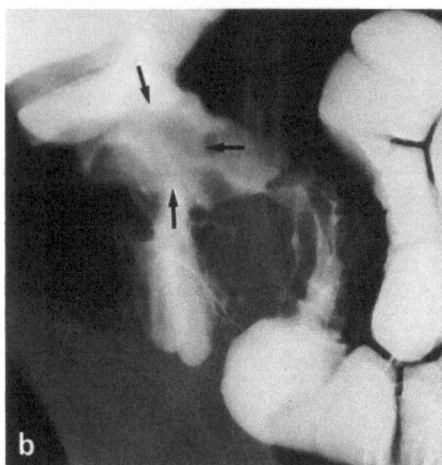

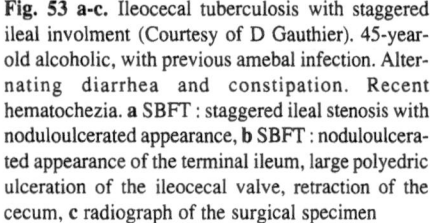

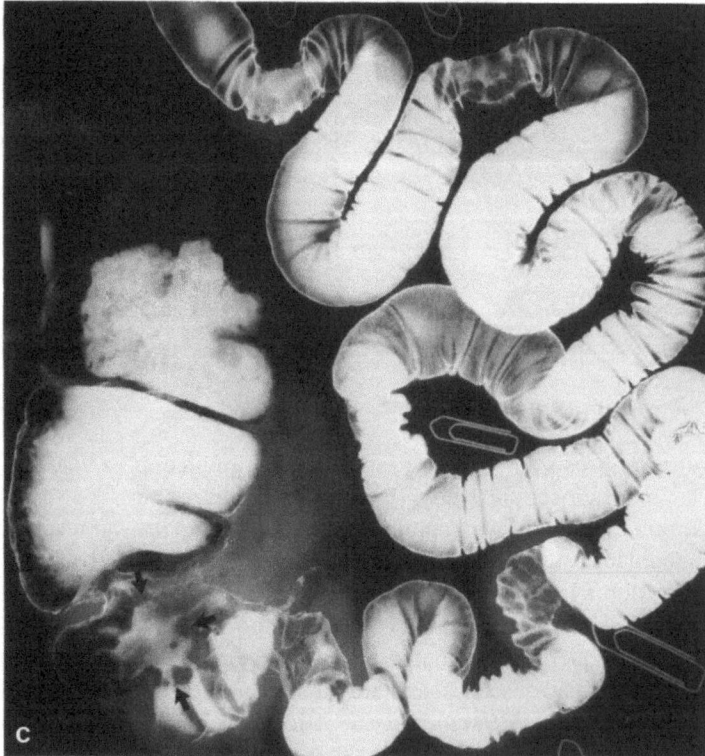

Fig. 53 a-c. Ileocecal tuberculosis with staggered ileal involment (Courtesy of D Gauthier). 45-year-old alcoholic, with previous amebal infection. Alternating diarrhea and constipation. Recent hematochezia. **a** SBFT : staggered ileal stenosis with noduloulcerated appearance, **b** SBFT : noduloulcerated appearance of the terminal ileum, large polyedric ulceration of the ileocecal valve, retraction of the cecum, **c** radiograph of the surgical specimen

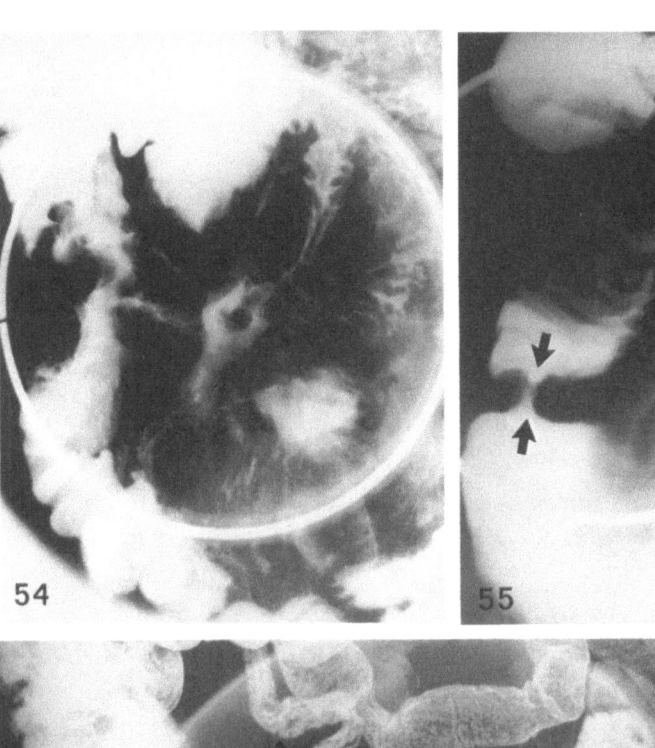

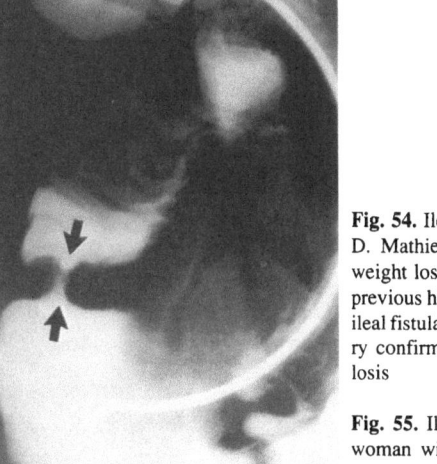

Fig. 54. Ileal tuberculosis (Courtesy od D. Mathieu). 39-year-old man. Fever, weight loss, poor general condition. no previous history of tuberculosis. SBFT : ileal fistula in the right iliac fossa. Surgery confirmed enteroperitoneal tuberculosis

Fig. 55. Ileal tuberculosis. 35-year-old woman with partial bowel obstruction and weight loss. SBFT : short ileal stenosis in the right iliac fossa

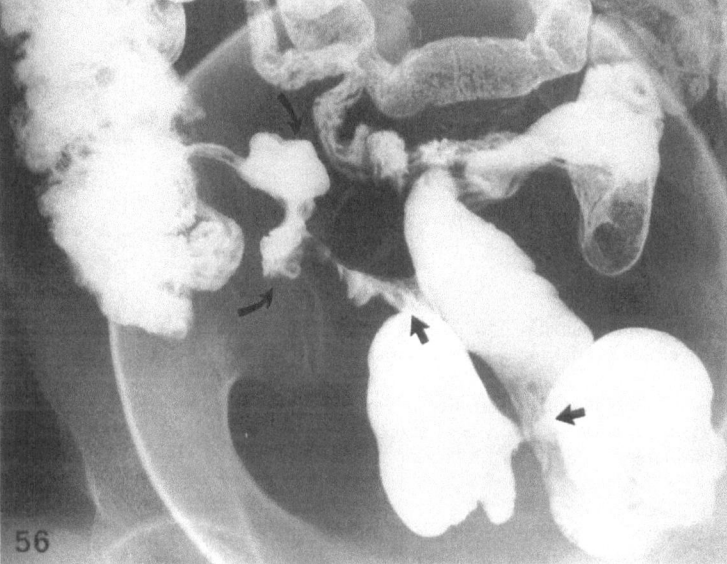

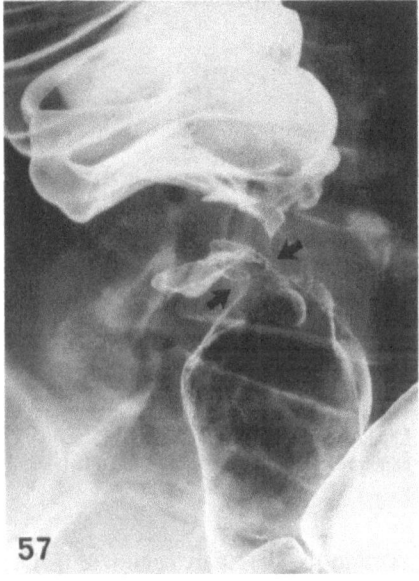

Fig. 56. Ileocecal tuberculosis. 61-year-old man. Previous history of tuberculous pleurisy, subocclusive episode and weight loss. SBFT : fixed, angulated terminal ileal loops with staggered stenoses and proximal saccules

Fig. 57. Ileocecal tuberculosis. 45-year-old man . Diarrhea for 6 months. DCBE : dilatation of the terminal ileum with sacculations, retraction of the cecum and stenosis above the ileocecal valve. Calcifications in the neighbouring lymph nodes

sis may occur. Peripheral adenopathy is frequent. Anal fistulae are rare. The laboratory evaluation may show an anemia, a leucocytosis, signs of malabsorption or decreased serum protein levels. Pulmonary radiographs showing active or old tuberculosis are very helpful. PPD skin tests are most often positive. The diagnosis of intestinal tuberculosis may be made on stool cultures in the absence of active pulmonary tuberculosis. The diagnosis is obviated if Koch's bacillus or caseating necrosis in the intestinal wall or lymph nodes are demonstrated. Biopsies performed during colonoscopy or laparoscopy sometimes suggest the diagnosis, but it is not always possible to demonstrate the bacilli and caseating necrosis,

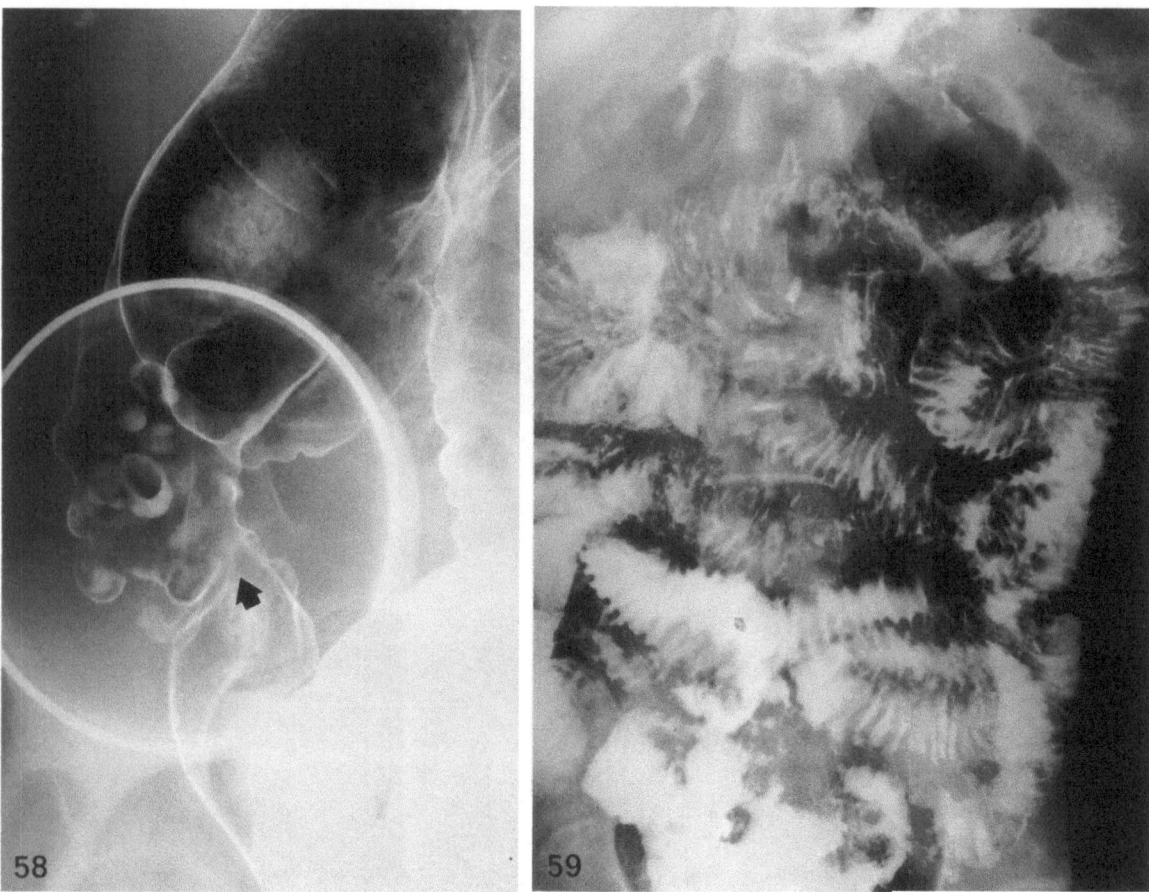

Fig. 58. DCBE : Ileocecal tuberculosis. 81-year-old woman. Chronic diarrhea. SBFT : moderate increase in the caliber of the terminal ileum, gaping ileocecal valve, retraction and sacculations of the cecum and right colon

Fig. 59. Diffuse tuberculosis. 40-year-old man. Previous history of tuberculosis. Recent febrile episode with diarrhea and weight loss. Laparoscopy : granulation tissue and peritoneal adhesions. Duodenoscopy : villous atrophy and ulcerated duodenitis. SBFT : diffuse abnormalities with contrast medium dilution and thickened folds

even in the surgical specimen, if the disease is old, or if previous antituberculous treatment has been administered.

Radiological findings

Elementary images

The analysis of the elementary images on small bowel follow-through reveals the following:
- inconstant functional disorders (hypermotility, hypertonia, dilution),
- fixed or angulated loops, extrinsic compression images, widened interloop gaps,
- short stenosis with gradual transition and smooth or ulcerated margins,
- nodulation evoking lymphoid hyperplasia or cobblestoning,
- multiple star-shaped or transverse ulcerations with convergent folds or circumferential around a stenosis or transmural and sometimes producing fistulae,
- thickened folds or with abnormal direction.
- There may also be calcifications in the neighbouring lymph nodes.

Progression of the radiological lesions

The most specific and frequent form involves the ileocecal area. It combines a short stenosis of the terminal ileum with or without ulceration, to a stiff and gaping ileocecal valve, with a deep notch in the cecum opposite the ileocecal valve and retraction of the cecal fundus, sometimes with saccules. When the retraction extends to the right colon, the latter organ ascends to the subhepatic region and the junction with the terminal ileum is angulated at 180°.

In other cases, the disease appears as an isolated involvement of the terminal ileum, which is then spastic. Palpation with antispasmodics reveals an ulceronodular appearance. The local increase in the interloop space demonstrates the thickening of the intestinal wall and the presence of adenopathy.

The intestinal disease is rarely more diffuse. If it is the case, the appearance is either that of a nonspecific «inflammatory» small intestine with contrast medium dilution and the presence of large folds without ulcerations, or that of abrupt staggered stenoses, which may be mistaken for primary or metastatic malignant tumours, Crohn's disease or chronic ulcerated jejunoileitis.

It is difficult to distinguish intestinal tuberculosis from Crohn's disease. Radiological signs favoring tuberculosis include a short length of terminal ileal involvement in the presence of a relatively extensive cecal retraction, a stiff and gaping ileocecal valve, the absence of tapered and asymmetric lesions, the transverse orientation of ileal ulcerations, the rarity of aphtoid ulcerations, rhagades, fissures and fistulae and the short length of the stenosis. The differential diagnosis is often not possible solely on the basis of radiographs, and is made only after clinical, radiological and laboratory data is integrated. Sometimes the correct nature of the lesions is only determined at laparotomy.

Progression of the disease

The outcome of digestive tuberculosis when treated usually results in healing of the lesions. The small bowel follow-through demonstrates tiered stenoses in the small intestine and, more importantly, scarring of the ileocecal region, with associated cecal retraction and distention of the terminal ileum, occasionally with saccules on both sides of a gaping ileocecal valve. Such a radiographic appearance is sometimes discovered during examination after the disease has spontaneously healed. If left untreated, digestive tuberculosis tends to spread and become generalized with abscess and fistulous formation, and the development of enteroperitoneal tuberculosis.

Complementary imaging

Ultrasound and computed tomography demonstrate a mass with intestinal gas in its center, as well as mesenteric adenopathy. These techniques are useful because they detect the involvement of neighbouring organs (liver, spleen, adnexa) or peritonitis in the form of ascites associated with subparietal masses, which may simulate peritoneal metastases.

Yersiniosis (figs. 60 to 62)

Yersiniosis is an infection caused by the Gram-negative bacteria *Yersinia enterocolitica* and *Yersinia pseudotuberculosis*, and which can present predominantly with intestinal and articular involvement. It is most often an acute infection with a self-limited course. Sometimes it may lead to a long-lasting subacute or even a severe, sometimes lethal disease. Since many benign infections are not diagnosed, the frequency of the disease is considerably underestimated but seems to keep increasing. The disease affects mainly the small intestine and the mesenteric lymph nodes, but autopsies of lethal forms show ulcerations in the entire digestive tract. Although yersiniosis exhibits similarities to Crohn's disease, they are not related diseases. Both sexes are equally affected at any age. The bacterium develops in animals or in man, with the possiblility of healthy carriers. The contamination route seems to be oral, via water or food. The disease is not highly contagious but limited epidemics are possible. Incubation occurs over a couple of days. The bacteria thrive at low temperatures.

Pathology

The mucosal surface of the intestine is covered with round or longitudinal ulcers on an erythematous background. Mesenteric adenopathy is a sine qua non of the disease when clinically present. Peripheral adenopathy may sometimes be observed, as can peritoneal exudation.

The histological appearance is that of an acute inflammation predominating in the mucosa. Ulcerations, sometimes extending into the muscularis, are often located over lymphoid follicles. Areas of necrosis are visible within edematous tissue infiltrated by polymorphonuclear and mononuclear cells. Gram-negative bacilli are found in the intestinal wall

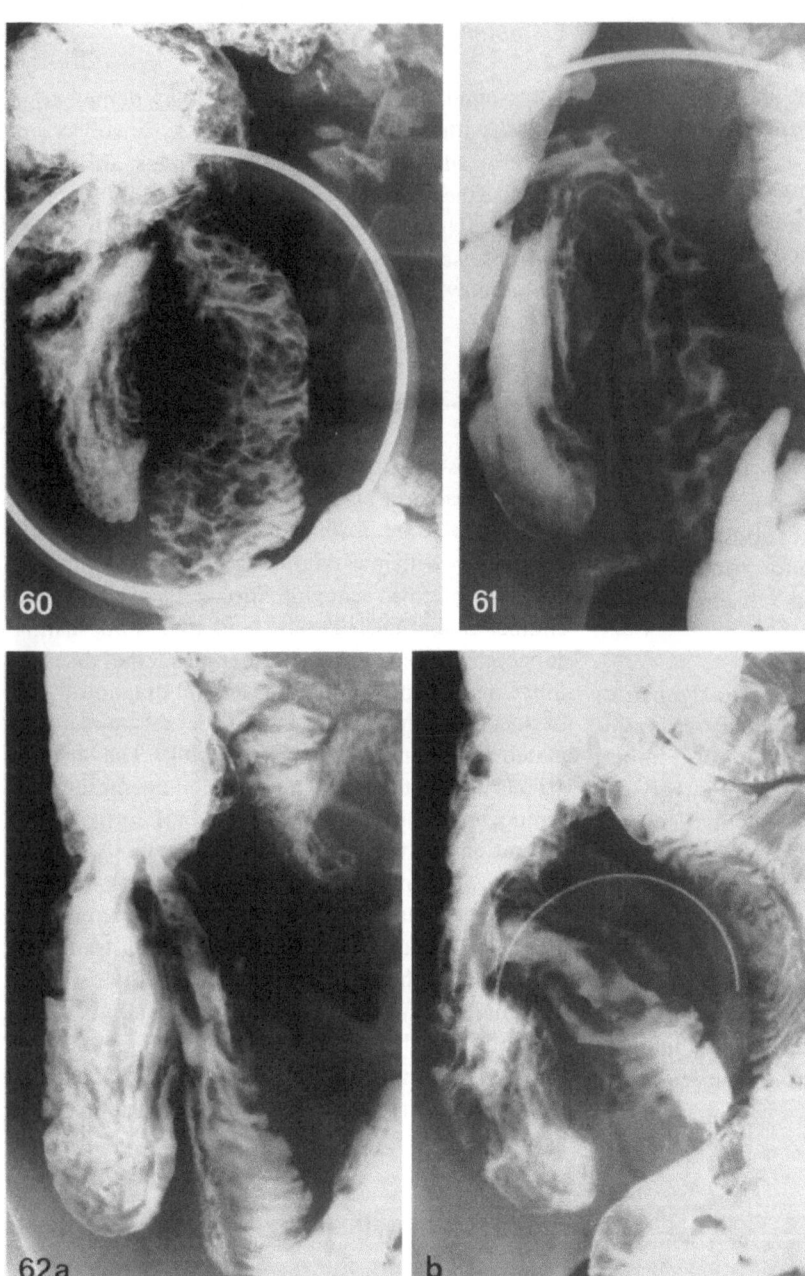

Fig. 60. Yersiniosis. 16-year-old girl. Right iliac pain and diarrhea. SBFT : nodulation of the terminal ileum and hypertrophy of one of Peyer's patches

Fig. 61. Yersiniosis. 28-year-old man. Epigastric pain. SBFT : nodulation and large folds in the terminal ileum

Fig. 62 a, b. Yersiniosis (Courtesy of P Mahieu). 43-year-old woman. Right iliac pain and fever. SBFT : **a** linear ulcer and **b** aphtoid ulcerations bordered by large inflammatory folds

at early stages of the disease. No granulomas and no giant cells are found.

Clinical findings

The disease may run an acute or subacute course with diarrhea, sometimes with fever, or it may mimick appendicitis, with right iliac pain, liquid stool, nausea and fever. *Yersinia enterocolitica* is responsible for an enterocolitic pattern of involvement, frequent in infants and young children, and which may cause dehydration. Hematochezia and perforation may occur in adults. Ulcerated colitis is sometimes seen in yersiniosis but is seldom symptomatic. Adenopathy sometimes may cause intussusception, especially in children. Healing is spectacular following the administration of tetracyclines.

Erythema nodosum, arthralgias with arthritis and sacroileitis may appear in time in the subacute forms, especially in patients carrying the HLA B27 antigen of the histocompatibility complex. Involvement of other organs, including pharyngitis, myocarditis, dematitis, glomerulonephritis, urethritis, hepatitis, osteitis or iritis (which thus produces a pattern similar to Reiter's syndrome in association with articular and urethral involvement) may rarely occur. Septicemia and death may result in chronically ill or immunocompromised patients.

Laboratory findings may yield an elevated sedimentation rate, and a leucocytosis. The absence of leucopenia differentiates the diarrheic forms of yersiniosis from typhoid fever. The diagnosis is made in the first few days after isolation of the bacteria in the stools, and the histological examination of mesenteric lymph nodes after surgery for presumed appendicitis. The levels of serum agglutinins increase over time, reaching their peak concentrations after 15 days, and then decreasing progressively over a couple of months. Acute and convalescent titres are therefore required for making the diagnosis.

Radiological findings

The disease predominates in, or is confined to the terminal ileum. The latter is spastic and shows a 10 to 20 cm long nodulation made up of round, juxtaposed or conglomerated elements, several millimeters to one centimeter in diameter, which are characteristic of lymphoid hyperplasia. Punctiform, aphtoid or longitudinal ulcerations are frequent and may be 1 to 2 cm long. The folds are irregularly thickened. Extrinsic compression due to adenopathy may be seen coupled to a slightly widened interloop gap. No stenosis, angulation or fissures are observed. The nodulation may persist for several months after the disappearance of the clinical and laboratory abnormalities. However, the radiological signs of improvement on two successive examinations usually occur earlier than in Crohn's disease with appropriate therapy.

Practical conclusion

This common disease goes often undiagnosed. It may follow an acute or subacute course, presenting with diarrhea alone, or it may mimic appendicitis. It may be accompanied by fever and arthralgias. Despite its benign course, it may initially be mistaken for Crohn's disease.

Intestinal infections (figs. 63 to 65)

Independently of those infections connected with tuberculosis, yersiniosis, Whipple's disease, tropical sprue, alpha-chain disease or immune deficiency other infections are frequently found in the small bowel.

The small intestinal infections are most often caused by exogenous organisms such as coliforms, staphylococci, shigellae, salmonellae, campylobacters, vibrio cholera, anaerobic bacteria or viruses (enterovirus, adenovirus, myxovirus, Norwalk-type virus, rotavirus, Epstein-Barr virus, etc.). These diseases have not been well characterized radiologically as they present as acute short lived diarrheal illnesses. Hemorrhage and perforation have been described in the severe forms. The radiological assessment most often consists only of plain radiographs, which may show a moderate distention of the bowel loops, air-fluid levels, a widened interloop gap due to intestinal wall thickening or peritoneal effusion, and broadened folds. Gas in the intestinal walls and the portal vein may be seen in necrotizing enterocolitis. A small bowel follow-through carried out in cases of typhoid fever, measles, scarlet fever or shigellosis demonstrates terminal ileitis with nodulation due to lymphoid hyperplasia and displaced loops suggesting the presence of adenopathy. Ulcerations, sometimes aphtoid in type, may be observed, but stenosis, angulation and fistulae are absent.

Subacute or chronic infectious jejunoileitis due to endogenous bacterial overgrowth may develop. Predisposing factors include previous hepatobiliary disease, hypochorhydria (e.g. following stomach surgery) and, most importantly, intestinal stasis.

These disorders are all characterized by stasis which contributes to bacterial proliferation. Some of the bacteria take up vitamin B12, thus preventing its absorption in the ileum, and deconjugate bile salts which are essential for proper fat absorption.

The bacterial overgrowth syndrome presents with pain, diarrhea, meteorism, a deterioration in the general condition of the patient, and signs of malabsorption. Treatment includes antibiotics and in some cases surgery aimed at removing a diverticulum, or correcting a defective previous surgical hook-up. The laboratory studies demonstrate macrocytic anemia, which is suggestive of the disease in this context, and sometimes hypoproteinemia or steatorrhea. A Schilling's test is usually abnormal. A jejunal biopsy will show inflammatory infiltration of the mucosa and sometimes partial villous atrophy.

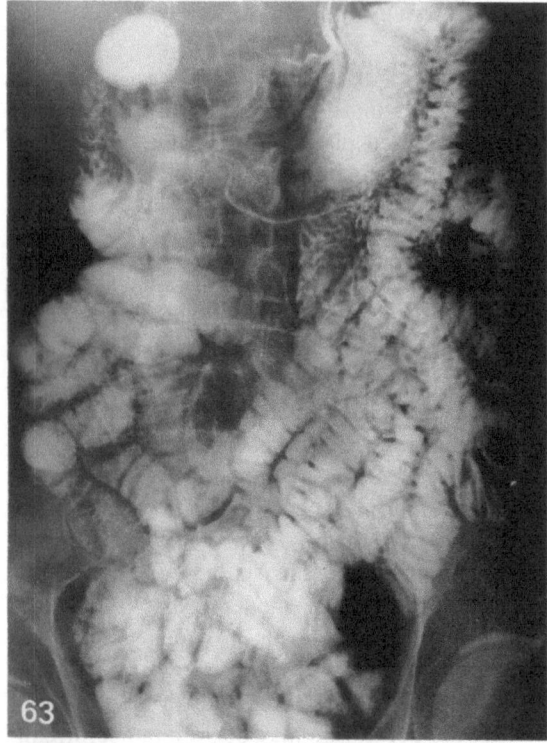 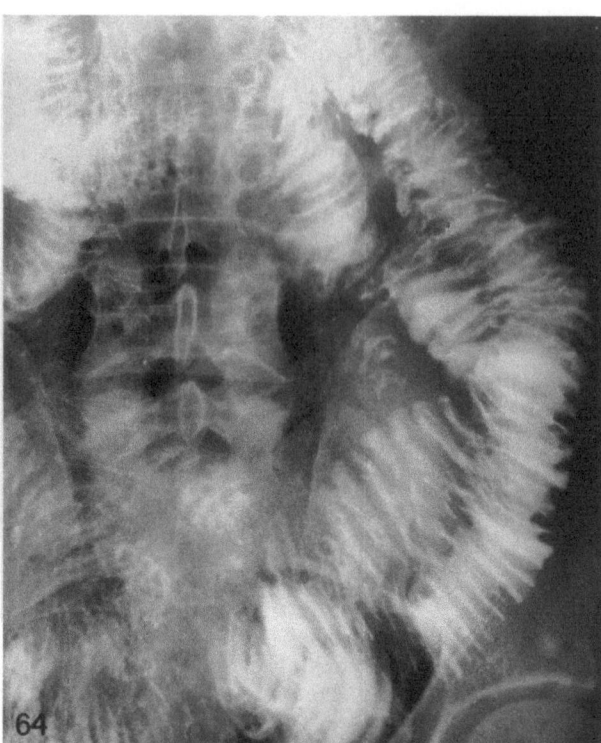

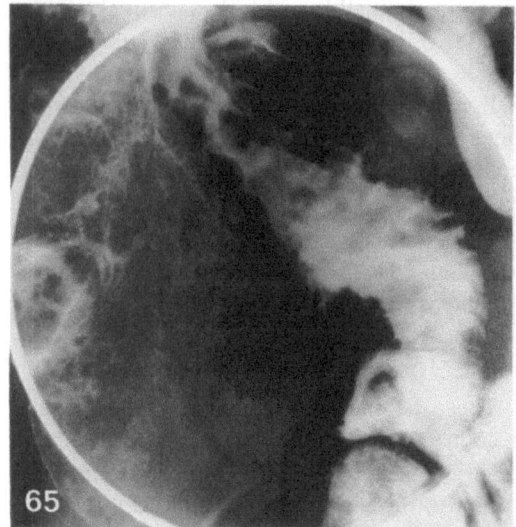

Fig. 63. Infectious jejunoileitis. 56-year-old diabetic man. Diarrhea. laboratory data : malabsorption, abnormal respiratory tests. SBFT :contrast medium dilution, moderates increase in the interloop gap, thickened and rarefied jejunal folds

Fig. 64. Infectious jejunoileitis. 44-year-old man. Chronic diarrhea two years after a lateral ileocolic anastomosis. Abnormal respiratory tets.
SBFT : contrast medium dilution, widened loop caliber and thickened folds

The diagnosis of bacterial overgrowth is made by a sheathed jejunal intubation and a breath test. Jejunal intubation collects Gram-negative and anaerobic bacteria, whose presence is abnormal in the jejunum.

Barium studies yield only nonspecific signs. The contrast medium is somewhat diluted, and the folds are moderately and regularly thickened. The major use of radiology is in the detection of stasis as the cause of the disease such as seen in chronic stenoses of any origin (in particular Crohn's disease), in atonia (scleroderma, visceral neuropathy, diabetes, vagotomy, etc.), in the presence of diverticula or a blind or stagnant loop following a surgical anastomosis.

Practical conclusions

Although a barium study is not indicated in acute intestinal infections, it is very useful in chronic in-

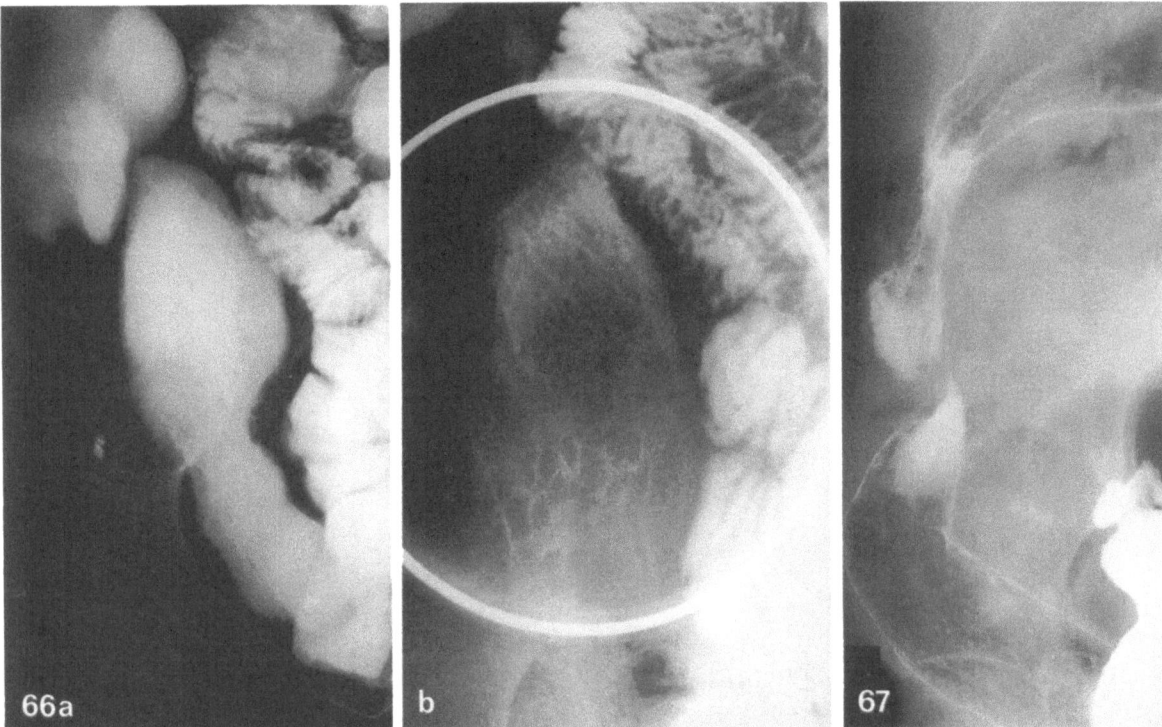

Fig. 66 a, b. Backwash ileitis. 27-year-old woman. Ulcerative colitis with pancolitis having evoluted over 15 years. SBFT : thin reticulation of the terminal ileum

Fig. 67. Backwash ileitis. 60-year-old woman. Disease caused by chronic laxative abuse. Double-contrast barium enema : thin reticulation of the colon and the terminal ileum

fections as radiology demonstrates the cause of the stasis which is most often responsible for the associated bacterial overgrowth syndrome.

Backwash ileitis (figs. 66 and 67)

Lesions of the terminal ileum are observed in chronic laxative abuse and in 75% of cases of ulcerative pancolitis. These are less frequent if the ulcerative colitis is confined to the left colon. The common anatomical feature of these diseases is the infiltration of the ileocecal valve, which causes its incompetence. The wall is edematous and acutely inflammed, but contains no granulomas or fibrotic areas, unlike what is observed in Crohn's disease.

Small bowel follow-through and ileal backwash during a barium enema demonstrate the gaping ileocecal valve and distended terminal ileum. The dilution of the contrast medium does not always permit a proper study of the mucosal alterations which includes reticulation, flat nodulation, or a punctated appearance with marginal microspiculation. Microulcerations or inflammatory pseudopolyps can be observed. The gaping ileocecal valve, the absence of stenosis or fistulae, the symmetry of the lesions, as well as their limited extent differentiate backwash ileitis from Crohn's disease, whose presence might be suggested in cases of colitis with terminal ileal involvement.

Whipple's disease (figs. 68 and 69)

Whipple's disease is a rare entity of unknown etiology, exhibiting a chronic course which leads to death in the absence of antibiotic therapy. However, the origin of the disease is not strictly speaking infectious. It is characterized by the proliferation of macrophages containing partially phagocytosed bacilli. This finding suggests an immune etiology to the disease, in particular a disorder of phagocytosis. The autopsy of subjects having died of the disease shows macrophage infiltration in several organs (intestine, joints, skin, lymph nodes, liver, heart,

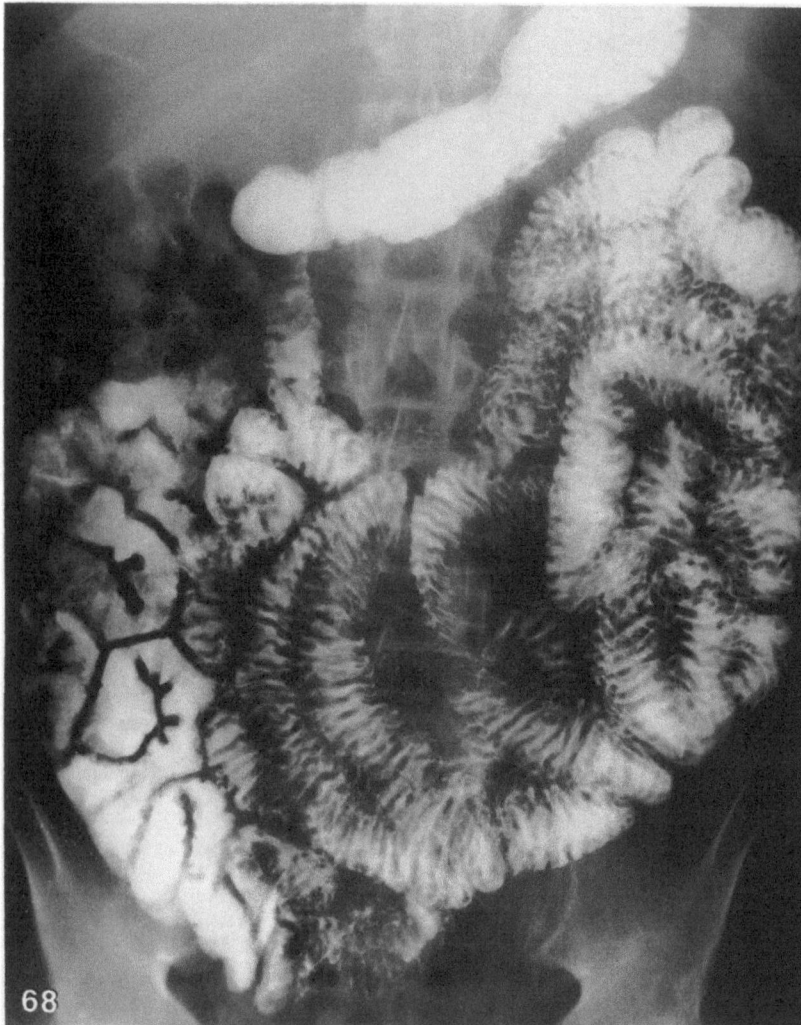

Fig. 68. Whipple's disease (Courtesy of J Pringot). 40-year-old man. Polyarticular pains. Deterioration in his general condition, intermittent diarrhea. SBFT : nodular folds of the jejunum, contrast medium dilution, widened interloop in the ileum

lungs and pleura, nervous system, etc.). The intestinal involvement often occurs late on. The disease occurs mostly in the fifth decade of life with a marked male predominance.

Pathology

The macroscopic study of the small intestine shows diffuse disease. The wall is thickened and the folds enlarged. The villi are broadened and flattened. The lymph vessels are distended. The mesentery contains many lymph nodes that are sometimes pseudotumoral.

Microscopic study demonstrates the characteristic lesion in Whipple's disease, i.e. the massive mucosal and submucosal infiltration of PAS-positive macrophages with a foamy cytoplasm, contai-

ning corpuscules which electron microscopy identifies as partially phagocytized bacteria. Great quantities of bacilli of various types are also found in the intestinal wall. Paradoxically, there are few polymorphonuclear cells and plasmacytes. The lymph vessels contain many lipid vacuoles, and are dilated and plugged. The macrophages are also found in the mesenteric lymph nodes where fibrosis may be present.

Clinical findings

Intestinal involvement appears rather late on in the evolution of Whipple's disease and manifests as intermittent diarrhea, meteorism and abdominal pain. The poor prognosis is due to the associated steatorrhea, which leads to cachexia. Hemorrhage is uncommon. Weight loss is usually prominent. The di-

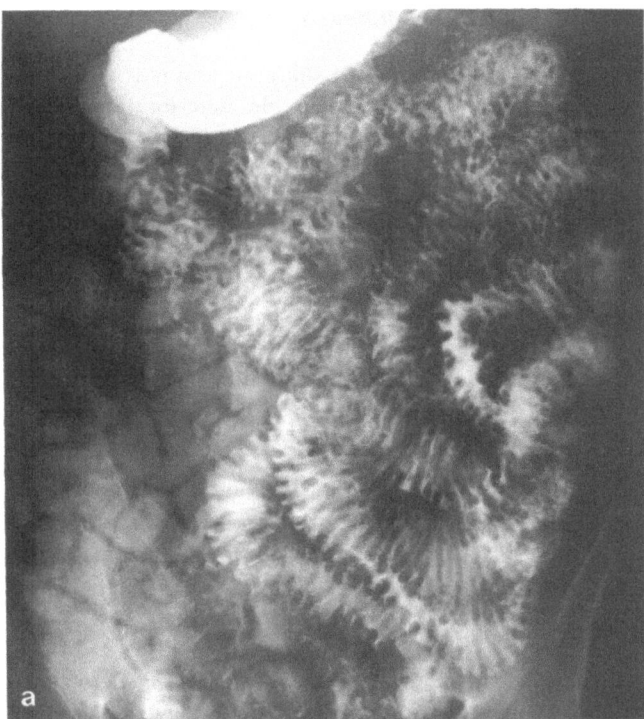

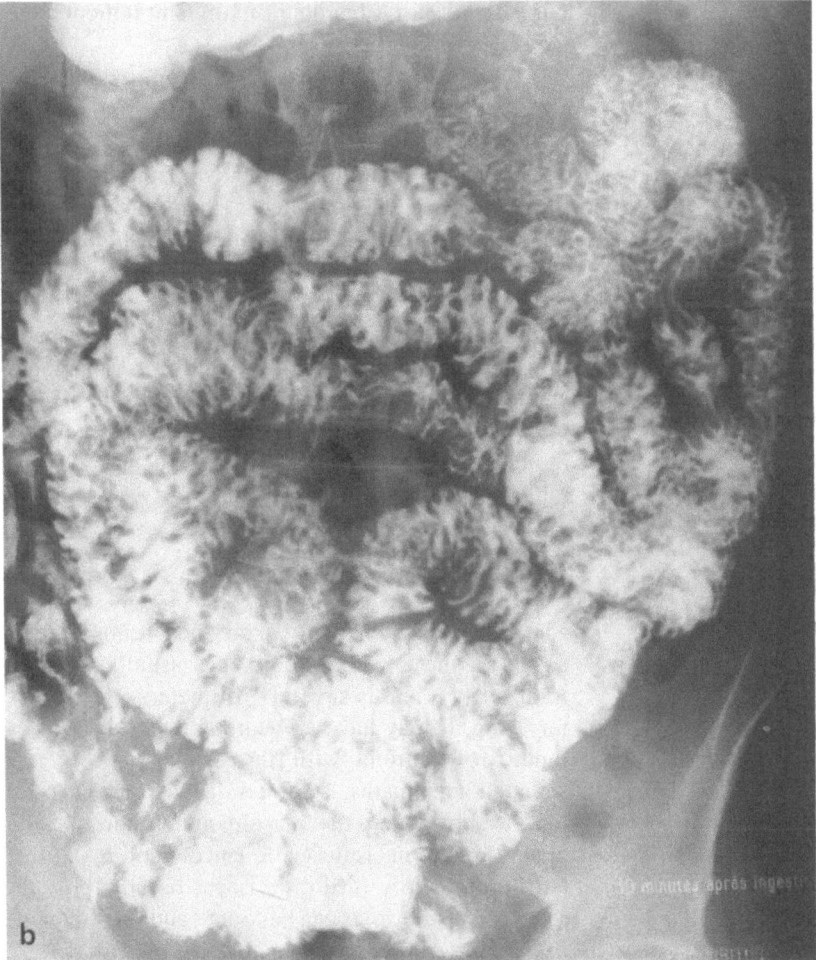

Fig. 69 a, b. Whipple's disease. 46-year-old man . Deterioration in his general condition, diarrhea, arthralgias. SBFT : **a** nodular thickening of the jejunal folds and contrast medium dilution, **b** after a 2-year treatment, persistent moderate nodulation with marginal microspiculation

sease often evolves insidiously over several months or even years as a long-lasting constant, or relapsing fever, or as mono- or polyarthritis producing transient, recurrent pain without radiological changes or deformity. The resulting arthritis may mimic rheumatoid arthritis or sacroileitis. Other signs may include skin hyperpigmentation, edema, purpura, a low-grade fever and a low blood pressure. Peripheral adenopathy is not always present but is suggestive of the disease when associated with fever, diarrhea and arthralgias. The involved abdominal lymph nodes are sometimes large enough to be palpated. Several other signs may occur during activity of the disease, including erythema nodosum, mediastinal adenopathy, endomyocarditis, pericarditis, peripheral ischemia, pleurisy, ascites or encephalopathy.

Untreated, the disease results in death. Improvement and cure with antibiotics occurs over several months. Although complete clinical resolution is the rule, histological abnormalities persist. Recurrence leading eventually to amyloidosis may occur.

Laboratory studies show a moderate increase in the sedimentation rate, an anemia, sometimes a leucocytosis, as well as decreased cholesterol, calcium and electrolyte levels. The glucose tolerance test curve is flat. Serum protein levels are decreased, but mucoproteins are typically increased. Steatorrhea and D-xylose malabsorption are present.

The diagnosis is based on a duodenojejunal biopsy even in the absence of clinical signs, and on rectal or nodal biopsies.

Radiological findings

Secretory functional alterations (dilution) are rare. Duodenal and jejunal involvements predominate. They are characterized by an increase in the height and width of the folds, which are often nodular but retain their winding appearance. The caliber and curvature of the loops are normal and the interloop gap is not widened. There are no nodules or ulcerations. A careful study of the jejunum shows a punctated appearance with microspiculation on tangential views produced by the broadened villi. Extrinsic compression by lymph nodes sometimes occurs.

Complementary imaging

Lymphangiography can opacify large, heterogeneous lymph nodes or demonstrate lymphatic blockage, but these signs are not specific.

Practical conclusions

The syndrome of fever, diarrhea, articular pains, adenopathy and a considerable deterioration in the patient's general condition must lead to a suspicion of Whipple's disease. This diagnosis is confirmed by large, winding folds in the duodenum and the jejunum, with broadened duodenojejunal villi. Biopsies demonstrate the disease. A correct diagnosis is vital since the disease can be cured in many with antibiotics, but if left untreated is lethal.

Nonspecific ulcers (figs. 70 to 72)

Ulcers in the small intestine may stem from various etiologies which include gastroenteric anastomoses, ingestion of potassium chloride tablets, ectopic gastric mucosa (in particular in a Meckel's diverticulum), ischemia (e.g. in contact with a foreign body), stasis (ileus, scleroderma), inflammatory disease (in particular Crohn's disease), infection (tuberculosis, yersiniosis, typhoid fever, bacillary dysentery, etc.), parasitic diseases, benign or malignant tumours, the Zollinger-Ellison syndrome, etc.

A «nonspecific» ulcer is a diagnosis of exclusion when no etiology can be found. Several mechanisms are postulated: ischemia due to local vascular disease, or to excitation of the sympathetic system, alimentary trauma or mucosal heterotopia. These ulcers arise at any age, and equally in both sexes. They mainly appear in the ileum and the proximal jejunum. They are usually isolated. Two or three lesions sometimes appear at some distance from each other in the small intestine. Multifocal ulcerated stenosing enteritis, which includes multiple ulcerated and recurrent stenoses, may present as such, although its relapsing course carries a much less favourable prognosis.

Pathology

The ulcer is often located on the antimesenteric aspect of the intestinal loop. It is usually oriented transversely, and is several millimeters to centimeters long. It may have an acute and slashed appearance, or be chronic with fibrosis and stenosis. Associated adenopathy is sometimes visible. The histology shows that the margin and fundus of the ulceration are necrotic while surrounded by a limited inflammatory infiltrate. Local polymorphic lesions of the arterioles can be found, and less frequently, edema or hemorrhages are also present.

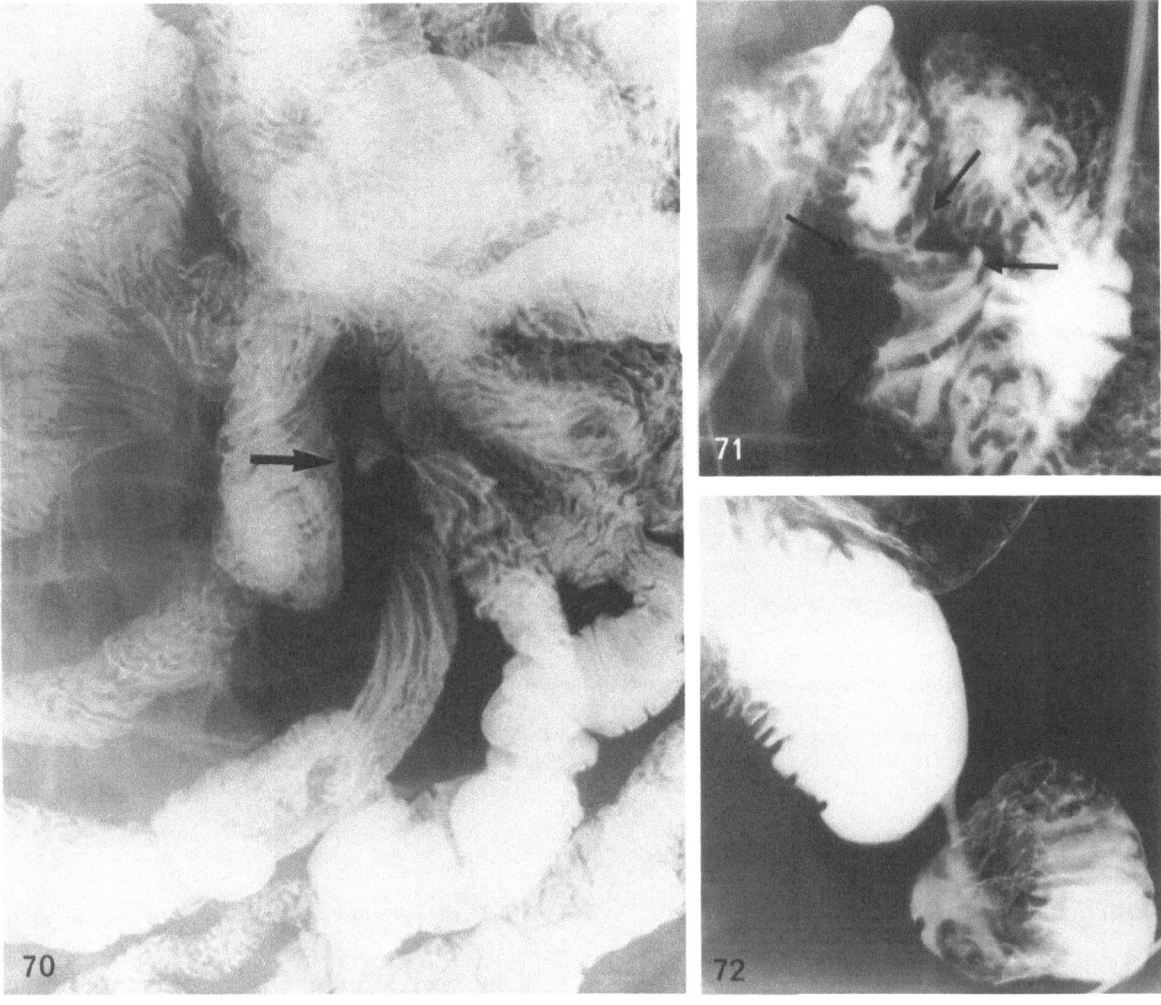

Fig. 70. Nonspecific ulcer. 56-year-old man. Repeated episodes of partial bowel obstruction 5 years after surgery for rupture of an aortic aneurysm. Anticoagulation therapy. SBFT : fixed and anguled distal jejunal loop, the apex of which shows an ulceration

Fig. 71. Nonspecific ulcer. 34-year-old woman. Diarrhea, poor general condition. Malabsorption syndrome and anemia. Oral birth-control pill. SBFT : narrowing with locally thickened folds in the first jejunal loop. The study of the surgical specimen reveals an ulcer that may have been ischemic

Fig. 72. Ulcer and foreign-body granuloma (Courtesy of J P Moiroud). 31-year-old woman. Postprandial pain and vomiting. SBFT : short stenosis of the first jejunal loop ; with smooth contours and an infundibular transition with the distended proximal segment.Surgical findings: ulcerated stenosis with a foreign-body granuloma in the fundus of the ulceration

Clinical findings

The clinical signs include pain, meteorism, diarrhea, but more importantly symptoms of partial obstruction and rarely malabsorption. Complications in the form of anemia, hemorrhage, occlusion or perforation are frequent. Surgery is necessary to the diagnosis and most often is the definitive treatment.

Radiological findings

Small bowel follow-through demonstrates the short annular stenosis outlined by proximal dilatation. The margins of the stenosis are most often smooth. The ulcer is rarely demonstrated. No contiguous abnormalities, such as angulated or fixed loops, are noted. Aphtoid ulcerations like those observed in Crohn's disease are absent.

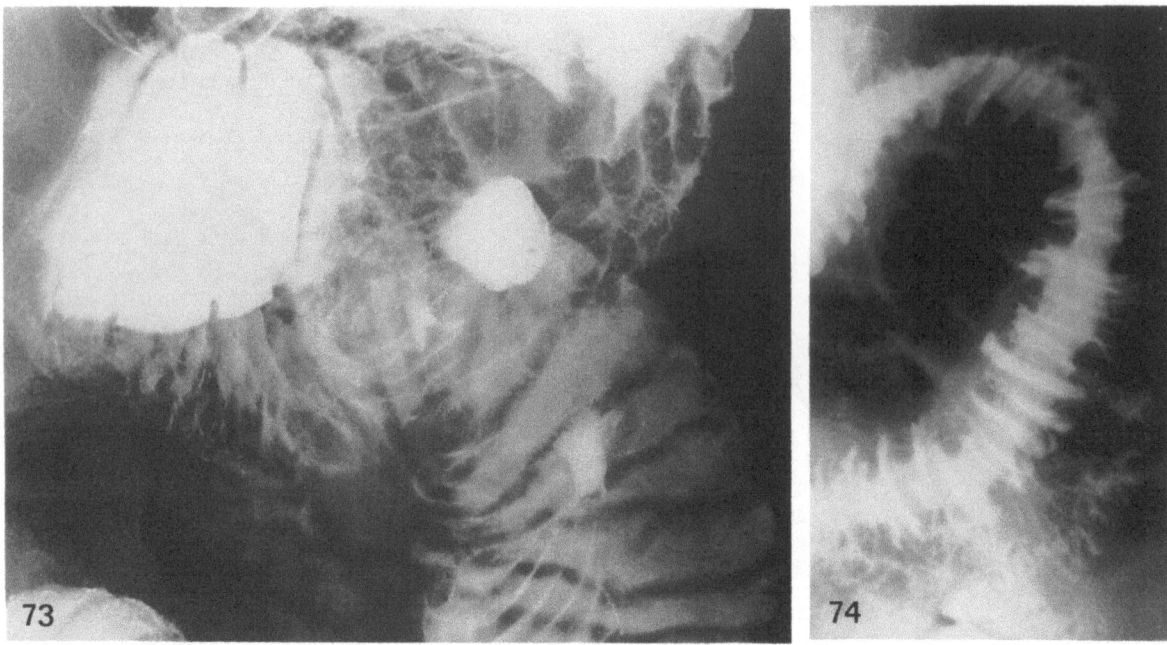

Fig. 73. Zollinger-Ellison syndrome. 34-year-old man. Recurrent postoperative peptic ulcer. SBFT : two ulcers in the efferent loop

Fig. 74. Ulcerate jejunitis secondary to nesiodioblastome. 57-year-old man. Abundant diarrhea and deterioration in the general condition. SBFT: unfoled first jejunal loop. Large, thickened and tall folds with scalloped contours. Endoscopy : multiple jejunal ulcerations

Practical conclusions

The diagnosis of a nonspecific ulcer of the small intestine is not always made on radiologic studies. Radiologists observing a short stenosis of the small intestine should know that it may be benign and attributable to no detectable cause.

The Zollinger-Ellison syndrome
(figs. 73 and 74)

The Zollinger-Ellison syndrome is caused by non-beta endocrine tumors of the pancreas secreting large quantities of gastrin. Such tumors are malignant in over 50% of cases and hepatic or nodal metastases are detected in 2/3 of patients at the time of diagnosis. This disease affects men and women equally and occurs at any age, but especially around forty years of age.

The disease most often appears as multiple, recurrent ulcers, mainly in the duodenum, sometimes in the jejunum and rarely in the stomach and the esophagus. They always recur after partial gastrectomy.

In 40 % of patients, diarrhea occurs due to acid hypersecretion.

In one out of five patients, the pancreatic tumor is associated with a suprarenal or parathyroid tumor or with a familial multiple endocrine neoplastic syndrome (Wermer's syndrome), with pituitary, parathyroid and pancreatic involvement.

Pathology

The pancreatic tumor is an adenocarcinoma in 60% of cases, an adenoma in 30% and represents diffuse hyperplasia in the other 10%. The tumor is most often small and difficult to demonstrate even on macroscopic examination. In the case of a malignant tumor, the lymph nodes are often more visible than the tumor itself, which is rarely larger than several centimeters in diameter. In addition, it is often ectopic and located in the duodenum, jejunum, stomach or in the hilum of the spleen.

The wall of the small intestine is thickened because of edema, inflammatory phenomena and hemorrhages around the ulcers. Partial villous atrophy may also be present.

Clinical findings

The occurrence of the ulcers is often preceded by diarrhea, either mild and semi-formed, or watery and abundant. It is the only symptom in some cases. When abundant, it leads to a deterioration in the patient's general condition. Water and electrolyte losses often occur, especially potassium and sodium. Dehydration and sometimes steatorrhea may follow.

The prognosis, either untreated or following partial gastrectomy, is poor because of the development of hemorrhage or perforation of the ulcers, or because of water and electrolyte losses. Complete gastrectomy has been replaced by the use of antisecretory agents. H2 blockers and omiprazole permit proper control of acid hypersecretion in almost all patients.

The diagnosis is made by measurement of the volume of gastric secretions, which exceeds 1 l in 12 h in 90% of all cases, coupled to the secretion of free hydrochloric acid, exceeding 60 mEq per litre in 95% of patients, in the presence of an inappropriate increase in serum gastrin levels.

Radiological findings

The characteristic appearance includes abnormalities of the stomach, duodenum and jejunum, as these decrease progressively towards the ileum, which itself is rarely affected. Considerable dilution or even flocculation of the contrast medium is noted. Peristalsis is rare in the stomach and the duodenum, with stasis of the barium solution contrasting sharply with the hypermotility of the jejunum. The caliber of the duodenal and jejunal loops is increased. The folds are thickened in the vertical portion of the stomach, where they can have a pseudolymphomatous appearance, as well as in the duodenum and jejunum. The jejunal folds are poorly delineated because of barium solution dilution, but may be as large as 4 to 5 mm in width. The interfold gaps are short and spiculated. The image is similar to that observed in hypoproteinemic edema. An associated ulcer is of great diagnostic value and should be searched for primarily in the superior part of the duodenum. Lower duodenal or jejunal ulcers suggest a Zollinger-Ellison syndrome. However, jejunal ulcerations are difficult to demonstrate because of dilution of the contrast medium.

Complementary imaging

The localization of the gastrinoma is often difficult. It requires imaging by ultrasound, computed tomography, selective arteriography and sometimes phlebography with venous sampling.

Practical conclusions

The presence of contrast medium dilution, stasis and duodenal dilatation, large gastric and upper intestinal folds, and especially the detection of duodenojejunal ulcers, all together should make the radiologist suspect a Zollinger-Ellison syndrome.

Chronic ulcerative jejunoileitis (fig. 75)

Chronic ulcerative jejunoileitis or Jeffries' disease is an exceptional disease of unknown origin. The diagnosis is made in cases where multiple ulcerations of the small intestine are associated with villous atrophy not cured by a gluten-free diet. No findings support the diagnosis of Crohn's disease, lymphoma, ischemia, infection, Whipple's disease or the Zollinger-Ellison syndrome, and there is no history of previous administration of potassium. Nonspecific ulcers and multifocal ulcerated stenoses are different from this condition as they do not exhibit villous atrophy. If resistance to a gluten-free diet occurs in a proven case of celiac disease with ulcers, the distinction between the two conditions may be difficult to make.

The disease carries a poor prognosis and is often lethal. Both sexes are equally affected, especially between the ages of 30 and 60. No treatment is of proven efficacy.

Pathology

The disease may be diffuse but usually predominates in the jejunum. Macroscopic study shows plaques of bowel wall thickening and an edematous, hypervascular serosa. The loops are sometimes dilated, with short successive stenoses. Cutting open a loop often will demonstrate the multiple transverse or longitudinal ulcerations that are often superficial but may be transmural. The mucosa between the ulcers shows villous atrophy, only partial while preserving normal areas, often extending into the ileum. Mul-

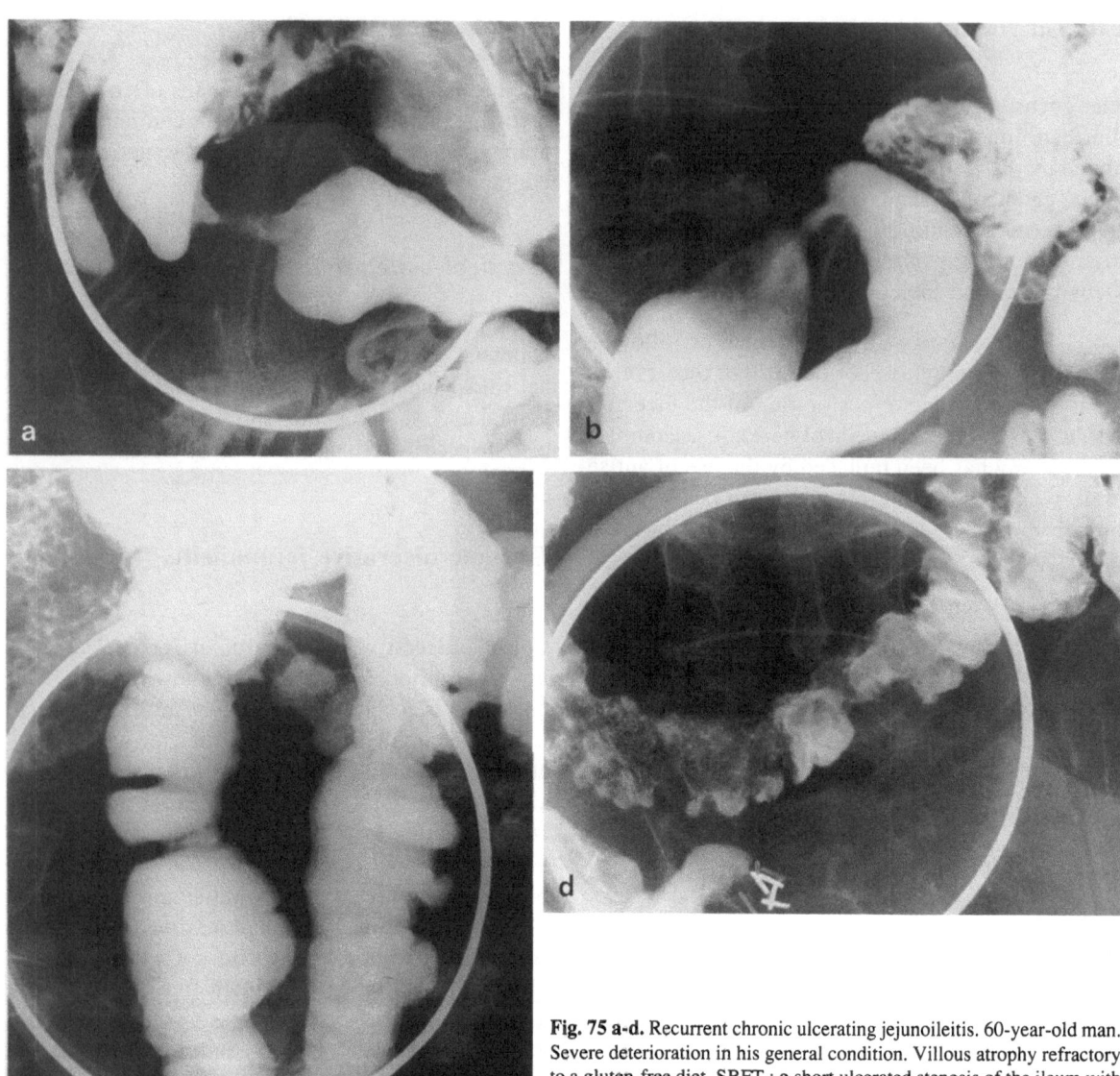

Fig. 75 a-d. Recurrent chronic ulcerating jejunoileitis. 60-year-old man. Severe deterioration in his general condition. Villous atrophy refractory to a gluten-free diet. SBFT : **a** short ulcerated stenosis of the ileum with an infundibular transition, **b** similar image with neighbouring aphtoid ulceration, **c** asymetric sacculation of a jejunal loop, **d** sacculation and punctated appearance of a jejunal loop. Surgical finding : nonspecific multiple ulcerations with inflammatory mesenteric adenopathy

tiple adenopathy is observed and the mesentery may be edematous.

Microscopic study shows that the lesions involve principally the mucosa and submucosa. The nonspecific ulcers are surrounded by inflammatory tissue containing numerous lymphocytes and monocytes as well as neutrophilic and eosinophilic polymorphonuclear cells. No granulomas, siderophages, bacteria or parasites are found.

Clinical findings

The condition displays a uniform pattern, associating periumbilical colicky pains, diarrhea, fever and an overall deterioration in the patient's general status. The severity of the disease is determined by both the presence of massive malabsorption (steatorrhea and loss of proteins) which is unaltered by a gluten-free diet, and frequent serious complications including perforation and hemorrhage.

Laboratory studies reflect a malabsorptive state. Anemia is invariably present, while leucocytosis and eosinophilia are sometimes observed. Cases of hypogammaglobulinemia have also been reported. The diagnosis is sometimes made at endoscopy but more often at laparotomy.

Radiological findings

The appearance combines the signs of celiac disease and ulcerated stenoses. Contrast medium dilution is seen with an increased caliber of loops, and rarified, thickened folds and with successive stenoses due to ulcers often invisible because of a significant secretory disorder. After some time, asymmetric segmental retractions occur with saccular images and distorted folds, which are perhaps due to healing of the ulcers.

Practical conclusions

Chronic ulcerative jejunoileitis is a rare disease with a very poor prognosis, which associates ulcers, stenoses, retractions and the usual findings of celiac disease, of which it might be a more severe form.

Behçet's disease (fig. 76)

Behçet's disease is a systemic disease which may be autoimmune in origin. It is characterized by aphtosis due to a nonspecific vascularity. The diagnosis is purely clinical. Some familial cases have been reported, which may indicate a hereditary tendency, or at least a predisposition since the disease affects the subjects of the HLA B5 group more often and, to a lesser extent, those of the HLA B12, B27 and A2 groups. This condition is rare in Europe and most frequent in Japan. It occurs at any age, especially in adults, and affects men more than women, although this difference disappears when the intestinal form alone is considered.

The most specific signs are buccal, genital and ocular (iridocyclitis, uveitis) aphtous ulcers. Other lesions may be cutaneous (dermatitis, pseudo-folliculitis, hypersensitivity to insect stings and skin tests), articular (arthritis without radiological signs), cardiovascular (phlebitis) and visceral (digestive, renal, pulmonary, pancreatic, neurological). Digestive involvement is observed in 10% of cases only, and its main manifestation is an ulcerating colitis. The ileum is sometimed involved as well as the

esophagus and the stomach. The disease is chronic and is manifested by intermittent flare-ups. The various lesions are not concomitant but appear in turn, sometimes over several years. The course is benign in the incomplete forms but may be downhill in some cases of ocular involvement and even lethal in some visceral forms, especially those with intestinal involvement. Only symptomatic treatment is available at present.

Pathology

The digestive lesions are extensive, and deep, round or oval ulcerations which are rarely linear or superficial and sometimes have detached margins. They are located on the antimesenteric side of a bowel loop. The neighbouring mucosa is normal or moderately inflamed. The histology shows that the ulceration is transmural and often extends into the serosa. The neighbouring tissue contains an inflammatory cell infiltrate (lymphocytes, polymorphonuclears, histiocytes and plasmocytes) in a typical perivascular distibution. Vascular thrombosis, lymph vessel dilatation and fibrinoid necrosis are sparse. No epithelioid granulomas are found. Fibrosis may remain after healing of the ulcers.

Clinical findings

The intestinal involvement causes a hemorrhagie diarrhea, pain, fever and weight loss. Perforation with peritonitis or abscess formation is frequent in the ileal forms and is an index of the severity of the disease. The course of the disease is chronic and recurrent despite surgery.

No laboratory abnormalities are noted besides an increased sedimentation rate during the acute exacerbations.

Radiological findings

The disease in the small intestine mainly involves the ileum with large aphtoid ulcerations, which sometimes appear as true ulcerated nodules outlined by converging folds. Peyer's patches are hypertrophied. Contrast medium dilution, widened loops and broadened folds are observed. There is neither stenosis nor bowel wall thickening (except in cases complicated by abscesses and fistulae). The ileal lesions are most often associated with an ulcerating colitis. The

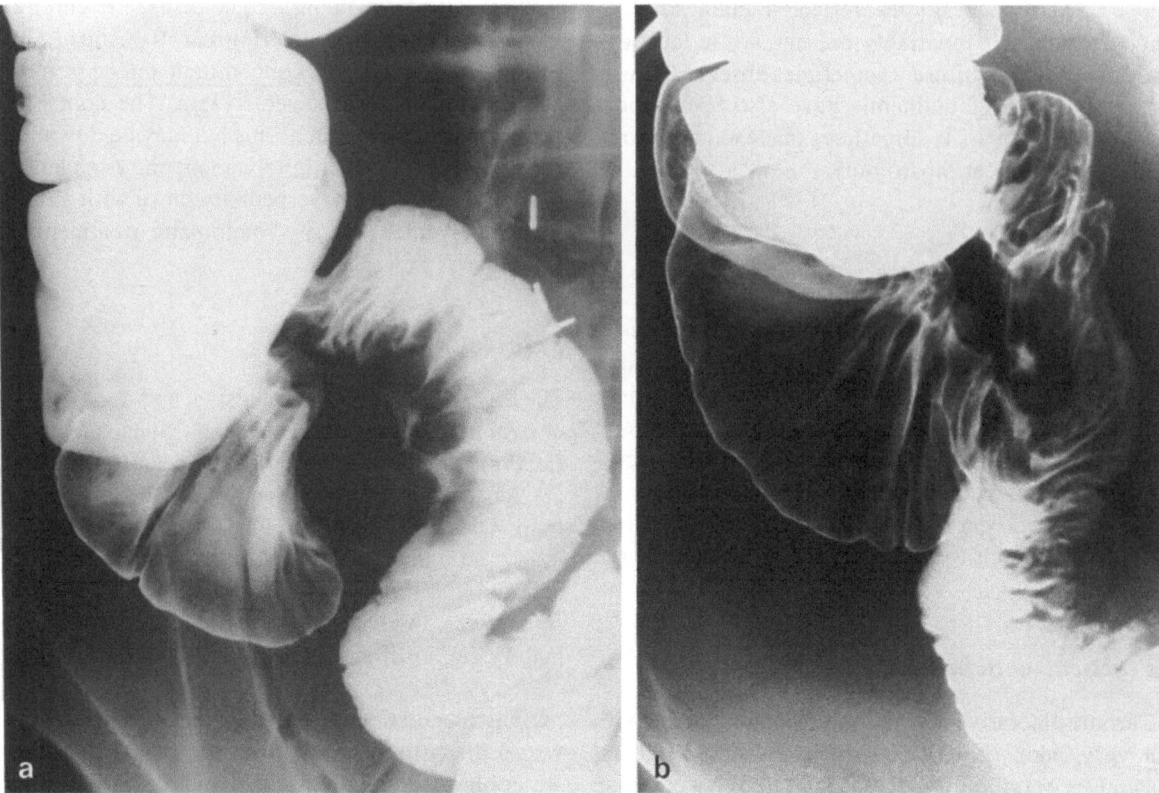

Fig. 76 a, b. Behçet's disease. 60-year-old man. Arteritis in the lower limbs. Lumbar sympathectomy. Epigastric and abdominal pain. Noduloulcerated lesion of the upper third of the esophagus seen at endoscopy. SBFT : **a, b** ulceration of the terminal ileum, outlined by convergent folds.

radiological appearance may be mistaken with Crohn's disease.

Practical conclusions

Behçet's disease is a rare entity which presents as diffuse, variably distributed aphtous ulcers with intermittent flare-ups. Its origin is unknown; it is a purely clinical diagnosis. Visceral, and in particular intestinal involvement carries a poor prognosis. The radiological appearance may be mistaken for Crohn's disease.

Eosinophilic gastroenteritis (figs. 77 to 80)

Eosinophilic gastroenteritis is characterized by a massive eosinophil infiltration of the wall of the small intestine. In half of all cases it occurs in the context of an allergic condition (rhinitis, eczema, asthma). An alimentary allergen (e.g. raw fish) can sometimes be identified, but its withdrawal does not always result in complete improvement. This condition is most often benign, with a chronic and recurrent course; it responds to steroid therapy. It affects both sexes equally at any age.

The infiltrate is diffuse or predominates in the jejunum. One of the specific features of the disease is the very frequent (90% of all cases) gastric involvement, in particular antral and pyloric. Eosinophilic gastritis without involvement of the small intestine is more frequent than the full gastroenteritis. A possible association with eosinophil infiltration of the colon, gallbladder, esophagus and liver has been reported. Other diseases with eosinophil tissue infiltration may also be observed in various parasitic infections and locally with inflammatory polyps and foreing-body granuloma reactions. A malignant form possessing the features of a plurifocal sarcoma must be distinguished.

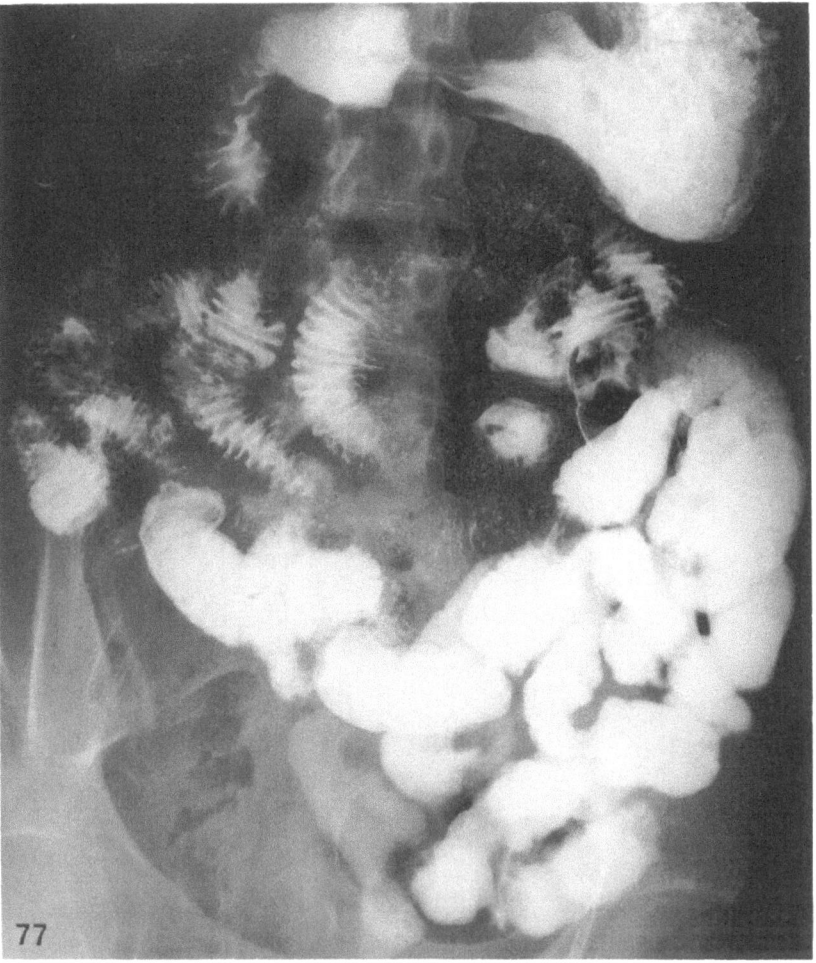

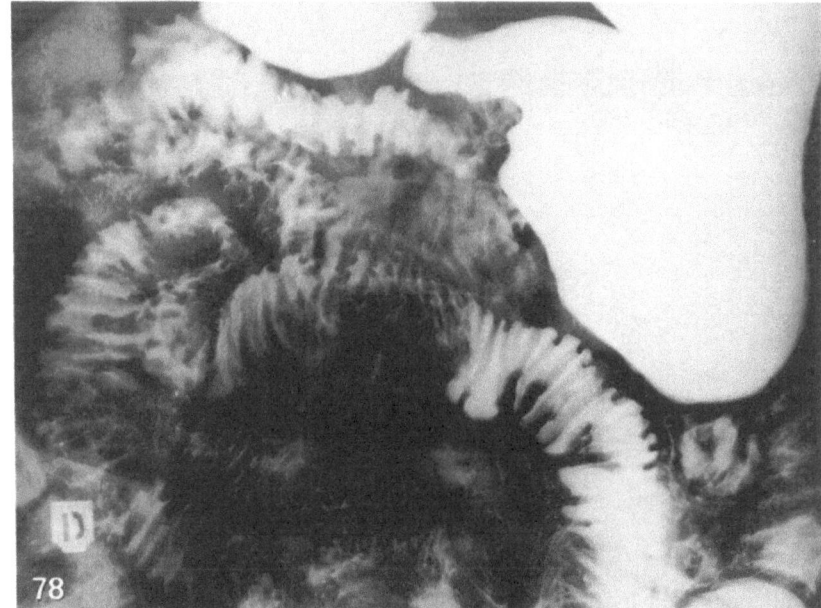

Fig. 77. Eosinophilic gastroenteritis. 21-year-old woman. Multiple allergies. Diarrhea. Blood count : 45,000 white blood cells with 83 % eosinophils. Eosinophil infiltrates of bone marrow and muscles. SBFT : segmental hypertonia and contrast medium dilution, moderate increase in the interloop gap, unfolded jejunal loops and large folds

Fig. 78. Eosinophilic gastroenteritis. 39-year-old woman. Multiple allergies. Chronic diarrhea. 50 % blood eosinophilia. Malabsorption. SBFT : segmental hypertonia and contrast medium dilution, irregularly broadened and nodular jejunal folds of increased height

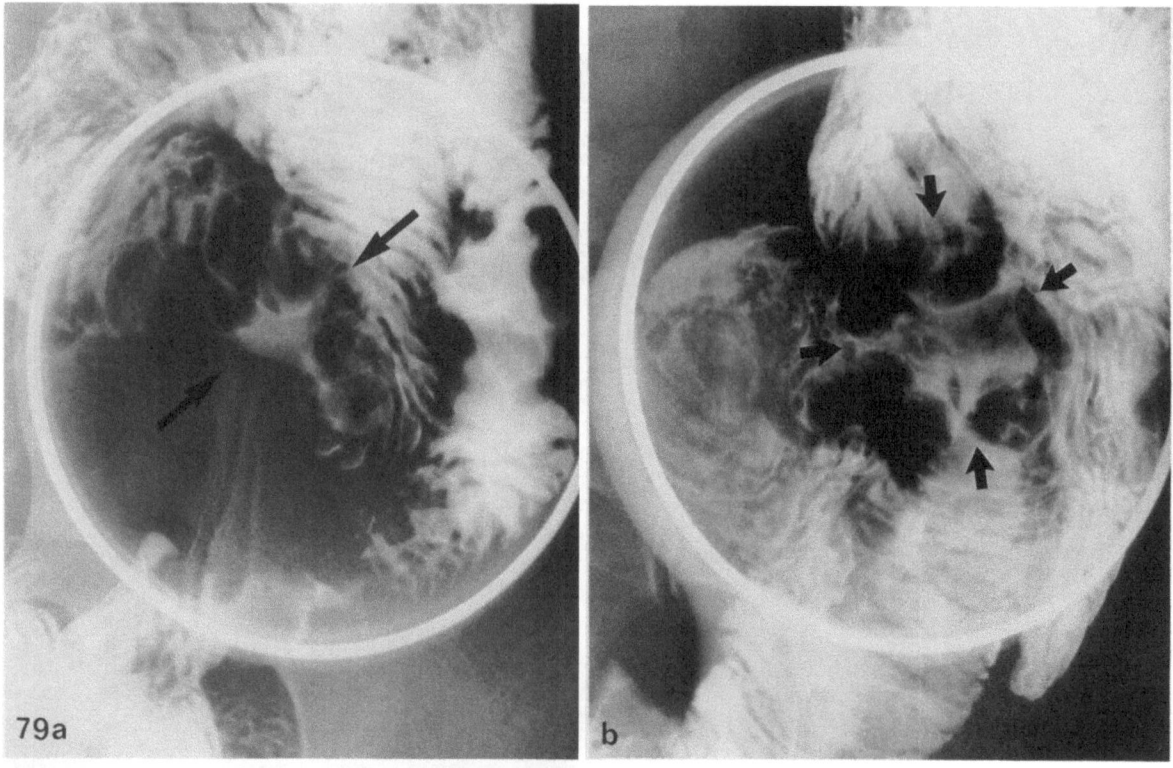

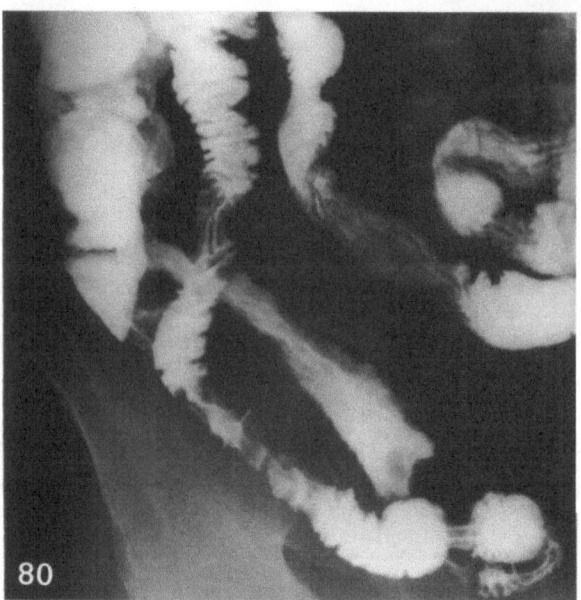

Fig. 79 a, b. Eosinophilic gastroenteritis (malignant form). 63-year-old man. Fever and poor general condition. Minor digestive symptoms, 31 % blood eosinophilia. SBFT : quadrangular jejunal ulcerations with a nodular ridge. Lethal outcome

Fig. 80. Eosinophilic ileitis. 64-year-old man. Epigastric pain, 12 % blood eosinophilia. SBFT : noduoulcerated appearance of the terminal ileum. Surgical findings : lymphoplasmocytic infiltration with numerous eosinophilis

Pathology

The macroscopic examination shows an intestinal wall thickened by hard plaques. The mucosa may show partial villous atrophy. Adenopathy and ascites are sometimes observed. The essential feature of the microscopic appearance is the massive eosino-phil infiltration predominating in the submucosa and often extending to the serosa, but more rarely to the mucosa. The eosinophils are clustered in perivascular sheaths. The wall is edematous and sometimes contains macrophages, giant cells or fibrosis. Necrosis is usually not seen. Ulcers are rare, except in the case of a malignant eosinophilic tumor.

Clinical findings

The disease causes nausea and vomiting, epigastric pain, meteorism and diarrhea, progressing by acute or subacute exacerbations which are sometimes triggered or aggravated by certain foods. Less frequent complications include obstruction, gastrointestinal hemorrhage, malabsorption, and a protein-losing enteropathy, growth retardation in children.

The laboratory studies demonstrate a leucocytosis due to eosinophilia, eosinophils sometimes comprising more than 50% of the blood smear. Eosinophilic gastroenteritis without blood eosinophilia is very rare. Albumin and gammaglobulin levels are sometimes decreased and immunoglobulin E levels are increased. Gastroscopy shows a thickened gastroduodenal wall but biopsies are often too superficial to yield a diagnosis. They often show partial or focal villous atrophy. The diagnosis can be made by laparoscopy but this modality is used only when the presentation is atypical, i.e. when no blood eosinophilia is noted.

Radiological findings

The lesions present with an extensive decrease in the caliber of intestinal loops, which is partially functional, and coupled to an increase in the interloop gap. The curvature of the loops is increased, thus completing the illusion of thickened walls. The folds are irregularly broadened and tall; although sometimes sparse, they are still sinuous. Their margins exhibit a double convexity on tangential views. Dilution occurs frequently. The appearance is characteristic when gastric abnormalities are also present. These latter include expansion defects and pseudotumoral stiffness of the antrum, with delayed evacuation due to partial pyloric stenosis, the presence of thickened and nodular folds, and irregular antral areolas in children.

Eosinophilic gastroenteritis may also rarely present with malignant appearing ulcerations dispersed throughout the small intestine, suggesting a diagnosis of lymphoma, sarcoma or metastases.

Practical conclusions

The radiological images associated with blood eosinophilia can usually yield the diagnosis of eosinophilic gastroenteritis, a most often benign disease of possibly allergic origin.

References

Crohn's disease

Symposium (1987) La maladie de Crohn. Diagnostic et thérapeutique. Acta Gastroent Belgica 50 : 481-648

Bodart P, Dive C, De Groote J, Van Trappen G, Vandenbroucke J (1959) Le diagnostic radiologique de l'iléite de Crohn. Arch Fr Mal App Dig 48 : 1672-1683

Bodart P, Dive C, Van Trappen G (1961) Radiologic differences between ileocecal tuberculosis and Crohn's disease. Am J Dig Dis 6 : 604-621

Bodart P, Pringot J (1977) Radiology of Crohn's disease. J. Belge Radiol 60 : 83-101

Brahme F, Hildell J (1976) Angiography in Crohn's disease revisited. AJR 126 : 941-951

Bray JF (1983) Filiform polyposis of the small bowel in Crohn's disease. Gastrointest Radiol 8 : 155-156

Chang SF, Burrell MI, Belleza NA, Spiro HM (1978) Borderlands in the diagnosis of regional enteritis. Trends in overdiagnosis and value of therapeutic trial. Gastrointest Radiol 3 : 67-72

Clavadetscher P, Deyhle P (1975) Diagnosis of Crohn's recurrence after surgery. Endoscopy 7 : 27-29

Chérigié E, Monnier JP, Donelli G (1973) Les aspects radiologiques des récidives de l'iléocolite granulomateuse. Ann Radiol 16 : 433-447

Crama-Bohbouth GE, Arndt JW, Pena AS, Verspaget HW, Tjon A Tham RT, Weterman IT, Pauwels EKJ, Lamers C (1988) Value of indium 111 granulocyte scintigraphy in the assessment of Crohn's disease of the small intestine : prospective investigation. Digestion 40 : 227-236

Crohn BB, Ginzburg L, Oppenheimer GD (1932) Regional ileitis pathological and clinical entity. JAMA 99 : 1323-1329

Dicandio G, Mosca F, Campatelli A, Bianchini M, D'Elia F, Dellagiovampaola C (1986) Sonographic detection of postsurgical recurrence of Crohn disease. AJR 146 : 523-526

Ekberg O (1977) Crohn's disease of the small bowel examined by double contrast technique. A comparison with oral technique. Gastrointest Radiol 1 : 355-359

Ekberg O, Baath L, Sjöström B, Lindhagen T (1984) Are superficial lesions of the distal part of the ileum early indicators of Crohn's disease in adult patients with abdominal pain ? A clinical and radiologic long term investigation. Gut 25 : 341-346

Ekberg O, Lindström C (1979) Superficial lesions in Crohn's disease of the small bowel. Gastrointest Radiol 4 : 389-393

Ekberg O, Fork F Th, Hildell J (1980) Predictive value of small bowel radiography for recurrent Crohn disease. AJR 135 : 1051-1055

Engelholm L, Mainguet P, Potvliège P (1976) Radiology in early Crohn's disease of the small bowel in : Weterman IT, Pena AS, Both CC (eds) The management of Crohn's disease. Excerpta Medica, Amsterdam, pp 73-76

Farmer RG, Hawk WA, Turnbull RB (1975) Clinical patterns in Crohn's disease : a statistical study of 615 cases. Gastroenterology 68 : 627-635

Fausa O, Nigaard K, Elgjo K (1977) Amyloidosis and Crohn's disease. Scand J Gastroenterol 12 : 657-662

Feczko PJ, Halpert LD (numéro spécial préfacé par) (1987) Radiology of inflammatory bowel disease. Radiol Clin N Am Janvier : 1-233

Fishman E, Wolf E, Jones B, Bayless Th, Siegelman S (1987) CT evaluation of Crohn's disease : effect on patient management. AJR 148 : 537-540

Fresko D, Lazarus SS, Dotan J, Reingold M (1982) Early presentation of carcinoma of the small bowel in Crohn's disease (Crohn's carcinoma), case reports and review of the literature. Gastroenterology 82 : 783-789

Gallego MS, Pulpeiro JR, Arenas A, Colina F (1986) Primary adenocarcinoma of the terminal ileum simulating Crohn's disease. Gastrointest Radiol 11 : 355-356

Ginzburg L, Marshak RH, Eliasoph J (1960) Regional jejunitis. Surg Gynecol Obstet 111 : 626-632

Glick SN, Teplick SK (1985) Crohn disease of the small intestine : diffuse mucosal granularity. Radiology 154 : 313-317

Goldberg HI, Caruthers SB, Nelson JA, Singleton JW (1979) Radiographic findings of the National Cooperative Crohn's disease study. Gastroenterology 77 : 925-937

Goldberg H, Gore R, Margulis A, Moss A, Baker E (1983) Computed tomography in the evaluation of Crohn's disease. AJR 140 : 277-282

Gottlieb C, Alpert S (1937) Regional jejunitis. AJR 38 : 881-883

Greenstein AJ, Janowitz HD, Sachar DB (1976) The extraintestinal complications of Crohn's disease and ulcerative colitis : a study of 700 patients. Medicine 55 : 401-412

Greenstein AJ, Wertkin M, Doughlin G, Sicular A (1979) Enteroenteric intussuception in Crohn's disease. Mount Sinai J Med 46 : 69-73

Greenstein AJ, Sachar DB, Greenstein RJ, Janowitz HD, Aufses AH (1982) Intra-abdominal abscess in Crohn's ileocolitis. Am J Surg 143 : 727-730

Herlinger H (1982) The small bowel enema and the diagnosis of Crohn's disease. Radiol Clin North Am 20 : 721-742

Herlinger H, O'Riordan D, Saul S, Levine MS (1986) Nonspecific involvement of bowel adjoining Crohn disease. Radiology 159 : 47-51

Hildell J, Lindström C, Wenckert A (1979) Radiographic appearances in Crohn's disease. I. Accuracy of radiographic methods. Acta Radiol Diagn 20 : 609-625

Hildell J, Lindström C, Wenckert A (1980) Radiographic appearances in Crohn's disease. IV. The new distal ileum after surgery. Acta Radiol 21 : 221-229

Higgens CS, Allan RN (1980) Crohn's disease of the distal ileum. Gut 21 : 933-940

Hillemand B (1971) La maladie de Crohn du grêle. Gaz Med France 78 : 2211-2224

Holt S, Samuel E (1979) Grey-scale ultrasound in Crohn's. Gut 20 : 590-595

Katzen BT, Sprayregen S, Chisolm A, Rossi P (1976) Angiographic manifestations of regional enteritis. Gastrointest Radiol 1 : 271-274

Khera DC, Shenai BU, Gelzyad EA, Maas LC, Karo JJ (1980) Ultrasound of the abdomen in Crohn disease. Gastroenterology 76 : 1168

Keller RJ, Hertz I, Zimmerman M, Geller S (1982) Carcinoma of the ileum simulating Crohn disease. AJR 138 : 151-153

Kerber GW, Frank PH (1984) Carcinoma of the small intestine and colon as a complication of Crohn disease : radiologic manifestations. Radiology 150 : 639-645

Kerber G, Greenberg M, Rubin J (1984) Computed tomography evaluation of local and extraintestinal complications of Crohn's disease. Gastrointest Radiol 9 : 143-148

Laufer I, Costopoulos L (1978) Early lesions of Crohn's disease. AJR 130 : 307-311

Louvel P, Benozio M, Guiller P, Challine B, Lérisson JA (1986) Evolution des images radiologiques élémentaires de l'iléite de Crohn, étude rétrospective d'une série homogène de 238 transits du grêle en double contraste. J Radiol 87 : 863-869

Marshak RH (1975) Granulomatous disease of the intestinal tract (Crohn's disease). Radiology 114 : 3-22

Miller T, Skucas J, Gudex D, Listinsky C (1987) Bowel cancer characteristics in patients with regional enteritis. Gastrointest Radiol 12 : 45-52

Milman PJ, Gold BM, Bagla S, Thorn R (1980) Primary ileal adenocarcinoma simulating Crohn's disease. Gastrointest Radiol 5 : 55-58

Modigliani R (1988) Maladies inflammatoires de l'intestin. Doin Paris

Nolan DJ, Piris J (1980) Crohn's disease of the small intestine : a comparative study of the radiological and pathological appearances. Clin Radiol 31 : 591-596

Nolan DJ (1987) The radiological appearances of small intestinal Crohn's disease with the enteroclysis technique. Acta Gastroenterol Belgica L : 513-518

Nolan DJ, Gourtsoyiannis NC (1980) Crohn's disease of the small intestine : a review of the radiogical appearances in 100 consecutive patients examined by a barium infusion technique. Clin Radiol 31 : 597-603

Papp JP, Pollard HM (1971) Adenocarcinoma occuring in Crohn's disease of the small intestine. Am J Gastroenterol 56 : 149-156

Pringot J, Goncette L, Mahieu P, Boverie J, Haot J (1984) Classification des lésions et critères radiologiques d'activité de la maladie de Crohn; corrélation avec l'anatomie pathologique. Acta Gastroent Belgica 47 : 289-297

Rickert RR, Carter HW (1980) The « early » ulcerative lesion of Crohn's disease : correlative light and scanning electron-microscopic studies. J Clin Gastroenterol 2 : 11-19

Ross D, Deininger HK (1979) Der morbus Crohn des Dickdarms. Fortschr Geb Roentgenstr Nuklearmed Ekganzungsband 131 : 169-173

Sartoris DJ, Harell GS, Anderson MF, Zboralske FF (1984) Small bowel lymphoma and regional enteritis : radiographic similarities. Radiology 152 : 291-296

Saverymuttu SH, Peters AM, Hodgson HJ, Chadwick VS, Lavender JP (1983) Indium leucocyte scanning in small bowel Crohn's disease. Gastrointest Radiol 8 : 157-161

Schmutz G, Drapé JL, Benhaim M, Jahn CH, Chapuis A, Degeorges A (1986) Aspect échographique de la maladie de Crohn, à propos de 42 examens. J Radiol 67 : 697-706

Schmutz G, Kempf F, Schutz JF, Riwer B (1980) Le transit du grêle en double contraste dans la maladie de Crohn, à propos de 32 examens. J. Radiol 61 : 235-241

Schölmerich J, Schmidt E, Schümichen C, Billmann P, Schmidt H, Gerok W (1988) Scintigraphic assessment of bowel involvement and disease activity in Crohn's disease using Technetium 99 m hexamethyl propylane amine oxyne as leucocyte label. Gastroenterology 95 : 1287-1293

Sonnenberg A, Erckenbrecht J, Peter P, Niederau C (1982) Detection of Crohn's disease by ultrasound. Gastroenterology 83 : 430-434

Warren S, Sommers SC (1947) Cicatrizing enteritis (regional ileitis) as a pathologic entity. Analysis of 120 cases. Am J Pathol 24 : 475-499

Welin S, Welin G (1973) A pathognomonic roentgenologic sign of regional ileitis (Crohn's ileitis). Dis Col Rect 16 : 473-478

Wellmann VN, Gebel M, Freise J, Groetz R (1980) Sonographic in der Diagnostik der Ileitis terminalis Crohn. Fortschr Röntgenstr 133 : 146-148

Wilhelm JP, Bresson A, Claudon M, Régent D, Champigneulle B, Bigard MA, Gaucher P (1988) Etude des anses grêles et du mésentère au cours de la maladie de Crohn : confrontation entre l'échographie, la tomodensitométrie et le transit du grêle chez 18 patients. Ann Gastroent Hepat 24 : 2

Yeh H, Rabinowitz JG (1983) Granulomatous enterocolitis : findings by ultrasonography and computed tomography. Radiology 149 : 253-259

Tuberculosis

Abrams JS, Holden WD (1964) Tuberculosis of the gastrointestinal tract. Arch Surg 89 : 282-293

Amerson JR, Martin JD (1964) Tuberculosis of the alimentary tract. Am J Surg 107 : 340-345

Archane MI, Hamani A, Bouziane M, Ohayon V, Touloune F, Hachim M (1983) La tuberculose iléo-cæcale. Ann Gastroenterol Hépatol 19 : 103-109

Bentley G, Webster JHH (1967) Gastro-intestinal tuberculosis. Br J Surg 54 : 90-96

Bernier JJ (1960) La tuberculose intestinale. Concours Med pp 5063-5067

Boddaert JC (1967) Tuberculose intestinale. Acta Gastroenterol Belgica 30 : 122-128

Boles RS, Gershon-Cohen J (1934) Intestinal tuberculosis. J Am Med Ass 103 : 1841-1844

Bondurant RE, Reid D (1975) Ileocecal tuberculosis. Am J Gastroenterol 63 : 58-65

Brombart M, Massion J (1961) Radiologic differences between ileocecal tuberculosis and Crohn's disease. Am J Dig Dis 6 : 589-603

Brombart M, Massion J, Bodart P, Dive C, Van Trappen G (1961) Radiologic differences betwen ileocecal tuberculosis and Crohn's disease. Am J Dig Dis 6 : 622

Burke GJ, Zafar SA (1975) Problems in distinguishing tuberculosis of bowel from Crohn's disease in Asians. Br Med J 4 : 395-397

Byrom HB, Mann CV (1969) Clinical features and surgical management of ileocaecal tuberculosis. Procr Soc Med 62 : 1230-1233

Carrera FG, Young S, Lewicki AM (1976) Intestinal tuberculosis. Gastrointest Radiol 1 : 147-155

Chawla S, Bery K, Indra KJ (1966) Enterolithiasis complicating intestinal tuberculosis. Clin Radiol 17 : 274-279

Chazelet C, Deixonne B, Eledjam JJ, Sawan S, Ould Said H, Baumel H (1988) A propos d'un cas de péritonite par perforation du grêle d'origine tuberculeuse. Revue de la littérature. Ann Gastroent Hepat 24 : 5

Chérigié E, Hillemand P, Proux Ch, Bourdon R (1955) Tuberculose de l'intestin grêle et de la région iléocæcale. Sem Hôp Paris, pp 1373-1388

Das P, Shukla HS (1976) Clinical diagnosis of abdominal tuberculosis. Br J Surg 63 : 941-946

Fung WP, Tan KK, Yu SF, Kho KM (1970) Malabsorption and subtotal villous atrophy secondary to pulmonary and intestinal tuberculosis. Gut 11 : 212-216

Gastli H, Hassine W, Abdesselem K, Gharbi HA (1983) Aspects échographiques de la tuberculose péritonéale, à propos de 14 cas. J Radiol 64 : 325-329

Gershon-Cohen J (1930) The diagnosis of early ileocecal tuberculosis. AJR 24 : 367-388

Gershon-Cohen J, Kremens V (1954) X-ray studies of the ileocecal valve in ileocecal tuberculosis. Radiology 62 : 251-254

Herlinger H (1978) Angiography in the diagnosis of ileocecal tuberculosis. Gastrointest Radiol 2 : 371-376

Howell JS, Knapton PJ (1964) Ileo-caecal tuberculosis. Gut 5 : 524-529

Levrat M, Despierres G, Wégelin JE (1950) Fausses appendicites et manifestations abdominales douloureuses de la primo-infection tuberculeuse. J Med Lyon, pp 457-464

Mitchell RS, Bristol LJ (1954) Intestinal tuberculosis : an analysis of 346 cases diagnosed by routine intestinal radiography on 5 529 admissions for pulmonary tuberculosis. Am J Med Sci, pp 241-249

Moss JD, Knauer CM (1973) Tuberculous enteritis. Gastroenterology 65 : 959-966

Ravault PP, Fraisse H, Loisy C (1950) La péritonite tuberculeuse du vieillard. J Med Lyon, pp 453-456

Paustian FF, Bockus HL (1959) So-called primary ulcerohypertrophic ileocecal tuberculosis. Am J Med, pp 509-518

Perreau P, Joubaud F, Boyer J, Plane P, Simard C (1972) Lithiase primitive du grêle et tuberculose intestinale. Sem Hôp Paris 48 : 2665-2670

Prout WG (1968) Multiple tuberculous perforations of ileum. Gut 9 : 381-382

Sankale M, Diop B, Frament V, Ancelle JP (1969) La tuberculose dans un service de médecine générale en Afrique noire. Sem Hôp Paris, pp 2155-2168

Scully RE, Galdabini JJ, Mc Neely BU (1980) Case records of the Massachusetts general hospital. N Engl J Med 303 : 445-451

Shah IC (1973) Ileocecal tuberculosis and Crohn's disease. NY St J Med 73 : 949-951

Tabrisky J, Lindstrom RR, Peters R, Lachman RS (1975) Tuberculous enteritis. Am J Gastroent 63 : 49-57

Tandon HD, Prakash A (1972) Pathology of intestinal tuberculosis and its distinction from Crohn's disease. Gut 13 : 260-269

Werbeloff L, Novis BH, Bank S, Marks IN (1973) The radiology of tuberculosis of the gastro-intestinal tract. Br J Radiol 46 : 329-336

Zeit M, Cope C (1983) Angiographic, radiographic, and computed tomographic findings in tuberculosis of the jejunum. Am J Gastroenterol 78 : 339-340

Yersiniosis

Bories P, Michel H (1981) Infections à yersinia enterocolitica. Nouv Presse Med 10 : 3613-3615

Bories P, Veyrac M (1983) Yersinioses et maladie de Crohn. Gastroent Clin Biol 7 : 570-572

Bradford WD, Noce PS, Gutman LT (1974) Pathologic features of enteric infection with yersinia enterocolitica. Arch Pathol 98 : 17-22

Chessum B, Frengley JD, Fleck DG, Mair NS (1971) Case of septicaemia due to yersinia enterocolitica. Br Med J 3 : 466

Delchier JC, Constantini D, Soule JC (1983) Présence d'agglutinines anti« yersinia pseudo-tuberculosis » lors d'une poussée de maladie de Crohn iléale, à propos de 3 cas. Gastroenterol Clin Biol 7 : 580-584

Ekberg O, Sjöström B, Brahme F (1977) Radiological findings in yersinia ileitis. Radiology 123 : 15-19

Keet EE (1974) Yersinia enterocolitica septicemia, source of infection and incubation period identified. N Y St J Med 74 : 2226-2230

Lacut JY (1977) Diagnostic et traitement des pasteurelloses. Cah Med 99 : 2959-2972

Leino R, Kalliomäki JL (1974) Yersiniosis as an internal disease. Ann Int Med 81 : 458-461

Mollaret HH (1971) L'infection humaine à « yersinia enterocolitica » en 1970, à la lumière de 642 cas récents. Pathol Biol 19 : 189-205

Pibarot ML, Carbon C (1984) Mise au point sur les « yersinioses ». Concours Med 1061-31 : 2941-2955

Sjöström B, Nilehn B (1968) Some aspects of the inflammation of the ileocæcal region with special reference to yersinia enterocolitica. Bull Soc Int Chir pp 386-392

Vantrappen G, Ponette E, Geboes K, Bertrand P (1977) Yersinia enteritis and enterocolitis : gastroenterological aspects. Gastroenterology 72 : 220-227

Van Wiechen PJ (1974) Radiological changes in the distal part or the ileum in association with yersinia enterocolitica infections. Radiol Clin Biol 43 : 242-253

Winblad S, Nilehn B, Sternby NH (1966) Yersinia enterocolitica (pasteurella X) in human enteric infections. Br Med J 2 : 1363-1366

Intestinal infections

Arnulf G, Buffard P (1953) L'iléite lymphoïde terminale. Presse Med 61 : 107-108

Brodey PA, Fertig S, Aron JM (1982) Campylobacter enterocolitis : radiographic features. AJR 139 : 1199-1201

Butler ML, Carlton L, DeGreen HP, Teplick ST, Metz JR (1974) Transient malabsorption in infectious mononucleosis. AJR 122 : 241-245

Cattan R (1959) Les jéjuno-iléites infectieuses subaiguës et chroniques de l'adulte. Sem Hôp Paris 51 : 2959-2963

Chérigié E, Tavernier C, Dupas, Raynal (1955) Les iléites terminales aiguës et subaiguës. Sem Hôp Paris 41 : 2417-2426

Chérigié E, Deporte A, Tavernier C, Pradel-Raynal Mme (1959) Iléites folliculaires et invagination intestinale. Ann Pediatr 54/11 : 3177-3192

Denoyel GA, Cloppet H (1977) La maladie des inclusions cytomégaliques. Cah Med 2 : 1821-1832

Francis RS, Berk RN (1974) Typhoid fever. Radiology 112 : 583-585

Gardiner R, Smith C (1987) Infective enterocolitides. Radiol Clin N Am Janvier : 67-78

Grundy A, Gilks CF (1984) Typhoid : an unusual cause of gastro-intestinal bleeding. Br J Radiol 57 : 344-346

Knapp AB, Horst DA, Eliopoulos G, Gramm HF, Gaber LW, Falchuk KR, Falchuk M, Trey C (1983) Widespread cytomegalovirus gastroenterocolitis in a patient with acquired immuno-deficiency syndrome. Gastroenterology 85 : 1399-1402

Lambert R, Marchat F (1975) Manifestations pathologiques de l'anse borgne. Concours Med 97-46 : 7474-7483

Levine RS, Warner NE, Johnson CF (1964) Cytomegalic inclusion disease in the gastro-intestinal tract of adults. Ann Surg 159 : 37-48

Loygue J, Dubois F, Pottiée-Sperry F (1964) Conséquences générales des laparotomies et des interventions portant sur le tube digestif. Rev Prat XIV : 719-734

Marsh PK, Gorbach SL (1982) Invasive enterocolitis caused by edwardsiella tarda. Gastroenterology 82 : 336-338

Petrella R, Young EJ Acute brucella ileitis. Amer J Gastroent 83 : 80-82

Ploussard JP (1971) Fièvre typhoïde, infections à entéro-virus. Concours Med 19 : 76-93

Richard C (1964) Les séquelles de la chirurgie du grêle. Rev Prat XIV : 779-787

Rosen P, Armstrong D, Rice N (1973) Gastrointestinal cytomegalovirus infection. Arch Intern Med 132 : 274-276

Roux M, Hillemand P, Delavierre Ph, Vayre P (1966) Iléites segmentaires aspécifiques. Presse Med 74 : 61-62

Schwöbel M, Hirsig J, Stauffer UG (1985) Contaminated small bowel syndrome presenting as an abdominal emergency in infants and children. Z kinderchir 40 : 228-232

Underwood JCE, Corbett CL (1978) Persistent diarrhoea and hypoalbuminaemia associated with cytomegalovirus enteritis. Br Med J 2 : 1029-1030

Backwash ileitis

Geoffrey A, Gardiner (1977) Backwash ileitis with pseudopolyposis. AJR 129 : 506-507

Whipple's disease

Barbotte P (1973) Aspect actuel de la maladie de Whipple. Lyon Méditerranée Médical IX : 1949-1961

Benozio M, Legendre H, Rymer R, May JP (1977) Diagnostic radiologique de la maladie de Whipple, à propos de 8 observations. Ann Radiol 20 : 461-468

Boddaert JC (1967) La maladie de Whipple. Acta Gastroenterol Belgica 30 : 132-139

Cerf M (1972) La maladie de Whipple, étude clinique, bactériologique et biologique. Ann Gastroenterol Hepatol 8 : 253-266

Dobbins WO (1981) Is there an immune deficit in Whipple's disease ? Dig Dis Sci 26 : 247-252

Enzinger FM, Helwig EB (1963) Whipple's disease, a review of the literature and report of fifteen patients. Virchows Arch Pathol Anat 336 : 238-269

Ganter P, Marche Cl, Delesque M, Laumonier R, Métayer J, Cerf M (1974) Etude histoenzymologique de la muqueuse intestinale dans 5 cas de maladie de Whipple, évolution sous traitement antibiotique. Ann Anat Pathol Paris 19 : 97-116

Matuchansky C, Lenormand Y (1976) La maladie de Whipple. Concours Med 98 : 5049-5057

Metman EH, Bertrand J (1979) La maladie de Whipple. Rev Fr Gastroenterol 151 : 49-64

Philips RL, Carlson HC (1975) The roentgenographic and clinical findings in Whipple's disease, a review of 8 patients. AJR 123 : 268-273

Rice RP, Roufail WM, Reeves RJ (1967) The roentgen diagnosis of Whipple's disease (intestinal lipodystrophy). Radiology 88 : 295-301

Tucat G (1982) La maladie de Whipple. Gastroenterologie 32 : 2379-2384

Nonspecific ulcers

Alexander HC, Schwartz GF (1966) Nonspecific jejunal ulceration : in search of an etiology. Gastroenterology 50 : 224-229

Billig DM, Jordan GL (1965) Nonspecific ulcers of the small intestine. Am J Surg 110 : 745-749

Boydstun JS, Gaffey TA, Bartholomew LG (1981) Clinicopathologic study of nonspecific ulcers of the small intestine. Dig Dis Sci 26 : 911-916

Chagnon JP, Devars du Mayne JF, Marche C, Vissuzaine C, Cerf M (1984) L'entérite sténosante multifocale crypto-génétique : une entite autonome ? Gastroenterol Clin Biol 8 : 808-813

Colin R (1981) Ulcères de l'intestin grêle. Ann Gastroenterol Hepatol 17 : 419-421

Davies DR, Brightmore T (1970) Idiopathic and drug-induced ulceration of the small intestine. Br J Surg 57 : 134-139

Gioanni T (1965) A propos des ulcères primitifs du grêle, une maladie du progrès médical. Marseille Med 7 : 613-617

Grosfeld JL, Schiller M, Weinberger M, Clatworthy WH (1970) Primary nonspecific ileal ulcers in children. Am J Dis Child 120 : 447-450

Karz S, Guth PH, Polonsky L (1971) Chronic ulcerative jejunoileitis. Am J Gastroenterol 56 : 61-67

Lawrason FD, Alpert E, Mohr FL, McMahon FG (1965) Ulcerative-obstructive lesions of the small intestine. JAMA 191 : 641-644

Maratka Z (1981) L'ulcère du colon et du grêle. Ann Gastroenterol Hepatol 17 : 123-129

Paille F, Champigneulle B, Brucker P, Bigard MA, Gaucher P (1981) L'entérite sténosante ulcéreuse plurifocale cryptogénétique, à propos de 2 observations. Ann Gastroenterol Hepatol 17 : 405-409

Porchet A (1962) Ulcère primitif de l'intestin grêle, à propos d'une observation inédite. Presse Med 70 : 1886-1887

Shah MJ (1968) Primary nonspecific ulcer of ileum presenting with massive rectal haemorrhage. Br Med J 3 : 474

Watson MR (1963) Primary nonspecific ulceration of the small bowel. Arch Surg 87 : 600-603

Wilson IH, Cooley NV, Luibel FJ (1968) Nonspecific stenosing small bowel ulcers. Am J Gastroenterol 50 : 449-455

The Zollinger-Ellison syndrome

Amberg JR, Ellison EH, Wilson SD, Zboralske FF (1964) Roentgenographic observations in the Zollinger-Ellison syndrome. JAMA 190 : 185-187

Bernstein JS, Groisser VW, Lawrence Lr (1963) Abnormal small-bowel X-ray patterns associated with active duodenal ulcer. Am J Dig Dis 8 : 174-190

Christoforidis AJ, Nelson SW (1966) Radiological manifestations of ulcerogenic tumors of the pancreas. JAMA 198 : 511-517

Ellison EH, Wilson SD (1964) The Zollinger-Ellison syndrome : re-appraisal and evaluation of 260 registered cases. Ann Surg 160 : 512-530

Herrington JL (1965) A teen-age boy with the Zollinger-Ellison syndrome presenting multiple ulcerations including perforation of a colonic ulcer. Surgery 58 : 442-447

Missakian MM, Carlson HC, Huizenga KA (1965) Roentgenographic findings in Zollinger-Ellison syndrome. AJR 94 : 429-437

Pagès JM (1974) Les formes diarrhéiques non ulcérogènes du syndrome de Zollinger-Ellison. Thèse, Lyon

Parrish JA, Rawlins DC (1965) Intestinal mucosa in the Zollinger-Ellison syndrome. Gut 6 : 286-289

Singleton JW, Kern F, Waddell WR (1965) Diarrhea and pancreatic islet cell tumor, report of a case with a severe jejunal mucosal lesion. Gastroenterology 49 : 197-208

Weber JM, Lewis S, Heasley KH (1959) Observations on the small bowel pattern associated with the Zollinger-Ellison syndrome. AJR 82 : 973-977

Zboralske FF, Amberg JR (1968) Detection of the Zollinger-Ellison syndrome : the radiologist's responsability. AJR 104 : 529-543

Zollinger RM, Ellison EH (1955) Primary peptic ulcerations of the jejunum associated with islet cell tumors of the pancreas. Ann Surg 142 : 709-728

Chronic ulcerative jejunoileitis

Armstrong BK, Ammon RK, Finlay-Jones LR, Joske RA, Vivian AB (1973) A further case of chronic ulcerative enteritis. Gut 14 : 649-652

Belaiche J, Modigliani R, Modigliani E, Galian A, Bernier JJ (1977) Jéjuno-iléite ulcéreuse chronique nonspécifique. Gastroenterol Clin Biol 1 : 553-560

Cerf M, Gouerou H, Marche C, L'Hirondel C, Debray C (1977) Jéjuno-iléite ulcéreuse diffuse : intérêt diagnostique de la jéjunoscopie. Gastroenterol Clin Biol 1 : 571-575

Gouerou H, Redelsperger PY, Galian A, Dervichian M, Pappo E, Cattan D (1977) Jéjuno-iléite ulcéreuse chronique avec malabsorption. Gastroenterol Clin Biol 1 : 561-570

Gouffier E, Phan A, Paraf A, Boddaert A, Chevrel JP (1977) Jéjuno-iléite ulcéreuse d'évolution récurrente, étude opératoire et endoscopique d'un nouveau cas. Gastroenterol Clin Biol 1 : 545-552

Jeffries GH, Steinberg H, Sleisenger MH (1968) Chronic ulcérative (non-granulomatous) jéjunitis. Am J Med 44 : 47-59

Klaeveman HL, Gebhard RL, Sessoms C, Strober W (1975) In vitro studies of ulcerative ileojejunitis Gastroenterology 68 : 572-582

Lamont CM, Adams FG, Mills PR (1982) Radiology in idiopathic chronic ulcerative enteritis. Clin Radiol 33 : 283-287

Mills PR, Brown IL, Watkinson G (1980) Idiopathic chronic ulcerative enteritis, report of 5 cases and review of the literature. Quart J Med XLIX : 133-149

Modigliani R (1977) Les duodéno-jéjuno-iléites chroniques non spécifiques, une entité anatomo-clinique de nosologie discutée. Gastroenterol Clin Biol 1 : 501-506

Modigliani R, Poitras P, Galian A, Messing B, Guyet-Rousset P, Libeskind MM, Piel-Desruisseaux JL, Rambaud JC (1979) Chronic nonspecific ulcerative duodenojejunoileitis : report of 4 cases. Gut 20 : 318-328

Modigliani R, Poitras P, Galian A, Messing B, Guyet-Rousset P, Libeskind MM, Piel-Desruisseaux JL, Rambaud JC (1979) Chronic nonspecific ulcerative duodenojejunoileitis : report of 4 cases. Gut 20 : 318-328

Moritz M, Moran JM, Patterson JF (1971) Chronic ulcerative jejunitis, report of a case and discussion of classification. Gastroenterology 60 : 96-102

Behcet's disease

Asakura H, Morita A, Morishita T, Tsuchiya M, Watanabe Y, Enomoto Y (1973) Histopathological and electron microscopic studies of lymphangiectasia of the small intestine in Behcet disease. Gut 14 : 196-203

Baba S, Maruta M, Ando K, Teramoto T, Endo I (1976) Intestinal Behcet's disease : report of 5 cases. Dis Col Rect 19 : 428-440

Baba S (1979) Clinical studies on intestinal Behcet disease. Stomach Intest 14 : 885-892

Boe J, Dalgaard JB, Scott D (1958) Mucocutaneous-ocular syndrome with intestinal involvement, a clinical and pathological study of 4 fatal cases. Am J Med, pp 857-867

Debray Ch, Paolaggi JA, Couturier D, Crespon B (1973) Colite ulcéreuse et syndrome de Behcet, intérêt de la coloscopie. Ann Med Int 124 : 931-935

Dowling GB (1961) Behcet disease. Proc R Soc Med 54 : 101-107

Fromer JL (1970) Behcet's syndrome. Arch Dermatol 102 : 116-117

Hamza M, Ben Ayed H (1981) Maladie de Behcet. Concours Med 103 : 841-856

Hamza M, Wechsler B, Hamza H, Ayed K, Godeau P (1988) Intestinal amyloidosis : an unusual complication of Behcet's disease. Amer J Gastroent 83 : 793-794

Hamza M, Zribi A, Chadli A, Benayed H (1975) La maladie de Behcet, étude de 22 cas. Presse Med 4 : 563-566

Hewitt J, Escande JP, Lauret Ph, Perlemutier L (1969) Critères de prévision du syndrome de Behcet. Bull Soc Fr Dermatol 76 : 565-568

McLean AL, Simms DM, Homer MJ (1983) Ileal ring ulcers in Behcet syndrome. AJR 140 : 947-948

O'Duffy JD, Carney JA, Deodhar S (1971) Behcet's disease, report of 10 cases, 3 with new manifestations. Ann Int Med 75 : 561-570

Rogé J (1985) Atteinte intestinale du syndrome de Behcet. Press Med 14 : 537-541

Rogé J, Fabre M, Durand B, Durand J, Benichou J, Paillas J, Roge F (1982) Les localisations intestinales du syndrome de Behcet, étude anatomo-clinique de 2 cas avec lésions vasculaires. Gastroenterol Clin Biol 6 : 872-878

Rogé J, Durand B (1982) Syndrome de Behcet et intestin. Gastroenterol Clin Biol 6 : 886-891

Schmutz G, Doffoel M, Zeller C, Coumaros D, Kempf F, Bockel R (1981) Localisations digestives de la maladie de Behcet, à propos d'une observation. J Radiol 62 : 515-520

Schnitzler L, Fortier P (1980) Maladie de Behcet. Rev Prat 30 : 3699-3704

Smith GE, Kime LR, Pitcher JL (1973) The colitis of Behcet's cet's disease : a separate entity ? Colonoscopic findings and literature review. Am J Dig Dis 18 : 987-1000

Wechsler B, Godeau P (1981) La maladie de Behcet. Gaz Med France 88 : 237-239

Eosinophilic gastroenteritis

Bogomoletz WV (1976) Les gastroentérites à ésosinophiles. Arch Fr Mal App Dig 65 : 357-360

Bogomoletz WV (1977) Eosinophilic gastroenteritis. Gastroenterology 73 : 191

Burhenne HJ, Carbone JV (1966) Eosinophilic (allergic) gastroenteritis. AJR 96 : 332-338

Chateau P (1978) Gastroentérite à éosinophiles, à propos de 2 cas qui sortent du cadre habituel de la maladie. Thèse, Lyon

Dalinka MK, Masters CJ (1970) Eosinophilic enteritis, report of a case whithout gastric involvement. Radiology 96 : 543-544

Edelman MJ, March TL (1964) Eosinophilic gastroenteritis. AJR 91 : 773-778

Goldberg HI, O'Kieffe D, Jenis EH, Boyce HW (1973) Diffuse eosinophilic gastroenteritis. AJR 119 : 342-351

Haberkern CM, Christie DL, Haas JE (1978) Eosinophilic gastroenteritis presenting as ileocolitis. Gastroenterology 74 : 896-899

Leinbach GE, Rubin CE (1970) Eosinophilic gastroenteritis : a simple reaction to food allergens ? Gastroenterology 59 : 874-889

Marshak RH, Lindner A, Maklansky D, Gelb A (1981) Eosinophilic gastroenteritis. JAMA 245 : 1677-1680

McNabb PC, Fleming CR, Higgins JA, Davis GL (1979) Transmural eosinophilic gastroenteritis with ascites. Mayo Clin Proc 54 : 119-122

Schulman A, Morton PCG, Dietrich BE (1980) Eosinophilic gastroenteritis. Clin Radiol 31 : 101-104

Teele RL, Katz AJ, Goldman H, Kettell RN (1979) Radiographic features of eosinophilic gastroenteritis (allergic gastroenteropathy) of childhood. AJR 132 : 575-580

Ureles AL, Alschibaja T, Lodico D, Stabins SJ (1961) Idiopathic eosinophilic infiltration of the gastrointestinal tract, diffuse and circumscribed. Am J Med, pp 899-909

Waldmann TA, Wochner RD, Laster L, Gordon RS (1967) Allergic gastroenteropathy, a cause of excessive gastrointestinal protein loss. N Engl J Med 276 : 761-769

Wehunt WD, Olmsted WW, Neiman HL, Phillips JF (1976) Eosinophilic gastritis, RPC from the AFIP. Radiology 120 : 85-89

Weisberg SC, Crosson JT (1973) Eosinophilic gastroenteritis, report of a case of 32 year's duration. Dig Dis 18 : 1005-1014

Celiac disease and malabsorption

Celiac disease (figs. 1 to 8)

Celiac disease or sprue is a malabsorptive syndrome caused by the atrophy of duodenojejunal mucosa which is cured by a gluten-free diet. It is the most common cause of chronic diarrhea of small intestinal origin. The disease is much more frequent in children (1 in 3,000) than in adults (1 in 100,000). In the latter, it can occur at any age, but usually manifests by age 50. Whereas in children, females are affected twice as often as males, there is no such difference in adults. Celiac disease is a genetic disease which occurs sporadically, affecting one child out of 50 in predisposed families. Several factors indicate an immunoallergic etiology. The allergen is the gliadin of gluten contained in some types of flour. Many of the affected subjects belong to the histocompatibility groups HLA B8 and DRW3.

Pathology

Atrophy of the duodenojejunal mucosa appears grossly as flattened, broadened villi, which disappear in case of complete atrophy. Histology reveals a decrease in the height of the epithelium, lengthened crypts and rarefied goblet cells. The mucosa and the submucosa are infiltrated by inflammatory cells. Associated lymph nodes are sometimes hyperplastic.

Clinical findings

In children, the disease begins a couple of weeks or months after the flour has first been ingested. The triggering factor is not identified in adults, but previous history of digestive symptoms during childhood are often elicited. The study of family members may reveal latent forms of the disease.

The main feature is diarrhea, which occurs in 80% of cases in children, but only in 50% of adult patients. It is rarely acute and profuse, and more frequently is made up of abundant, pasty stools 3 to 10 times heavier than normal. The diarrhea is sometimes associated with anorexia, vomiting, abdominal pain and meteorism. It may go unnoticed, whereas signs of malabsorption are reported. These include anemia, osteomalacia, hemorrhages, infections, edema, tetany, neuropathies and, in children, growth retardation and behavioral disorders.

Untreated, celiac disease leads to a malnourished state. A gluten-free diet produces considerable clinical improvement within a couple of weeks. If not definite, the diagnosis is confirmed by relapse if gluten is reinstalled too early in the diet. A normal diet can often be returned to progressively, after a two-year avoidance of gluten. In other cases, a milk-free diet and even steroid therapy must be associated to the gluten-free diet because the lesions of the intestinal wall sometimes cause associated lactase deficiency. A poor response to the gluten-free diet may be caused by the development of ulcers, which may lead to obstruction, hemorrhage or perforations and carry a poor prognosis. These ulcers appear in the duodenum, the small intestine and even the colon. Cancers, especially digestive tumors and in particular lymphomas, appear in 10 to 15% of patients with celiac disease. The risk may be associated with a particular genetic predisposition. Lymphomas occur more frequently in older subjects, regardless of the

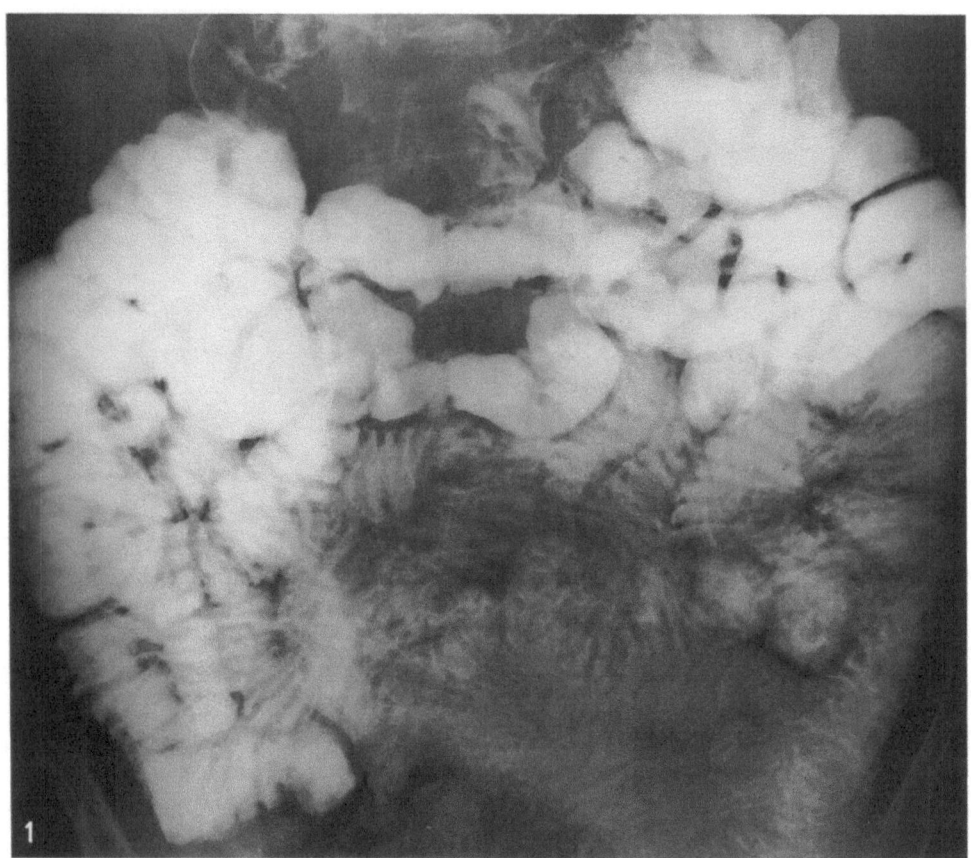

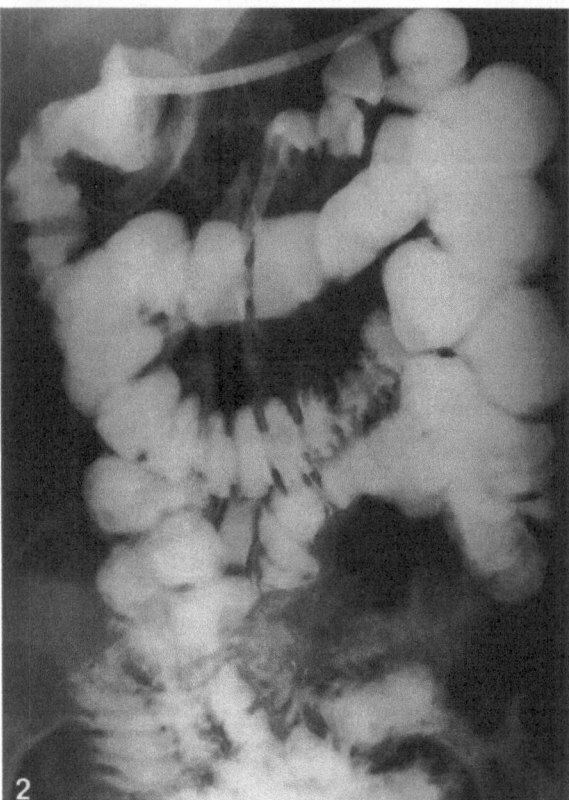

Fig. 1. Celiac disease. 51-year-old man. Chronic diarrhea. Weight loss. Malabsorption syndrome. Type V villous atrophy. SBFT : contrast medium dilution, atonia, disappearance of the jejunal folds

Fig 2. Celiac disease. 39-year-old woman. Recent diarrhea. Hypokalemia. Total villous atrophy improved by a gluten-free diet. SBFT: increased caliber and rarefaction of the jejunal folds

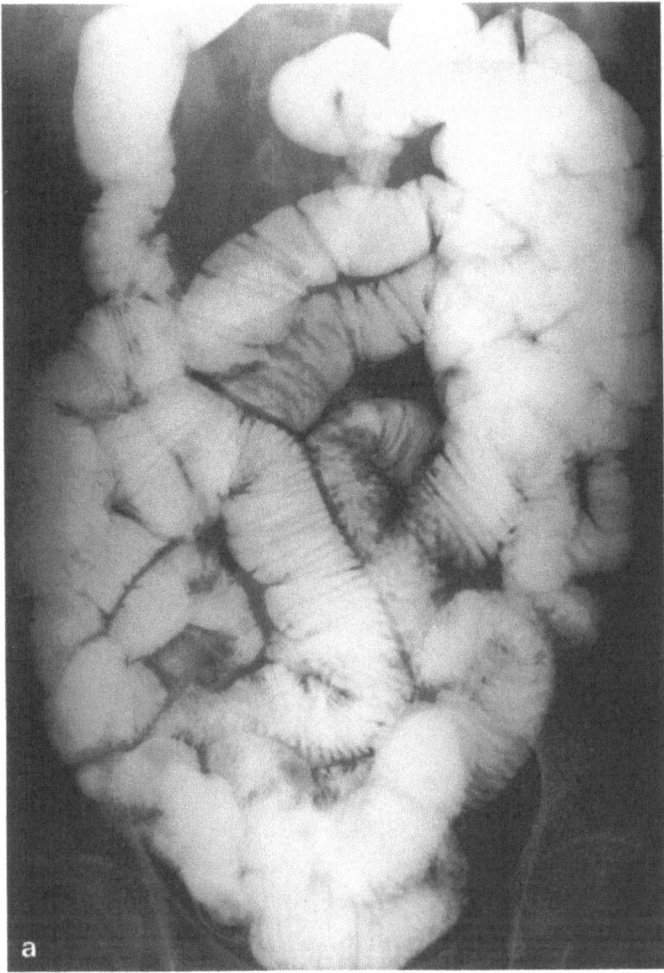

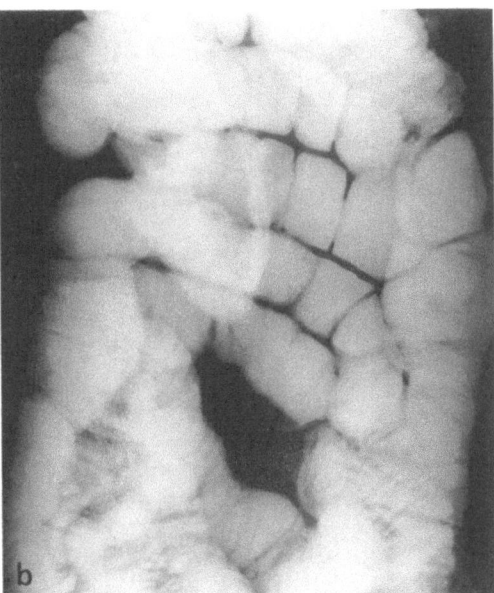

Fig. 3 a, b. Celiac disease. 49-year-old woman. Chronic diarrhea for 2 years. Malabsorption syndrome. Total villous atrophy. SBFT : a, b increased caliber, rarefaction of the jejunal folds, jejunal transformation of the ileum

duration of the disease. It may originate in or outside the bowel; the lymphoma is often located in the jejunum, and of the histiocytic type. Indications that a tumour has arisen include resistance to the diet, deterioration of the patient's general status, fever, obstruction, or perforation.

The diagnosis of celiac disease is confirmed by laboratory tests if a micro-, normo- or macrocytic anemia is associated with decreased levels of calcium and electrolytes, folate and proteins, especially albumin and gammaglobulins. Many tests of absorption indicate a small bowel disorder, including steatorrhea in 75% of all patients and carbohydrate malabsorption in 80%. Direct or magnified images of the duodenum and jejunum show villous atrophy, which is graded on biopsy from I, corresponding to an almost normal appearance, to V, i.e. complete atrophy. Grade IV or V villous atrophy in the duodenum needs to be present for a diagnosis of celiac disease.

The absorptive impairment is related to the spread of the lesions rather than to the degree of atrophy. In 10% of cases, villous atrophy is caused by another condition than celiac disease. The latter can only be diagnosed with confidence after a therapeutic trial.

Radiological findings

Plain films often reveal a great quantity of gas in the intestinal loops and sometimes jejunal distention. Air-fluid levels are observed during acute exacerbations. Other signs described include a megacolon, renal stones and gallstones.

A small bowel follow-through (SBFT) is useful when the clinical, laboratory or histological data is not typical, and also when it is necessary to rule out other pathologic entities once the diagnosis of villous atrophy has been made. A SBFT is normal in

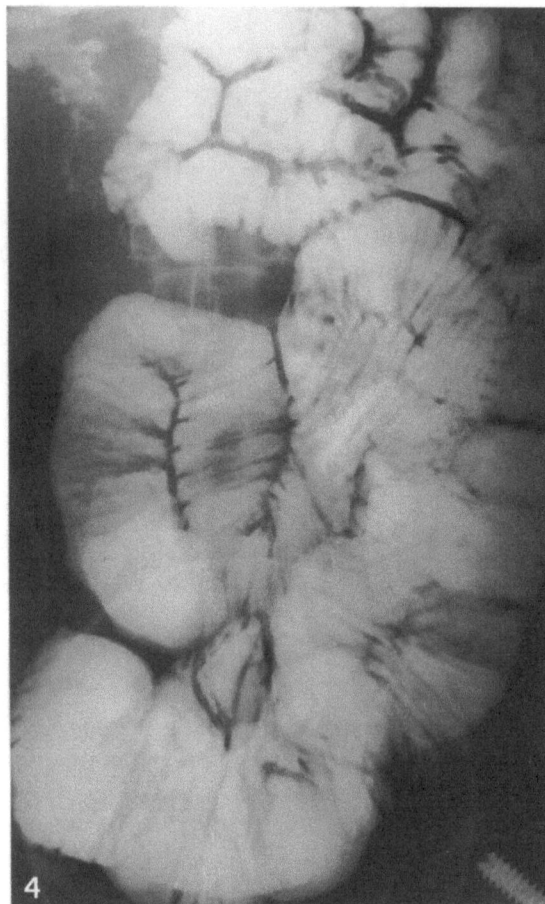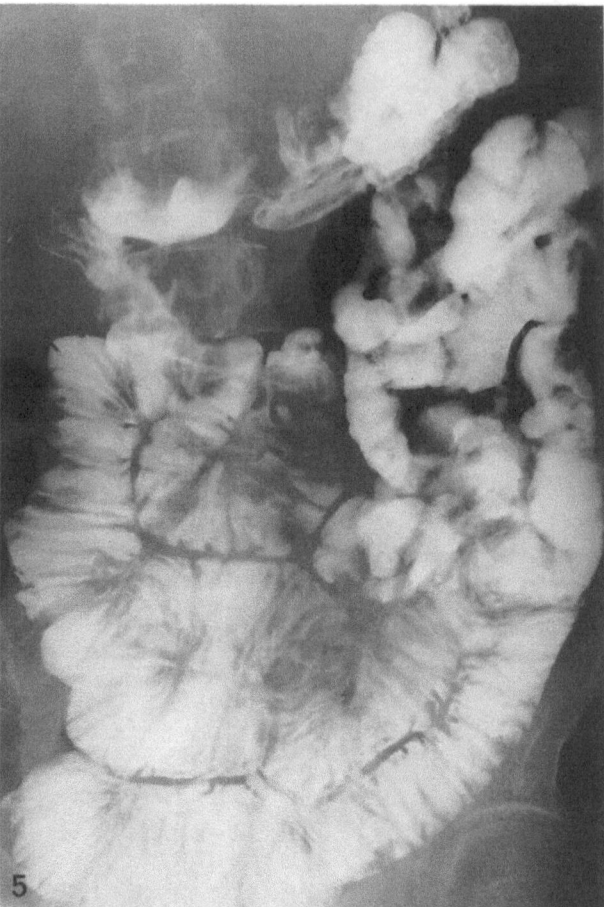

Fig. 4. Celiac disease. 45-year-old man. Mild chronic diarrhea since childhood, worse for the last 3 months with weight loss. Type V villous atrophy. SBFT : jejunal atony with widened distal loops, increased interloop gap, and rarefied folds in the proximal jejunum

Fig. 5. Celiac disease. 51-year-old woman. Chronic diarrhea. Recent abdominal pain. Type V villous atrophy. SBFT : Disappearance of folds in the proximal jejunum with the image of intestinal wall coalescence distally

5 to 10% of patients with celiac disease. *Nonspecific abnormalities* are observed in other cases with associated contrast medium dilution and dilatation of jejunal loops. This malabsorptive pattern is not specific as to its cause. It is due to celiac disease in 60% of instances, to another cause of malabsorption (discussed below) in 30% and reflects no specific disease in the remaining 10%. In celiac disease, the severity of the abnormalities is proportional to that of the clinical and laboratory signs, and not to the degree of the villous atrophy.

Contrast medium dilution mainly occurs in the distal jejunum and ileum and may be associated with fragmentation of the barium column. This appearance is in part avoided by enteroclysis. Jejunal dilatation is assessed by measuring 3 filled loops perpendicularly to the axis of their lumen. Dilatation is

moderate when the average caliber is 30 to 35 mm and marked if it exceeds 35 mm. Haworth's tables must be referred to for children. Dilatation is segmental and discontinuous and does not increase progressively as in a dilatation proximal to an obstruction. The duodenum may be dilated or narrowed and the ileum may be dilated in the diffuse forms. Dilatation is usually associated with stasis in the duodenum and in the first intestinal loops. The interloop gap is slightly widened.

The most specific signs of celiac disease include functional intussusceptions, with flaccidity of the bowel wall, coupled to an alteration of the folds. Transient and sometimes multiple, nonobstructive intussusceptions are observed in 20% of cases, especially in the jejunum. Other than in celiac disease, they have been reported rarely in adults with tropical sprue, parasitic diseases, cow milk intole-

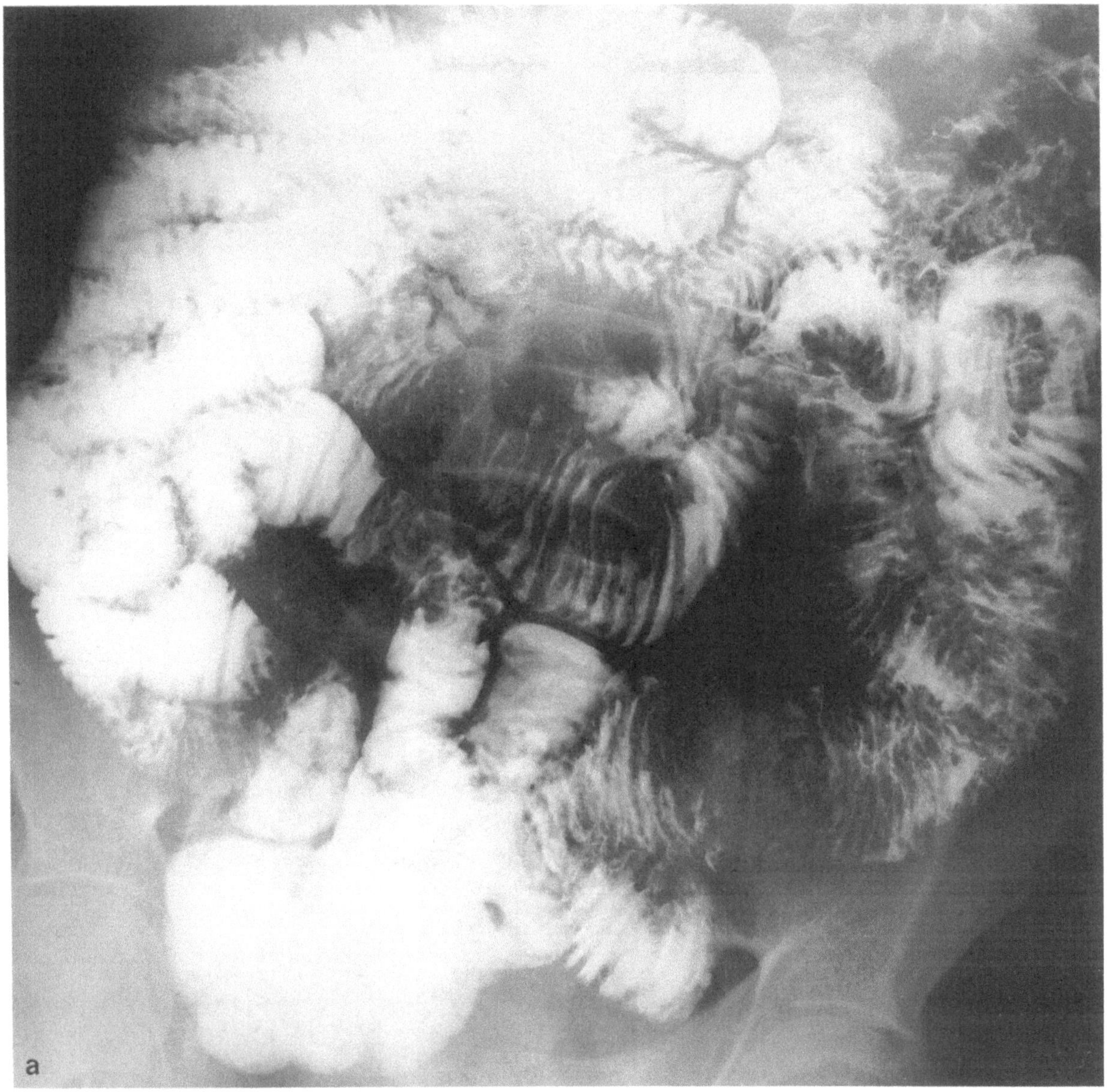

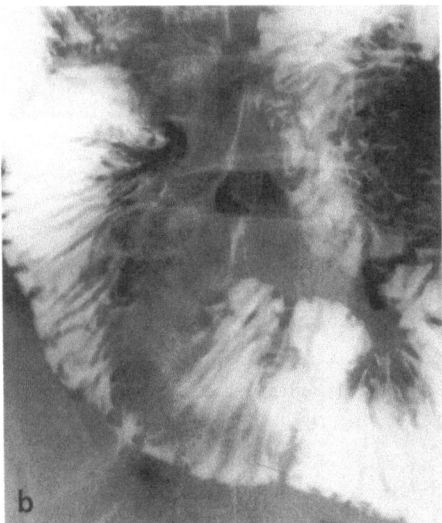

Fig. 6 a, b. Celiac disease. Two examples of pseudonodular opacification defects caused by the coalescence of the walls of a hypotonic loop

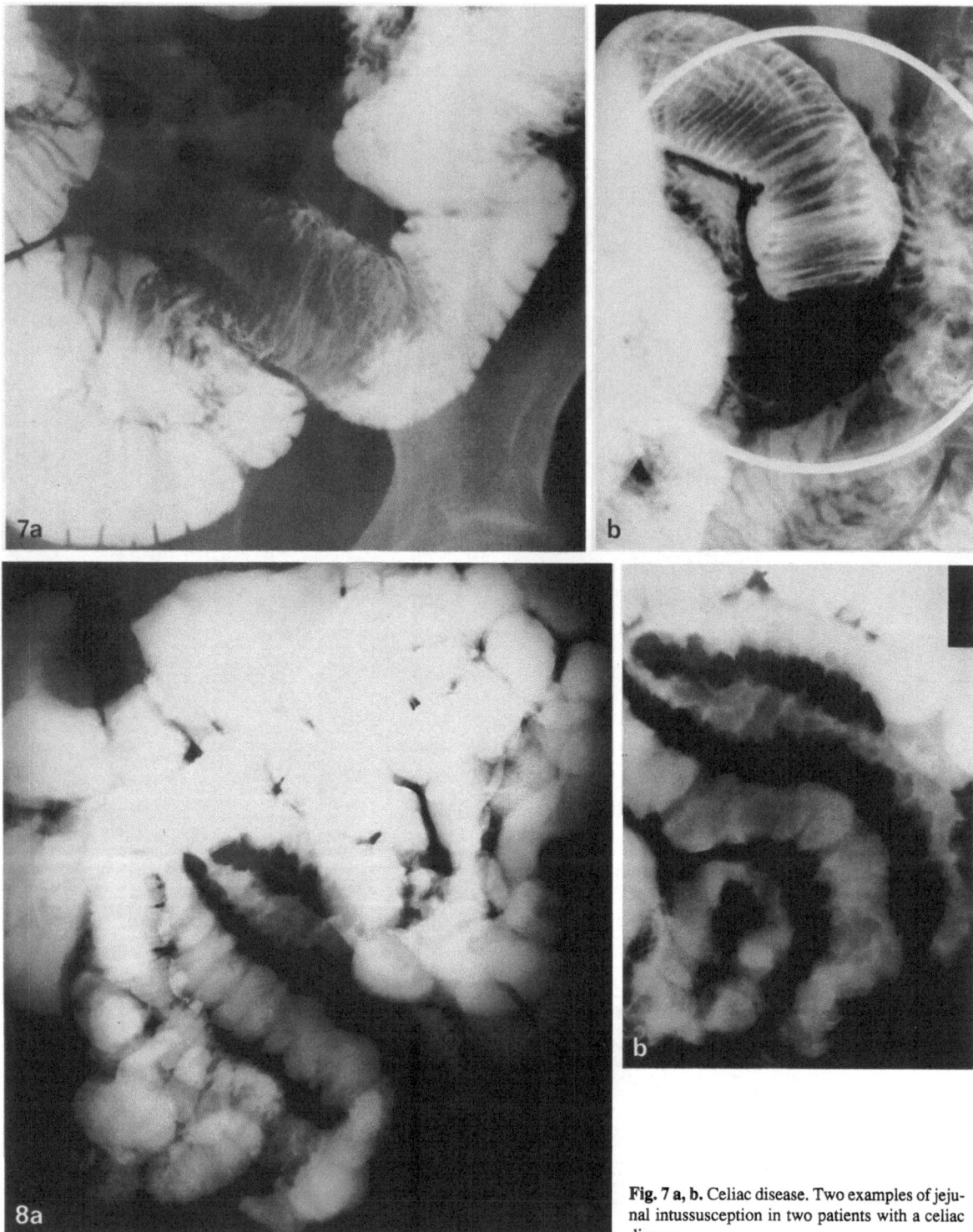

Fig. 7 a, b. Celiac disease. Two examples of jejunal intussusception in two patients with a celiac disease

Fig. 8 a, b. Lymphoma associated with celiac disease. 71-year-old man. Progression of celiac disease over 20 years. Refractoryness to a gluten-free diet. Poor general health. SBFT : a, b "inverted" small intestine due to celiac disease. Widened interloop gap and segmental nodulation of the proximal ileum (lymphoma)

rance and scleroderma. The flaccidity of the intestinal wall is a consequence of hypotonia and causes intermittent coalescence of the walls. This in turn produces notches or filling defects with indistinct contours, which disappear or increase according to the position of the loop and to the amount of compression. Such images can be regarded as the first stage of intussusception. The duodenal folds are thickened in 75% of cases and those of the jejunum are thicker than 2 mm in 50%. The interloop gap is moderately widened. One sign of celiac disease is the decreased height of the folds, which is measured along the margins of the jejunal loops. Fold rarefaction is the most typical sign demonstrated if the size of the interfold gap, which normally ranges from 2 to 8 mm after small bowel follow through, varies between 3 and 16 mm. Herlinger considers that the disease is very likely if less than 3 folds per inch (25 mm) are visible after enteroclysis. In the severe forms, the duodenal folds are thickened and rarefied, while the jejunal folds have completely disappeared. Abnormally dense ileal folds are observed late in the disease and are usually associated with a considerable rarefaction of jejunal folds. This produces a highly specific «inverted bowel» image. This «jejunal transformation» of the ileum is probably caused by functional adaptation aimed at compensating the acquired jejunal absorptive deficiencies.

Villous atrophy is sometimes seen on double contrast studies as a reticular pattern with meshes smaller than 1 mm in diameter.

To summarize, the most typical image includes contrast medium flocculation, widened jejunal loops, rarefied or absent jejunal folds, transient intussusceptions, bowel wall flaccidity, large jejunal folds and an «inverted bowel» image.

The complications of celiac disease must be systematically looked for and are often difficult to demonstrate. Lymphoma is often undetected by radiological techniques because of its diffuse, infiltrating character, hence the importance of repeated jejunal biopsies. The radiologist's attention is sometimes drawn to rigidity along the margins of the duodenum or the jejunum, the appearance of localized large, nodular folds, the extension of changes into the ileum, the presence of a stenosis or an increase in the interloop gap. The discovery of ulcers in association with findings suggestive of celiac disease raises the problem as to whether the condition is a complicated celiac disease or a different disease altogether.

Complementary imaging

Ultrasound and computed tomography can demonstrate the widened loops and, in severe cases, the presence of associated adenopathy which may be pseudocystic, as well as the fibroinflammatory involvement of the mesentery.

Disorders causing villous atrophy other than celiac disease

The aforementioned radiological abnormalities including villous atrophy are not specific for celiac disease and may be found in other conditions.

Duhring's disease or herpetiform dermatitis appears as a variant of celiac disease, as bullae and skin erythema are associated with subtotal villous atrophy, which responds to a gluten-free diet. The clinical and radiological signs of malabsorption are not prominent.

Collagenous sprue (fig. 9) has many points in common with celiac disease but biopsies reveal a collagenous strip between the epithelium and the lamina propria, in addition to villous atrophy. The prognosis is poor. The radiological appearance is similar to celiac disease.

Tropical sprue is rare in France but frequent in some tropical areas. It may be the consequence of malnutrition and chronic intestinal infections. It occurs at any age, but more in adults. Villous atrophy is incomplete and focal. The classic signs include buccal aphtous ulcers and a megaloblastic anemia. Other signs include diarrhea with steatorrhea, vitamin deficiencies and weight loss. Fat and D-xylose absorption tests are abnormal, as is a Schilling's test. Treatment includes antibiotics, folic acid and vitamin B12. The small bowel follow-through appearance can be normal or reveal moderate dilatation of the loops as well as contrast medium flocculation and fragmentation without fold rarefaction or bowel wall flaccidity.

Lymphoma and alpha-chain disease sometimes occur in a diffuse form with subtotal villous atrophy shown on biopsies. They exhibit radiological appearances quite similar to that of celiac disease. The diagnosis of lymphoma must be suggested if the disease does not improve with a gluten-free diet.

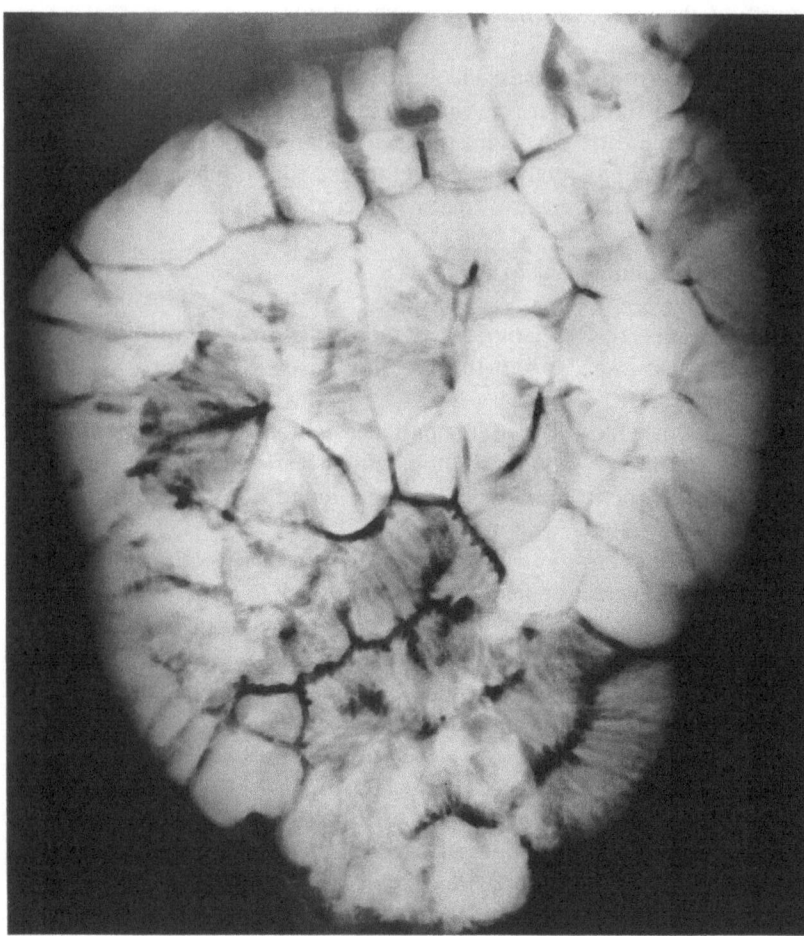

Fig. 9. Collagenous sprue. 10-year-old boy. Chronic diarrhea for 3 years. poor general condition. Type V villous atrophy, not cured by a gluten-free diet. SBFT : atonia, rarefied jejunal folds, jejunal transformation of the ileal folds with marginal microspiculation and discrete widening of the interloop gaps

Immuno-deficient states, especially when complicated by intestinal infections, can be associated with total villous atrophy and radiological signs of malabsorption.

Several diseases can present with incomplete, focal mucosal atrophy. In addition to the specific signs of these diseases, when present, a small bowel follow-through shows nonspecific abnormalities including contrast medium flocculation, and both distended loops and thickened folds. This is the case in chronic infectious jejunoileitis, chronic ulcerative jejunoileitis, milk protein intolerance, ischemia, parasitic infections, drug intoxication, Whipple's disease, the Zollinger-Ellison syndrome, eosinophilic gastroenteritis, consequences of radiation therapy, etc.

Mucosal atrophy has also been reported in severe malnutrition (kwashiorkor), ulcerative colitis and cystic fibrosis with pancreatic involvement. Atrophy frequently occurs in lactose intolerance, either primary and hereditary or secondary to acute insults of the intestinal mucosa. The diagnosis is made with a lactose tolerance test and the measurement of lactase activity in the intestinal mucosa. The radiological abnormalities are increased by adding lactose to the barium solution.

Functional small intestine

The nonspecific radiological abnormalities of the «functional small intestine» include contrast medium dilution with a moderate, intermittent and irregular increase in the caliber of the loops. This appearance is due to disorders other than celiac disease in one-third of cases. In addition to the other causes of villous atrophy mentioned above, any diffuse disease of the small intestine without villous atrophy can cause malabsorption and produce the image of a «functional small intestine».

Practical conclusions

The combination of contrast medium dilution and the presence of distended jejunal loops is a sign of celiac disease more than half the time. The diagnosis is very likely if rarefied jejunal folds, transient intussusceptions, bowel wall flaccidity and an «inverted» small intestine appearance are also present. Radiologists must suggest duodenojejunoscopy to prove villous atrophy, even in the presence of a negative initial routine endoscopic study.

References

Celiac disease

Al-Kawas FH, Murgo A, Foshag L, Sheils W (1988) Lymphadenopathy in celiac disease : not always a sign of lymphoma. Amer J Gastroent 83 : 301-303

Baer AN, Bayless TM, Yardley JH (1980) Intestinal ulceration and malabsorption syndromes. Gastroenterology 79 : 754-765

Bayless TM, Kapelowitz RF, Shelley WM, Ballinger WF, Hendrix TR (1967) Intestinal ulceration, a complication of celiac disease. N Engl J Med 276 : 996-1002

Bernier JJ, Soule C, Galian A, Rambaud JC, Modigliani R, Matuchansky C (1975) Etude de l'absorption intestinale de l'eau, des électrolytes et du glucose dans la maladie cœliaque de l'adulte par la méthode de la perfusion intestinale. Arch Fr Mal App Dig 64 : 495-506

Bova JG, Friedman AC, Weser E, Hopens TA, Wytock DH (1985) Adaptation of the ileum in nontropical sprue : reversal of the jejunoileal fold pattern. AJR 144 : 299-302

Brauner-Karray R, Montagné JPh, Fontaine JL (1980) Place des examens radiologiques dans le diagnostic et la surveillance des intolérances au gluten de l'enfant. Ann Pediatr 27 : 223-226

Bret P, Francoz JB, Bret Pa, Cuche C, Gérard C (1980) Images lacunaires et invaginations dans 25 cas de maladie cœliaque. J Radiol 61 : 723-727

Brunton FJ, Guyer PB (1983) Malignant histiocytosis and ulcerative jejunitis of the small intestine. Clin Radiol 34 : 291-295

Cerf M, Marche C, Fremont A, Eugène C, Paolaggi JA, Leymarios J, Couturier D, Debray C (1975) Régime sans gluten et évolution de la maladie cœliaque de l'adulte. Arch Fr Mal App Dig 64 : 483-493

Collins SM, Hamilton JD, Lewis TD, Laufer I (1978) Small-bowel malabsorption and gastrointestinal malignancy. Diagn Radiol 126 : 603-609

Cooke WT, Fone DJ, Cox EV, Meynell MJ, Gaddie R (1963) Adult coeliac disease. Gut 4 : 279-291

Cooper BT, Holmes GKT, Cooke WT (1982) Lymphoma risk in coeliac disease of later life. Digestion 23 : 89-92

Cosnes J, Modigliani R, Rambaud JC, Matuchansky C, Galian A, Pariente A, Bernier JJ (1979) Maladie coeliaque de l'adulte, relation entre l'étendue des lésions anatomiques et la sévérité de la maladie. Gastroenterol Clin Biol 3 : 521-530

Déchavanne M, Barthe J (1971) L'intolérance au gluten de l'adulte (à propos de 15 observations). Lyon Med 225 : 411-417

Delamarre J, Capron JP, Joly JP, Rémond A, Audebert M, Murat JL, Revert R, Trinez G (1984) Atonie vésiculaire et maladie cœliaque de l'adulte, étude radiographique et échographique de 15 cas. J Radiol 65 : 133-136

Dharmsathaphorn K, Freeman DH, Binder HJ, Dobbins JW (1982) Increased risk of nephrolithiasis in patients with steatorrhea. Dig Dis Sci 27 : 401-405

Dowling RH, Henry K (1972) Non-responsive coeliac disease. Br Med J 3 : 624-631

Fortier-Beaulieu M, Frézal J, Rey J (1964) Modifications radiologiques de l'intestin grêle au cours des maladies cœliaques de l'enfant. Ann Radiol 7 : 422-428

Fortier-Beaulieu M, Labrune M, Capdeville R (1966) Invaginations fonctionnelles et organiques du jéjunum chez le nourrisson et l'enfant. J Radiol 47 : 277-282

François R, Pouillaude JM, Cret L, Neyron de St-Julien Ch (1972) Maladie cœliaque, intolérance à la gliadine. Concours Med 94 : 3897-3910

Frank PH, O'Connell D (1977) Pneumatosis cystoides intestinalis and obstructing intussusception in celiac disease. Gastrointest Radiol 2 : 109-111

Freeman HJ, Weinstein WM, Shnitka TK, Piercey JRA, Wensel RH (1977) Primary abdominal lymphoma, presenting manifestation of celiac sprue or complicating dermatitis herpetiformis. Am J Med 63 : 585-594

Gefter WB, Evers KA, Malet PF, Kressel HY, Thompson JJ (1981) Nontropical sprue with pneumatosis coli. AJR 137 : 624-625

Ghisolfi J, Rieu D (1981) Aspects actuels de l'intolérance au gluten chez l'enfant. Gastroenterol Pediatr 31 : 1229-1242

Girard M, Bel A (1965) La sprue nostras et les steatorrhées idiopathiques d'origine intestinale. Rev Prat XV : 577-587

Gough KR, Read AE, Naish JM (1962) Intestinal reticulosis as a complication of idiopathic steatorrhoea. Gut 3 : 232-239

Haworth EM, Hodson CJ, Pringle EM, Young WF (1968) The value of radiological investigations of the alimentary tract in children with the coeliac syndrome. Clin Radiol 19 : 65-76

Herlinger H, Maglinte DT (1986) Jejunal fold separation in adult celiac disease : relevance of enteroclysis. Radiology 158 : 605-611

Jabbari M, Wild G, Goresky CA, Daly DS, Lough JO, Cleland P, Kinnear DG (1988) Scalloped valvulae conniventes : an endoscopic marker of celiac sprue. Gastroenterology 95 : 1518-1522

Jones B, Bayless TM, Fishman EK, Siegelman SS (1984) Lymphadenopathy in celiac disease : computed tomographic observations. AJR 142 : 1127-1132

Jos J, De Tand MF, Arnaud-Battandier F (1985) Etiopathogénie de la maladie cœliaque : attrait et fragilité des hypothèses. Presse Med 14 : 1027-1030

Kappelman NB, Burrell M, Toffler R (1977) Megacolon associated with celiac sprue, report of 4 cases and review of the literature. AJR 128 : 65-68

Kumar P, Bartram CI (1979) Relevance of the barium follow-through examination in the diagnosis of adult celiac disease. Gastrointest Radiol 4 : 285-289

Labrune M, Guinard J, Bocquet F, Dommergues JP (1978) Indications actuelles du transit baryté de grêle dans les malabsorptions de l'enfant. J Radiol 59 : 407-411

Mainguet P (1984) L'abord diagnostique des syndromes de malabsorption de l'adulte. Tempo Med 165 : 57-70

Marn CS, Gore RM, Ghahremani GG (1986) Duodenal manifestations of nontropical sprue. Gastrointest Radiol 11 : 30-35

Masterson JB, Sweeney EC (1976) The role of small bowel follow-through examination in the diagnosis of coeliac disease. Br J Radiol 49 : 660-664

McCrae WM, Sweet EM (1964) Radiology in diagnosis of coeliac disease. Br Med : 163-164

McLean AM, Farthing MJG, Kurian G, Mathan VI (1982) The relationship between hypoalbuminaemia and the radiological appearances of the jejunum in tropical sprue. Br J Radiol 55 : 725-728

Modigliani R, Matuchansky C, Galian A, Poupon R, Rambaud JC, Bernier JJ (1975) Maladie cœliaque de l'adulte (48 cas). Arch Fr Mal App Dig 64 : 465-481

Modigliani R (1977) La maladie cœliaque de l'adulte. Concours Med 99-47 : 7357-7365

Moss AA (1976) Postvagotomy unmasking of nontropical sprue. Gastrointest Radiol 1 : 173-175

Nisard A, Lecharpentier Y, Louvel A, Galian A, Bleichner G, Boisson J, Rambaud JC (1976) Etude anatomo-pathologique d'un lymphome malin compliquant une maladie cœliaque de l'adulte. Arch Fr Mal App Dig 65 : 295-305

Paliard P, Riou JP, Lesbros F, Abdessemed H (1976) Maladie cœliaque de l'adulte et lymphome malin jéjunal, présentation d'un cas. Lyon Med 236 : 581-584

Porcher P, Chenderovitch J (1953) La radiologie de l'intestin grêle au cours des diarrhées graisseuses idiopathiques. Sem Hop Paris, pp 3730-3739

Rubin CE (1970) Sprue by any other name. Gastroenterology 58 : 409-527

Ruoff M, Lindner AE, Marshak RH (1968) Intussusception in sprue. AJR 104 : 525-528

Sackier JM, Smith EJ, Wood CB (1988) Cystic pneumatosis in celiac disease. Gut 29 : 852-855

Sanderson MC, Davis LR, Mowat AP (1975) Failure of laboratory and radiological studies to predict jejunal mucosal atrophy. Arch Dis Child 50 : 526-531

Swinson CM, Coles EC, Slavin G, Booth CC (1983) Coeliac disease and malignancy. Lancet I : 111-115

Scott BB, Losowsky MS (1976) Patchiness and duodenal-jejunal variation of the mucosal abnormality in coeliac disease and dermatitis herpetiformis. Gut 17 : 984-992

Seliger G, Goldman AM, Firooznia H, Lawrence LR (1973) Ulceration of the small intestine complicating celiac disease. Dig Dis 18 : 820-823

Smith SEW, Littlewood JM (1977) The two-film barium meal in the exclusion of coeliac disease. Clin Radiol 28 : 629-634

Thompson H (1974) Necropsy studies on adult coeliac disease. J Clin Pathol 27 : 710-721

Trier JS, Falchuk ZM, Carey MC, Schreiber DS (1978) Celiac sprue and refractory sprue. Gastroenterology 75 : 307-316

Vachon A, Lejeune E, Astruc H (1954) La sprue essentielle, notions cliniques et thérapeutiques récentes, à propos de 4 observations. Rev Lyon Med, pp 383-397

Vachon A, Berger M, Yves A, Cornut H (1961) Exploration de l'absorption intestinale par les isotopes radioactifs et son application à la pathologie de l'intestin grêle. Rev Lyon Med, pp 757-765

Vachon A, Paliard P, Abry M, Barthe J (1968) La biopsie jéjunale dans les syndromes de malabsorption et les diarrhées chroniques de l'adulte. J Med Lyon 1146 : 1211

Wackenier JP, Simar J, Goor M, Houcke M, Farriaux JP, Fontaine G, Meresse-Rougee F, Sturque MN (1975) Etude de la maladie cœliaque, à propos de 68 observations. Rev Pediatr XI : 21-34

Weill J (1980) L'évolution nosologique de la maladie cœliaque. Ann Gastroenterol Hepatol 16 : 347-350

The others malabsorptions

Barry RE, Morris JS, Read AE (1971) Collagenous sprue. N Engl J Med 284 : 1041

Berk RN, Lee FA (1973) The late gastrointestinal manifestations of cystic fibrosis of the pancreas. Radiology 106 : 377-381

Caldwell WL, Swanson VL, Bayless TM (1965) The importance and reliability of the roentgenographic examination of the small bowel in patients with tropical sprue. Radiology 84 : 227-240

Cattan R (1953) Introduction à l'étude des stéatorrhées. Sem Hop Paris 72 : 3721-3724

Cockel R, Hill EE, Rushton DI, Smith B, Hawkins CF (1973) Familial steatorrhea with calcification of the basal ganglia and mental retardation. Q J Med XLII : 771-783

Collins JR, Isselbacher KJ (1965) The occurence of severe small intestinal mucosal damage in conditions other than celiac disease (nontropical prue), report of 2 cases. Gastroenterology 49 : 425-431

Cortner JA (1959) Giardiasis, a cause of celiac syndrome. Am J Dis Child 98 : 311-316

Creyssel R, Replumaz PR, Pinet F, Bosson P, Payen P (1953) La sprue chirurgicale, l'anémie mégaloblastique carentielle des anastomoses intestinales. Rev Med Lyon, pp 189-200

Descos L, Minaire Y, Lambert R (1980) Le point sur les malabsorptions. Lyon Med 243 : 693-703

Duchier J (1974) Intolérance au lactose par déficit en lactase. Arch Fr Mal App Dig 63 : 513-531

Eckstein RP, Dowsett JF, Riley JW (1988) Collagenous enterocolitis : a case of collagenous colitis with involvement of the small intestine. Amer J Gastroent 83 : 767-771

Floch MH, Caldwell WI, Sheehy TA (1962) A histopathologic basis for the interpretation of small bowel roentgenography in tropical sprue. AJR 87 : 709-716

Friedman J (1954) Roentgen studies of the effects on the small intestine from emotional disturbances. AJR 72 : 367-379

Gardner FH (1958) Tropical sprue. N Engl J Med 258 : 791-796

Gawkrodger DJ, Blackwell JN, Gilmour HM, Rifkind EA, Heading RC, Barnetson RStC (1984) Dermatitis herpetiformis : diagnosis, diet and demography. Gut 25 : 151-157

Horswell RR, Hargrove MD, Peete WP, Ruffin JM (1961) Scleroderma presenting as the malabsorption syndrome, a case report. Gastroenterology 40 : 580-582

Isbell RG, Carlson HC, Hoffman HN (1969) Roentgenologic-Pathologic correlation in malabsorption syndromes. AJR 107 : 158-169

Kermarec J, Schenowitz G (1981) Pour une interprétation fonctionnelle des atrophies villositaires de l'intestin grêle. Ann Gastroenterol Hepatol 17 : 79-85

Laws JW, Booth CC, Shawdon H, Stewart JS (1963) Correlation of radiological and histological findings in idiopathic steatorrhoea. Br Med J : 1311-1314

Laws JW, Neale G (1966) Radiological diagnosis of disaccharidase deficiency. Lancet I : 139-143

Leneman F, Fierst S, Gabriel JB, Ingegno AP (1962) Progressive systemic sclerosis of the intestine presenting as malabsorption syndrome. Gastroenterology 42 : 175-180

McCarthy DM, Katz SI, Gazze L, Waldmann TA, Nelson DL, Strober W (1978) Déficit isolé en IgA avec atrophie villositaire et auto-anticorps anti-cellule épithéliale. J Immunol 120 : 932-938

McClelland HA, Lewis MJ, Naish JM (1962) Idiopathic steatorrhoea with intestinal pseudo-obstruction. Gut 3 : 142-144

Mignon F (1977) Orientations diagnostiques devant une stéatorrhée. Concours Med 99-17 : 2674-2680

Pepper HW, Brandborg LL, Shanser JD, Goldberg HI, Moss AA (1974) Collagenous sprue. AJR 121 : 275-282

Rogé J, Delavierre Ph, Lagrue G, Durand H, Silvereano de Roissard F (1973) Amylose du grêle responsable d'un syndrome sévère de malabsorption intestinale. Sem Hop Paris 49 : 3147-3150

Rosenthal FD (1957) Small intestinal lesions with steatorrhea in diffuse systemic sclerosis (scleroderma). Gastroenterology 32 : 332-341

Salem SN, Truelove SC, Richards WCD (1964) Small-intestinal and gastric changes in ulcerative colitis : a biopsy study. Br Med J 1 : 394-398

Salem SN, Truelove SC (1965) Small-intestinal and gastric abnormalities in ulcerative colitis. Br Med J 1 : 827-831

Salen G, Goldstein F, Wirts CW (1966) Malabsorption in intestinal scleroderma, relation to bacterial flora and treatment with antibiotics. Ann Int Med 64 : 834-841

Sava G, Marescaux J, Grenier JF (1979) Les diarrhées consécutives aux interventions chirurgicales. Ann Gastroenterol Hepatol 15 : 209-220

Shiner M, Doniach I (1960) Histopathologic studies in steatorrhea. Gastroenterology 38 : 419-440

Shiner M, Pearson JR (1981) Abnormalities in the jejunal mucosa in arab children. Gastroenterol Clin Biol 5 : 663-673

Sloper KS, Dourmashkin RR, Bird RB, Slavin G, Webster ADB (1982) Chronic malabsorption due to cryptosporidiosis in a child with immunoglobulin deficiency. Gut 23 : 80-82

Swischuk LE, Welsh JD (1968) Roentgenographic mucosal patterns in the « malabsorption syndrome ». Am J Dig Dis 13 : 59-77

Tête R, Boyer JD, Slaoui H, Mas R (1979) Diarrhée chronique avec malabsorption par amylose intestinale secondaire à une polyarthrite rhumatoïde au cours d'un diabète. Lyon Med 242 : 283-288

Trier JS (1971) Diagnostic value of peroral biopsy of the proximal small intestine. N Engl J Med 285 : 1470-1473

Tully TE, Feinberg SB (1974) A roentgenographic classification of diffuse diseases of the small intestine presenting with malabsorption. AJR 121 : 283-290

Vachon A, Lejeune E, Grivet A (1954) Les stéatorrhées en dehors de la sprue. Rev Lyon Med, pp 399-413

Vinnik IE, Kern F, Struthers JE (1962) Malabsorption and the diarrhea of diabetes mellitus. Gastroenterology 43 : 507-519

Warter J, Storck D, Christmann D, Meyer F (1979) Syndrome de malabsorption à la phase initiale d'un purpura rhumatoïde sévère. Nouv Presse Med 8 : 1245-1248

Weinstein WM, Saunders DR, Tytgat GN, Rubin CE (1970) Collagenous sprue, an unrecognized type of malabsorption. N Engl J Med 283 : 1298-1301

Weizman Z, Stringer DA, Durie PR (1984) Radiologic manifestations of malabsorption : a nonspecific finding. Pediatrics 74 : 530-533

Woods CA, Foutch PG, Kerr DM, Haynes WC, Sanowskir A (1988) Collagenous sprue as a cause for malabsorption in a patient with myotonic dystrophy : a new association. Amer J Gastroent 83 : 765-766

Parasitic infections

Parasitic diseases of the small intestine are usually not detected by radiology. Parasitic studies of stools, duodenal intubation, and serodiagnosis are needed. However, a number of parasitic infections produce digestive symptoms that lead the physician to request a barium study of the small intestine. Radiologists must therefore be familiar with the appearance of such diseases.

Parasitic diseases can present in three different ways in the small intestine:
- As an endoluminal foreign body when the parasite is large,
- As nonspecific inflammation of the intestinal wall, or
- with lymphoid nodular hyperplasia.

The parasites of the small intestine belong to 3 groups:
- protozoa: *Giardia lamblia, Isospora belli, Cryptosporidium* sp.,
- helminths: *Ascaris lumbricoides, Strongyloides stercoralis, Ankylostoma duodenale, Anisakis, Taenia saginata*,
- fungi: *Candida, Histoplasma, Paracoccidioides, Mucorreceae* (rarely).

Giardia lamblia (fig.1) is a widely distributed protozoon with flagellae. Two to 10% of the world population are infected by this parasite. The infection is often associated with a general or selective (IgA) deficiency. Patients with gastrectomy or blood group A are more susceptible to infection. Contamination occurs via water and is favoured by poor hygiene. The infectious form adheres to the walls of the jejunum and causes focal villous atrophy or a mechanical barrier due to mucus hypersecretion.

The clinical sign of contamination is a diarrheal episode which is self-limited and lasts 2 to 3 weeks. There are many healthy carriers. Chronic giardial manifestations including asthenia, dyspepsia, epigastric pain, diarrhea and, in one-third of cases, malabsorption. The diagnosis is made on stool cultures or with the study of duodenal fluid, and possibly on intestinal biopsy.

The radiological abnormalities are neither constant nor specific. They may appear either as functional abnormalities (hypersecretion, hypermotility) and thickened jejunal folds, or as lymphoid hyperplasia appearing as multiple round nodules of the same size, 2 to 5 mm in diameter, scattered from the duodenum to the ileum. The intestinal wall is not thickened.

Isospora belli is a sporozoon of animals developing within intestinal cells. The diagnosis can be made only on a jejunal biopsy because the oocytes are not readily demonstrated in the stools.

The main clinical sign is diarrhea which stops without therapy. However, serious forms present with severe diarrhea, steatorrhea and a deterioration in general status. These are observed in one-third of infected patients, especially in the case of a genetic or acquired immunodeficient state.

The radiological signs present as functional abnormalities and large folds in the duodenum and jejunum.

Cryptosporidium sp. is a protozoon belonging to the Coccidia. Transmission is indirect through soiled foods but can also be direct, for instance in homosexual subjects. One third of the infections

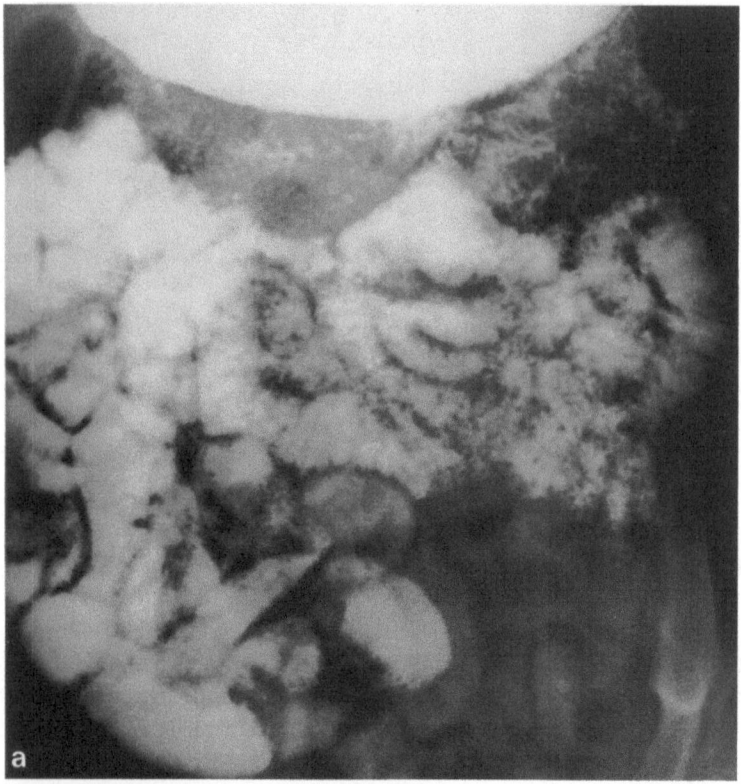

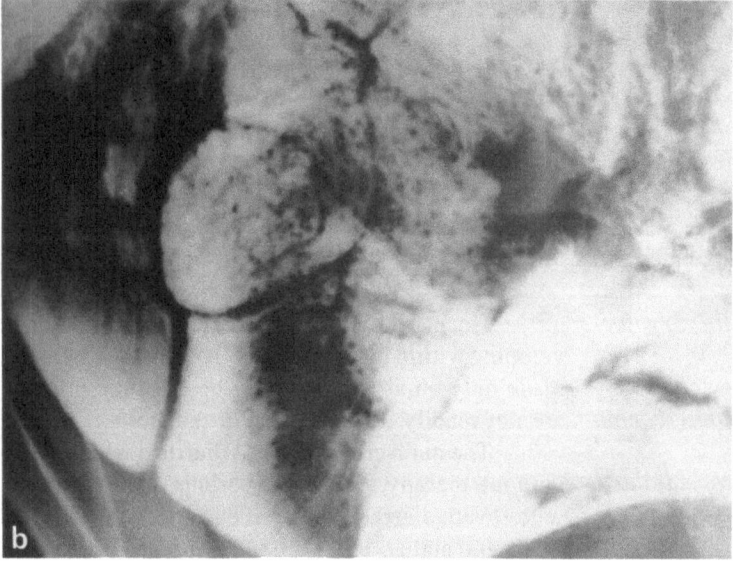

Fig. 1 a, b. Giardiasis. 10-year-old boy. Chronic diarrhea. Jejunal biopsy : giardiasis and lymphoid hyperplasia. SBFT : contrast medium dilution, diffuse micro-nodulation

caused by this parasite now occur in patients with AIDS.

The clinical signs include an abundant, watery diarrhea similar to that observed in cholera, fever, a deterioration in the patient's general condition, and abdominal cramps.

Radiologic studies show diffuse enteritis with considerable functional abnormalities (contrast me-dium dilution, spasm) and thickened folds in the je-junum and ileum.

Ascaris lumbricoides (nematode or round worm) (figs. 2 and 3) is the most frequent parasite to cause infection, since it affects 30% of the world population, in particular children in areas with poor hygiene. Contamination occurs via food. The parasite migrates into the duodenal mucosa, through the liver and into the lung. It then moves upwards in the tracheobronchial tree and back to the digestive tract. This migration explains the clinical signs: cough, asthma (pulmonary infiltration with eosinophilia), rash, pruritus, insomnia, nausea, vomiting and abdominal pain. The worms can cause obstruction by assembling in clusters. Other complications are possible and include appendicitis, peritonitis, jaundice and pancreatitis. Peripheral eosinophilia is common. Stool cultures make the diagnosis possible.

The clusters of worms are sometimes visible on plain radiographs as a heterogeneous, plurinodular opacity in a distended loop. The worm becomes visible on small bowel follow-through because it is 10 to 30 cm long and at least 5 mm wide. It appears as a radiotransparent line in the intestinal lumen. Since the worm absorbs the baryta solution, an opaque line representing its intestine can sometimes be demonstrated on late images (a small bowel follow-through of a parasite's intestine!!).

Strongyloides stercoralis (eelworm) is a 2 to 3 mm long round worm whose larvae develop in warm water (tropical climate). It migrates into the digestive tract after a transcutaneous, and then pulmonary penetration.

The clinical signs include ulcer-like pain in half the cases and diarrhea in 20% of infected patients. The infection causes blood eosinophilia. Severe infections occur in immunocompromised patients, or those on steroid therapy and present with intense diarrhea, a protein-losing enteropathy, and respiratory disorders. The diagnosis is based on the study of stools or a duodenal aspirate.

Radiology shows the involvement of the duodenum and of the jejunum. The folds are thickened or disappear. Multiple ulcerations and sometimes stenoses can be observed.

Ankylostoma duodenale is a 5 to 20 mm long worm which penetrates through the skin into the lung, and then migrates into the duodenum. It causes ulcer-like abdominal symptoms, decreased appetite, a microcytic iron deficency anemia, and a marked blood eosinophilia. Duodenal intubation and stool cultures yield the diagnosis.

Radiology shows distended duodenojejunal loops and rarefied folds.

Anisakis infects sea fish (mackerel, herring). The ingested larvae cause abdominal pain, a change in bowel habits, obstructive episodes, gastrointestinal bleeding, and a marked eosinophilia.

Radiology shows the lesions in the stomach or in the ileum. They form either an extensive nodulation associated with thickened folds, or an isolated pseudotumoral nodule due to the formation of an eosinophilic granuloma. The relation with eosinophilic gastroenteritis is still unknown.

Taenia saginata (cestode or tapeworm) (fig. 4) is the most widespread parasite in France. It is a very long worm (4 to 5 m) with a diameter ranging from 1 to 5 mm. Contamination occurs with the ingestion of raw beef which contains the larvae. Raw pork causes infection with the smaller *Taenia soleum.*

There are few clinical signs, but abdominal pain and vomiting may be present. The infection causes blood eosinophilia. The shedding of metameres in stool is intermittent. Serodiagnosis is sometimes useful.

Radiologically, the tapeworm forms a long, continuous, radiotransparent ribbon from the jejunum to the ileum. Since it lacks a digestive tract, it never presents with an opaque central line such as with the Ascaris. Mucosal alterations of the small intestine seldom occur.

Candida albicans is a yeast that can cause severe digestive disease, especially in case of an immune deficiency, diabetes or cachexia. Involvement of the small intestine is often associated with diffuse disease of the digestive tract and is manifested as intense diarrhea.

Radiologic studies show a nonspecific jejunoileitis with contrast medium dilution, distended loops and thickened folds. Ulcerations may also be visible.

Histoplasma capsulatum affects mainly the respiratory organs and causes histoplasmosis. Other visceral lesions, especially in the ileum and the colon, can also appear.

Radiology shows superficial (sometimes deep) ulcers, nodulations and strictures in the ileum and colon.

Paracoccidioides brasiliensis causes blastomycosis, a Central and South American disease. This disease involves the skin alone or multiple organs, lymph nodes and bones. Digestive involvement causes chronic diarrhea, abdominal pain and sometimes a palpable mass.

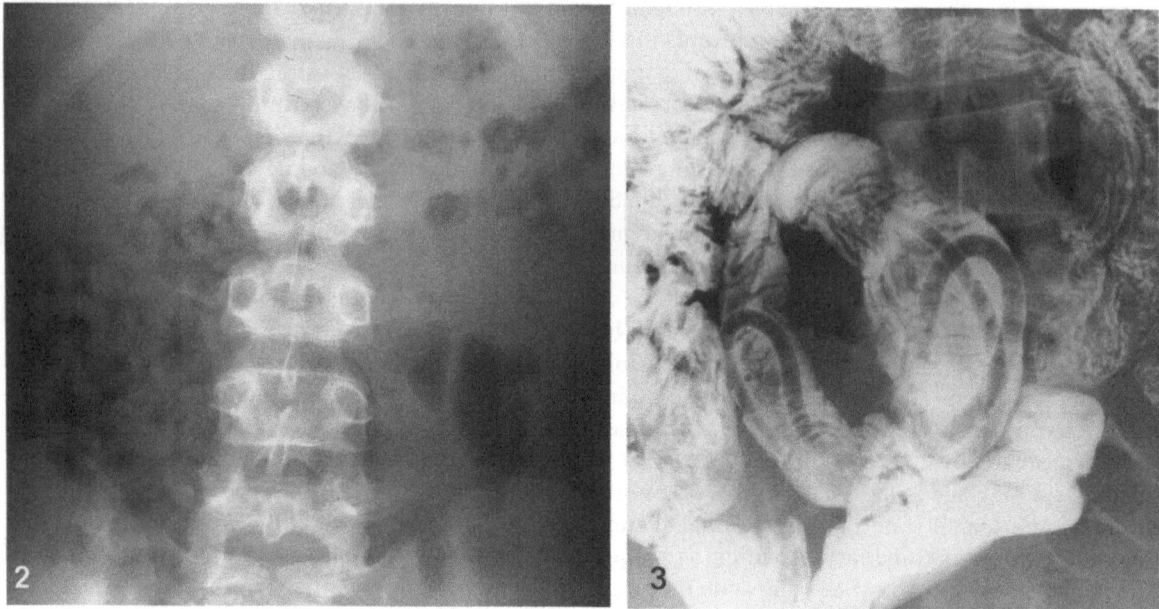

Fig. 2. Ascariasis (Courtesy of D Gauthier). Plain film of the abdomen : cluster of vermicular images on the right side

Fig. 3. Ascariasis. 30-year-old woman. Mild digestive symptoms. SBFT : ribbon images with regular contours

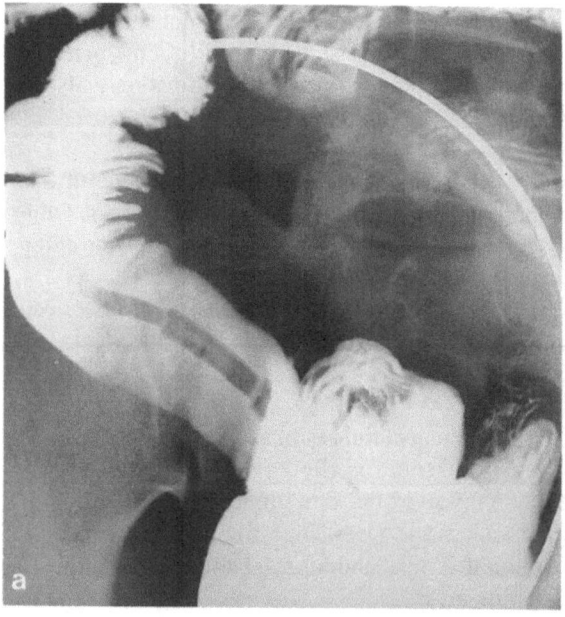

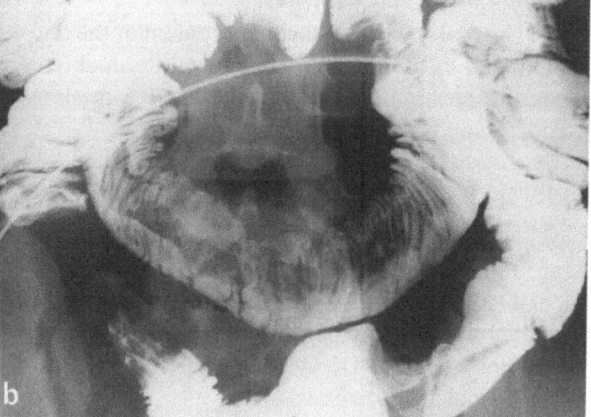

Fig. 4 a, b. Taenia (Courtesy of D Gauthier). 20-year-old woman. Appendiceal symptoms. SBFT : ribbon-shaped vermicular images made up of segments of varying caliber

The radiological appearance of the lesions mimicks Crohn's disease or tuberculosis because they predominate near the ileocecal junction and combine stenosis to the presence of large folds.

Mucoraceae is the agent of mucormycosis, an African disease affecting mainly immunosuppressed, cachectic and diabetic patients. The fungus causes thrombosis and infarction as well as ulcers and perforations in the digestive tract. The condition often presents acutely and dramatically.

The radiological appearance is that of acute ischemia.

Practical conclusions

Parasitic diseases are sometimes demonstrated incidentally on small bowel follow-through. Endoluminal worms must not be mistaken for other foreign bodies, nor clusters of worms with nodulations such as may be encountered in malignant non-Hodgkin's lymphomas. This diagnosis is sometimes mistakingly questioned in the presence of diffuse parasitic micronodulations. Lastly, parasitic infections sometimes have the appearance of acute nonspecific enteritis, in particular in an immunosuppressed host.

References

Avritchir Y, Perroni AA (1978) Radiological manifestations of small intestinal South American blastomycosis. Radiology 127 : 607-609

Berk RN, Wall SD, McArdle CB, McCutchan JA, Clemett AR, Rosenblum JS, Premkumer A, Megibow AJ (1984) Cryptosporidiosis of the stomach and small intestine in patients with AIDS. AJR 143 : 559-564

Brandon J, Glick SN, Teplick SK (1985) Intestinal giardiasis : the importance of serial filming. AJR 144 : 581-584

Cortner JA (1959) Giardiasis, a cause of celiac syndrome. J Dis Child 98 : 311-316

Current WL, Reese NC, Ernst JV, Bailey WS, Heyman MB, Weinstein WM (1983) Human cryptosporidiosis in immunocompetent and immunodeficient persons, studies of an outbreak and experimental transmission. N Engl J Med 308 : 1252-1257

Dallemand S, Waxman M, Farman J (1983) Radiological manifestations of Strongyloides stercoralis. Gastrointest Radiol 8 : 45-51

Danis M, Gentilini M (1979) Les diarrhées parasitaires. Ann Gastroenterol Hepatol 15 : 385-389

Fischer D, Labayle D, Versapuech JM, Grange D, Kemeny F (1987) Atteinte candidosique de l'intestin grêle compliquée de perforation. Un cas d'évolution favorable. Gastrointest Clin Biol 11 : 514-517

Haws CC, Long RF, Caplan GE (1977) Histoplasma capsulatum as a cause of ileocolitis (case report). AJR 128 : 692-694

Liepman M (1975) Disseminated Strongyloides stercoralis, a complication of immunosuppression. JAMA 231 : 387-388

Matheron S, Girard PM (1987) La cryptosporidiose. Concours Med 190 : 1829-1835

Matsui T, Iida M, Murakami M, Kimura Y, Fujishima M, Yao Y, Tsuji M (1985) Intestinal anisakiasis : clinical and radiologic features. Radiology 157 : 299-302

Megibow AJ, Balthazar EJ, Hulnick DH (1987) Radiology of non neoplastic gastrointestinal disorders in acquired immune deficiency syndrome. Semin Roentgen 22 : 31-41

Merrouche Y, Royer I, Gobert JG, Guillevin L (1987) Infestation digestive à Taenia saginata compliquée d'enteropathie exsudative. Gastroent Clin Biol 11 : 526

Neefe LI, Pinilla O, Garagusi VF, Bauer H (1973) Disseminated strongyloidiasis with cerebral involvement, a complication of corticosteroid therapy. Am J Med 55 : 832-838

Penalba CH, Cerf M, Bigot JM, Edouard A, Rieux D (1983) Aspects radiologiques du duodénum et du grêle dans l'anguillulose sévère, à propos de 4 observations. J Radiol 64 : 241-248

Powell RW, Moss JP, Nagar D, Melo JC, Boram LH, Anderson WH, Cheng SH (1980) Strongyloidiasis in immunosuppressed hosts, presentation as massive lower gastrointestinal bleeding. Arch Intern Med 140 : 1061-1063

Purtilo DT, Meyers WM, Connor DH (1974) Fatal strongyloidiasis in immunosuppressed patients. Am J Med 56 : 488-493

Randall Radin D, Fong T, Halls JM, Pontrelli GN (1983) Monilial enteritis in acquired immunodeficiency syndrome. AJR 141 : 1289-1290

Roussin-Bretagne S, Devars Du Mayne JF, Cerf M (1988) L'anguillulose. Ann Gastroent Hepat 24 : 7

Schulman A, Bornman P, Kaplan C, Morton P, Rose A (1979) Gastrointestinal mucormycosis. Gastrointest Radiol 4 : 385-388

Sloper KS, Dourmashkin RR, Bird RB, Slavin J, Webster ADB (1982) Chronic malabsorption due to cryptosporidiosis in a child with immunoglobulin deficiency, case report. Gut 23 : 80-82

Strijk SP, Rosenbush G (1981) Radiologic findings in parasitic infection of the small bowel. J Belge Radiol 3 : 233-239

Weissberg DL, Berk RN (1978) Ascariasis of the gastrointestinal tract. Gastrointest Radiol 3 : 415-418

Weisburger WR, Hutcheon DF, Yardley JH, Roche JC, Hillis WD, Charache P (1979) Cryptosporidiosis in an immunosuppressed renal-transplant recipient with IgA deficiency. Am J Clin Pathol 72 : 473-478

Wynne JM, Ellman BAH (1983) Bolus obstruction by ascaris lumbricoides. S Afr. Med J 63 : 644-646

Yoshida T, Nozaki F, Tanaka K, Ebihara H, Shimayama T, Katsuki T (1981) Strongyloides stercoralis hyperinfection : sequential changes of gastrointestinal radiology after treatment with Thiabendazole. Gastrointest Radiol 6 : 223-225

Zimbalist E, Gettenberg G, Brejt H (1987) Ileocolonic schistosomiasis presenting as lymphoma. Amer J Gastroent 82 : 476-478

Vascular diseases

Nongangrenous intestinal ischemia
(figs. 1 to 11)

The small intestinal vascular supply stems from the superior mesenteric artery, which anastomoses extensively with the celiac and inferior mesenteric artery. In addition, arterioles form anastomoses which interconnect the straight vessels of the intestinal wall. Mesenteric ischemic accidents are frequent in spite of this dense vascularity. This is explained by both the preferential reduction in splanchnic blood flow to maintain cerebral and cardiac perfusion in cases of systemic hypovolemia or decreased heart rate, and by the fragile vasculature of the villi. Like the other organs, the small intestine may develop ischemia following a decrease in arterial supply due to several causes:
- arterial stenosis caused by atherosclerosis, a volvulus, adhesions, tumoral infiltration of the mesentery, primary or radiation-induced mesenteric fibrosis or compression,
- a vascular embolism or
- vasculitis due to connective tissue disease, Henoch-Schönlein purpura, obliterating thromboangeitis or Degos' disease.

In addition, ischemia may appear in the absence of obstructive vascular lesions, especially with congestive heart failure or shock. Previous atheromatous lesions aggravate the effects of such nonobstructive ischemia.

Nongangrenous intestinal ischemia represents a subacute or chronic, not an acute, condition. The outcome depends on the duration and the degree of the decrease in mesenteric blood flow. Initially there is superficial hemorrhagic necrosis of the mucosa, which may either disappear within a couple of days or, evolve and become transmural over a long segment of bowel resulting in infarction. If the ischemic transmural lesions remain local, they may disappear completely or lead to stricture formation.

Pathology

The lesions are confined to the mucosa and submucosa at first. The mucosa is necrotic and ulcerated. The villi disappear. The inflammatory reaction is not very extensive initially but progresses with the action of intraluminal bacteria. The submucosa is edematous, with congested vessels. Granulation tissue containing macrophages and fibroblasts appear with healing or they may result in stricture formation. The submucosa is replaced by hyaline connective tissue with few blood vessels, while fibrosis extends into the serosa and the mesentery. The ischemic origin of such a stenosing lesion is not readily demonstrated. Transmural infiltration by iron-laden macrophages, the destruction of the muscularis by mutilating fibrosis and the lesions caused by endarteritis or arteriolar obliteration are characteristic but not always present.

Clinical findings

The onset of pain may be acute or chronic, sometimes atypical and ill-defined, in the form of an abdominal ache. The resulting epigastric pain radiates to the entire abdomen, occurring 30 to 60 min after meals and increasing with the quantity of nutrients ingested. Food restriction reduces pain but

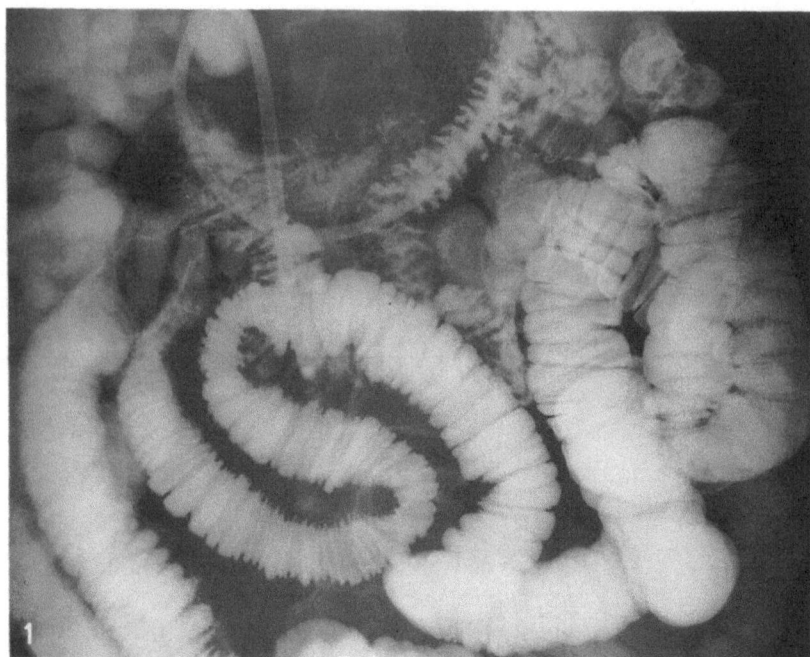

Fig. 1. Ischemia. 50-year-old woman. Cardiac failure, subacute onset of abdominal pain. SBFT : unfolded loops, widened interloop gap, palisading folds in the and proximal distention distal jejunal, with a decreased caliber and proximal distension

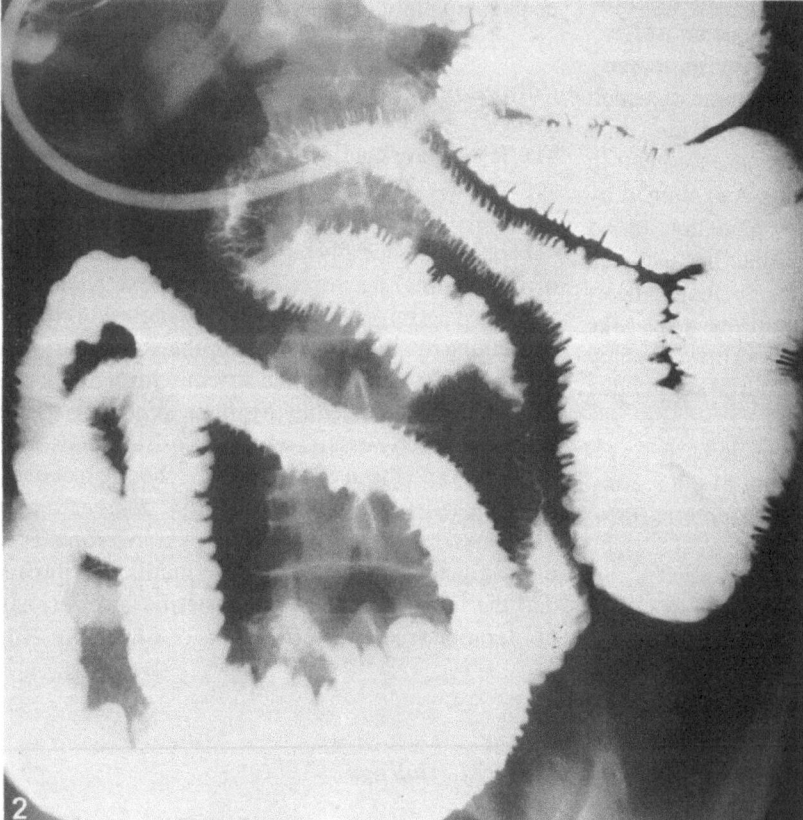

Fig. 2. Ischemia. 54-year-old woman. Abdominal pain and diarrhea 2 weeks after cholecystectomy. SBFT : alternate hypotonic and spastic segments, widened interloop gap, palisading folds with marginal microspiculation

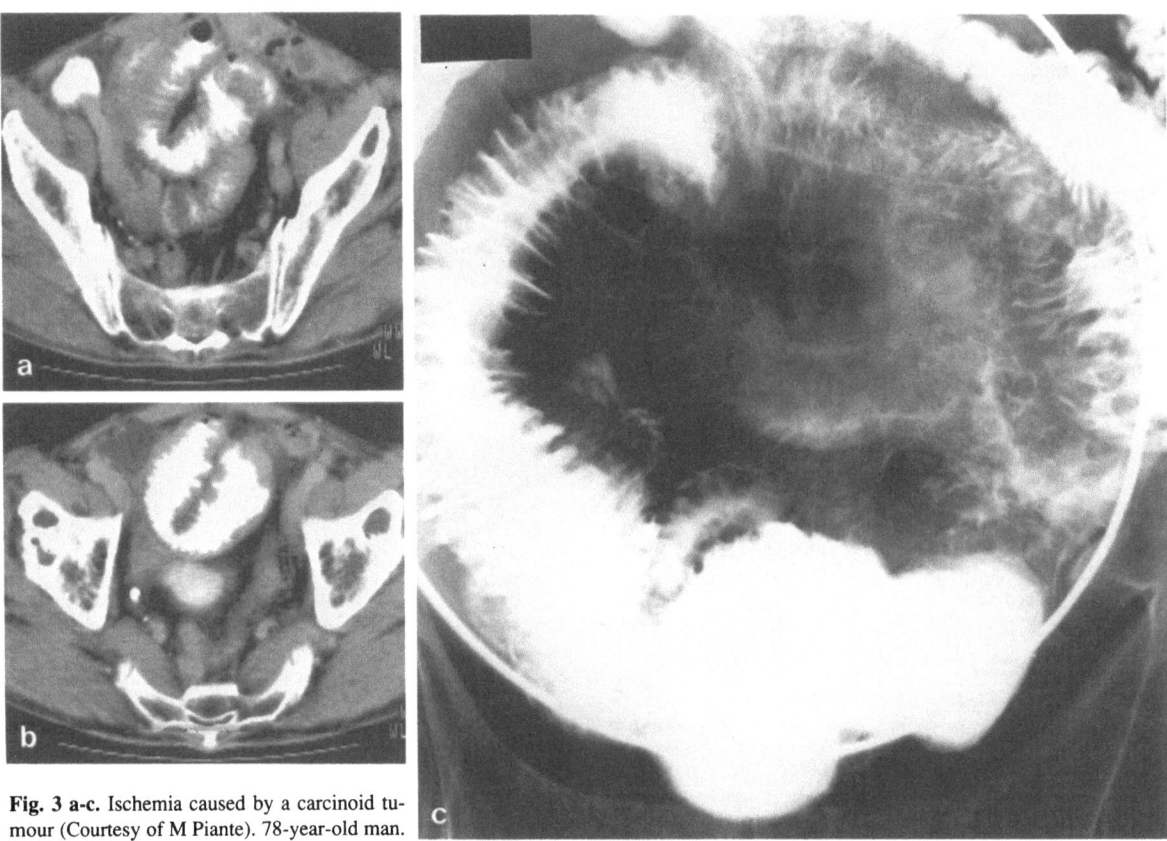

Fig. 3 a-c. Ischemia caused by a carcinoid tumour (Courtesy of M Piante). 78-year-old man. Long-standing abdominal pain. Mass on the right side. **a, b** CT scan : increased loop caliber, wall thickening, palisading folds **c** SBFT : unfolded ileal loops, and surrounding concentrically a lucent area. Thickened, lengthed, and stiffend folds

causes weight loss. Associated factors include advanced age, diabetes, hyperlipemia, the use of tobacco and lower limb arteritis.

Mild episodes of diarrhea are sometimes noted. Intestinal obstruction due to ischemic stenosis causes changes in bowel habits that worsen progressively, as well as Koenig's syndrome and sometimes diarrhea due to bacterial overgrowth proximal to the stenosis. Acute obstruction may also occur. The history sometimes is that of painful episodes followed by a symptom-free period lasting a couple of days or months.

The diagnosis is made using all the clinical, radiological and arteriographic data available.

Radiological findings

The plain abdominal radiographs sometimes reveal nonspecific aortic calcifications and air in the small intestine. In case of obstruction, air-fluid levels are visible in the small intestine. The gas pattern sometimes displays a stenosis or thumbprinting.

A small bowel follow-through (SBFT) is very often performed after negative gastric and colonic endoscopic studies. And it is sometimes normal. In the subacute form, the SBFT often demonstrates a moderate decrease in the caliber of one or several loops of the small intestine. This narrowed area is centered, symmetric and regular, and causes moderate distention of the proximal loops. The folds are thickened and taller, straight and parallel, producing a «palisade» appearance with spiculated margins (decreased interfold gaps). The margins of the opaque barium column are indistinct , indicating the inflammatory character of the lesion. Frequent spastic phenomena increase the stenosis and make it difficult for the contrast medium to fill the loop. Thumbprinting is sometimes demonstrated, especially along the antimesenteric margin. The folds may disappear completely. The opacity of the contrast medium displays reticulated positive images along the smooth

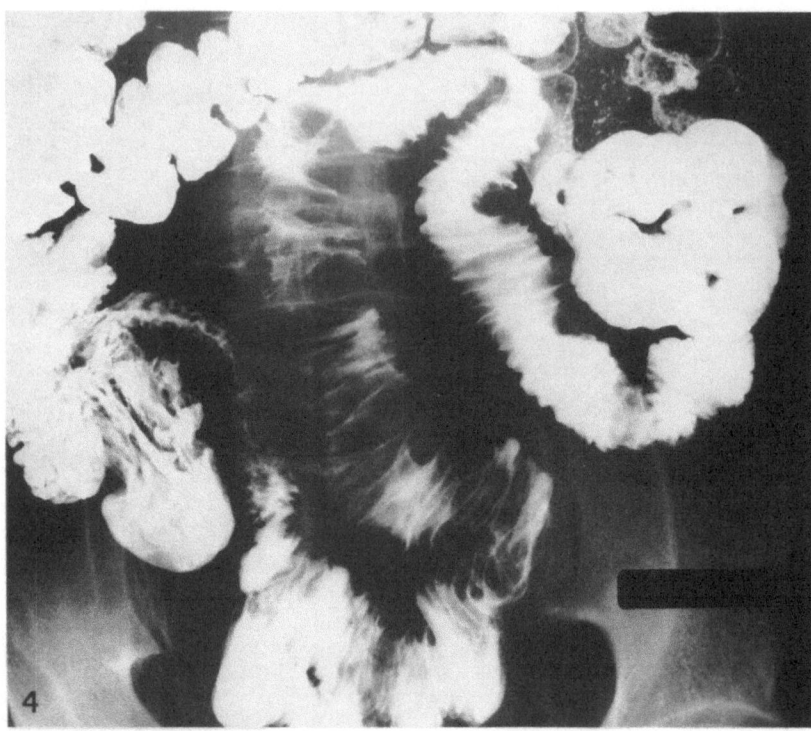

Fig. 4. Ischemia. 29-year-old man. Sub-occlusive episode. Polycythemia (6 ,500,000 red blood cells). No laboratory evidence of inflammation. SBFT : widened interloop gap, palisading folds and marginal notches in a distal loop

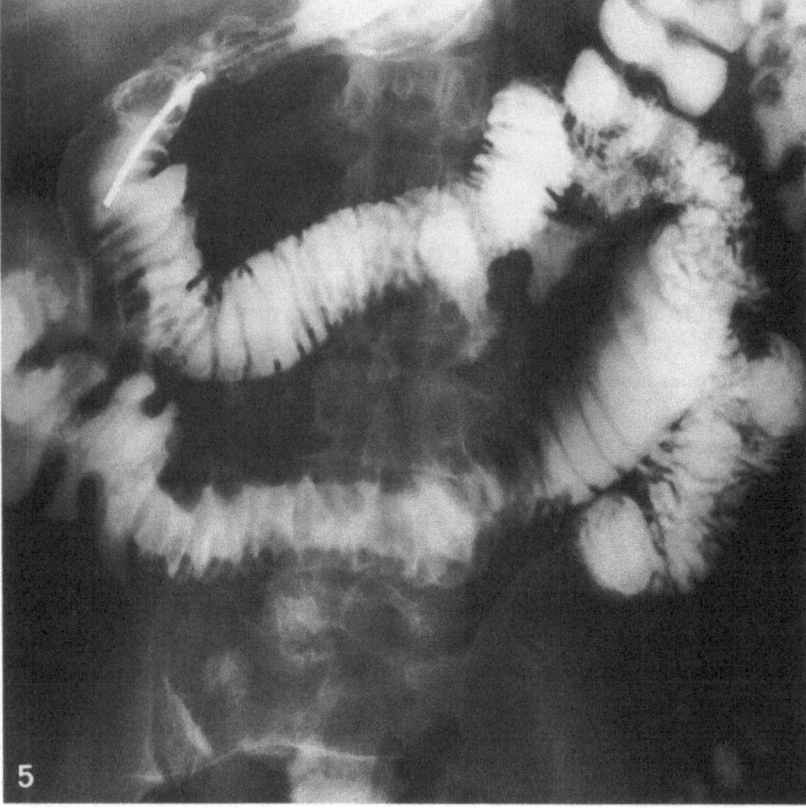

Fig. 5. Ischemia. 60-year-old man. Arteritis and diabetes. Ileal resection for bowel infarction. SBFT : marginal notches and thickened folds in the terminal loop

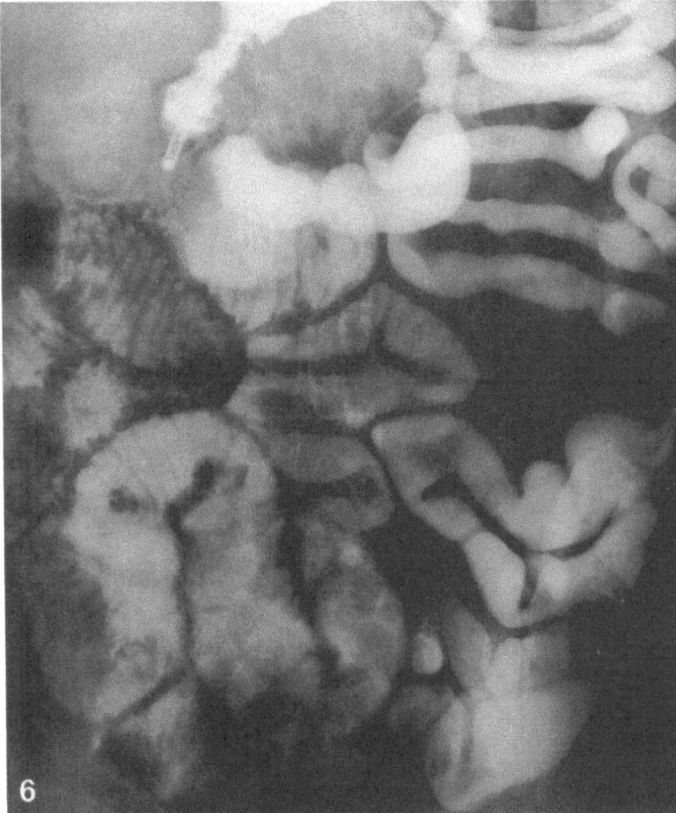

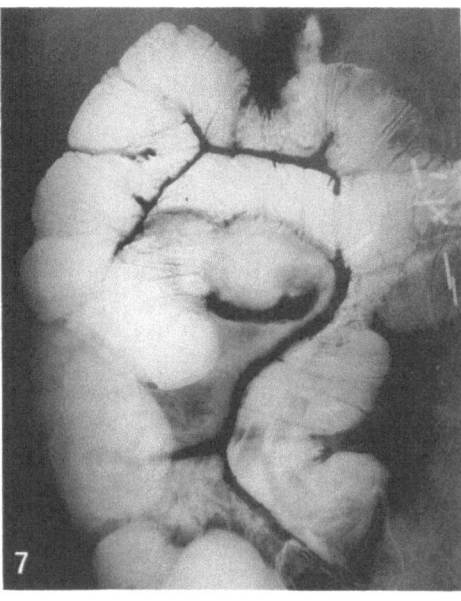

Fig. 7. Ischemia. 67-year-old man. Changes in bowel habits and weight loss following aortofemoral bypass surgery. SBFT : short jejunal stenosis with smooth margins and a gradual transition, widened interloop gap

Fig. 6. Ischemia. 70-year-old man with arteritis. Chronic diarrhea with malabsorption. Arteriography : abrupt cut-off of the 3rd jejunal artery. SBFT : ribbon-like appearance of the jejunal loops with widened interloop gaps, disappearance of the folds and jejunal transformation of the ileum

intestinal wall, indicating superficial ulcerations. These are visible on tangential views as marginal microspiculation.

Narrowing is maximal in its central portion, with contiguous ulcerations and marginal notches, and broadened folds at its proximal and distal ends. The intestinal wall is thickened but the loop is still relatively mobile in the peritoneal cavity.

Signs of ischemia (rectilinear folds, decreased and spiculated interfold gaps, marginal notches) on a widened loop must lead to a distal search for obstruction due to an adhesion or tumour. Signs of ischemia proximal to an obstructive lesion require urgent surgery.

Signs of an extensive enteropathy are observed in some cases. The involved loops are hypotonic. The normal mucosal pattern is replaced by a thin reticulated appearance due to superficial ulcerations. These mucosal abnormalities are usually associated with moderate thickening of the bowel wall, sometimes with mesenteric abnormalities such as fixed, stiff or abnormally separated loops. These lesions

can involve all the loops of the small intestine, but the proximal jejunal loops are rarely affected. The intermediate segments are most frequently involved. The predominating midintestinal location of the lesions and the possible concomitant mesenteric abnormalities rule out celiac disease.

If another barium examination is performed after some time, it can demonstrate either the complete disappearance of the abnormalities or, on the contrary, the occurrence of stricture formation, which is always shorter than the initially involved segment.

A resulting ischemic stricture is characteristically regular, short, centered and exhibits a gradual proximal and distal transition, most often with a smooth central part. Irregularly scattered, linear or broad superficial ulcerations are sometimes observed and more easily visualized in the proximal aspect of the stricture. No fistulae are seen. In some cases, the stenosing lesion is extensive and causes a tight narrowing of several loops. This stenosis is irregular and includes narrow segments in some portions, and small saccules in others. Barium studies rarely show

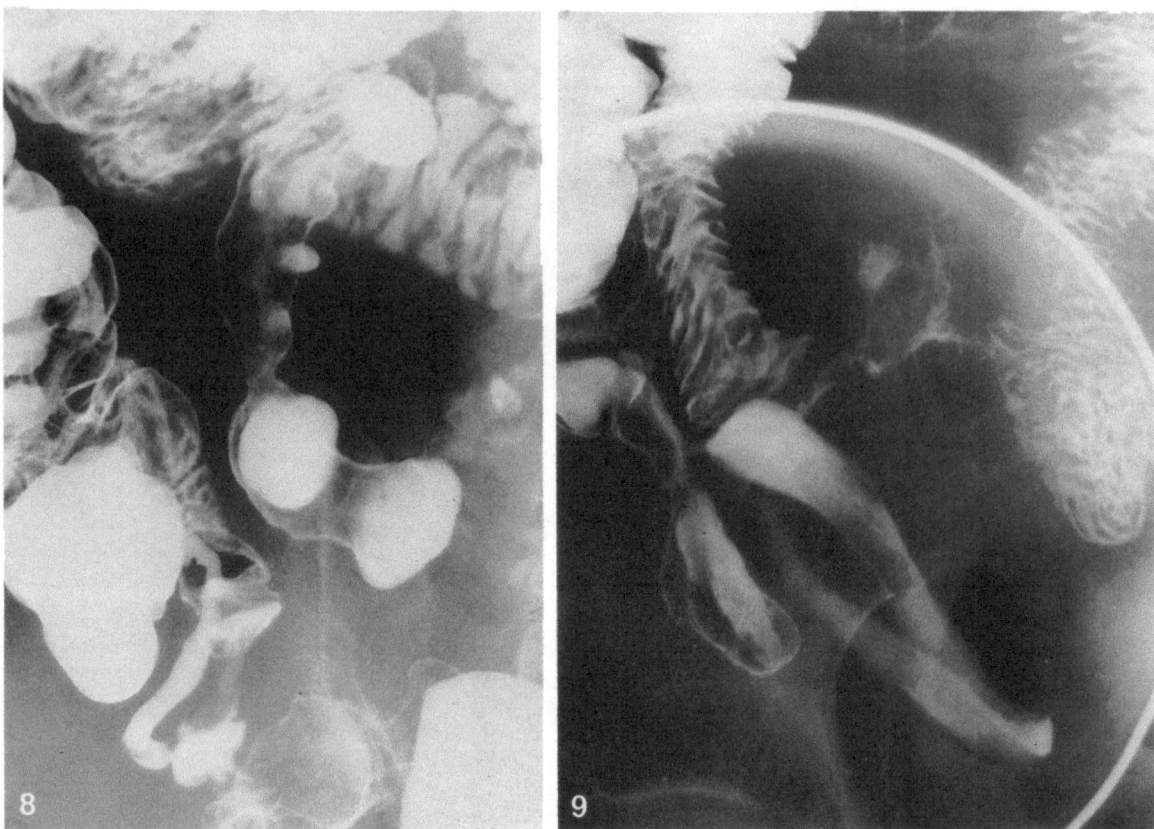

Fig.8. Ischemia. 64-year-old man with hypertension and cardiac failure. Subocclusion. SBFT : irregular narrowing of the last ileal loops with sacculation

Fig. 9. Ischemia. 71-year-old woman. Diarrhea and malabsorption after extensive resection for ileomesenteric infarction. SBFT : stenosis with smooth margins and angulated last loop. Fistula beginning at the anastomosis

a series of ulcerated stenoses. Proximal dilatation of the small intestine reflects a chronic appearance with rare, thickened folds. The narrowed segment is very often fixed due to mesenteric retraction, but the proximal and distal loops conserve their mobility and flexibility.

The diagnosis of ischemia is sometimes difficult. Straight, lengthened and parallel folds with or without marginal notches are also present with intramural hematomas. The notches of hematomas appear in the mesenteric aspect of the loop, whereas those of ischemia are seen in its antimesenteric border. An underlying vascular disorder is often noted in cases of intramural hematoma but the obstructive event is more acute. The most important factor to allow its identification is an increase in the prothrombin time.

Ischemic stenosis is not always easy to differentiate from tumoral and inflammatory stenosis, in particular from Crohn's disease. The stricture in ischemia is rarely asymmetric. No rhagade or aph-toid ulcerations are observed and the saccules are usually not found on the antimesenteric aspect. The diagnosis of radiation-induced enteritis is based on the patient's history. A tumoral origin is ruled out because of the regular, centered, gradual and smooth character of the ischemic stricture. However, primary or metastatic cancers of the small intestine may also have this appearance.

Complementary imaging

Arteriography is performed because of a high degree of clinical suspicion seldom reveals distal or trunk obstruction in the intestinal arteries, the mesenteric arches or the straight vessels. Extensive atherosclerosis is most often noted. Given the frequency of such atherosclerosis, the diagnosis of mesenteric ischemia is made only when at least two out of three large mesenteric vessels, including the celiac artery,

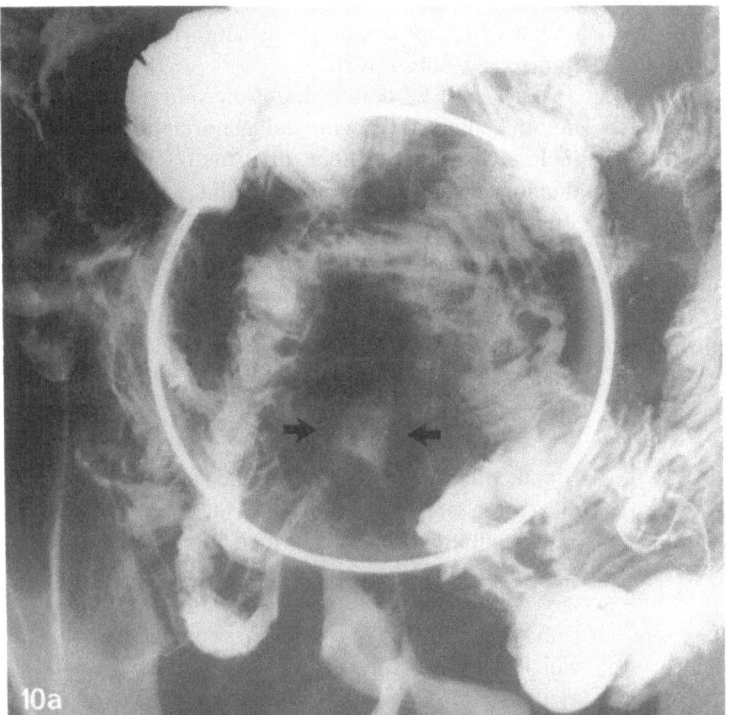

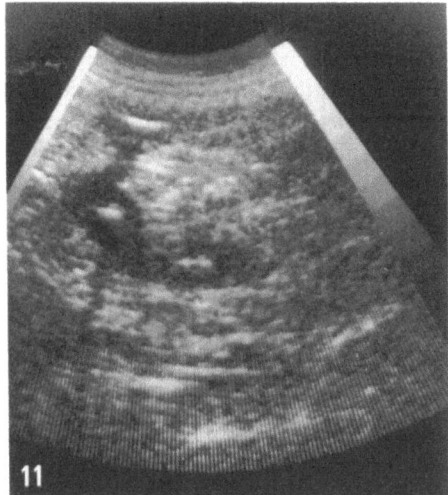

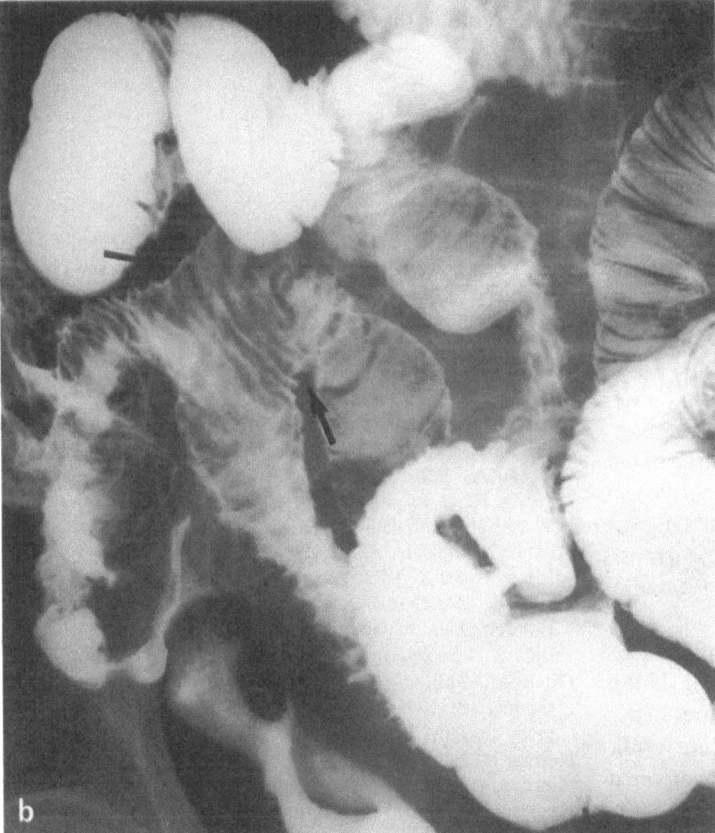

Fig. 10 a, b. Ischemia. 74-year-old woman. Alternating diarrhea and subocclusion 2 months after abdominal trauma with hemoperitoneum and injurius of the omentum and mesentery which were overseen. SBFT : **a** Long ribbon stenosis of an angular fixed pelvic loop with blind fistula. **b** Accessorily Meckel's diverticulum on a neighbouring loop

Fig. 11. Ischemia. 70-year-old man, known vascular disease. Subocclusion. Ultrasound : regular, circumferential, hypoechogeneic thickening of the wall of several loops of the small intestine

the superior mesenteric artery and the inferior mesenteric artery, are decreased by more than 50%.

In the acute stage, ultrasound reveals a moderate (less than 1 cm), regular, hypoechogenic thickening of the wall of an intestinal loop, in line, and showing a smooth transition with the neighbouring segments, usually without associated peritoneal fluid. In some cases, it demonstrates several atonic, crowded loops with thin walls (under 2 mm), filled with fluid, sometimes with moderate ascites. In the chronic stage of an intestinal stricture, ultrasound demonstrates stasis and sometimes the stenosis as a concentric image, with a regular, circumferential thickening of the intestinal wall.

Ultrasound can demonstrate alterations of the aorta or of the superior mesenteric artery.

Computed tomography provides information similar to that of ultrasound which may however be more explicit.

Practical conclusions

The radiological diagnosis of nongangrenous mesenteric ischemia of the small intestine is important because the clinical findings are misleading and atypical. The diagnosis is often made on SBFT. Arteriography is rarely diagnostic in this subacute or chronic condition, but must be performed rapidly in the case of an acute clinical presentation because of the high risk of subsequent rapid progression to bowel infarction. The discovery of ischemic strictures will almost always necessitate surgical repair.

Venous thrombosis

Thrombosis of the superior mesenteric vein or of one of its branches can occur with oral contraceptive use, hyper coagulable status (e. g. Waldenström's disease or paroxysmal nocturnal hemoglobinuria), cirrhosis or obstruction to mesenteric blood flow (volvulus, adhesions, nodal or tumoral compression).

Thrombosis can be acute and dramatic, causing bowel wall infarction and perforation. If less severe, it favours the formation of intramural hematomas. If the venous obstruction is subacute, collateral circulation develops sometimes with varices in the mesentery or the intestinal wall.

Thrombosis causes variably acute and intense abdominal pain and intestinal bleeding. The diagnosis is based either on the patient's history or on arteriography, (where collateral vessels are opacified on late films), or at emergency surgery. Recanalization occurs only rarely.

The SBFT demonstrates the signs of an intramural hematoma: segmental abnormalities which include decreased caliber, thickened, tall folds and thumbprinting. Varices are sometimes observed as a sinuous network enmeshed in the mucosal folds. The demonstration of varices may be seen with portal hypertension as well.

Intramural hematomas of the small intestine

Blood collection in the wall of the small intestine is most often seen by radiologists in the context of over-anticoagulation. The appearance observed on SBFT is described in Chapter VIII. We will only mention the other causes of small intestinal intramural hematomas in this chapter. These include trauma, which may be surgical or endoscopic, vascular malformations, coagulation disorders such as hemophilia, leukemia, disseminated intravascular coagulation, multiple myeloma, dialysis, Henoch-Schönlein purpura and venous thrombosis.

References

Ischemia

Alpern MB, Glazer GM, Francis IR (1988) Ischemic or infarcted bowel : CT findings. Radiology 166 : 149-152

Alschibaja T, Morson BC (1977) Ischaemic bowel disease. J Clin Pathol (Suppl) 11 : 68-77

Baxter R, Nino-Murcia M, Bloom RJ, Kosek J (1988) Gastrointestinal manifestations of essential mixed cryoglobulinemia. Gastrointest Radiol 13 : 160-162

Boley SJ, Brandt LJ, Veith FJ (1978) Ischemic disorders of the intestines. Curr Probl Surg 15 : 4

Corbeau A, Félix M, Gioan JM, Burelle H, Clément JP (1977) Rétrécissement post-traumatique de l'intestin grêle avec étude radiologique en double contraste après intubation duodénale, à propos d'une observation. J Radiol Electrol 58 : 827-831

Druart F, Morichau-Beauchant M, Matuchansky C (1979) Entéropathies ischémiques de l'adulte. Gastroenterol Clin Biol 3 : 683-694

Gillet M, Philippe E, Stoebner P, Sava G, Viville C, Grenier JF (1969) Les sténoses cicatricielles de l'intestin grêle d'origine ischémique. Ann Chir 23 : 481-491

Hertzer NR, Beven EG, Humphries AW (1977) Chronic intestinal ischemia. Surg Gynecol Obstet 145 : 321-328

Jacobson ED (1973) Mesenteric circulatory regulation in normal and ischemic states. In : Sadek K (ed) Hilal : Small vessel angiography. Mosby, Saint-Louis, pp 434-437

Joffe N, Goldman H, Antonioli DA (1977) Barium studies in small bowel infarction, radiological pathological correlation. Radiology 123 : 303-309

Kieny R, Cinqualbre J, Eisenmann B, Tongio J (1976) Ischémie mésentérique chronique. Ann Radiol 19 (3) : 371-375

Kieny R, Cinqualbre J, Wenger JJ, Tongio J (1979) Les ischémies intestinales aiguës. Expansion Scientifique Française, Paris

Le Thi Huong Du, Wechsler B, Bletry O, Guillevin L, Langlois P, Tran Ba Loc P, Godeau P (1985) Angéites nécrosantes et manifestations abdominales. Ann Gastroenterol Hepatol 21 : 153-158

Marshak RH, Lindner AE, Maklansky D (1976) Ischemia of the small intestine. Am J Gastroenterol 66 : 390-400

Meyers MA, Kaplowitz N, Bloom AA (1973) Malabsorption secondary to mesenteric ischemia. AJR 119 : 352-358

Saegesser F, Borgeaud J, Schnyder P, Tabrizian M, Richon CA (1976) Les sténoses de l'intestin grêle d'origine ischémique de l'adulte (lésions segmentaires et transmurales). Schweiz Med Wschr 106 : 367-376

Schmutz G, Kempf F, Wenger JJ, Tongio J (1980) Le transit du grêle dans l'ischémie mésentérique chronique, à propos d'une observation avec malabsorption. J Radiol 61 : 737-739

Schmutz G, Schutz JF, Kempf F, Baumann R, Weill JP (1980) Aspects radiologiques de l'ischémie colique non gangréneuse. J Radiol 61 : 603-609

Thomas ML (1972) Plain film and barium studies of the ischaemic bowel. Clin Gastroenterol 1 : 581-595

Williams LF (1971) Vascular insufficiency of the intestines. Gastroenterology 61 : 757-777

Wolf BS, Marshak RH (1956) Segmental infarction of the small bowel. Radiology 66 : 701-707

Venous thrombosis

Agarwal D, Scholz FJ (1981) Small-bowel varices demonstrated by enteroclysis. Radiology 140 : 350

Becquemin JP, Fagniez PL, Soule JC, Chapelier A, Bizard T, Julien M (1981) Infarctus veineux entéromésentérique, les difficultés d'un diagnostic précoce. Gastroenterol Clin Biol 5 : 992-997

Federle M, Clark RA (1979) Mesenteric varices : a source of mesosystemic shunts and gastrointestinal hemorrhage. Gastrointest Radiol 4 : 331-338

Gille P, Aubert D, Mourot M (1979) Sténose de la veine mésentérique supérieure par malposition intestinale et volvulus du grêle. Chir Pédiatr 20 : 41-42

L'Herminé C, Paris JC, Bergerp, Lemaitre L, Delemazureo (1981) Complications vasculaires des volvulus chroniques du grêle, intérêt de l'artériographie. Med Chir Dig 10 : 113-119

Park RW, Watkins JB (1979) Mesenteric vascular occlusion and varices complicating midgut malrotation. Gastroenterology 77 : 565-568

Soper NJ, Rikkers LF, Miller FJ (1985) Gastrointestinal hemorrhage associated with chronic mesenteric venous occlusion. Gastroenterology 88 : 1964-1967

Randall Radin D, Siskind BN, Alpert S, Bernstein RG (1986) Small-bowel varices due to mesenteric metastasis. Gastrointest Radiol 11 : 183-184

Verma TR, Bankole MA (1973) Lymphovenous obstruction in anomalous midgut rotation. Arch Dis Child 48 : 154-157

Hematoma

Dodds WJ, Spitzer RM, Friedland GW (1970) Gastrointestinal roentgenographic manifestations of hemophilia. AJR 110 : 413-416

Fingerhut A, Hillion D, Eugène C, Pourcher J, Fendler JP, Ronat R (1980) Hématome intra mural duodeno jejunal révélant une périartérite noueuse. Med Chir Dig 9 : 419-423

Kattan KR, Marsch JT (1988) Gastrointestinal manifestations in hemophilia. Radiol Clin N Am 6 : 1282-1283

Kolodny M, Mushlin AI, Baker WG, Sleisenger MH, Nachman RL (1968) Intramural small intestinal hematoma, a review and a report of a new case : uremia. Arch Intern Med 121 : 438-446

Monnier JM, Bigot JM, Chermet J, Fragoa M (1974) Les hématomes intrapariétaux du grêle. J Rad Electrol 55 : 217-222

Iatrogenic conditions

Iatrogenic lesions of the small intestine are caused by drugs, surgery or radiation therapy. Surgical accidents and complications are discussed in the chapter on the postoperative patient.

Drug-induced lesions

Some drugs can cause lesions of the small intestine, which may or may not disappear when treatment is stopped.

Hematomas caused by anticoagulant therapy (figs. 1 to 6)

Intramural hematomas occur in the small intestine due to overdosage during anticoagulant therapy which inhibits the synthesis of vitamin K-dependent coagulation factors. The diagnosis must be made in order to avoid unnecessary surgery.

Pathology

The most frequent sites for intramural hematomas are the duodenum, and next the jejunum. The hematoma appears in the submucosa, displaces the mucosa and progressively infiltrates the muscularis. It soon becomes circumferential and extends along the intestinal axis, involving one or several loops.

Clinical findings

The patient may present because of a gastrointestinal hemorrhage and also display ecchymoses, epis-taxis, bleeding of the gums and hematuria indicating a bleeding tendency. The clinical signs include colicky pains or subocclusion in the absence of hemorrhage. The diagnosis is made with the measurement of prothrombin levels, which are often lower than 10% of control (but can exceptionally be normal), coupled to the radiological findings. The hematoma disappears without residual signs when the anticoagulated state is reversed.

Radiological findings

Plain films can demonstrate a visible loop with thickened walls or gas distention proximal to the lesion.

The small bowel follow throught (SBFT) reveals a 10 to 30 cm long narrowed segment, most often in a moderately fixed, unfolded jejunal loop with thickened walls (increased interloop gap). The folds of the loop are tall, broadened, straight and dense. On tangential views, the reduced interfold gap produces spiculations (the «stacked coin» appearance). The course of the folds is either parallel (palisading folds) or irregular, with possible nodular folds which then alternate with marginal «thumbprints». The abnormal region displays sharply delineated margins. No functional alterations are noted in the other loops, but distention is sometimes observed proximally. The lesions are relatively malleable on palpation. The evolution of the radiological appearance usually results in complete healing without stricture formation within a couple of weeks after discontinuation of therapy.

The radiological lesion is nonspecific. It can be observed after trauma, in any disease causing coagulation disorders, in venous thrombosis or in ische-

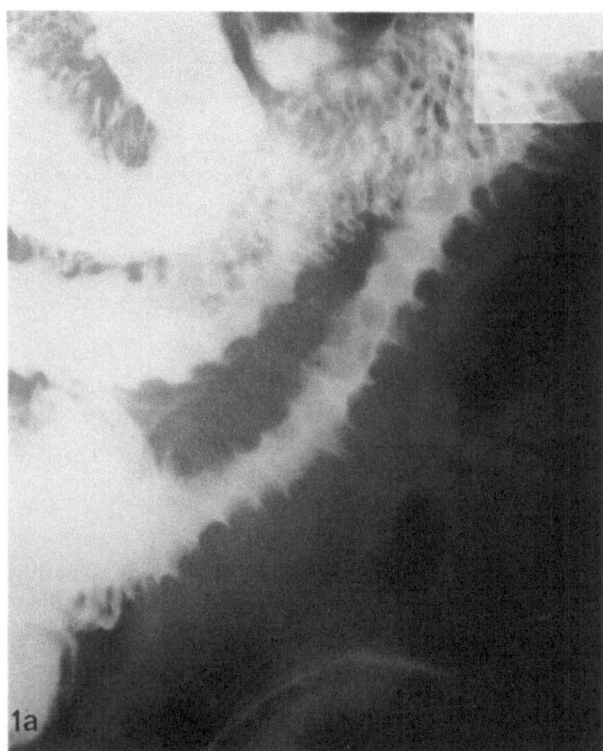

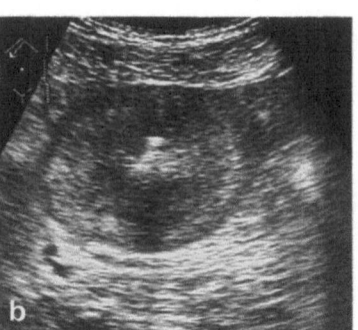

Fig.1 a, b. Hematoma. 65-year-old man. Cardiac failure. Anticoagulant therapy. Abnormal prothrombin time. **a** SBFT : tall, broadened, nodular folds in a narrowed jejunal loop. **b** ultrasound: homogeneous mural thickening (2cm)

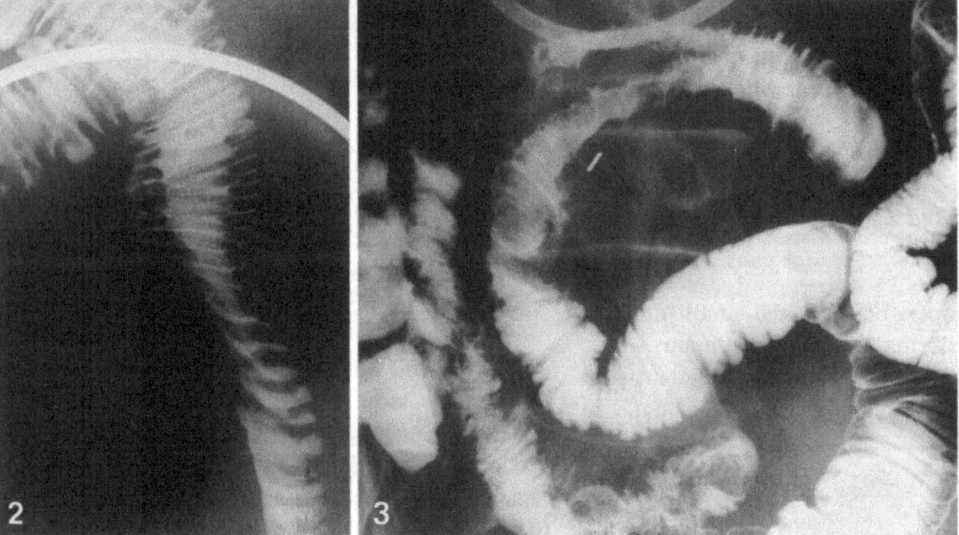

Fig. 2. Hematoma. 65-year-old woman. Cardiac failure. Anticoagulant therapy. Proctorrhagia and melena. Abnormal prothrombin time SBFT : tall rectilinear, parallel folds in a narrowed jejunal loop

Fig. 3. Hematoma. 70-year-old man. Infarct. Anticoagulant therapy. Abnormal prothrombin time. SBFT : segmental decrease in the caliber of an ileal loop, marginal notches, broadened, tall, rectilinear and parallel folds

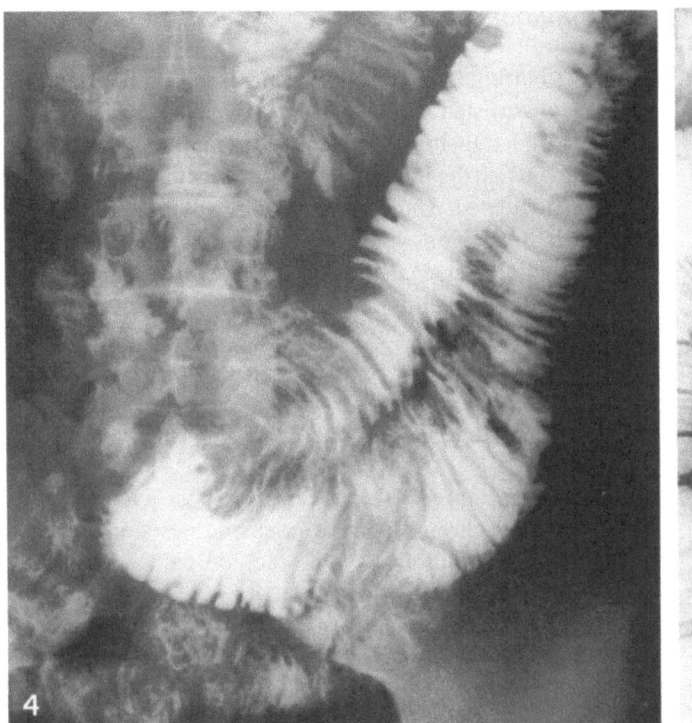

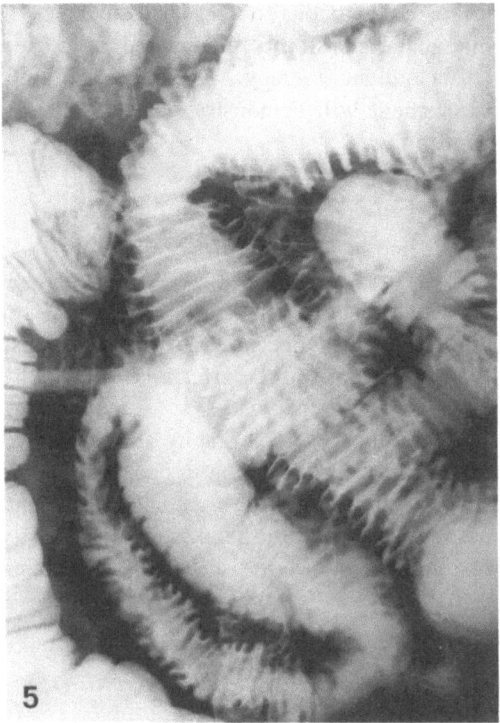

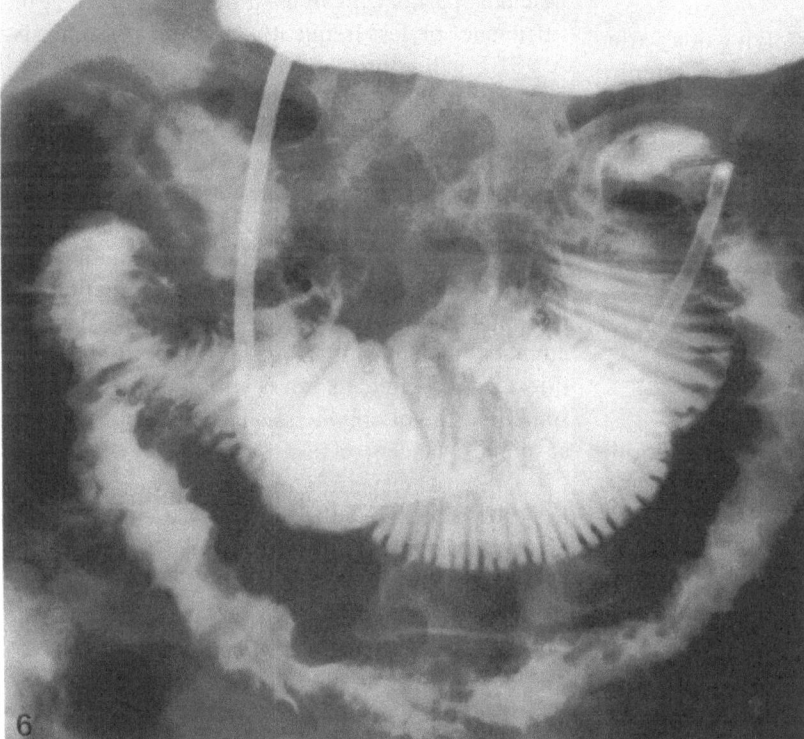

Fig. 4. Hematoma. 47-year-old man. Myocardial infarction. Anticoagulant therapy. Painful episode with proctorrhagia and anemia. Abnormal prothrombin time. SBFT : increased caliber of a jejunal loop with tall rectilinear folds

Fig. 5. Hematoma. 66-year-old man. infarction treated with anticoagulants. Abnormal prothrombin time . SBFT : increased caliber of a jejunal loop with broadened, tall, parallel and rectilinear folds

Fig. 6. Hematoma. 72-year-old man. Infarct. Anticoagulant therapy. SBFT : stiffened, narrowed jejunal loop bordered showing thumbprinting

mia. Accidents due to overdosage must be the first diagnostic possibility considered in a patient on anticoagulant therapy. An ensuing radiological assessment will demonstrate the absence of other conditions.

Complementary imaging

Ultrasound shows fluid in the peritoneal cavity, in addition to the hypoechogenic, homogeneous thickening of the wall of the affected loop which corresponds to the hematoma.

Computed tomography sometimes confirms the bowel wall thickening in one loop and demonstrates an adjacent mass formed by the presence of an associated mesenteric hematoma. The density of the lesions varies with the age of the hematoma.

Ulcer induced by potassium chloride tablets (figs. 7 and 8)

Tablets of potassium chloride dissolving at a variable rate in the intestine are sometimes used to replenish the potassium loss caused by diuretic therapy, especially in cardiac patients. The intestinal lesion seems to appear because of the high local potassium concentration which causes paralysis and slowing of the blood flow in the affected areas. The risk increases with the amount ingested but exists even at low doses.

Pathology

The absorption of concentrated potassium chloride can cause localized infarction due to regional venous thrombosis, with a rapidly stenosing circumferential ulceration. The ulcer then extends into the markedly edematous submucosa.

Clinical findings

The patient may present with episodes of subocclusion or with pain alone, hemorrhage, anemia, and less often with diarrhea or a perforation. Healing of the ulcer may result in stricture formation, so that the symptoms sometimes arise several months after the treatment has been stopped. The lesions then require surgical correction.

Radiological findings

A barium study will show one or rarely several short annular stenoses, usually in line and exhibiting a tapered transition with the proximal and distal segments, in the jejunum or ileum. Ulceration goes often undetected. The degree of proximal dilatation is variable. Lesions suggestive of associated ischemia including marginal defects with thickened, straight and tall folds and thumbprinting are sometimes seen near the ulcerations.

Other drug-induced lesions

Contraceptives taken recently or in the past can cause acute or chronic, local or extensive mesenteric thrombosis. The clinical signs include pain, nausea and diarrhea which is sometimes bloody. Radiological studies reveal signs of ischemia. The condition may be lethal.

The vasoconstriction caused by ergotamine derivatives in the treatment of migraines can induce vascular spasms with signs of intestinal vascular insufficiency or, less frequently, arteriolar thrombosis. A SBFT will confirm an ischemic appearance.

High doses of digitalis sometimes aggravate the existing vascular pathology due to its splanchnic vasoconstrictive action.

Ganglioplegics, psychoactive drugs with anticholinergic effects (antidepressants, phenothiazines, etc.), a number of antimitotic drugs, muscle relaxants, treatments causing potassium depletion and morphine derivatives may all induce dilatation and atonia of small intestinal loops. Electrolyte abnormalities and ischemic disorders with intestinal paresis, sometimes involving the stomach and colon, appear at more advanced stages.

Fibrosing peritonitis with subocclusion has been described after the long-term use of the beta-blocker practotol. The SBFT shows fixed, distorted or dilated loops.

A number of drugs (cholestyramine, albumin) can cause complete or partial mechanical obstruction due to a volume effect.

Gold salts sometimes cause ileal wall lesions which may induce diarrhea.

Intestinal hypersensitivity can be observed, in particular with penicillins.

Mucosal atrophy has been reported after a number of treatments, including neomycin and antimitotic drug use.

Anti-inflammatory drugs used for a long pe-

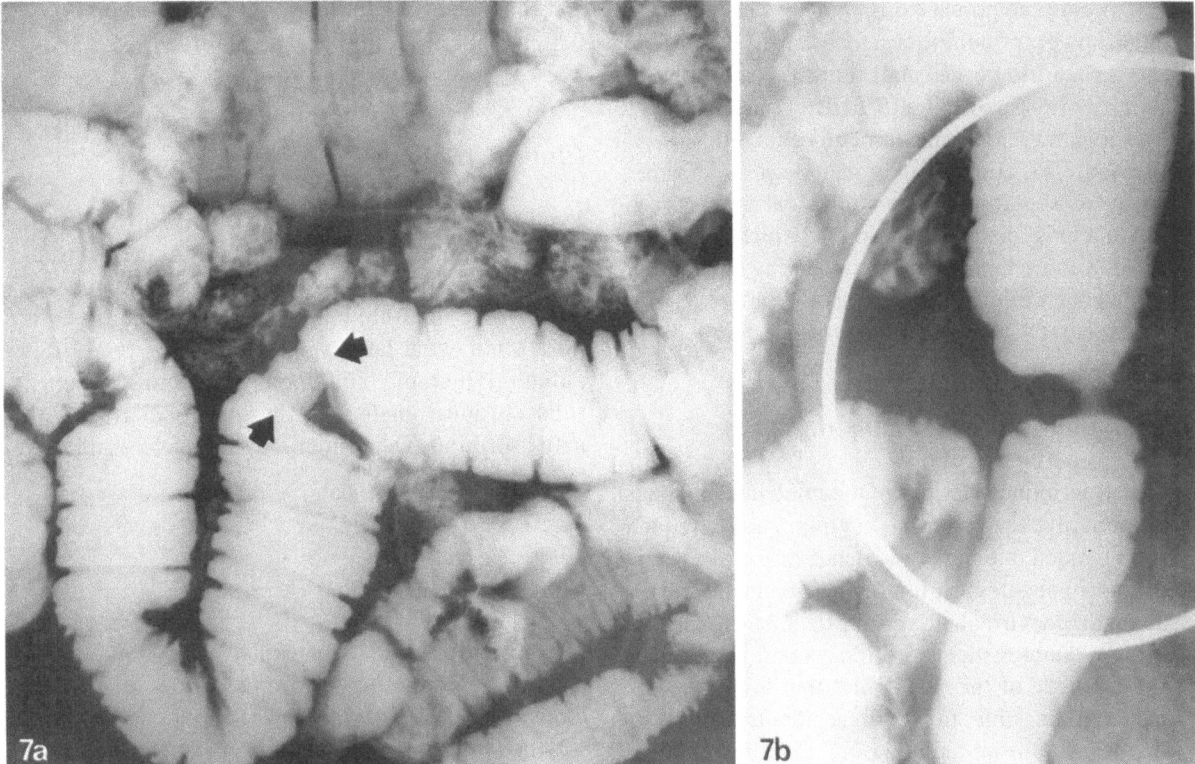

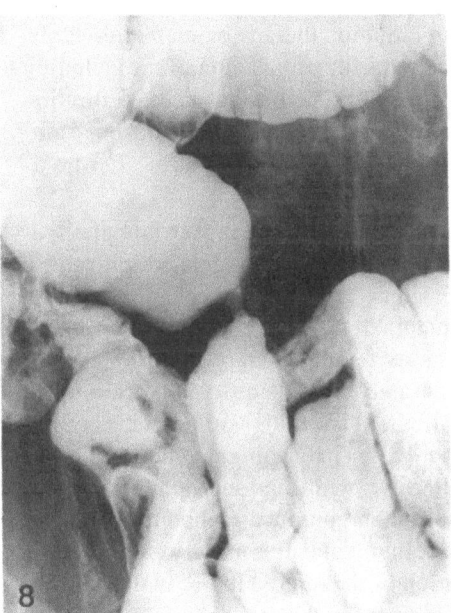

Fig. 7 a, b. Drug-induced ulcer. 60-year-old woman. Daily ingestion of potassium chloride tablets for 5 years, abdominal pain, vomiting. SBFT : two sites of short jejunal narrowing with local disappearance of the folds

Fig. 8. Drug-induced ulcer. 66-year-old woman. Potassium chloride tablets taken during 6 weeks two months before the examination. Abdominal pain followed by a subocclusive episode. SBFT : short annular stricture centered on a small ulceration, with distention of the proximal loop, at the junction of the jejunum and ileum

riod of time can produce inflammatory lesions of the small bowel, protein loss, stenosis or perforation.

Stenosis of the small intestine caused by the toxicity of 5-fluxoridine (5 FUDR) has been noted after its intravenous and sometimes its intra-arterial infusion. The clinical signs include pain, diarrhea, nausea and vomiting. The radiological appearance is that of a long, distal ileal stricture, which can extend over the entire ileum, with disappearing or irregularly thickened folds. The signs usually improve when chemotherapy is stopped.

Radiation-induced lesions (figs. 9 to 17)

Radiation-induced lesions of the small intestine most often involve the ileum and are found more frequently in women due to the incidence of pelvic irradiation for gynecological tumours. The small intestine also undergoes irradiation during treatment for cancers of the rectum, testicles or kidneys and lymphomas. The mobility of the small intestinal loops usually makes it possible to avoid accidents caused by overdosage during radiotherapy. Fixed loops are at considerably higher risk. Pre-existing tables allow for the assessment of risk according to the dose and to its distribution. The risk is increased when the fields of treatment overlap, when radium implants and radiation therapy are associated, or with adjuvant chemotherapy. Radiation enteritis is observed in 10% of the patients treated with radiotherapy. Late lesions, occurring up to 25 years after radiation therapy, may occur in 25 to 50% of patients having received a total of 60 Gy.

Pathology

Acute lesions develop during the course of radiation and in the following two months. Since the ionizing action is proportional to the rate of cell multiplication, the epithelium is the most fragile layer. Its destruction leads to transient or persistent villous atrophy. The lesions depend on the degree of bowel wall involvement, from simple edema to necrosis with fistula and abscess formation. The prognosis also depends on the associated mesenteric lesions, especially the vascular changes. These occur from the 3rd month onwards as an obliterating endarteritis causes mesenteric and intestinal ischemic fibrosis. The intestinal mucosa is atrophied and displays telangectasiae while the submucosa and the serosa are thickened. In addition to strictures, ulcerations, fistulae and infarction can be observed.

Clinical findings

Symptoms of intolerance (pain, diarrhea, vomiting) may develop during the treatments. Acute obstruction, abscess formation or a perforation sometimes appear over the following weeks. The clinical signs most often occur later, within months of years after radiation therapy, and include abdominal pains, subocclusion, sometimes hemorrhage or diarrhea with malabsorption. The lesions are often severe and may be lethal.

Radiological findings

In addition to a small intestinal occlusion pattern, plain radiographs may show gas in one or several loops, which are fixed, with abnormal curvatures, a widened interloop gap and thickened mucosal folds.

A small bowel follow-through is rarely performed during radiation therapy or soon afterwards. It then demonstrates functional alterations including hypertonia, hyperkinesia, contrast medium dilution and segmentation with the presence of thickened mucosal folds. The abnormalities disappear after treatment has ceased.

These findings can also appear late after radiation therapy and are then associated with more severe local lesions. The most typical appearance is that of an ischemia. It displays abnormal positioning which presents as regular juxtaposition of distant, parallel, moderately stiffened loops, often of a decreased caliber. The folds are either parallel, rectilinear and dense (palisading), sometimes broadened and alternate with marginal notches, or are completely absent and produce a ribbon appearance within the loop. Involvement is usually circumferential. The position of the injured loops, which corresponds to the fields of irradiation, helps in making the diagnosis, as can associated rectocolic or bony radiation injuries.

The lesions rarely improve, and on the contrary most often lead to the formation of straight, curved or angulated strictures, usually centered on the bowel lumen and several centimeters long, sometimes multiple (staggered in the same segment). The margins are smooth, producing tubular strictures, or covered with spicules if ulcerations are present. The

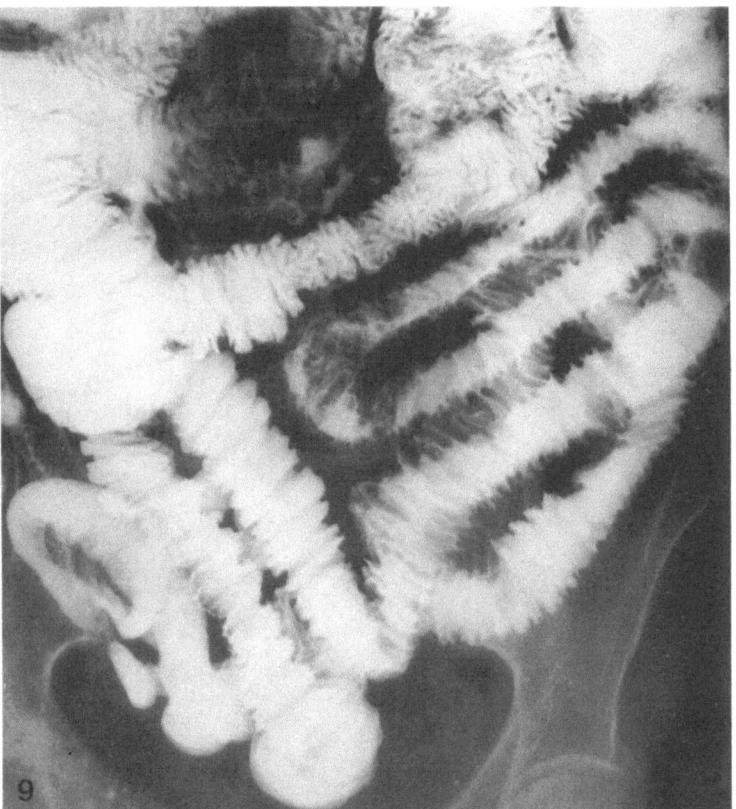

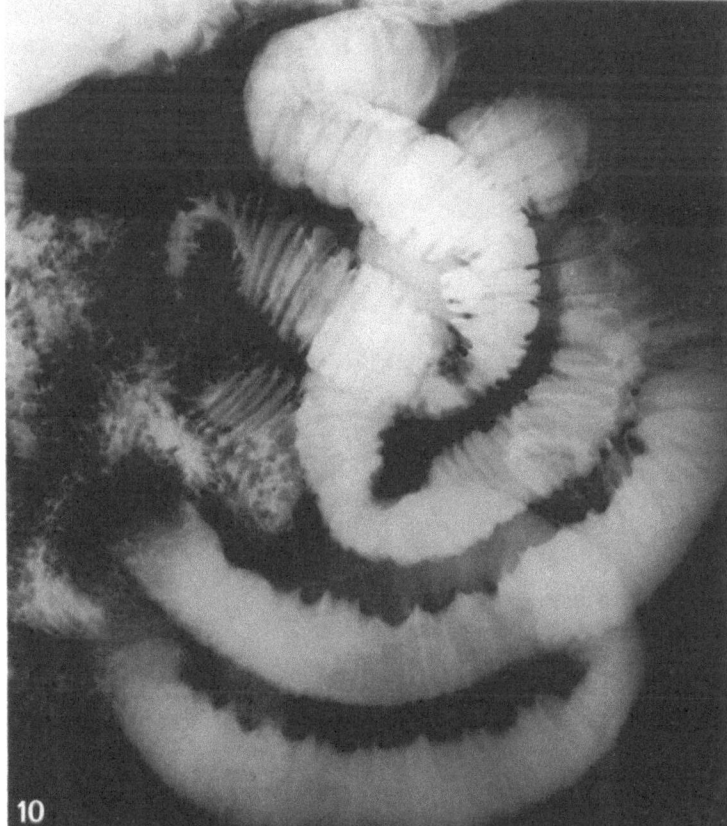

Fig. 9. Radiation enteritis. 62-year-old woman. Subocclusive episode 3 years after hysterectomy and cobalt therapy for cancer of the cervix. SBFT: parallel and relatively fixed distal loops, widened interloop gap and broadened, tall, rectilinear folds

Fig. 10. Radiation enteritis. 43-year-old woman. Diarrhea and meteorism 18 months after surgery and cobalt therapy for a cancer of the ovary. SBFT: unfoled relatively fixed loops, widened interloop gap, marginal notches and broadened, tall, rectilinear and parallel folds

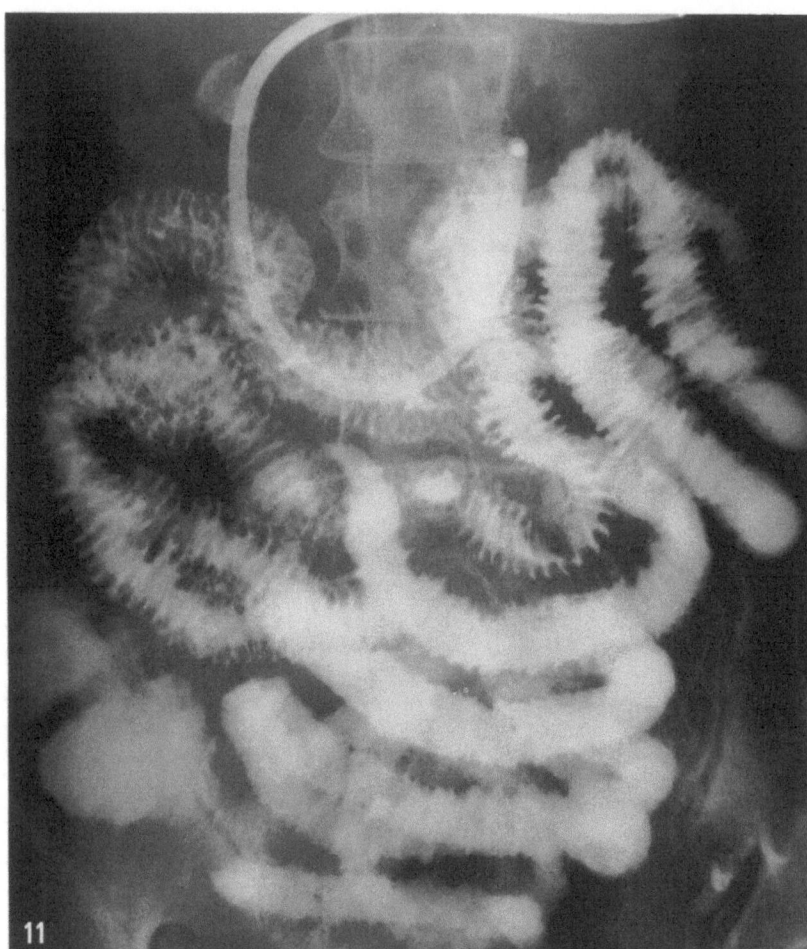

Fig. 11. Radiation enteritis. 38-year-old woman. Diarrhea and malabsorption 6 months after cobalt therapy for a cancer of the cervix. SBFT : diffuse involvement of the small intestine, contrast medium dilution, widened interloop gap, increased height of jejunal folds and marginal spiculation of the ileum with a parallel orientation of ileal folds

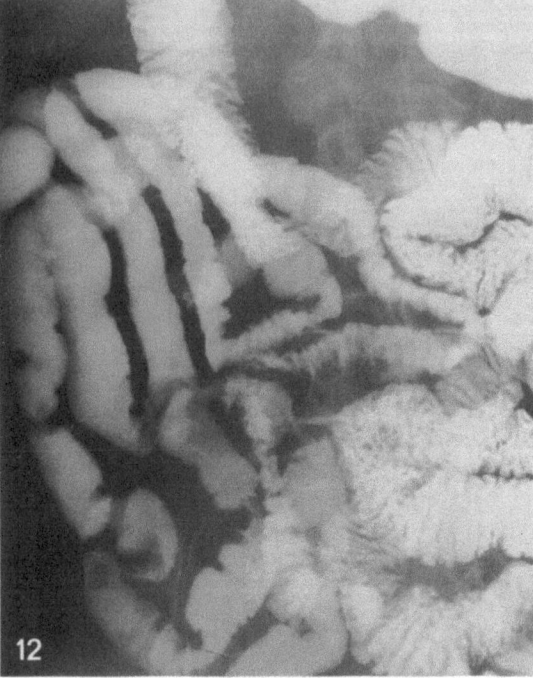

Fig. 12. Radiation enteritis. 62-year-old woman. Subocclusion 9 years after surgery and radiation therapy for cancer of the ovary. SBFT : parallel ileal loops on the right flank with widened interloop gaps, and disappearance of the folds

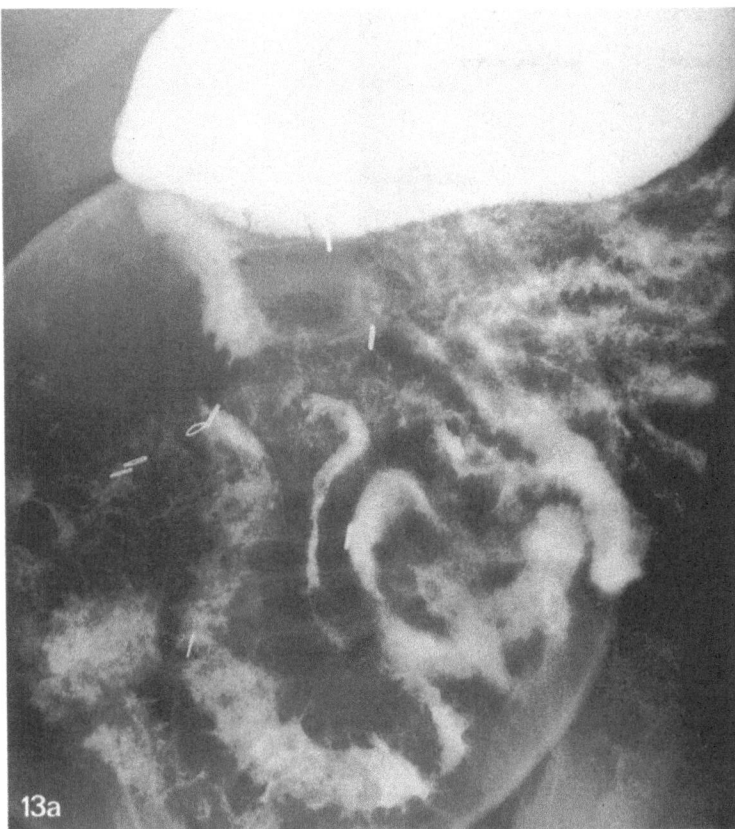

Fig. 13 a, b. Radiation enteritis. 13-year-old child. Diarrhea, malabsorption and retarded growth 8 years after partial left nephrectomy and cobalt therapy for a Wilms' tumour, also 3 years post-right nephrectomy, cobalt therapy and chemotherapy. SBFT : diffuse involvement of the small intestine, contrast medium dilution and flocculation, increased curvature and widened interloop gap, fixed loops and tall, broadened folds obliterated by hypersecretion

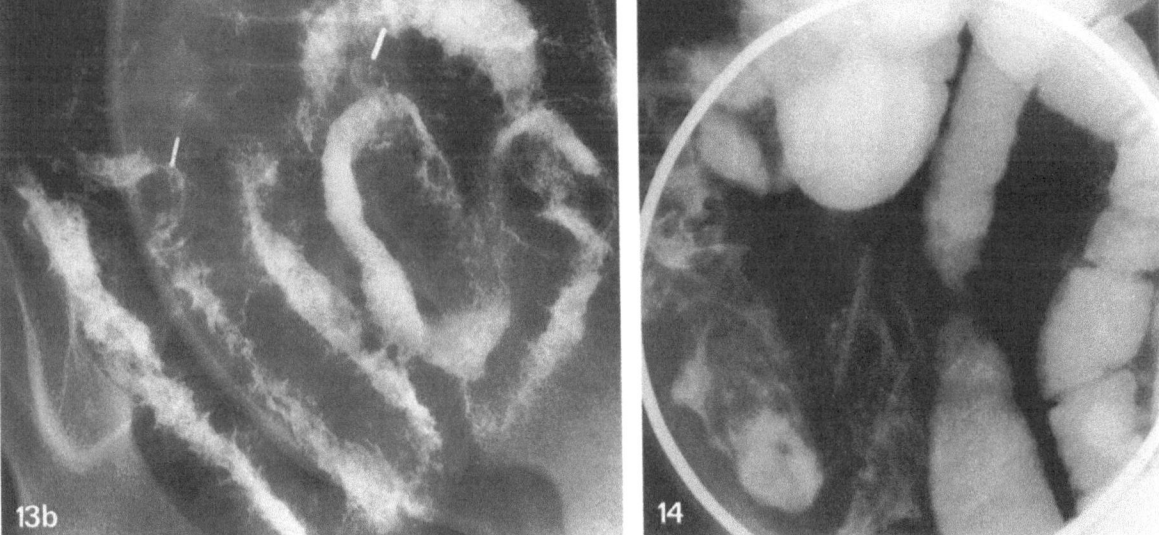

Fig. 14. Radiation stricture. 71-year-old woman. Subocclusion 4 years after radiation therapy for cancer of the cervix. SBFT : short ileal stricture with gradual and smooth transition with distal and proximal segments

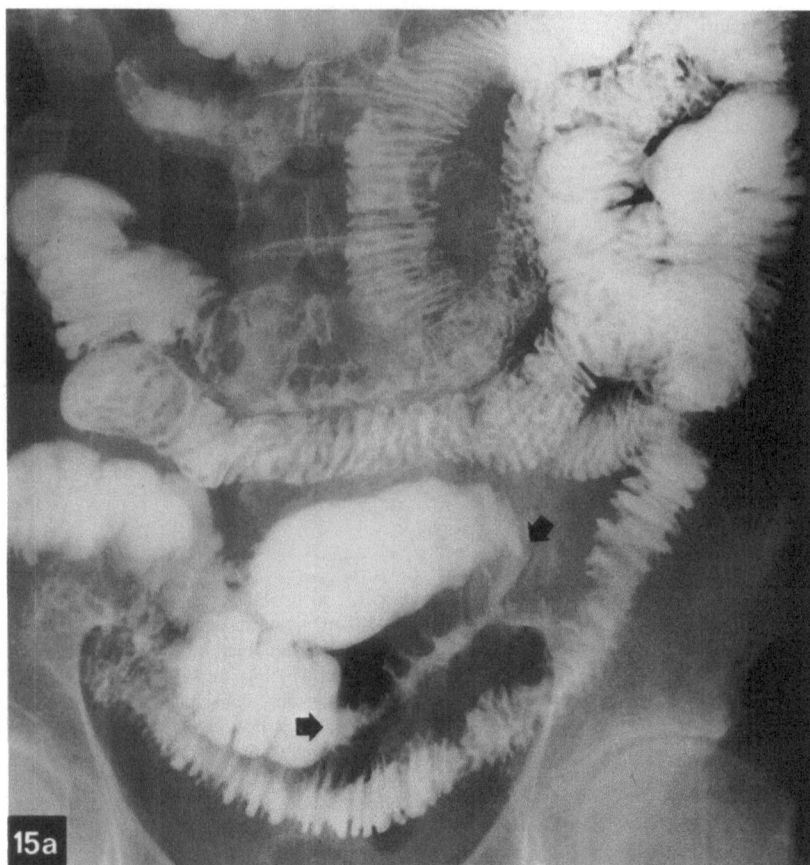

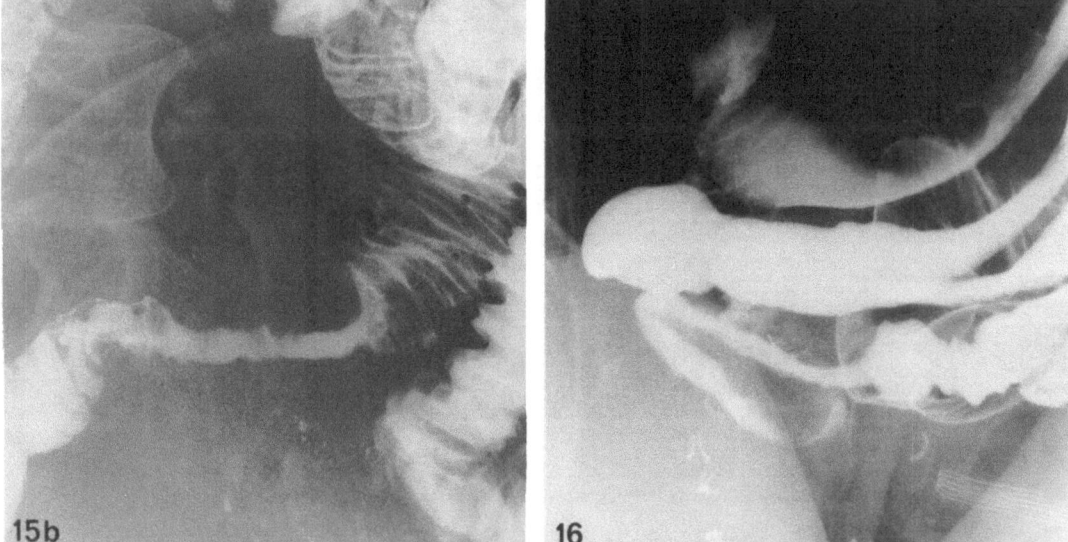

Fig. 15 a, b. Radiation stricture. 54-year-old man. Subocclusive syndrome one year after cobalt therapy for Hodgkin's disease. SBFT : a unfolded pelvic loops, widened interloop gap, straight tall folds and segmental narrowing with broadened folds, b long stricture of a foldless ileal loop

Fig. 16. Radiation stricture. 61-year-old man. Subocclusive episode after prostatectomy and cobalt therapy for cancer of the rectum. SBFT: fixed, angulated pelvic loops with long stricture of the most inferior loop

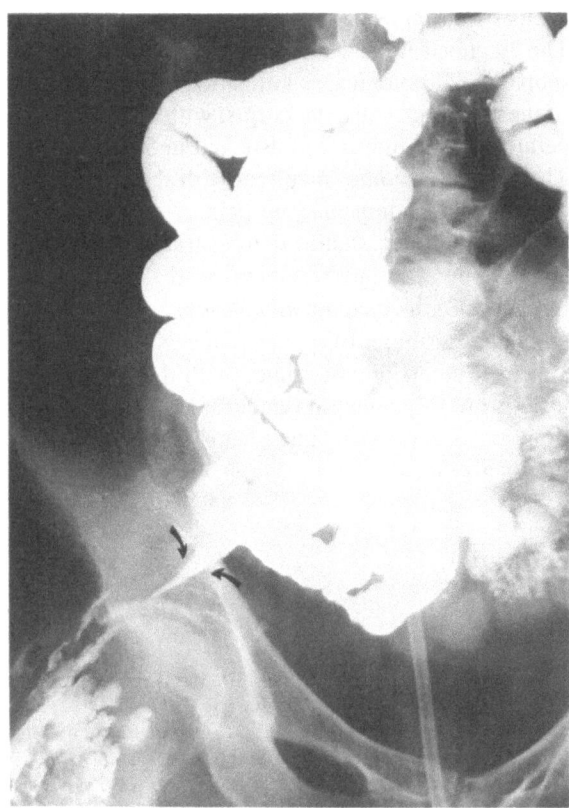

Fig. 17. Radiation fistula. 62-year-old woman. Inguinal abscess 3 years after cobalt therapy for cancer of the cervix. SBFT : fistula beginning in the ileum and leading to a fluid collection near the inguinal canal

severe forms are complicated by local, mainly ileoi-leal or ileosigmoid fistulae.

Complementary imaging

Arteriography is not particularly helpful. Computed tomography is more useful to assess the extent of the lesions. It demonstrates the thickness of the intestinal wall and the extent of the associated mesenteric lesions. It can be useful to differentiate the lesions from postoperative adhesions, tumoral recurrence and, more importantly, peritoneal metastases, which are difficult to exclude. In the acute stage, computed tomography reveals edema causing thickening of the walls of the involved loops, with considerable contrast enhancement in the mucosa. In the chronic forms, the regular, concentric bowel wall thickening caused by fibrosis does not exceed 15 mm. Hypodense images are sometimes observed in the submucosa. The mesenteric fat may exhibit an abnormal density due to fibrosis. The absence of a tumour mass rules out a recurrence or metastases.

Practical conclusions

Radiation lesions bear no specific signs. Their appearance is the same as in ischemia. The etiological diagnosis is made by considering the patient's history and the location of the lesions (ileal more often than jejunal), which corresponds to the fields of the radiotherapy. Radiotherapists and radiologists must try to prevent such iatrogenic lesions with appropriate radiotherapeutic and surgical techniques aimed at excluding the small intestine from the area receiving radiation or at protecting it.

Graft-versus-host disease

Graft-versus-host disease is often observed a few weeks after bone marrow grafting for aplasia or leukemia. It is caused by damage from the donor lymphocytes, contained in the graft, directed against the tissue of the immunosuppressed recipient. The lymphocytes, skin (eruption), liver (hepatitis) and intestines are involved. The disease often regresses on its own, but it may become chronic or be lethal. The diagnosis is made by cutaneous, rectal or hepatic biopsies. Pathological examination shows necrosis of the epithelial cells, the crypts, with edema and ulcerations. The intestine is affected in 50% of cases. The disease becomes manifest with the appearance of diarrhea accompanied by pain.

Radiologic studies demonstrate a rapid transit and loops with increased curvature. The folds are thickened in the jejunum and disappear in the ileum, which has a ribbon-like appearance. Nodulation can appear if ulcers are associated with the edema. The lesions are segmental in the chronic form. Sacculations and exceptionally pneumatosis cystoides intestinalis are noted.

References

Hematomas

Balthazar J, Einhorn R (1976) Intramural gastrointestinal hemorrhage. Gastrointest Radiol 1 : 229-239

Hugues C, Conn J, Sherman J (1977) Intramural hematoma of the gastrointestinal tract. Am J Surg 133 : 276-279

Klepping C, Martin F, Villand J, Baudet JG (1973) Hématome intra-mural du jéjunum sous traitement anticoagulant, intérêt diagnostique du transit baryté. Rev Fr Gastroenterol 87 : 85-91

Lichtenstein H, Capelle Ph, Bognel JC, Conte M (1972) Les hématomes intra-pariétaux du grêle au cours de traitement anticoagulant. Sem Hôp Paris 48 : 183-187

Plojoux O, Hauser H, Wettstein P (1982) Computed tomography of intramural hematoma of the small intestine. Radiology 144 : 559-561

Schmutz G, Kempf F, Charbel P, Bareiss P (1980) Hématome intramural de l'iléon sous traitement anticoagulant exploré par transit du grêle en double contraste. J Radiol 61 : 287-289

Schutz JF, Baumann R, Constantinesco A, Kerschen A, Kempf F, Weill JP (1977) Hématome intramural du grêle sous traitement anticoagulant : évolution radiologique, à propos d'un cas. J Radiol Electrol 58 : 221-226

Senturia H, Susman N, Shyken H (1961) The roentgen appearance of spontaneous intramural hemorrhage of the small intestine associated with anticoagulant therapy. AJR 86 : 62-69

Wiot J, Weinstein A, Felson B (1961) Duodenal hematoma induced by coumarin. AJR 86 : 70-75

Ulcer induced by potassium chloride tablets

Albot G, Olivier Cl, Baruchel Y (1981) L'ulcère sténosant et l'ulcère perforant de l'intestin grêle dus aux comprimés à délitement intestinal de chlorure de potassium. Ann Gastroenterol Hépatol 17 : 423-430

Allen A, Boley J, Schultz L, Schwartz S (1965) Potassium-induced lesions of the small bowel. JAMA 193 : 86-89

Baker D, Schrader W, Hitchcock Cl (1964) Small-bowel ulceration apparently associated with thiazide and potassium therapy. JAMA 190 : 586-590

Bismuth H, Cartier F, Hepp J (1966) Les sténoses ulcéreuses du grêle après absorption de comprimés de potassium. Arch Fr Mal App Dig 55 : 1058-1060

Bismuth H, Samain H, Martin E (1966) Les sténoses ulcéreuses du grêle après absorption de comprimés de potassium. Presse Med 74 : 1801-1804

Boley J, Allen A, Schultz L, Schwartz S (1965) Potassium-induced lesions of the small bowel. JAMA 193 : 997-1000

Labram C (1970) Potassium et lésions de l'Intestin Grêle : Concours Médical, 92, 36, 6496-6499

Morgenstern L, Freilich M, Panish J (1965) The circumferential small-bowel ulcer : JAMA, 191, 8, 637-640

Sowka P (1988) Complications intestinales liées au Kalienor Thèse Nancy

Other drug induced lesions

Ansell G (1969) Radiological manifestations of drug-induced disease. Clin Radiol 20 : 133-148

Bjarnason I, Prouse P, Smith T, Gumpel MJ, Zanelli G, Smethurst P, Levi S, Levi AJ (1987) Blood and protein loss via small intestinal inflammation induced by non steroidal anti-inflammatory drugs. Lancet Septembre : 711-714

Ghahremani G, Meyers M, Farman J, Port R (1977) Ischemic disease of the small bowel and colon associated with oral contraceptives. Gastrointest Radiol 2 : 221-228

Hyson E, Burrell M, Toffler R (1977) Drug-induced gastrointestinal disease. Gastrointest Radiol 2 : 183-212

Kelvin FM, Gramm HF, Gluck WL, Lokich JJ (1986) Radiologic manifestations of small bowel toxicity due to floscuridine therapy. AJR 146 : 39-43

Radiation induced lesions

Bories-Azeau A, Castel C, Grasser M, Dayan L (1981) Les lésions radiothérapiques de l'intestin. Cah Méd 6 : 1863-1868

Carr ND, Pullen BR, Hasleton PS, Schofield PF (1984) Microvascular studies in human radiation bowel disease. Gut 25 : 448-454

Cohen N, Creditor M (1983) Iso-effects tables for tolerance of irradiated normal human tissues. Int J Radiat Oncol Biol Phys 9 : 233-241

Cosset JM, Le Bourgeois JP, Eschwege F (1977) Complications digestives tardives de la radiothérapie. Concours Médical 99 : 1422-1430

De Poerck AF, Engelholm L, De Tœuf J, Barbier P, Guien C, Jeanmart L (1980) Radiation enteritis of small intestine. J Belge Radiol 63 : 573-579

Fishmann E, Zinreich E, Jones B, Siegelman S (1984) Computed tomographic diagnosis of radiation ileitis. Gastrointest Radiol 9 : 149-152

Gendre JP, Cosnes J, Le Quintrec Y (1983) L'entérite radique chronique. 1. La malabsorption intestinale, corrélations anatomo-fonctionnelles. Gastroenterol Clin Biol 7 : 664-670

Laugier A, Cosser JM (1979) Diarrhée et radiothérapie. Ann Gastroentérol 15 : 269-271

Le Quintrec Y, Vitaux J (1980) Complications intestinales de la radiothérapie abdomino-pelvienne. Concours Médical 102 : 1329-1343

Le Parco JC, Vitaux J, Fouet P (1977) Les complications intestinales de la radiothérapie abdomino-pelvienne, présentation de 5 cas avec étude de l'absorption intestinale. Gastroenterol Clin Biol 1 : 751-760

Mendelson RM, Nolan DJ (1985) The radiological features of chronic radiation enteritis. Clin Radiol 36 : 141-148

Potish RA, Twiggs LB, Adcok LL, Prem KA (1983) Logistic models for prediction of enteric morbidity in the treatment of ovarien and cervical cancers. Am J Obstet Gynecol 147 : 65-72

Rogers L, Goldstein H (1977) Roentgen manifestations of radiation injury to the gastrointestinal tract. Gastrointest Radiol 2 : 281-291

Rubin P, Casarett GN (1968) Alimentary tract. In : Clinical Radiation Pathology, Saunders, Philadelphia, 1 : 153-292

Schmutz G, Ridereau C, Beigelman C, Thibault F, Baumann R, Vaxman D (1988) L'entéroclyse dans l'entérite radique chronique. Etude de 43 observations. J Radiol 69 : 315-322

Stines J, Régent D, Barlier C, Verhaeghe JL, Becker S (1988) L'imagerie dans le grêle radique. Feuillets de radiologie 28 : 441-458

Van Haecke P, Vitaux J, Michot F, Hay JM, Flamant Y, Maillard JN (1981) Lésions radiques intestinales, critères pronostiques et attitude thérapeutique. Nouv Presse Med 10 : 879-883

Graft-versus-host disease

Belli AM, Williams MP (1988) Graft-versus-host disease : findings on plain abdominal radiography. Clin Rad 39 : 262-264

Fisk JD, Shulman HM, Greening RR, McDonald GB, Sale GE, Thomas ED (1981) Gastrointestinal radiographic features of human graft-vs-host disease. AJR 136 : 329-336

Maile CW, Frick MP, Crass JR, Snover DC, Weisdorf SA, Kersey JH (1985) The plain abdominal radiograph in acute gastrointestinal graft-vs-host disease. AJR 145 : 289-292

Rosenberg HK, Serota FT, Koch P, Borden S, August CS (1981) Radiographic features of gastrointestinal graft-vs-host disease. Radiology 138 : 371-374

Schimmelpenninck M, Zwaan F (1982) Radiographic features of small intestinal injury in human graft-versus-host disease. Gastrointest Radiol 7 : 29-33

Schuttevaer HM, Kroon HM, Shaw PC (1986) Graft-versus-host disease of the gastrointestinal tract. Diagn Imag 55 : 254-261

Immune-mediated disorders

Failure of immune function affects mainly cell-mediated immunity (T lymphocytes) and humoral immunity (immunoglobulins secreted by plasmacytes derived from B lymphocytes). Deficient cell-mediated immunity is assessed by direct cell count or after immunofluorescent studies and with functional tests in tissue cultures. The diagnosis of humoral immunodeficiency is made with electro- and immunoelectrophoresis.

Immune deficiency can be primary (congenital or acquired) or secondary.

Bruton's agammaglobulinemia is a sex-linked congenital disease, which usually does not cause intestinal disorders. It is different from the other conditions because lymphoid tissue (tonsils, Peyer's patches) is absent or scarce. Selective congenital deficiencies are more frequent, in particular immunoglobulin A deficiency (one individual out of 700 to 1000).

Primary hypogammaglobulinemia of the acquired type, i.e. detected in adults, may be congenital. Its onset is usually between 30 and 40 years of age and it is equally frequent in both sexes. The disease involves immunoglobulins G (the most abundant ones in serum), A (the most abundant ones in intestinal secretions) or M, either separately or simultaneously. Associated disorders of cell immunity are frequent.

Secondary deficiencies are caused by diseases of the immune system (leukemia, lymphoma, Waldenström's macroglobulinemia, alpha-chain disease) or by severe hypoproteinemia (malnutrition, protein-losing enteropathy, nephrotic syndrome). Both types of disease affect mainly humoral immunity, while the HIV virus, Hodgkin's disease, radiation therapy and immunosuppressive treatments (for an autoimmune disease, prior to bone marrow grafting or after organ transplantation) cause cell-mediated immunodeficiency. AIDS (the acquired immunodeficiency syndrome) has a special status because of its predisposing factors and of its spectacular spread. This disease caused by the HIV retrovirus is transmitted through blood and sexual intercourse. It mainly affects the population of certain countries (West Indies, central Africa), homosexual men, drug addicts, hemophiliacs and patients receiving blood transfusions. It occurs at any age, with a maximal incidence between 30 and 40 years of age. It is characterized by a decrease in cell immunity affecting helper T lymphocytes, with lymphopenia and anergy, while humoral immunity is relatively preserved.

Hypogammaglobulinemia causes repeated infections, especially of the nose and throat and in the lungs. Pneumonia can cause death. Other infections may involve the digestive tract, the skin or the joints or cause meningitis, hepatitis, nephritis or septicemia. The infectious agents (bacteria, parasites, viruses) are numerous and often multiple. Autoimmune diseases occur frequently. The illness is chronic and often well tolerated. However, amyloidosis can aggravate these. In addition, there is a considerable risk (10% of all cases) of digestive adenocarcinomas, or of lymphomas.

The risk of infection by various agents is increased in AIDS and with immunosuppressive treatments. These two diseases are characterized by uncommon parasitic infections (cryptosporidiosis, strongyloidiasis, *Pneumocystis carinii*) and mycoses (gastrointestinal candidiasis, aspergillosis, cryptococcosis). In addition to the risks of carcinoma and lymphoma, a frequent cause of death, especially in homosexual patients is the occurrence of Kaposi's

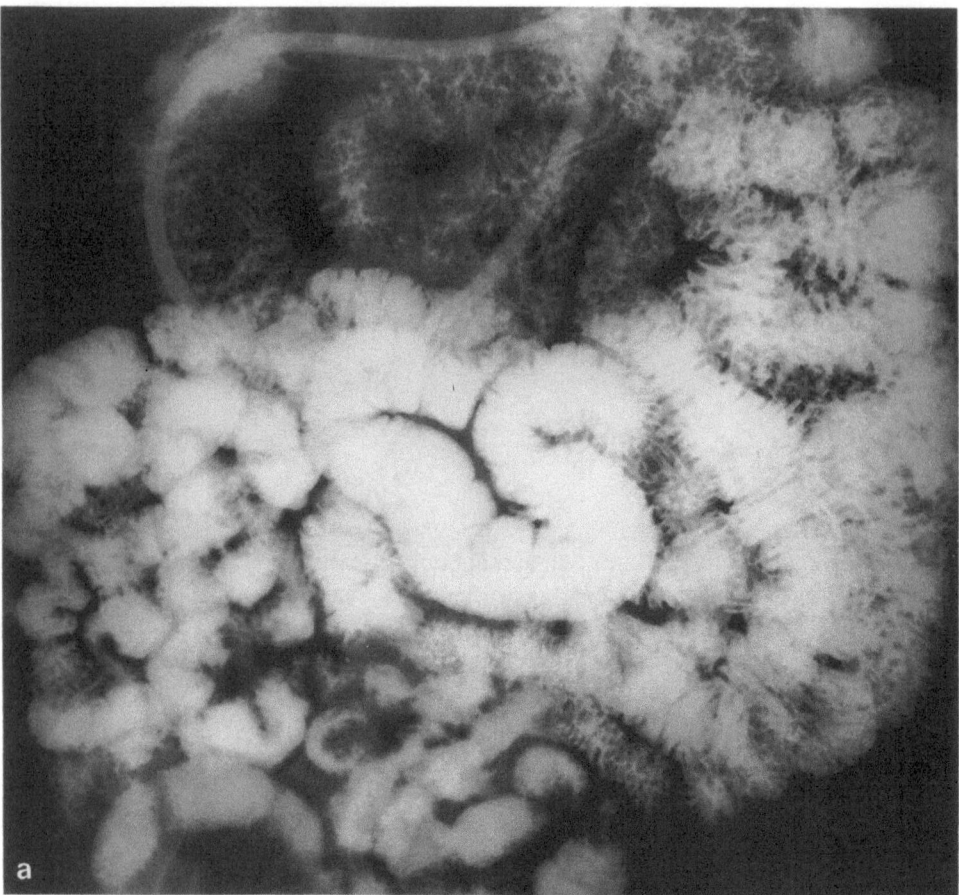

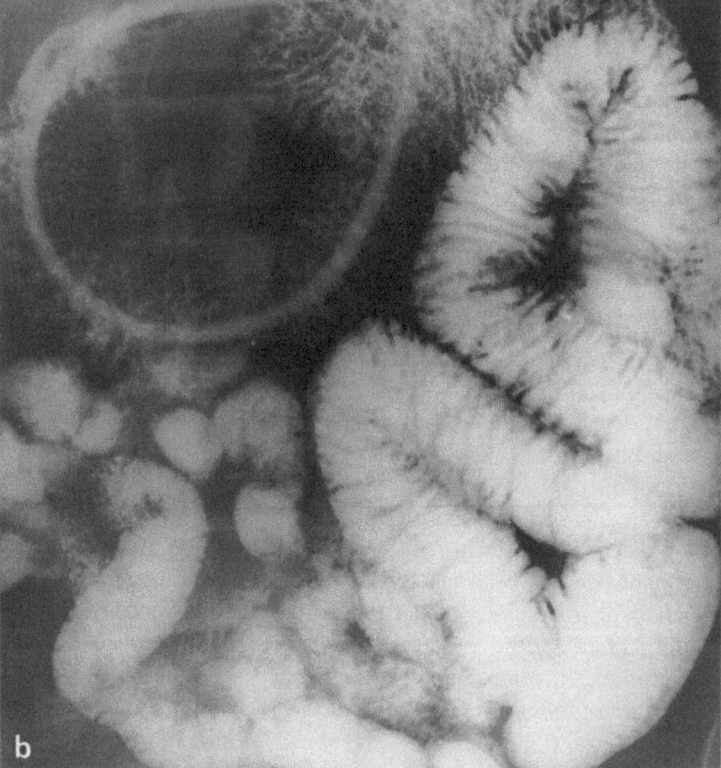

Fig. 1 a, b. Immune deficiency. 40-year-old woman. Recurrent giardiasis. Immunoglobulin G deficiency. Duodenal biopsy : lymphoid hyperplasia. SBFT: contrast medium dilution in the ileum, duodenojejunal micronodulation

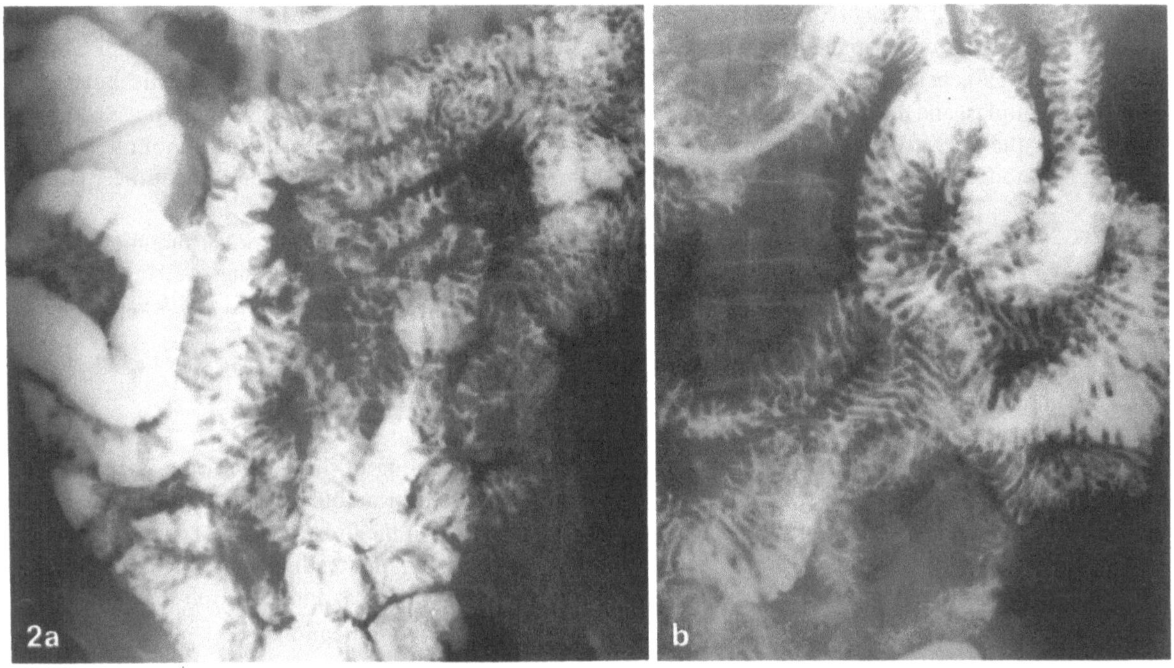

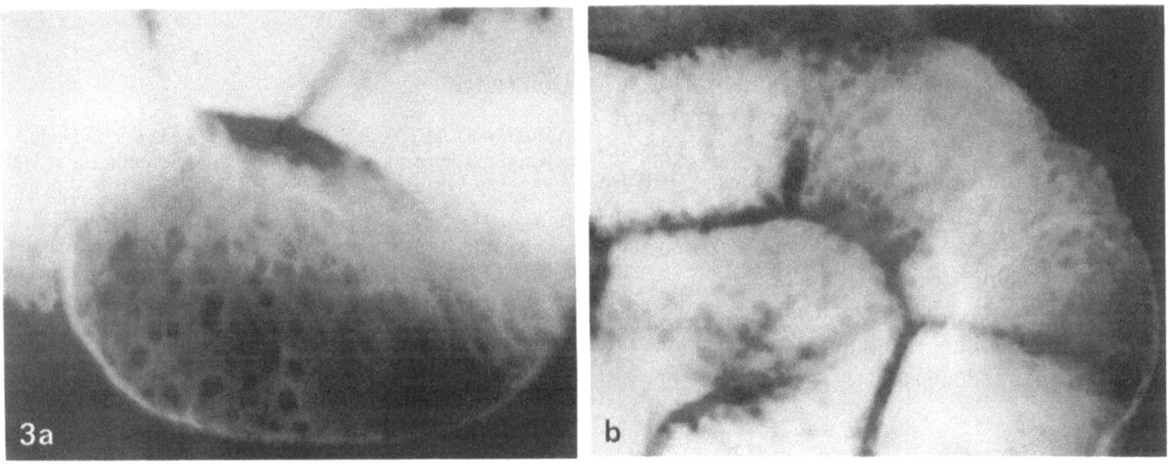

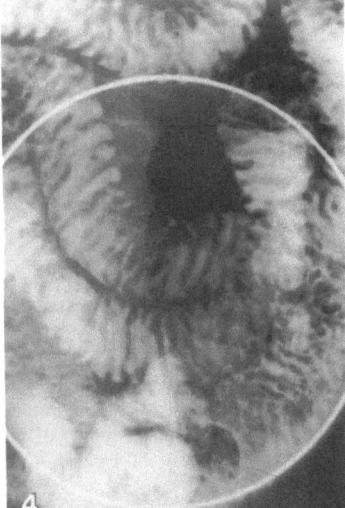

Fig. 2 a, b. Immune deficiency. 50-year-old man. Diarrhea, malabsorption, chronic hepatitis, hypogammaglobulinemia. SBFT : a, b nodular appearance of jejunal folds

Fig. 3 a, b. Immune deficiency. 29-year-old man. Chronic diarrhea since childhood. Endoscopy : subtotal villous atrophy. Ineffective gluten-free diet. Hypogammaglobulinemia. Giardiasis. SBFT : a, b ileal nodulation

Fig. 4. Immune deficiency. 28-year-old homosexual man. Diarrhea. Malabsorption. AIDS. SBFT : nodular appearance of the jejunal folds

sarcoma. The skin eruption typical of the disease (violaceous macules and papules) is diffuse. Involvement becomes general as a rule, with metastases to the lymph nodes, and the deep organs or the bones. Spread into the digestive tract produces multiple submucosal nodules.

Pathology

Intestinal biopsy reveals nonspecific inflammation or lymphocyte infiltration. In hypogammaglobulinemia, the submucosa contains few or no plasmacytes. Nodular lymphoid hyperplasia occurs in more than half of patients with symptomatic hypogammaglobulinemia. It is often observed in association with giardiasis. Incomplete, focal villous atrophy, rarely total, may occur. The mesenteric lymph nodes are hypertrophied.

Clinical findings

Infections of the small intestine are often due to staphylococci, salmonellae, shigellae or giardiae; rarely cytomegalovirus, *Cryptosporidium* or mycobacteria, and exceptionally candidiasis may cause diffuse digestive involvement. Infectious causes often cannot be found for the digestive disorders seen in hypogammaglobulinemia.

The most frequent sign is abundant or moderate diarrhea, with or without malabsorption. Fever, weight loss and adenopathy are also frequently noted.

Radiological findings

In most symptomatic cases, a small bowel followthrough reveals contrast medium dilution and thickened folds, either predominating in the jejunum or diffusely distributed, and less frequently, distended loops. This appearance of jejunoileitis is often caused by secondary infections. Other findings include ulcers (cytomegalovirus) or a punctated superficial appearance due to villous hypertrophy (Mycobacterium Avium Intracellulare).

In 25% of patients with symptomatic hypogammaglobulinemia, jejunal, ileal or diffuse micronodulation is visible as small, round, sessile elements, 2 to 3 mm in diameter, all similar to each other and uniformingly distributed. No associated abnormality, (i.e. functional disorders or large folds), is observed as a rule. The duodenum and the colon may

be involved. The diagnosis of nodular lymphoid hyperplasia is usually straightforward. This appearance suggests hypogammaglobulinemia but is not specific for this condition, since it has been reported in typhoid fever, giardiasis alone without hypogammaglobulinemia, lymphoma, and sometimes without any detectable pathology.

The study of the films must include a search for an associated malignant disease, including an epithelioma, a lymphoma or Kaposi's sarcoma.

Practical conclusions

The understanding of disorders of the immune system is improving. Radiologists must be able to consider such diseases in the presence of nonspecific inflammation of the small intestine, or of extensive nodular lymphoid hyperplasia, and to search for their possible malignant complications.

References

Ajdukiewicz AB, Youngs GR, Bouchier IAD (1972) Nodular lymphoid hyperplasia with hypogammaglobulinaemia. Gut 13 : 589-595

Berk RN, Wall SD, McArdle CB, McCutchan JA, Clemett AR, Rosenblum JS, Premkumer A, Megibow AJ (1984) Cryptosporidiosis of the stomach and small intestine in patients with aids. AJR 143 : 549-554

Bersani D, Mugel-Riwer B, Lallemand M, Diebolt M (1984) Hyperplasie lymphoïde nodulaire, forme diffuse étendue du bulbe duodénal au rectum, associée à une agammaglobulinémie. J Radiol 65 : 863-867

Bradford BF, Abdenour GE, Frank JL, Scott GB, Beerman R (1988) Usual and unusual radiologic manifestations of acquired immunodeficiency syndrome (AIDS) and human immunodeficiency virus (HIV) infection in children. Radiol Clin N Am 2 : 341-343

Bryk D, Farman J, Dallemand S, Meyers MA, Wecksell A (1978) Kaposi's sarcoma of the intestinal tract : roentgen manifestations. Gastrointest Radiol 3 : 425-430

Corlin RF, Pops MA (1972) Nongranulomatous ulcerative jejunoileitis with hypogammaglobulinemia, clinical remission after treatment with γ globulin. Gastroenterology 62 : 473-478

Coussement A, Dujardin P, Loubière M, Serres JJ (1977) Hyperplasie lymphoïde du grêle associée à une hypogammaglobulinémie primitive de l'adulte. J Radiol 58 : 527-530

Current WL, Reese NC, Ernst JV, Bailey WS, Heyman MB, Weinstein WM (1983) Human cryptosporidiosis in immunocompetent and immunodeficient persons, studies of an outbreak and experimental transmission. N Engl J Med 308 : 1252-1257

Davis TJ, Berk RN (1977) Immunoglobulin deficiency diseases of the intestine. Gastrointest Radiol 2 : 7-11

De Smet AA, Tubergen DG, Martel W (1976) Nodular lymphoid hyperplasia of the colon associated with dysgammaglobulinemia. AJR 127 : 515-517

Frager DH, Frager JD, Brandt LJ, Wolf EL, Rand LG, Klein RS, Beneventano TC (1986) Gastrointestinal complications of AIDS : radiologic features. Radiology 158 : 597-603

Friedman-Kien AE, Laubenstein LJ, Rubinstein P, Buimovici-Klein E, Marmor M, Stahl R, Spigland I, Kwang Soo Kim, Zolla-Pazner S (1982) Disseminated Kaposi's sarcoma in homosexual men. Ann Int Med 96 : 693-700

Hermans PE, Diaz-Buxo JA, Stobo JD (1976) Idiopathic late-onset immunoglobulin deficiency, clinical observations in 50 patients. Am J Med 61 : 221-237

Hermans PE, Huizenga KA, Hoffman HN, Brown AL, Markowitz H (1966) Dysgammaglobuninemia associated with nodular lymphoid hyperplasia of the small intestine. Am J Med 40 : 78-89

Hill CA, Harle TS, Mansell PWA (1983) The prodrome, Kaposi sarcoma, and infections associated with acquired immuno-deficiency syndrome : radiologic findings in 39 patients. Radiology 149 : 393-399

Hodgson JR, Hoffman HN, Huizenga KA (1967) Roentgenologic features of lymphoid hyperplasia of the small intestine associated with dysgammaglobulinemia. Radiology 88 : 883-888

Jaffe HW, Bregman DJ, Selik RM (1983) Acquired immune deficiency syndrome in the United States : the first 1 000 cases. J Infect Dis 148 : 339-345

Keller D, Piombini JL, Levy M, Hernandez N, Forster E (1980) Manifestations digestives de la maladie de Kaposi. Rev Fr Gastroent 162 : 11-16

Lamers CB, Wagener T, Assman K, Van Tongeren J (1980) Jejunal lymphoma in a patient with primary adult-onset hypogammaglobulinemia and nodular lymphoid hyperplasia of the small intestine. Dig Dis Sci 25 : 553-557

Liepman M (1975) Disseminated strongyloides stercoralis, a complication of immunosuppression. JAMA 231 : 387-388

Mackenzie Crooks DJ, Brown WR (1980) The distribution of intestinal nodular lymphoid hyperplasia in immunoglobulin deficiency. Clin Radiol 31 : 701-706

Marshak RH, Hazzi C, Lindner AE, Maklansky D (1974) Small bowel in immunoglobulin deficiency syndromes. AJR 122 : 227-239

Marshak RH, Lindner AE, Maklansky D (1976) Immunoglobulin disorders of the small bowel. Radiol Clin North Am 14 : 477-491

Marshak RH, Lindner AE, Maklansky D (1979) Lymphoreticular disorders of the gastrointestinal tract : roentgenographic features. Gastrointest Radiol 4 : 103-120

Matuchansky C, Duprey F, Briaud M, Babin P, Touchard G, Bloch P, Lenormand Y, Morichau-Beauchant M (1982) Hyperplasie nodulaire lymphoïde diffuse de l'intestin grêle chez l'adulte sans déficit reconnu de l'immunité générale ni digestive. Gastroenterol Clin Biol 6 : 239-248

Mayaud C, Touboul JL, Akoun G (1985) Les déficits immunitaires acquis. Rev Prat 35 : 1769-1779

Megibow AJ, Balthazar EJ, Hulnick DH (1987) Radiology of nonneoplastic gastrointestinal disorders in acquired immune deficiency syndrome. Semin Roentgen 22 : 31-41

Mildvan D, Mathur U, Enlow RW, Romain PL, Winchester RJ, Colp C, Singman H, Adelsberg BR, Spigland I (1982) Opportunistic infections and immune deficiency in homosexual men. Ann Int Med 96 : 700-704

Miniconi P, Dedieu Ph (1976) Entéropathies et carence primitive en IgA. Concours Med 98-40 : 5922-5926

Moneret-Vautrin DA, Belut D, Nicolas JP, Grilliat JP (1981) Déficit en IgAs intestinales chez les patients porteurs de candidose digestive chronique ou récidivante. Nouv Presse Med 10 : 1656

Morichau-Beauchant M (1985) SIDA. Gastroenterol Clin Biol 9 : 323-326

Neefe LI, Pinilla O, Garagusi VF, Bauer H (1973) Disseminated strongyloidiasis with cerebral involvement, a complication of corticosteroid therapy. Am J Med 55 : 832-838

Parnaud E, Bauer P (1985) Localisations digestives des maladies sexuellement transmissibles chez l'homosexuel mâle. Presse Med 14 : 1282-1286

Penny R (1969) Nodular lymphoid hyperplasia of the small intestine and hypogammaglobulinemia. Gastroenterology 56 : 982-984

Peterson R (1976) Gastrointestinal abnormalities in renal homotransplant patients. J Can Assoc Radiol 27 : 240-249

Powell RW, Moss JP, Nagar D, Melo JC, Boram LH, Anderson WH, Cheng SH (1980) Strongyloidiasis in immuno-suppressed hosts, presentation as massive lower gastrointestinal bleeding. Arch Intern Med 140 : 1061-1063

Purtilo DT, Meyers WM, Connor DH, (1974) Fatal strongyloidiasis in immunosuppressed patients. Am J Med 56 : 488-493

Quinn TC, Stamm WE, Goodell SE, Mkrtichian E, Benedetti J, Corey L, Schuffler MD, Holmes KK (1983) The polymicorbial origin of intestinal infections in homosexual men. N Engl J Med 309 : 576-582

Rambaud JC, De Saint-Louvent P, Marti R, Galian A, Mason DY, Wassef M, Licht H, Valleur P, Bernier JJ (1982) Diffuse follicular lymphoid hyperplasia of the small intestine without primary immunoglobulin deficiency. Am J Med 73 : 125-132

Randall Radin D, Fong T, Halls JM, Pontrelli GN (1983) Monilial enteritis in acquired immunodeficiency syndrome. AJR 141 : 1289-1290

René E, Marche C, Régnier B, Saimot AG, Vittecoq B, Matheron S, Le Port C, Bricaire F, Bure A, Brun-Vezinet C, Deluol AM, Coulaud JP, Modai J, Vilde JL, Vachon F, Cerf M, Bonfils S (1985) Manifestations digestives du syndrome d'immunodéficience acquise (SIDA) : étude chez 26 patients. Gastroenterol Clin Biol 9 : 327-335

Rose HS, Balthazar EJ, Megibow AJ, Horowitz L, Laubenstein LJ (1982) Alimentary tract involvement in Kaposi sarcoma : radiographic and endoscopic findings in 25 homosexual men. AJR 139 : 661-666

Roseau G (1985) Entéropathie du SIDA. Presse Med 14 : 9

Schaefer PS, Friedman AC (1981) Nodular lymphoid hyperplasia of the small intestine with Burkitt's lymphoma and dysgammablobulinemia. Gastrointest Radiol 6 : 325-328

Simmons RL, Matas AJ, Rattazzi LC, Balfour HH, Howard RJ, Najarian JS (1977) Clinical characteristics of the lethal cytomegalovirus infection following renal transplantation. Surgery 82 : 537-546

Sloper KS, Dourmashkin RR, Bird RB, Slavin G, Webster ADB (1982) Chronic malabsorption due to cryptosporidiosis in a child with immunoglobulin deficiency. Gut 23 : 80-82

Urmacher C, Myskowski P, Ochoa M, Kris M, Safai B (1982) Outbreak of Kaposi's sarcoma with cytomegalovirus infection in young homosexual men. Am J Med 72 : 569-575

234   Radiology of the small intestine

Vermess M, Waldmann TA, Pearson KD (1973) Radiographic manifestations of primary acquired hypogammaglobulinemia. Radiology 107 : 63-69

Vincent M, Robbins AH (1985) Mycobacterium avium-intracellulare complex enteritis : pseudo-Whipple disease in AIDS. AJR 144 : 922-924

Wall SD, Ominsky S, Altman DF, Perkins CL, Sollitto R, Goldberg HI, Margulis AR (1986) Multifocal abnormalities of the gastrointestinal tract in AIDS. AJR 146 : 1-5

Weisburger WR, Hutcheon DF, Yardley JH, Roche JC, Hillis WD, Charache P (1979) Cryptosporidiosis in an immunosuppressed renal-transplant recipient with IgA deficiency. Am J Clin Pathol 72 : 473-478

Connective tissue diseases

Scleroderma (figs. 1 to 5)

Scleroderma is a connective tissue disease, possibly of autoimmune origin, causing smooth muscle atrophy and collagen infiltration of tissues. This rare disease appears at any age and twice as often in women as in men. It occurs in local cutaneous forms and in diffuse forms involving all viscera.

Skin lesions (hard, thick skin) and vasomotor disorders (Raynaud's phenomenon) are the major clinical signs. Telangectasiae, calcium deposits in soft tissues (Thibierge-Weissenbach syndrome) and lysis of the bony extremities of the fingers occur frequently. The esophagus is involved in 80% of patients, sometimes as its first manifestation. Several other organs can be affected, including the heart, the lungs, the kidneys, the intestines, muscles and joints. There is no relation between the cutaneous and visceral lesions. The prognosis of the disease is very variable because there are stable, progressive forms, and fulminant forms leading to death.

Pathology

The intestinal wall is flaccid. Histology shows the atrophy of the muscular fibers in the muscularis mucosae and the circular layer of the muscularis. The intercellular space of the muscularis and the submucosa is invaded by collagen fibres and perivascular inflammatory cells. Blood vessels are blocked. The myenteric plexuses remain intact. The serosa is thickened and fibrosed. The mucosa is preserved or shows a decrease in the height of the villi.

Clinical findings

The clinical signs and symptoms of small intestinal involvement are not always observed. They sometimes exist prior to other signs, however concomitant esophageal abnormalities are almost always noted. The intestinal disease causes diarrhea and episodes of subocclusion, anorexia, vomiting, meteorism, malabsorption or steatorrhea due to bacterial overgrowth. Ulcerations and perforations can occur.

The laboratory findings are normal. A decreased alveolar diffusion of carbon monoxide is sometimes noted, as well as karyotypic abnormalities. The manometric studies of the esophagus demonstrate considerable atonia. The diagnosis of scleroderma is based on typical clinical signs combined to characteristic findings on cutaneous or intestinal biopsies.

Radiological findings

The appearance of the small intestine observed on plain films is quite similar to that of occlusion, with distended loops and air-fluid levels. Strings of bubbles have been described, evoking pneumatosis cystoides intestinalis or even a pneumoperitoneum without clinical symptoms.

The small bowel follow-through demonstrates the considerable atonia causing delayed evacuation of the loops, as well as segmental or extensive dilatation, in particular in the distal jejunum. Marginal sacculation and sometimes functional intussusceptions are observed. The rectilinear folds retain their normal thickness. The interfold gaps are redu-

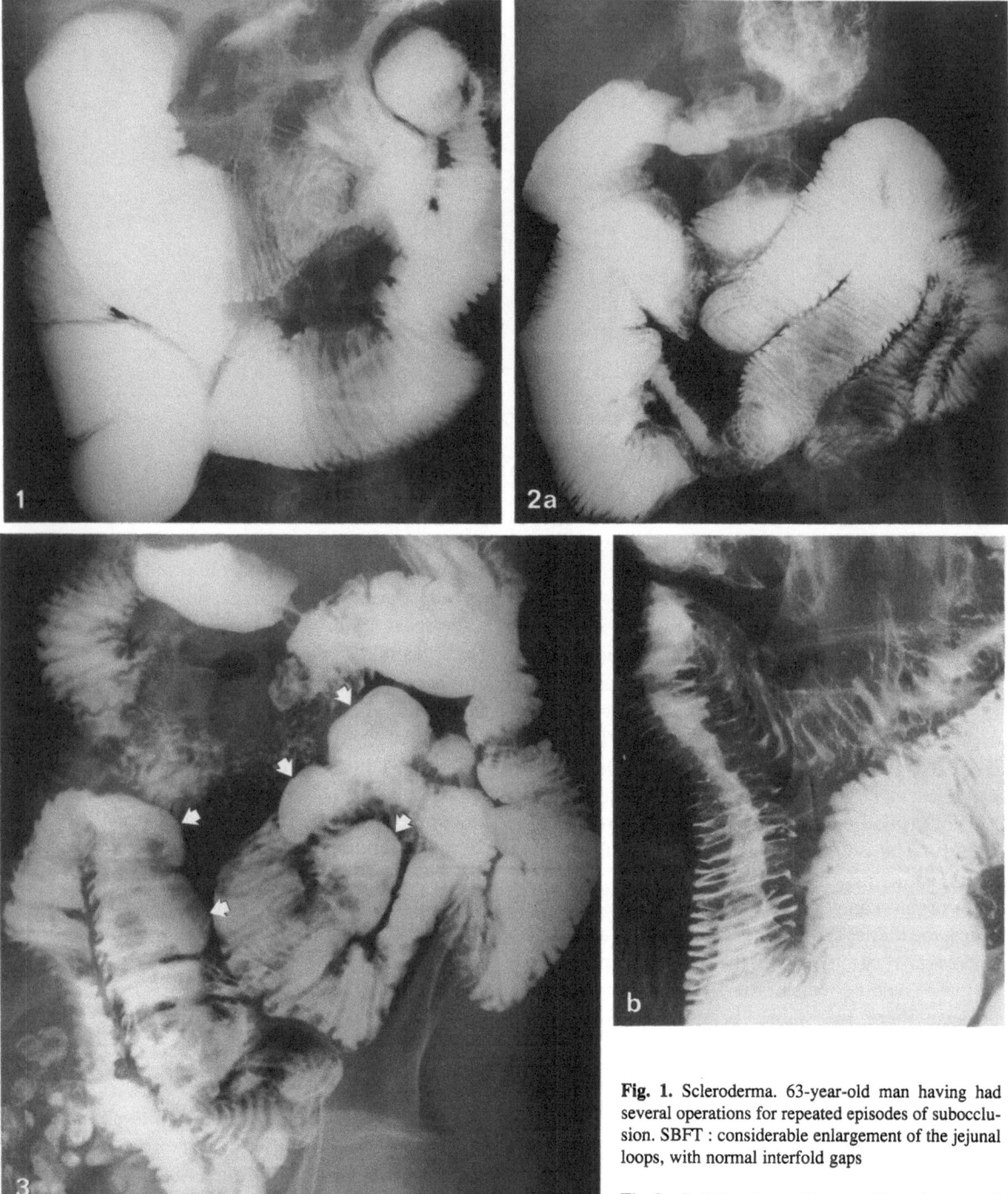

Fig. 1. Scleroderma. 63-year-old man having had several operations for repeated episodes of subocclusion. SBFT : considerable enlargement of the jejunal loops, with normal interfold gaps

Fig. 2 a, b. Scleroderma. 30-year-old man having had 3 operations for repeated episodes of subocclusion. SBFT : **a, b** increased jejunal caliber with normal interfold spaces. On one segment (**b**), increase in the height of the straight, parallel folds and narrowed lumen (transient appearance)

Fig. 3. Scleroderma (Courtesy of CL L'Herminé). 55-year-old woman. Scleroderma and Raynaud's phenomenon. SBFT : discontinous increase in jejunal caliber with saccules and diverticula

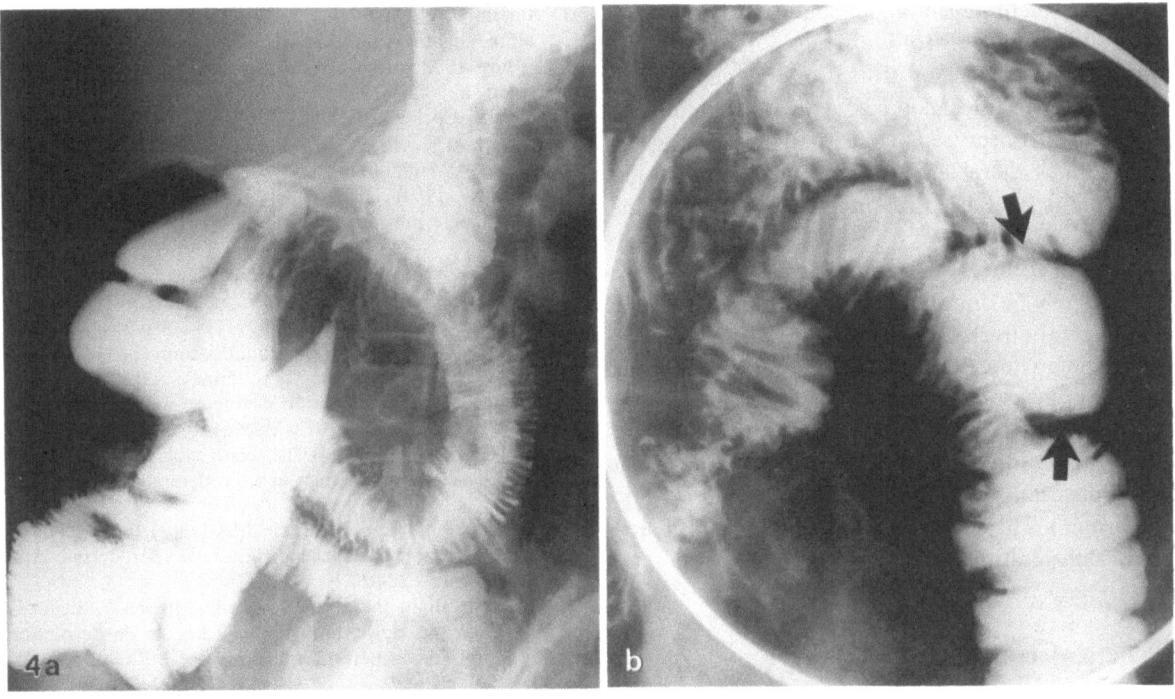

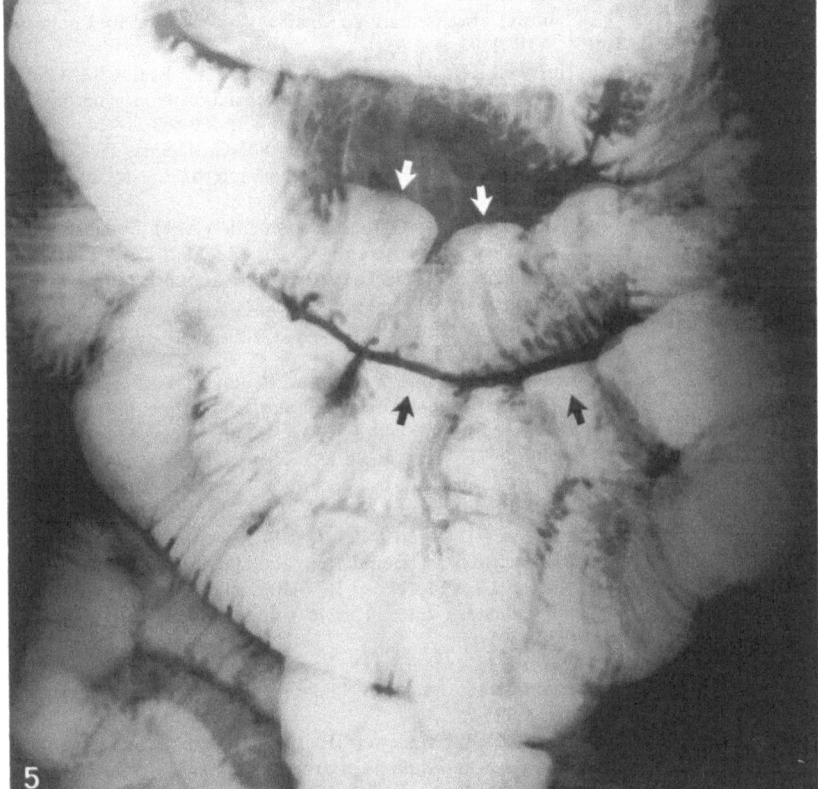

Fig. 4 a, b. Scleroderma. 29-year-old woman. Scleroderma evolving over 10 years. Refractory constipation. SBFT : **a** increased height of the straight, parallel jejunal folds with narrowed lumen (transient appearance). **b** jejunal sacculation

Fig. 5. Scleroderma. 40-year-old man. Diarrhea, deterioration of his general condition. Scleroderma. SBFT: beginning jejunal sacculation

ced, thus distinguishing the condition from celiac disease, in which the folds are rarefied. The contrast medium is usually not diluted or fragmented. Tall and thickened folds may be due to associated ischemia, and are observed in contracted loops. Images of gas bubbles characteristic of pneumatosis cystoides intestinalis have been reported along the intestinal walls.

The clinical and radiological signs of subocclusion may be mistaken for an obstruction and lead to useless, or even dangerous surgery. It is therefore important to note the lack of esophageal motility that characterizes scleroderma with its frequently associated reflux, delayed gastric evacuation and a significant dilatation of the duodenum even in the procubitus position (contrarily to the «mesenteric fork» syndrome). The colon is sometimes atonic or distended, with multiple sacculations.

Practical conclusions

The esophagus should be examined before a mechanical obstruction is diagnosed in presence of dilatation and delayed evacuation of loops of small intestine, since esophageal atonia is a sign of scleroderma. This cautious approach should prevent unnecessary and dangerous surgery.

Other connective tissue diseases (figs. 6 and 7)

Digestive disorders due to abnormal vascularization occur in 50% of cases of *systemic lupus erythematosus*, 16% of patients with *periarteritis nodosa* and some cases of *Horton's disease*. The clinical symptoms include pain, diarrhea and hemorrhage. Perforation or mesenteric infarction are sometimes observed.

Barium studies reveal typical signs of ischemia, including tall, broadened folds, thumbprinting, alternating narrowed and distended segments, contrast medium dilution and spasms.

Dermatomyositis exceptionally involves the small intestine and causes constipation, meteorism and hemorrhages. The small bowel follow-through shows a slow progress of the barium meal, as well as distended loops and in some cases, ulcerations.

References

Blau EB, Morris RF, Yunis EJ (1977) Polyarteritis nodosa in older children. Pediatrics 60 : 227-234

D'Angelo WA, Fries JF, Masi AT, Shulman LE (1969) Pathologic observations in systemic sclerosis (scleroderma), a study of 58 autopsy cases and 58 matched controls. Am J Med 46 : 428-440

Ferroir JP, Cocheton JJ (1982) Les atteintes du tube digestif au cours des collagénoses. Concours Med 104 : 5371-5381

Fingerhut A, Hillion D, Eugène C, Pourcher J, Fendler JP, Ronat R (1980) Hématome intramural duodéno-jéjunal révélant une péri-artérite noueuse. Med Chir Dig 9 : 419-423

Fujioka M, Bender T, Young LW, Girdany BR (1980) Polyarteritis nodosa in children : radiological aspects and diagnostic correlation. Radiology 136 : 359-364

Gondos B (1960) Roentgen manifestations in progressive systemic sclerosis (diffuse scleroderma). AJR 84 : 235-247

Guillevin L (1985) La périartérite noueuse systémique aujourd'hui. Concours Med 107 : 1429-1441

Hale CH, Schatzki R (1944) The roentgenological appearance of the gastrointestinal tract in scleroderma. AJR 51 : 407-420

Heinz ER, Steinberg AJ, Sackner MA (1963) Roentgenographic and pathologic aspects of intestinal scleroderma. Ann Int Med 59 : 822-826

Hélénon Ch, Bigot JM, Jacri P, Sraer D, Mignon F, Richet G (1977) Aspects de l'artériographie au cours de l'évolution des lésions de la péri-artérite noueuse. J Radiol 58 : 45-50

Horowitz AL, Meyers MA (1973) The « hide-bound » small bowel of scleroderma : characteristic mucosal fold pattern. AJR 119 : 332-334

Horswell RR, Hargrove MD, Peete WP, Ruffin JM (1961) Scleroderma presenting as the malabsorption syndrome, a case report. Gastroenterology 40 : 580-582

Huriez Cl, Bergoend H, L'Herminé C, Thomas P, Piette F, Brouet JF (1973) Manifestations intestinales des sclérodermies. Ann Dermatol 100 : 481-490

Kahn IJ, Jeffries GH, Sleisenger MS (1966) Malabsorption in intestinal scleroderma. N Engl J Med 274 : 1339-1344

Kleinman P, Meyers MA, Abbott G, Kazam E (1976) Necrotizing enterocolitis with pneumatosis intestinalis in systemic lupus erythermatosus and polyarteritis. Radiology 121 : 595-598

Leneman F, Fierst S, Gabriel JB, Ingegno AP (1962) Progressive systemic sclerosis of the intestine presenting as malabsorption syndrome. Gastroenterology 42 : 175-180

Meihoff WE, Hirschfield JS, Kern F (1968) Small intestinal scleroderma with malabsorption and pneumatosis cystoides intestinalis, report of 3 cases. JAMA 204 : 854-858

Miercort RD, Merrill FG (1969) Pneumatosis and pseudo-obstruction in scleroderma. Radiology 92 : 359-362

Mueller CF, Morehead R, Alter AJ, Michener W (1972) Pneumatosis intestinalis in collagen disorders. AJR 115 : 300-305

Oliveros MA, Herbst JJ, Lester PD, Ziter FA (1973) Pneumatosis intestinalis in childhood dermatomyositis. Pediatrics 52 : 711-712

Olmsted WW, Madewell JE (1976) The esophageal and small-bowel manifestations of progressive systemic sclerosis. Gastrointest Radiol 1 : 33-36

Peachey RDG, Creamer B, Pierce JW (1969) Sclerodermatous involvement of the stomach and the small and large bowel. Gut 10 : 285-292

Queloz JM, Woloshin HJ (1972) Sacculation of the small intestine in scleroderma. Radiology 105 : 513-515

Reinhardt JF, Barry WF (1962) Scleroderma of the small bowel. AJR 88 : 687-692

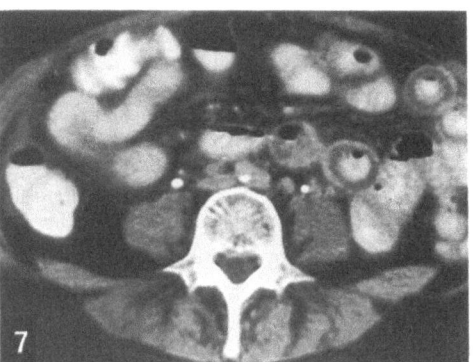

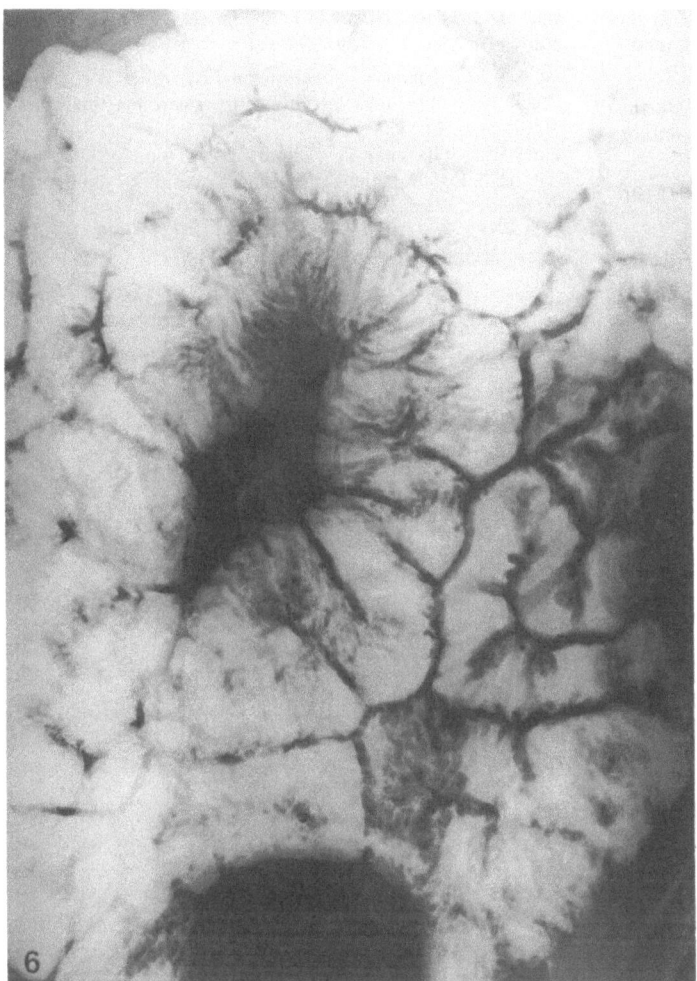

Fig. 6. Systemic lupus erythematosus. 45-year-old man. Chronic diarrhea, deterioration of his general condition. Cutaneous and serological diagnosis of systemic lupus erythematosus. Biopsy : total duodenojejunal atrophy. SBFT : moderately widened interloop gap in the distal jejunum, broadened and rarefied folds

Fig. 7. Systemic lupus erythematosus. 58-year-old woman treated for systemic lupus erythematosus with hemolytic anemia for 2 years. Computed tomography: regular thickening of the walls of the jejunal loops, producing a double contour

Richard M, Mario A, Fouillet JJ, Fresneau M (1976) Les complications digestives de la périartérite noueuse. Concours Med 98 : 7591-7595

Rosenthal FD (1957) Small intestinal lesions with steatorrhea in diffuse systemic sclerosis (scleroderma). Gastroenterology 32 : 332-341

Salem SN, Truelove SC (1965) Small-intestinal and gastric abnormalities in ulcerative colitis. Br Med J 1 : 827-831

Salem SN, Truelove SC, Richards WCD (1964) Small-intestinal and gastric changes in ulcerative colitis : a biopsy study. Br Med J 1 : 394-398

Shapeero LG, Myers A, Oberkircher PE, Miller WT (1974) Acute reversible lupus vasculitis of the gastrointestinal tract. Radiology 112 : 569-574

Steiner RM, Glassman L, Schwartz MW, Vanace P (1974) The radiological findings in dermatomyositis of childhood. Radiology 111 : 385-393

White WD, Treece TR, Juniper K (1970) Pneumatosis in scleroderma of the small bowel. JAMA 212 : 1068

Miscellaneous diseases

Lymphangiectasia (figs. 1 and 2)

The dilatation of the lymphatic vessels in the intestinal wall causes a protein-losing enteropathy, the major finding of which is hypoproteinemia. The disease can be primary or secondary. Primary lymphangiectasia (Waldmann's disease) is congenital and often familial, and associated with multiple malformations of the lymphatic system. It appears during childhood or adolescence. Secondary forms are more frequent, lymphatic dilatation being caused by an obstacle distally such as fibrosis, infiltration of the mesentery (adenopathy, primary tumour or metastasis, Crohn's disease, tuberculosis, Whipple's disease, parasitic infection, sarcoidosis, etc.), intestinal malrotation or chronic volvulus. It can also be the consequence of high venous pressure such as seen in constrictive pericarditis, cardiac failure, decompensated cirrhosis or nephrotic syndrome. Some of these causes can be cured and must be systematically searched for.

Pathology

Macroscopic studies show the lymphatic vessels of the mesentery and of the serosa as protruding pearly structures. The mesenteric lymph nodes are hypertrophied. The intestinal wall is thickened and the villi broadened. Microscopic study shows the considerable dilatation of the lymphatic vessels in the mucosa and submucosa, containing lipid-filled macrophages. The wall is infiltrated by edema.

Clinical findings

The intestinal symptoms are often minor. They include diarrhea, which is rarely severe, with intermittent steatorrhea, abdominal pains and vomiting. The main signs include massive peripheral edema, ascites and pleurisy, sometimes a sensitivity to infections, and disorders due to associated hypocalcemia including growth retardation in children. The outcome may be spontaneous regression, chronicity or deterioration. A protein-rich diet with few fats is advisable if no curable cause of the disease is identified. The laboratory assessment reveals hypoproteinemia with depressed levels of albumin and gammaglobulins, hypocalcemia, lymphopenia, sometimes a decrease in cholesterol, and anemia. Carbohydrate absorption tests are normal. The digestive loss of proteins is demonstrated by the measurement of the levels of radiolabelled albumin or polyvynilpyrrolidone absorbed after oral ingestion or, by the increased fecal clearance of alpha-1-antitrypsin. Jejunal biopsy is very useful if it includes the submucosa as it will demonstrate lymphangiectasia.

Radiological findings

Barium studies of the small intestine may be normal. They may also show diffuse abnormalities of the jejunum and ileum, including significant dilution of the contrast medium, an increase in the height and thickness of the folds, which are sometimes stiff and slightly nodular, increased curvature and widened

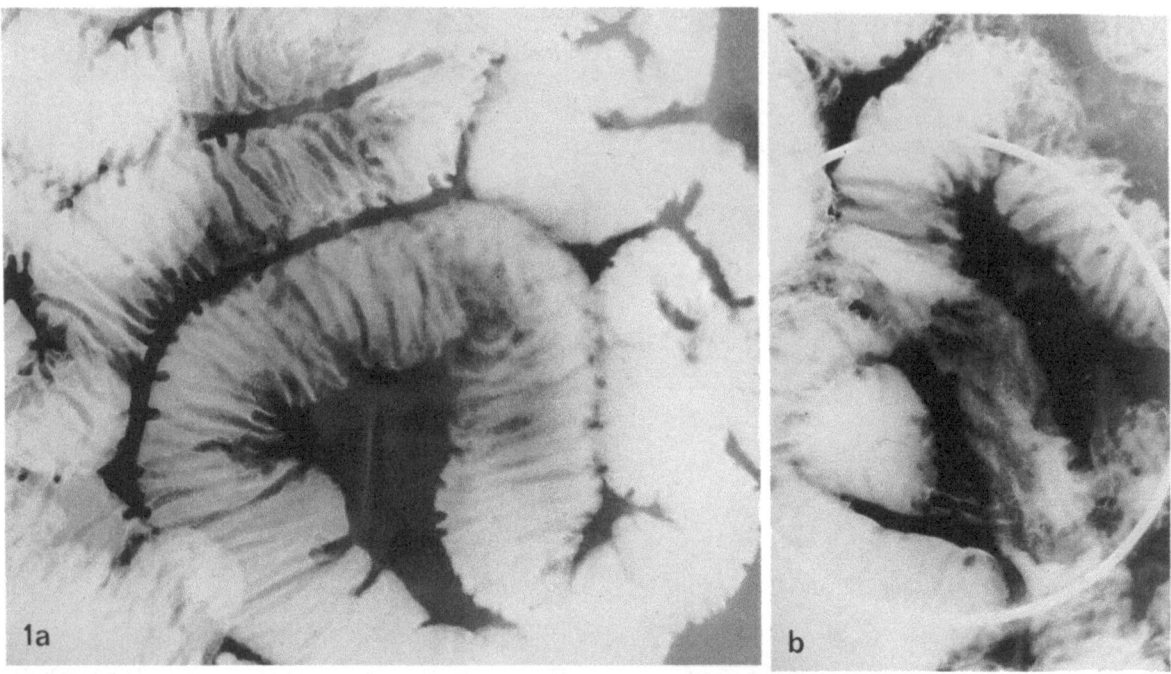

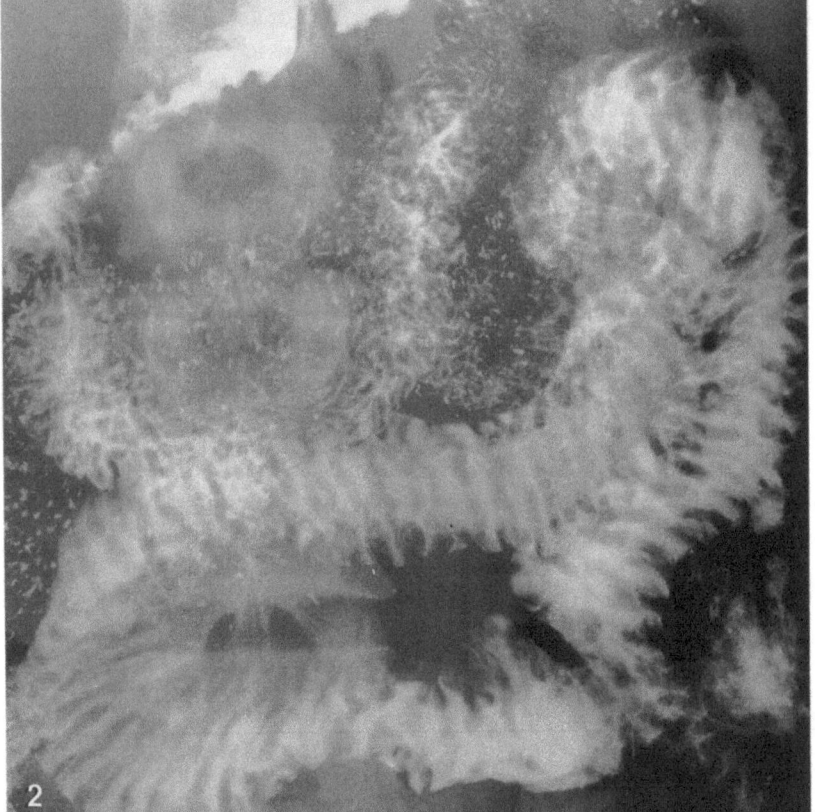

Fig. 1 a, b. Lymphangiectasia. 19-year-old woman. Post-hepatitis decompensated cirrhosis. SBFT : **a, b** superficial punctated appearance of the jejunum and ileum

Fig. 2. Lymphangiectasia. 27-year-old man. Intermittent diarrhea, hypoproteinemia with a laboratoryproven protein-losing enteropathy. SBFT : contrast medium dilution, moderate increase in the jejunal caliber, thickened folds and marginal spiculations which is difficult to see on the reproduction

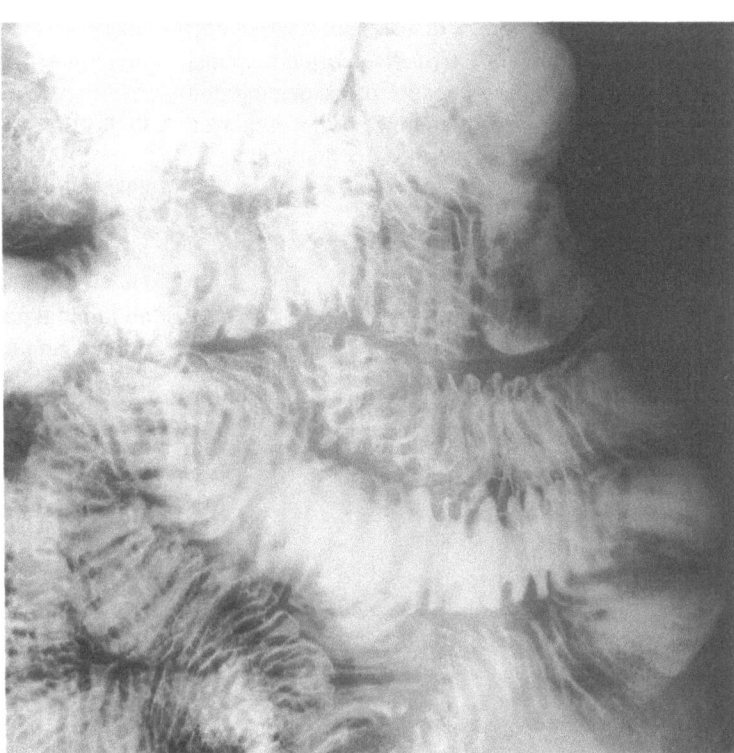

Fig 3. Hypoproteinemia. 46-year-old man. Alcoholism. Cirrhosis with hypoproteinemia. SBFT : moderate increase in the jejunal caliber. Tall thickened folds

interloop gaps. A closer examination of the films shows micronodulations with a diameter of about one millimeter, corresponding to the enlarged villi. Larger nodules due to true cystic lymphangiomas are sometimes observed. The caliber of the loops is normal or moderately increased. The interfold spaces are normal. The loops are neither stiff nor ulcerated.

The differential radiological diagnosis includes edema caused by hypoproteinemia of other origins, allergies or eosinophilic gastritis, although these occur in a different context.

Complementary imaging

In the primary forms, lymphangiography shows hypoplasia and diffuse malformations of the lymphatic system. In the secondary forms, the abnormalities are not constantly seen but other signs include stasis, obstruction, reflux of the contrast medium into the mesenteric ducts and the intestinal lumen, and dilatation of the lymphatic channel.

Practical conclusions

The diagnosis of intestinal lymphangiectasia should be considered by radiologists in the case of hypoproteinemia when large, straight folds and thickened intestinal walls are associated with marked dilution of the contrast medium and with micronodulation of the mucosal surface. Lymphangiography is very useful for assessing the disease.

Intestinal edema caused by hypoproteinemia (fig. 3)

Hypoproteinemia rarely causes abnormalities of the small intestine. The causes of hypoproteinemia include decompensated cirrhosis, the nephrotic syndrome, congenital metabolic defects (very rare), nutritional deficiency or protein-losing enteropathy. Protein-losing enteropathy in turn may have several etiologies, including Ménétrier's disease, infectious gastroenteritis, celiac disease, allergy, ischemia, agammaglobulinemia, lymphangiectasia, Whipple's,

Crohn's or Hirschsprung's diseases, ulcerative colitis or digestive cancers. Cirrhosis is often responsible for intestinal edema because of associated conditions such as: hypoproteinemia, portal hypertension and bacterial overgrowth.

Pathology

The wall of the loops is thickened and the blood vessels enlarged. Microscopic study shows edema and a cellular infiltrate, in particular in the submucosa.

Clinical findings

The digestive symptoms (diarrhea, abdominal pain) are sometimes attributed to those of the primary disease.

Radiological findings

The SBFT sometimes demonstrates disorders of tone. The interloop gaps are widened and the loops unfolded and moderately distended. The folds are tall, thickened, and straight. The interfold spaces are normal. The abnormalities are diffuse but predominate in the jejunum. The folds are often also broadened in the colon.

Practical conclusions

Radiologists cannot diagnose hypoproteinemia but they must be able to recognize its appearance in the small bowel.

Amyloidosis (figs. 4 and 5)

Amyloidosis is caused by the infiltration of amyloid in various tissues. The composition of this substance is not completely defined as yet, but it is akin to immunoglobulins. The disease can be *secondary* to chronic infection (bronchopulmonary, urinary, intestinal or osseous), chronic inflammation (rheumatoid arthritis, Crohn's disease, ulcerative colitis), a cancer, a hemopathy, connective diseases, and in general to any long-lasting immune stimulation. The disease is related to and often associated with multiple myeloma.

Amyloidosis can be *primary* as well, and is then often seen in subjects over age 70.

It is sometimes *familial*, in particular in many cases of «periodic disease». This hereditary disease with variable expression, also called familial Mediterranean fever, mainly affects certain ethnic groups (Jews, Armenians). It associates fever, articular and abdominal pains, sometimes mimicking an acute abdomen, and follows an intermittent course with exacerbations lasting for one or two days.

Amyloidosis is sometimes monovisceral but it most often affects several organs, including the kidneys, heart, muscles, liver, spleen, pancreas, brain, gingivae, tongue and salivary glands. The invasion of the digestive tract is almost always found at autopsy but causes symptoms in only one third of patients. The small intestine is then involved in half the cases. The disease is lethal, most often because of renal failure. Steroids are harmful. A number of cases of secondary amyloidosis can be cured if the causal disease is treated.

Pathology

Macroscopic study reveals stiff intestinal loops. The intestinal wall contains scattered whitish deposits. Microscopy shows that these homogeneous deposits are made up of amyloid . These are initially found exclusively in the vascular walls and around blood vessels, and only later invade the intercellular spaces of the muscularis, submucosa and mucosa to finally infiltrate the entire intestinal wall. The nerves and plexuses are destroyed. Inflammatory infiltration and edema occur, partial villous atrophy may develop as can infarction, ulceration and perforation.

Clinical findings

The involvement of the small intestine is most often silent, but it can also be the first manifestation of the disease. It causes dyspeptic disorders, diarrhea or constipation, sometimes simulating obstruction. The course of the disease may sometimes be complicated by malabsorption, a protein-losing enteropathy, hemorrhages or a perforation.

The diagnosis of amyloidosis is made on rectal, jejunal or renal biopsies or with a peritoneal fat pad aspirate.

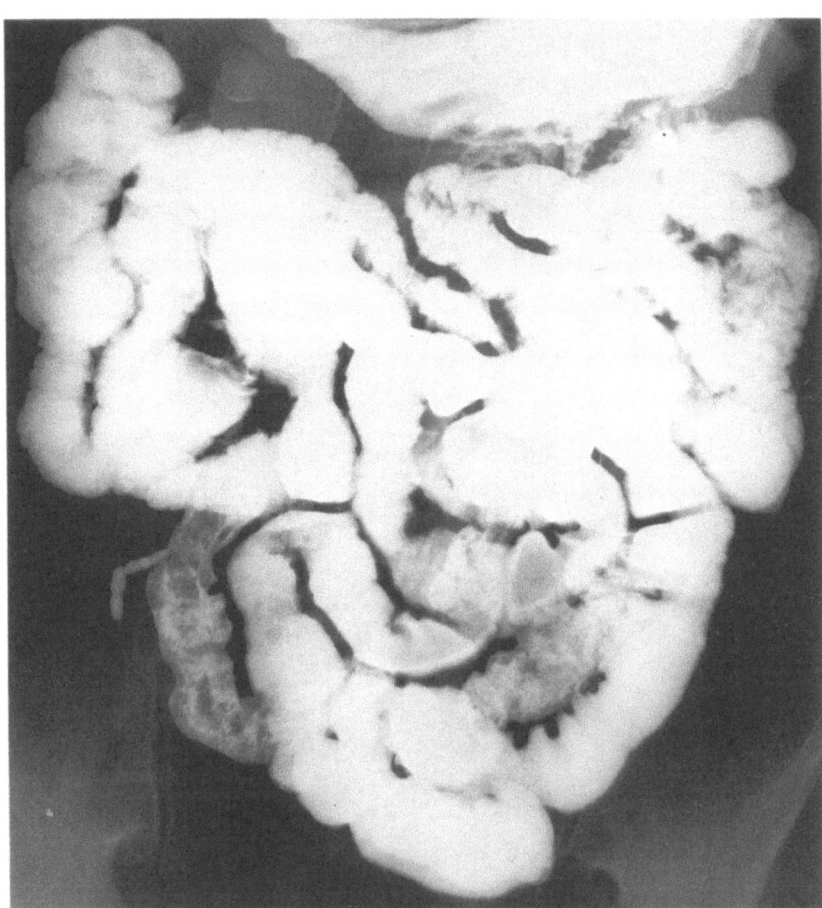

Fig. 4. Amyloidosis (Courtesy of D Régent). 53-year-old woman. Myeloma. Pain, vomiting and melena. Gastric biopsy : amylosis. SBFT : diffuse alterations including abnormal curvature, widened interloop gap and sparse folds

Radiological findings

Even when the small intestine is affected by the disease, the SBFT is normal in one out of 5 cases. In the others, extensive or diffuse abnormalities are found. Transit time is increased and the loops are atonic. Intermittent segmental dilatation and sometimes intussusceptions may be seen. Wall infiltration accounts for the increase in the interloop gap, the unfolded loops, thickened folds ; it rarely causes nodule formation. The number of folds is sometimes decreased in the jejunum and increased in the ileum (jejunal transformation). Contrast medium dilution does not occur. In half the cases, delayed evacuation of the esophagus and stomach may exist. The radiological appearance sometimes suggests scleroderma or ischemia. However, the intestinal wall is thicker than in scleroderma and the lesions are more diffuse than in ischemia.

Practical conclusions

In the clinical context, and in the presence of motor disorders and signs of extensive bowel wall infiltration of the small intestine, the diagnosis of amyloidosis must be considered. This may avoid unnecessary surgery for a disease with a poor prognosis.

Pneumatosis cystoides intestinalis

The specific finding of pneumatosis cystoides is the presence of gas bubbles in the intestinal wall. The term usually does not include necrotizing enteritis or ileomesenteric infarction, which also cause the appearance of intramural air but are accompanied by more severe signs and a worse outcome.

Pneumatosis cystoides of the small intestine is almost always benign, often with few signs, and

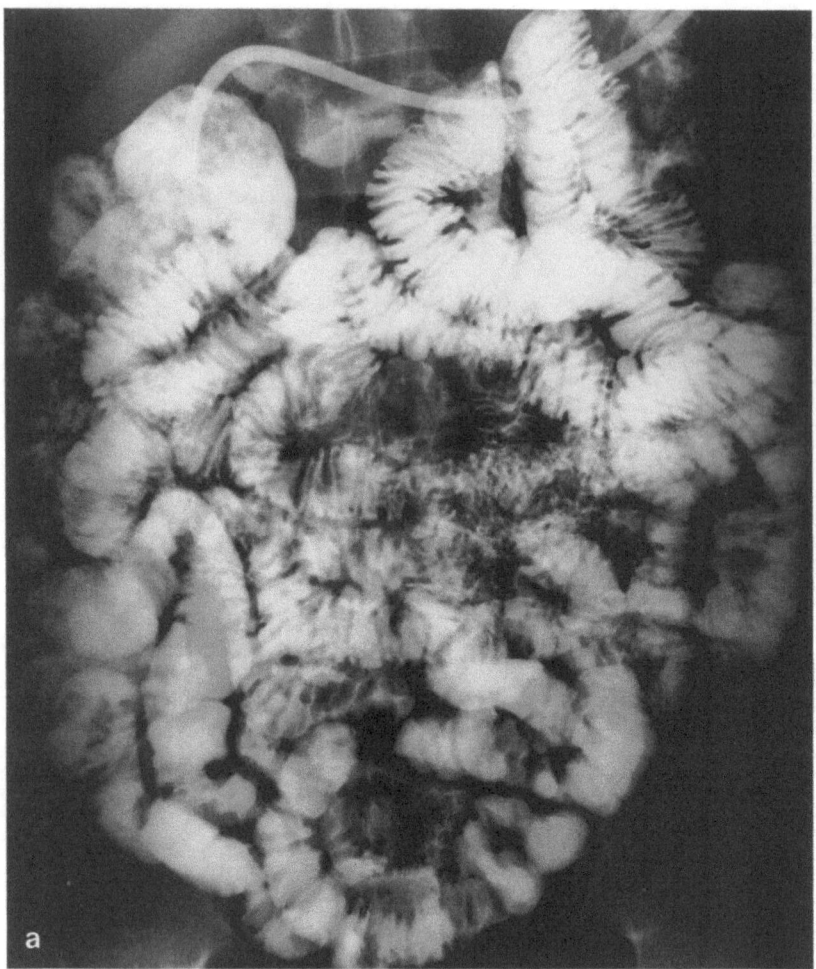

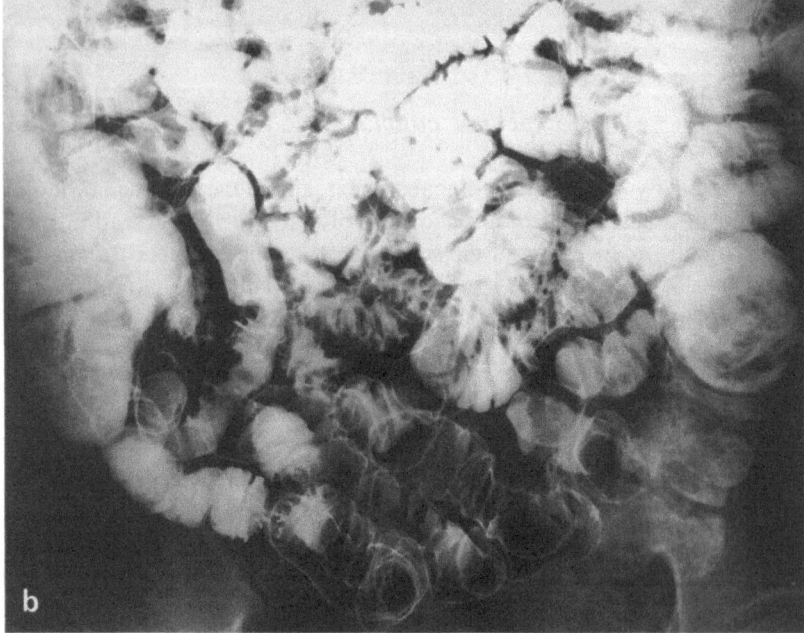

Fig. 5 a, b. Amyloidosis. 40-year-old man. Cutaneous Kaposi's ksyndrome slowly progressing over 12 years. Diarrhea and malabsorption. Jejunal biopsy : perivascular amyloid deposits. SBFT : moderately widened gap between the ileal loops and slightly broadened folds

much less frequent than its colonic counterpart. It occurs at any age, but especially in adults. The bubbles of gas appear in the jejunum more often than in the ileum. They can also be observed in the stomach or the mesocolon, and be associated with a pneumoperitoneum. Several factors can trigger the disease: emphysema with asthma, pulmonary fibrosis, bowel obstruction when associated with an ulceration (pyloric stenosis due to an ulcer, a volvulus, an obstruction caused by adhesions, Crohn's or connective tissue diseases), ischemia, sprue, lactose intolerance, steroid therapy or surgery such as intestinal bypass for obesity. The cause is not always identified. The formation of the bubbles has been explained by a mechanical theory according to which intestinal gas under high pressure penetrates into the intestinal wall through lesions of the mucosa. Some authors think that the forms occurring in patients with respiratory insufficiency are caused by the rupture of alveoli coupled to the mediastinal and retroperitoneal diffusion of air.

Pathology

The examination shows pearly bubbles, several millimeters to one or two centimeters in diameter, mainly in the subserosa and sometimes in the submucosa as well. These bubbles are more numerous along the antimesenteric aspect of the loops. They contain a mixed gas with a great quantity of nitrogen (70 to 90%). The microscopic study shows that they correspond to cavities that may be surrounded by epithelium, sometimes communicating with each other or with a dilated lymphatic vessel. The peripheral tissue is inflamed and contains multinucleated giant cells. Small fibrous scars, maybe due to the healing of cysts, are noted in some areas.

Clinical findings

In addition to the asymptomatic forms discovered at radiology, the disease can cause moderate diarrhea, meteorism and abdominal pains. The onset is usually acute with a short initial phase; the course lasts for a couple of days or weeks, and the disease resolves spontaneously or after oxygen therapy. The condition may rarely be chronic or complicated by malabsorption, perforation or obstruction. The prognosis depends on the precipitating cause.

Radiological findings

The diagnosis is made on plain films when these show clusters or strings of small gas bubbles, or even more so, a pneumoperitoneum without any clinical signs of perforation or shock. When the small intestine is opacified with barium, round or oval lesions appear with a size ranging from several millimeters to one or two centimeters, forming notches along the external contour of the lumen which are malleable on compression. Their characteristic gas content is not always obvious and must be carefully looked for. The bubbles are different from the intramural air observed in gangrene following acute ischemia or necrotizing enterocolitis, which forms a linear structure or very small bubbles (smaller than 5 mm). In addition, other concomitant abnormalities are observed with gangrene, such as thickened intestinal walls and folds, contrast medium dilution, intraperitoneal fluid or air in the portal vein. In fact, the clinical signs of gangrene and pneumatosis cystoides intestinalis can rarely be confused.

Complementary imaging

Computed tomography clearly demonstrates the gas bubbles within the wall of intestinal loops.

Practical conclusions

Radiologists must be able to identify pneumatosis cystoides intestinalis, a benign disease with a very typical appearance. Only in cases of gangrene is gas also found in the intestinal wall. But the clinical signs of the latter cannot be mistaken with those of pneumatosis cystoides. Small bowel involvement is much less frequent than its colonic counterpart.

Food allergies

Food allergies are still not well understood. The patient in whom it occurs may be atopic or not. Several food allergies have been identified, the most widely recognized ones being cow milk allergy of infants and young children, which may also occur later in life, and the allergies to soya proteins, celery salt, eggs, shellfish, etc.

While a number of allergies cause eosinophilic gastroenteritis, which we have already discussed, others present different signs and symptoms including:

- anaphylactic shock that may be lethal. Digestive symptoms are then minor,
- an acute abdominal syndrome associating pain, diarrhea and sometimes a hemorrhage due to vasculitis. The allergy can then be diagnosed by the concomitant presence of urticaria or Quincke's edema.
- malabsorption secondary to mucosal atrophy in the small intestine due to toxic or autoimmune phenomena. This mechanism may play a role in celiac disease.

The diagnosis is difficult if no peripheral signs of allergy are visible. The circumstances of occurrence and the immunological tests sometimes make it possible to identify the allergen, whose withdrawal leads to full resolution. If not, antiallergic therapy will help the patient. The allergen can sometimes be reintroduced without harm after several months of avoidance.

The radiological studies are most often normal. Contrast medium dilution, enlarged loops and broadened folds are observed in cases of mucosal atrophy. In this condition the radiological abnormalities may be markedly brought out by adding the allergen to the barium preparation.

Henoch-Schönlein purpura (fig. 6 and 7)

Purpura simplex (Henoch-Schönlein purpura) is a vasculitis, probably caused by a hypersensitivity phenomenon. Its diagnosis is clinical. The disease occurs in children, more often in boys than in girls, but in adults as well. A previous or concomitant infection occurs in 9 cases out of 10.

An episode of urticaria is followed by purpura in the lower limbs and by acral edema. The typical cutaneous signs are sometimes delayed, thus making the diagnosis difficult. Articular pain is usually noted. Glomerulonephritis occurs in 50% of patients and may carry a poor prognosis. Digestive signs occur in two-thirds of patients, and involve the stomach, small intestine or colon. Resolution is often rapid, most often taking two to four weeks and rarely several months. Recurrence is possible. The disease is lethal in 2% of all cases.

There are no specific laboratory findings for purpura simplex. Anemia and signs of inflammation are observed, without coagulation disorders.

Pathology

The wall of the intestinal loops is thickened, edema-tous and hemorrhagic. Microscopic study shows infarction, ulcerations, intramural hemorrhages and submucosal and mucosal edema. The blood vessels are thrombosed, partly due to endothelial proliferation indicating the presence of vasculitis.

Clinical findings

The digestive symptoms include abdominal pain, vomiting, intestinal bleeding, rarely hematemesis and sometimes changes in bowel habits. Low fever may be present. Laparotomy is performed in 10 to 20% of the cases because the delayed occurrence of purpura does not permit early diagnosis, and because of the possible development of intussusception and perforation. Healing is most often spontaneous in the other cases.

Radiological findings

The SBFT demonstrates a decrease in peristalsis and abnormalities either in the duodenojejunum, or in the terminal ileum, sometimes diffuse. They include: increased caliber, widened interloop gap and stiff, unfolded loops. The folds are broader and taller, and the interfold spaces are reduced in some segments. Thumbprinting indicating intramural hemorrhages are noted. Intussusception can occur. If the clinical diagnosis is doubtful, a second SBFT examination a few days later demonstrates the rapid improvement of the lesions.

Complementary imaging

Computed tomography confirms the presence of hematomas in the intestinal walls as lesions of liquid density along the loops.

Practical conclusions

The diagnosis of purpura simplex should be considered in children if the SBFT shows signs of intramural hemorrhages.

Sarcoidosis

Sarcoidosis, also called benign lymphogranulomatosis or Besnier-Boeck disease, is a disease of unk-

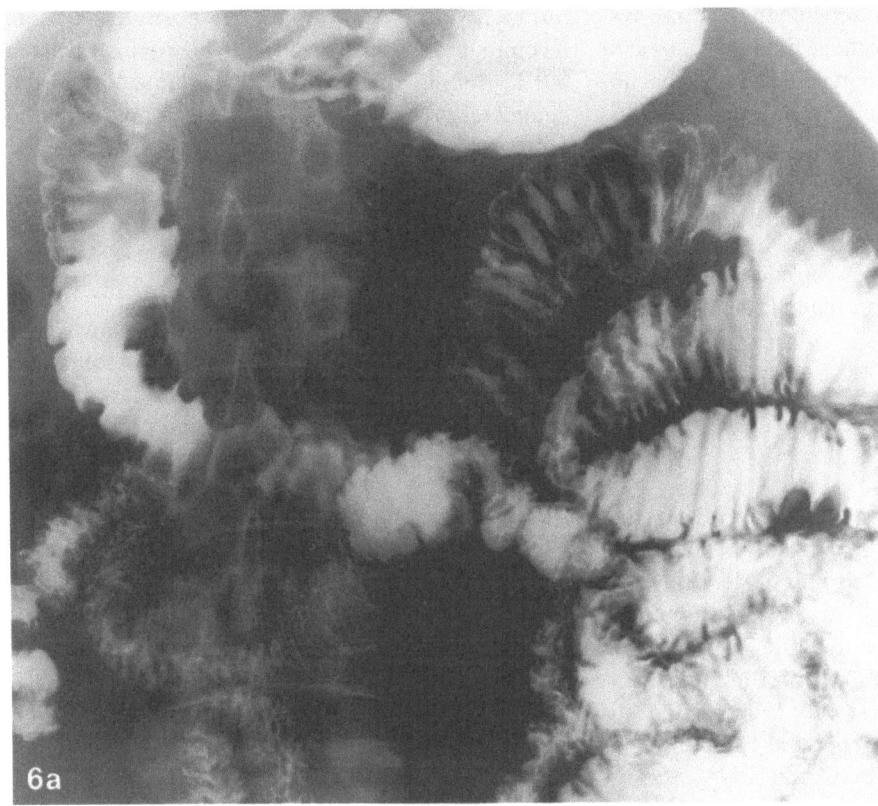

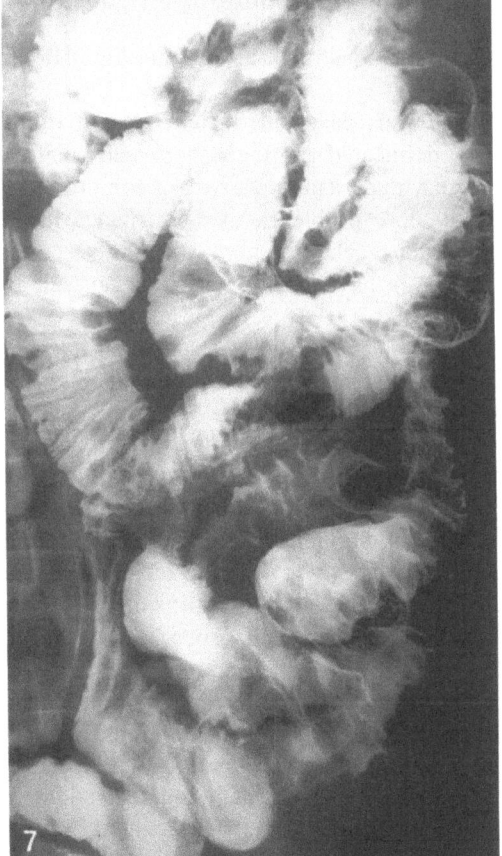

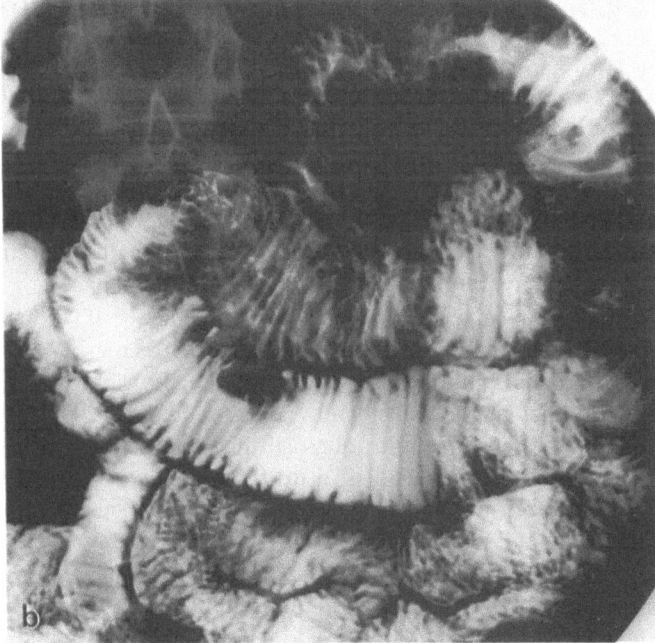

Fig. 6 a, b. Henoch-Schönlein purpura. 42-year-old man. Epigastric pain. SBFT : multifocal lesions, marginal notches, thickened and sometimes tall folds in the duodenum and the jejunum

Fig. 7. Henoch-Schönlein purpura (Courtesy of D Régent). Pain, diarrhea and melena 5 months after an accidental burn in a 43-year-old man. Cutaneous purpura, glomerulonephritis. Malabsorption and protein-losing enteropathy. SBFT : contrast medium dilution, moderately widened interloop gaps, marginal notches and nodules in the jejunum

nown origin affecting the reticuloendothelial system. It may be related to immune disorders, some of its signs suggesting delayed hypersensitivity phenomena. The disease has genetic or geographic contributing factors and mainly affects young adults, and women slightly more often. It usually presents with pulmonary, nodal, cutaneous and articular involvement. Its course is benign in 75% of cases. In a quarter, however, it becomes chronic with eventual cardiopulmonary and neurological complications which may lead to death.

Pathology

Macroscopic study of the small intestine reveals that its walls are thickened by submucosal and serosal nodules producing excentered sites of stenosis separated by normal segments. Ulceration is sometimes observed and adenopathy is the rule.

The histological abnormalities are nonspecific and are of diagnostic use only if associated clinical signs are typical. They appear as epithelioid nodules without necrosis, often coalescing and surrounded by somewhat inflammatory tissue. Giant cells are sometimes observed. All the lesions are at the same stage. The entire wall is involved, in particular the submucosa.

Clinical findings

Digestive involvement causing diarrhea, subocclusion and a hypoproteinemic syndrome is exceptionnal. We may suppose the existence of the disease if other, more frequent signs are observed, such as mediastinal and pulmonary involvement including bilateral mediastinal adenopathy, macronodular or miliary pulmonary infiltration or fibroemphysema. Cutaneous involvement is also frequent and is characterized by multiple small, deformable, painless, red and swollen spots on the face and limbs. Articular pain or inflammatory arthritis are frequent. Radiographs of the bony extremities sometimes show geodes with clear margins. The other organs involved are the peripheral lymph nodes, the liver, the spleen, the eyes, the salivary and endocrine glands, the central and peripheral nervous systems, the kidneys and the heart.

The laboratory findings include a normal sedimentation rate, high levels of serum globulins and hypercalciuria. A characteristic sign is tubercu-

lin anergy in cases of previous positive reaction. Kveim's intradermal reaction is positive, at least at the beginning of the disease, but this test is not completely specific. The diagnosis is mainly based on biopsy of the bronchi, lymph nodes, skin, liver, muscles, etc.

Radiological findings

The rare cases described in the literature show short, staggered stenoses, multiple nodules, or nodulations evoking lymphoid hyperplasia, and large folds. Contrast medium dilution is sometimes observed, as are ulcers.

Practical conclusions

Digestive radiology is not often used in sarcoidosis since intestinal involvement is rarely found in this disease. The diagnosis can be made if the other viscera are involved or, if the signs are nonspecific. by studying the histology of surgical specimens.

Intraluminal foreign bodies (figs. 8 to 10)

A SBFT can demonstrate various intraluminal foreign bodies.

Bubbles are easily identified. Their margins are clearly delineated and their shape and position both change with peristaltic waves and compression. They rarely pose problems, as for instance in an atonic loop not reached by compression.

Parasites have been previously studied in Chapter IV.

Food fragments or *phytobezoars* can stagnate in the intestinal lumen and cause partial or complete obstruction. The impaction may be caused by a stricture, diverticula and sometimes atonia (e.g. after vagotomy). It is often not possible to identify its cause. In 2/3 of the cases, fragmentation defects are accounted for by previous gastric surgery (gastrectomy), the absence of teeth or the excessively rapid ingestion of meals. In addition, alimentary foreign bodies are very often made of fibers (kaki, squash, cauliflower, beans, etc.) or of nondigestible elements (cherry pits). More than 60 different foods have been described. Symptoms occur usually a couple of hours after the meal, but may only manifest much later.

SBFT shows the image of a round lacuna with clear or irregular margins, often with a fibrillar structure, with or without proximal distention. The

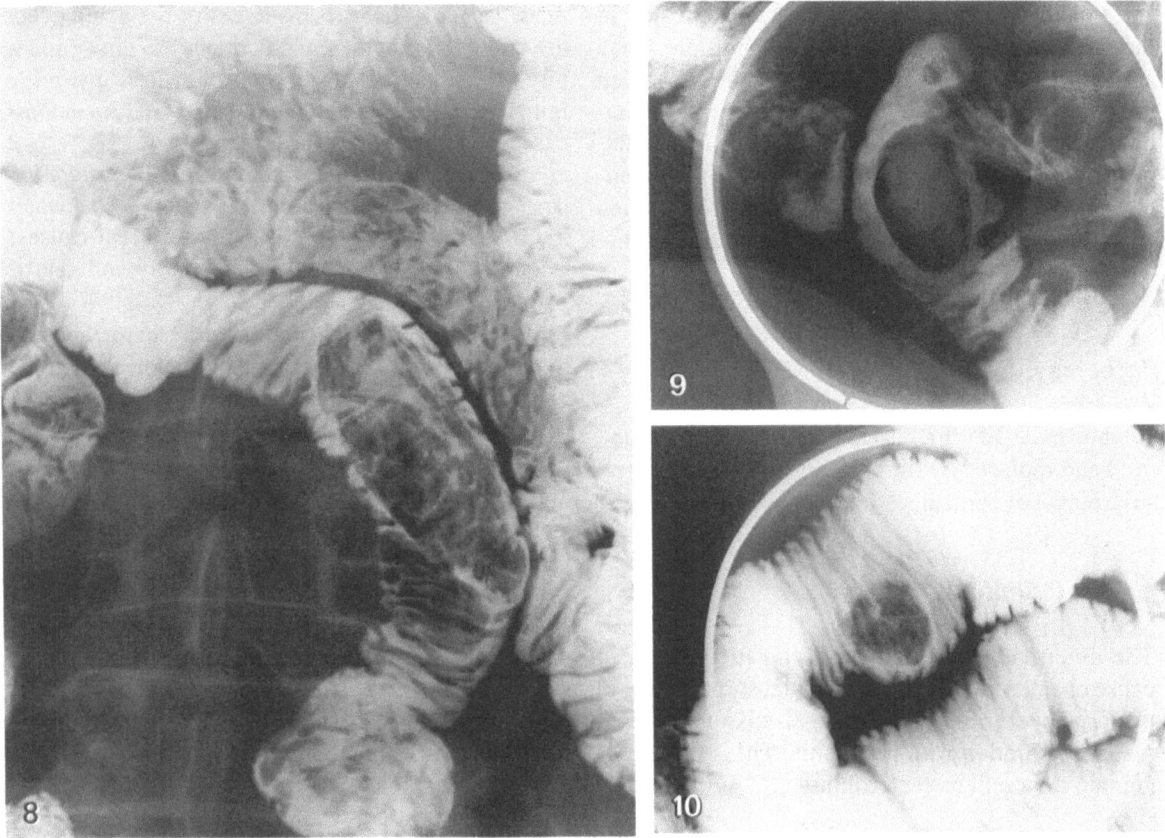

Fig. 8. Intraluminal foreign body. 60-year-old man. Recent abdominal pain. SBFT : ovoid intrajejunal nodule outlined by a dense rim, and fixed on palpation. A follow-up examination performed a few days later demonstrated the disappearance of the lesion

Fig. 9. Intraluminal foreign body. 30-year olf man. Abdominal pain 4 months after gastrectomy for an ulcer. SBFT : ovoid intrajejunal nodule with clear, slightly irregular margins, and fixed on palpation. Negative findings during surgery for eventration two months later

Fig. 10. Intraluminal foreign body. 45-year-old man. Acute intestinal obstruction recurring after medical treatment, 20 years after vagotomy. SBFT : jejunal atonia,. Round nodule, outlined by a dense slightly irregular rim. Surgical finding : bezoar

appearance can be mistaken for that of a tumoral obstruction.

Gallstone ileus due to perforation of the gallbladder into the intestine is a well-known occurrence. The stratified appearance of the calculi sometimes suggests the diagnosis on plain films, even more so if air is observed in the biliary duct. However, the calculus is not always calcified and aerobilia is not seen if the gallbladder is excluded.

Narcotics are sometimes packed in condoms and swallowed by smugglers. These produce oval nodules with a slightly irregular extremity corresponding to the sealed end.

Enterolithiasis is formed by the concretion of biliary salts and of calcium or other mineral salts due to stasis of any cause and favoured by an alkaline environment. It is most frequent in the ileum and is ob-

served in diverticula (in particular with a Meckel's diverticulum), proximal to a stricture (Crohn's disease, tuberculosis, congenital atresia, etc.) or in a blind loop following surgical anatomosis.

Practical conclusions

The presence of intraluminal foreign bodies can cause obstruction, mimick a tumour, or indicate another lesion.

Acquired diverticula (fig. 11)

Acquired diverticula are different from congenital diverticula in that they are associated with abnormalities of the tunica muscularis. They are located in the mesenteric aspect of the loop and multiple. They are most frequent in the jejunum and are observed in 1% of all SBFT examinations. As their implantation forms a neck smaller than their maximum diameter, they are easily distinguished from the saccules seen in Crohn's disease, ischemia, scleroderma and after ulcer healing or surgery (end to side or side to side anastomosis).

Pathology

The muscular fibers are sparse, atrophied or vacuolized and replaced by fibrosis. Lesions of the myenteric plexuses sometimes occur.

Clinical findings

The diverticula are often asymptomatic. They can cause changes in bowel habits, malabsorption due to bacterial overgrowth, hemorrhage, volvulus, abscesses or perforation with peritonitis. They sometimes contain concretions (enteroliths).

Radiological findings

Plain films can show the diverticula, filled with air or exhibiting air fluid levels, enteroliths or pneumatosis cystoides intestinalis.

The round or oval, rare or innumerable addition images, some millimeters to several centimeters in diameter are mainly found in the jejunum, and are readily opacified during SBFT. Contrast medium dilution and enlarged jejunal loops are often noted. An atypical diverticulum may rarely mimick an ectasiating tumour.

Pseudoobstruction

Several factors can slow transit time and cause intestinal dilatation in the absence of mechanical obstruction.

Acute *paralytic ileus* can occur in cases of shock (trauma, surgery, pancreatitis), intense pain (renal colic), acute anoxia (cardiac or respiratory failure, myocardial infarction, mesenteric thrombosis), severe infection (cholecystitis, pneumonia, peritonitis, septicemia), electrolyte disorders (hypokaliemia) or intoxication (amanitas). The diagnosis is

made easier if the circumstances of the acute event are known, if the intestinal contents are not completely blocked and if distention is diffuse, involving both jejunoileal and colic segments as it does in most cases of pseudoobstruction.

The signs of *chronic intestinal pseudoobstruction* are more misleading. Its overall frequency is low but it may be due to many different causes:
- congenital disease (visceral myopathy and neuropathy),
- idiopathic pseudoobstruction with steatorrhea and hypertrophy of the layers of the mesenteric plexuses, beginning in adults without any familial features,
- collagen vascular diseases, in particular scleroderma as well as systemic lupus erythematosus and dermatomyositis,
- amyloidosis,
- chronic ischemia of the small intestine,
- celiac disease,
- parasitic diseases (trypanosomiasis)
- vagotomy: transit is sometimes delayed, but diarrhea also occurs due to bile acid or pancreatic enzyme deficiencies, or to bacterial overgrowth. The intestinal loops are sometimes distended;
- drugs (psychoactive drugs, opiates, phenothiazines, anticholinergics, antimitotics),
- diabetes,
- hypoparathyroidism,
- myxedema: intestinal paralysis is usually associated with atonia of the entire digestive tract and sometimes with ascites. It may be the presenting symptom and is corrected by treatment ;
- the Ehler-Danlos syndrome, a hereditary disease with variable expression causing articular hyperlaxity and skin hyperelasticity.

Practical conclusions

In the case of small intestinal dilatation, a number of clinical and radiological signs make it possible to diagnose pseudoobstruction, thus avoiding unnecessary surgery.

Isolated transit time acceleration

A number of diseases cause transit time acceleration of the small intestine without other abnormalities. They result in diarrhea, which is often postprandial, urgent and not very abundant. Steatorrhea and water and electrolyte losses may occur, but malabsorption is not observed.

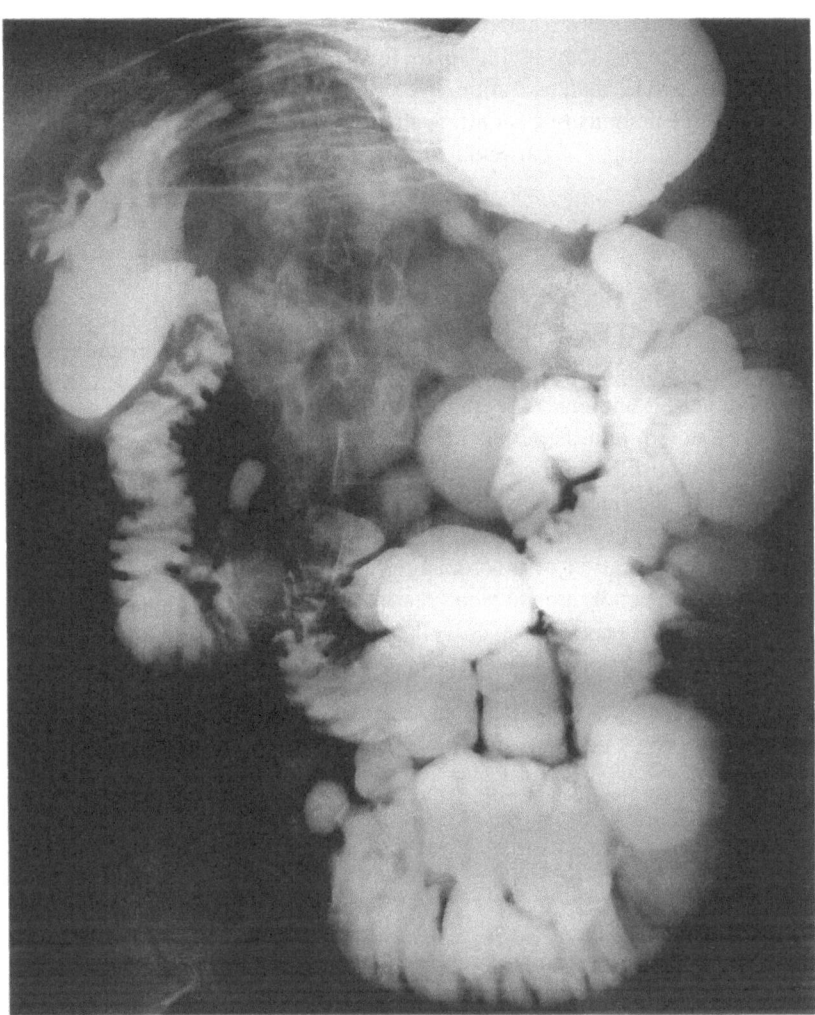

Fig. 11. Jejunal diverticulosis. 78-year-old man operated for obstruction due to an adhesion after cholecystomy. New subocclusive episode. SBFT : multiple diverticula with increased jejunal caliber, may be secondary to a postoperative adhesion

A SBFT is normal or accelerated. The average caliber is sometimes decreased due to hypertonia and, less frequently, increased.

Transit time acceleration has several causes, including:
- diabetes: the disorder is caused by neuropathy. Malabsorption can be caused by an associated secondary infection,
- pancreatic insufficiency,
- medullary cancers of the thyroid gland (30% of all cases),
- hyperthyroidism (40% of all cases),
- gastroenteric anastomoses,
- sympathectomy,
- intestinal resection,
- amyloidosis,
- diseases of the central nervous system,
- carcinoid tumours (in case of hepatic metastases),
- Verner-Morrison syndrome: VIP hypersecretion by an endocrine tumour of the pancreas, bronchi, adrenals or sympathetic ganglia resulting in an increased volume of intestinal secretion rather than in real transit time acceleration;
- idiopathic, maybe functional causes.

Fabry's disease

Fabry's disease is an exceptional hereditary disease due to alpha-galactosidase deficiency causing abnormal sphingolipid metabolism. The typical signs reflect ocular and cutaneous involvement (angiokeratoma), as well as infiltration of the lymph nodes, joints, kidneys, heart, nervous system and digestive system. Treatment is based on replacement of the missing enzyme. The histological examination shows lipid deposits in the arteries and the lymphatic vessels. The digestive symptoms include pain, fever, diarrhea and vitamin B12 malabsorption.

SBFT demonstrates contrast medium dilution and widened loops, in particular in the ileum.

Xanthomatosis

Xanthomatosis is caused by the infiltration of lipid-filled macrophages in the skin and viscera. Skin involvement (xanthoma) is typical. Cirrhosis is sometimes noted, and the levels of blood cholesterol and phospholipids are increased. Macroscopic examination of the intestinal walls shows that they are thickened by yellowish plaques. Histological study shows the infiltration of macrophages with foamy cytoplasm, especially around blood vessels and mainly in the submucosa and serosa, as well as the presence of multinucleated giant cells.

SBFT shows the diffuse and regular thickening of the folds of small intestine.

Mastocytosis (fig. 12)

Mastocytosis is caused by the infiltration of mast cells and fibrosis of the skin and the reticuloendothelial system. The systemic form is an adult disease, which, in children, is most often confined to the skin.

Skin lesions, including urticaria pigmentosa, pachydermia and erythroderma, are typical but not always observed. Hepatosplenic, and bony lesions (increased bone density, less frequently lacunae) and gastroduodenal ulcers appear. Digestive symptoms are frequent and may be caused by histamine release. Gastroscopy shows urticarial papules. The diagnosis is made with a bone marrow aspirate and skin biopsies.

The pathological examination requires specific dyes and reveals the infiltrate of mast cells in the submucosa. A great number of eosinophils, plasmacytes and lymphocytes are observed as well. The mucosa can undergo partial, focal atrophy and the villi may be broadened.

SBFT shows the thickened intestinal walls with broadened or disappearing folds. The typical appearance is that of small nodules, 2 to 5 mm in diameter, segmentally distributed, most often extending to the stomach and to the superior part of the duodenum. The nodules exceptionally are larger and centered on a pool of barium.

Abetalipoproteinemia (figs. 13 and 14)

Abetalipoproteinemia or acanthocytosis is a rare congenital disease accounting for the malabsorption of fats and of liposoluble vitamins (vitamin A, carotenoids). It causes growth retardation in children, nervous disorders (ataxia), muscle atrophy and retinitis pigmentosa. The biological studies show typical acanthocytosis and the absence of plasma betalipo-

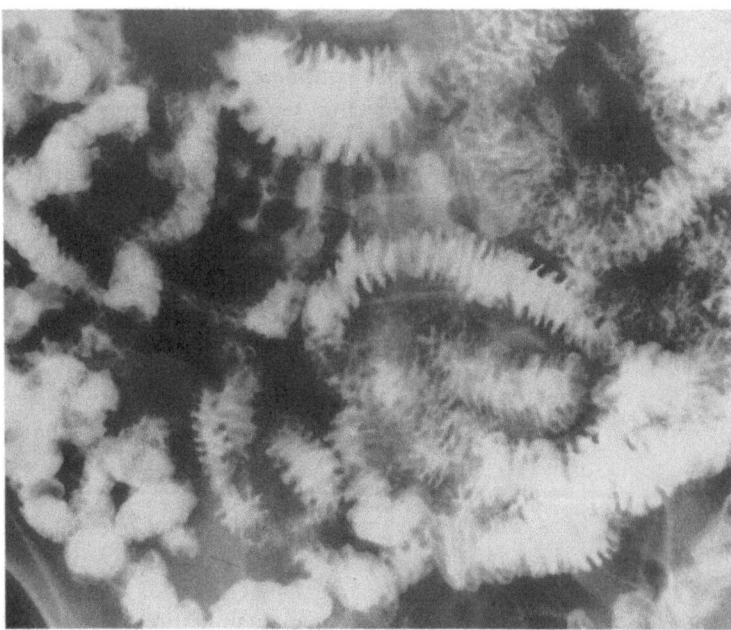

Fig. 12. Mastocytosis (Courtesy of P Mahieu). 60-year-old woman. Cutaneous mastocytosis, abdominal pain and vomiting. Biopsy showed duodenal and jejunal mastocytosis. SBFT : hypertonia with diffuse contrast medium segmentation. Nodular folds

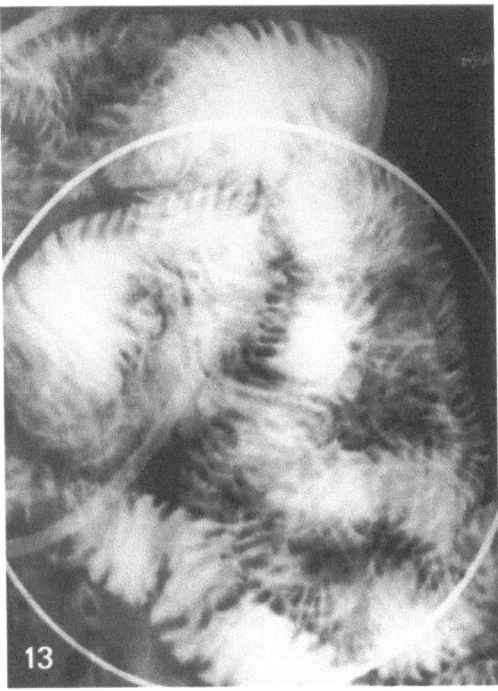

Fig. 13. Abetalipoproteinemia. 40-year-old woman. Mental retardation, malabsorption. SBFT : increased height of the jejunal folds

Fig. 14 a, b. Abetalipoproteinemia.(Courtesy of G. Gay). 21-year-old woman. Diarrhea and weight loss. SBFT : contrast medium dilution and segmentation, moderately widened interloop gap. Broadened jejunal folds

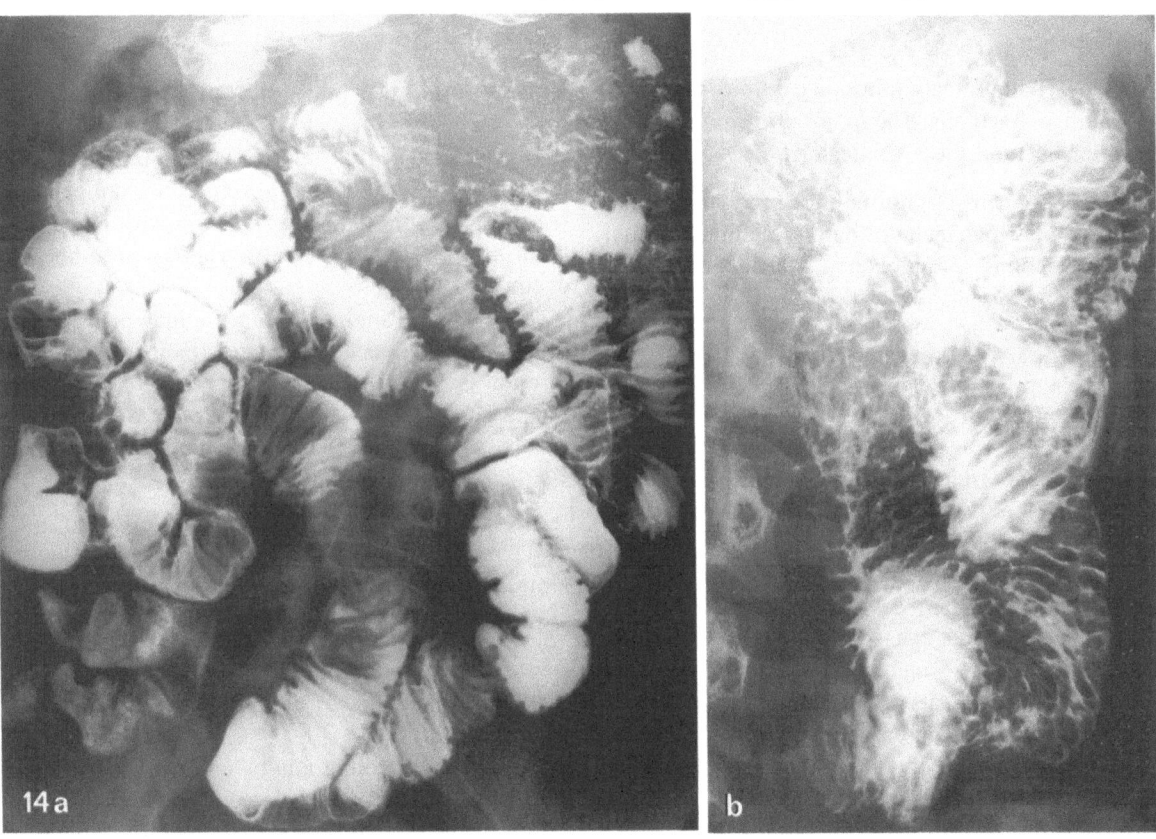

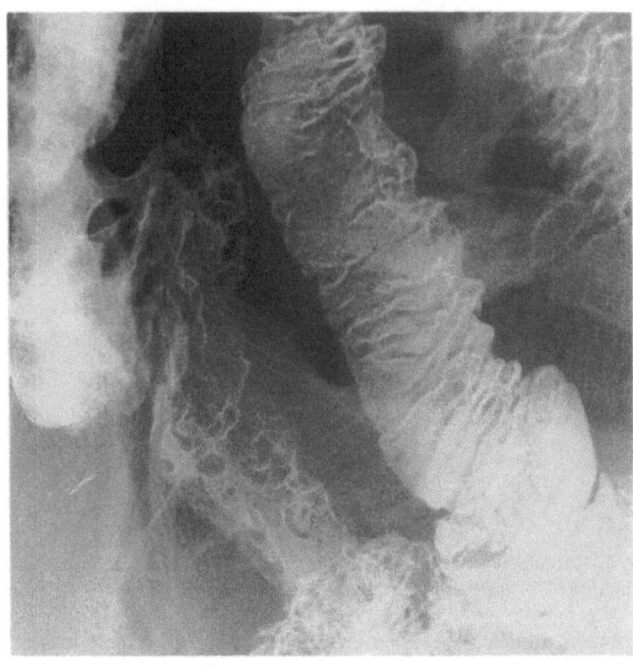

Fig. 15. Wegener's syndrome. 36-year-old woman. Sinusitis, conjonctivitis. Articular pains. Cutaneous, pulmonary and renal lesions. SBFT : nodulation of the terminal ileum

proteins. Histological studies reveal lipid infiltration of the digestive cells. The major clinical symptoms are diarrhea and those of steatorrhea.

SBFT shows abnormalities predominating in the jejunum which include contrast medium dilution, distended loops and thickened but sinuous folds.

Hereditary angioneurotic edema

The hereditary angioneurotic edema is a disease of dominant inheritance with variable penetrance, causing edema in the skin and mucosal surfaces in case of emotion or shock. The crises last for one to two days and end spontaneously only to reccur later. Laryngeal edema may develop and be lethal.

The disease is caused by deficiency in a factor inhibiting esterase, which controls the activity of the C1 and C4 components of the complement. It occurs at any age but most often begins in childhood. The digestive symptoms include abdominal pains and vomiting associated with malaise. Ascites with a fluid rich in eosinophils is sometimes noted.

The SBFT is abnormal only during the acute episodes, and reveals segmental abnormalities including thickened walls, broadened folds and thumb-printing. Their normal appearance returns after the crisis.

Paroxysmal nocturnal hemoglobinuria

Paroxysmal nocturnal hemoglobinuria is a disease of unknown etiology, which is sometimes congenital. It causes chronic hemolytic anemia with hemoglobinuria. Vascular, especially venous, thromboses occur.

The intestinal symptoms include pain, vomiting and digestive hemorrhage. Ileomesenteric infarction is often the cause of death.

The SBFT shows an appearance of intestinal ischemia: slow transit, abnormal bowell wall expansion and thumbprinting.

Degos' disease

Degos' disease or malignant atrophic papulosis is an obliterating angeitis of unknown, perhaps autoimmune, origin.

It affects young adults, and men more often than women. The cutaneous signs, sometimes very discrete, are typical for the disease. They include papules of several millimeters in diameter centered on hollow spots. The disease is likely to extend to other organs, in particular to the digestive tract.

The pathological examination shows diffuse submucosal lesions made up of local arterial thromboses with bowel wall necrosis. The digestive symptoms are not very specific except for the complications due to hemorrhage, perforation or obstruction. Evolution is often lethal because of recurrence and the lack of appropriate therapy.

The SBFT shows a specific appearance of small intestinal ischemia. Arteriography can demonstrate arteriolar stenoses.

Wegener's syndrome (fig. 15)

Wegener's syndrome is a granulomatous vasculitis causing lesions of the arterioles similar to those of periarteritis nodosa. The disease gives rise to diffuse fibrinoid lesions. Granulomas made up of fibro-inflammatory tissue are often centered on a necrotic area. Clinically, this rare adult disease affects the respiratory tract (sinuses, lungs) and sometimes the eyes, the nervous system and the joints. Renal involvement is extremely severe in the absence of immunosuppressive treatment. Digestive involvement causes ulcerations and sometimes perforation of the small intestine and colon.

The SBFT demonstrates the ulcerations or, after their healing, nodulation and abnormal bowel wall expansion.

References

Lymphangectasia

André C (1975) Les fuites protéiques digestives. Cah Med Lyon 51 : 627-630
Belaiche J, Vesin P, Chaumette MT, Julien M, Cattan D (1980) Lymphangiectasies intestinales et fibrose des ganglions mésentériques. Gastroenterol Clin Biol 4 : 52-58
Bernier JJ (1980) Comment et quand diagnostiquer une entéropathie exsudative ? Concours Med 102 : 55-57
Bujanover Y, Liebman WM, Goodman JR, Thaler MM (1981) Primary intestinal lymphangiectasia, case report with radiological and ultrastructural study. Digestion 21 : 107-114
Curet Ph, Waiss L, Wiart D, Grellet J (1983) Malabsorption et anomalies vasculaires mésentériques supérieures complexes, à propos d'un cas. J Radiol 64 : 69-72
Desprez-Curely JP, Bismuth V, Bourdon R (1965) Hypoprotéinémie « idiopathique » et stéatorrhée, démonstration lymphographique d'une fistule lympho-intestinale. Ann Radiol 8 : 1-16
Dobbins WO (1966) Electron microscopic study of the intestinal mucosa in intestinal lymphangiectasia. Gastroenterology 51 : 1004-1017

Fortas L, Frexinos J (1973) Les entéropathies exsudatives d'origine lymphatique, symptomatologie et explorations. Arch Fr Mal App Dig 62 : 501-512
Fortas L, Frexinos J (1973) Les entéropathies exsudatives d'origine lymphatique, aspects étiopathogéniques et notions thérapeutiques. Arch Fr Mal App Dig 62 : 685-696
Frexinos J (1974) Les entéropathies exsudatives. Nouv Presse Med 3 : 2568-2572
Goutet JM, Chaouachi B, Gruner M, Navarro J (1981) Les entéropathies exsudatives de l'enfant. Gastroenterol Pediatr 31 : 1159-1174
Hess J, Kruizinga K, Bijleveld CMA, Hardjowijono R, Eygelaar A (1984) Protein-losing enteropathy after Fontan operation. J Thorac Cardiovasc Surg 88 : 606-609
Hoang C, Halphen M, Galian A, Brouet JC, Marsan C, Leclerc JP, Rambaud JC (1985) Atteinte intestinale et entéropathie exsudative au cours de la macro-globulinémie de Waldenström, cas cliniques. Gastroenterol Clin Biol 9 : 444-448
Kingham JGC, Moriarty KJ, Furness M, Levison A (1982) Lymphangiectasia of the colon and small intestine. Br J Radiol 55 : 774-777
Kumpe DA, Jaffe RB, Waldmann TA, Weinstein MA (1975) Constrictive pericarditis and protein losing enteropathy, an imitator of intestinal lymphangiectasia. AJR 124 : 365-373
Ligny G, Van Cauter J, Engelholm L, Witterwulghe M (1981) Lymphangiectasies et entéropathie exsudative. Acta Gastroenterol Belg 44 : 69-482
Marshak RH, Wolf BS, Cohen N, Janowitz HD (1961) Protein-losing disorders of the gastrointestinal tract : roentgen features. AJR 77 : 893-905
Navarro J (1981) Les gastroentéropathies exsudatives en pédiatrie. Gastroenterol Pediatr 31 : 1255-1266
Nouel O, Eugène C, Gislon J, Marche C (1975) Entéropathie exsudative et mésentérite rétractile. Arch Fr Mal App Dig 64 : 233-238
Olmsted WW, Madewell JE (1976) Lymphangiectasia of the small intestine : description and pathophysiology of the roentgenographic signs. Gastrointest Radiol 1 : 241-243
Pock-Steen OCh (1966) Roentgenologic changes in protein-losing enteropathy. Acta Radiol Diagn 4 : 681-689
Rao SSC, Dundas S, Holdsworth CD (1987) Intestinal lymphangiectasia secondary to radiotherapy and chemotherapy. Dig Dis Sci 32 : 939-942
Roberts SH, Douglas AP (1976) Intestinal lymphangiectasia : the variability of presentation, a study of 5 cases. Q J Med XLV : 39-48
Rogé J, Marche C, Camilleri JP, Druet P, Silvereano-Roge F, Vernier G (1978) Entéropathie exsudative et macroglobulinémie, présentation d'1 cas suivi depuis 9 ans ; revue de la littérature. Gastroenterol Clin Biol 2 : 897-906
Schwarz Tiene E (1966) L'entéropathie exsudative en pathologie pédiatrique. Concours Med 88 : 1220-1226
Servelle M, Rouffilange F, Andrieux J, Soulie J, Seguin P, de Leersnider D (1968) Lymphographie des chyliferes intestinaux. Sem Hôp Paris 13/3 : 881-892
Shimkin PM, Waldmann TA, Krugman RL (1970) Intestinal lymphangiectasia. AJR 110 : 827-841
Strober W, Wochner RD, Carbone PP, Waldmann TA (1967) Intestinal lymphangiectasia : a protein-losing enteropathy with hypogammaglobulinemia, lymphocytopenia and impaired homograft rejection. J Clin Invest 46 : 1643-1656

Vardy PA, Lebenthal E, Shwachman H (1975) Intestinal lymphangiectasia : a reappraisal. Pediatrics 55 : 842-851

Verma TR, Bankole MA (1973) Lymphovenous obstruction in anomalous midgut rotation. Arch Dis Child 48 : 154-157

Vesin P (1977) Les gastro-entéropathies « exsudatives ». Cah Med Lyon 3 : 439-444

Waldmann TA (1966) Protein-losing enteropathy. Gastroenterology 50 : 422-443

Waldmann TA, Steinfeld JL, Dutcher TF, Davidson JD, Gordon RS (1961) The role of the gastrointestinal system. in : idiopathic hypoproteinemia. Gastroenterology 41 : 197-207

Intestinal edema caused by hypoproteinemia

Balthazar EJ, Gade MF (1976) Gastrointestinal edema in cirrhotics, radiographic manifestations and pathogenesis with emphasis on colonic involvement. Gastrointest Radiol 1 : 215-223

Farthing MJG, McLean AM, Bartram CI, Baker LRI, Kumar PJ (1981) Radiologic features of the jejunum in hypoalbuminemia. AJR 136 : 883-886

McLean AM, Farthing MJG, Kurian G, Mathan VI (1982) The relationship between hypoalbuminaemia and the radiological appearances of the jejunum in tropical sprue. Br J Radiol 55 : 725-728

Vachon MMA, Nové-Josserand G, Yves A, Cornut H (1961) L'intestin grêle au cours des hépatites alcooliques. Rev Lyon Med, pp 767-775

Amyloidosis

Chapuy P (1977) Sénescence et amyloïdose. Cah Med Lyon 2 : 2379-2382

Cordier JF, Creyssel R (1977) Gammapathie monoclonale et amyloïdose. Cah Med Lyon 2 : 2352-2353

Cordier JF, Rousset H (1977) Classifications des amyloïdoses. Cah Med Lyon 2 : 2345

Glenner GG, Ein D, Terry WD (1972) The immunoglobulin origin of amyloid. Am J Med 52 : 141-147

Godeau P, Frances C, Le Charpentier Y (1976) Amylose et pathologie digestive. Arch Fr Mal App Dig 65 : 5-8

Godeau P, Herson S, Herreman G (1980) La maladie périodique. Concours Med 102-10 : 1311-1321

Grimaud JA, Chevallier M (1977) Le diagnostic anatomopathologique de l'amyloïdose. Cah Med Lyon 2 : 2347-2351

Legge DA, Carlson HC, Wollaeger EE (1970) Roentgenologic appearance of systemic amyloidosis involving gastrointestinal tract. AJR 110 : 406-412

Pandarinath GS, Levine SM, Sorokin JJ, Jacoby JH (1978) Selective massive amyloidosis of the small intestine mimicking multiple tumors. Radiology 129 : 609-610

Raffi F, Lerat F, Cuillière P, Roudier JM, Le Bodic L, Rymer R (1985) Amylose péritonéale au cours d'une macroglobulinémie de Waldenström, aspect tomodensitométrique. J Radiol 66 : 735-738

Rogé J, Delavierre Ph, Lagrue G, Durand H, Silvereano de Roissard F (1973) Amylose du grêle responsable d'un syndrome sévère de malabsorption intestinale. Sem Hop Paris 49 : 3147-3150

Rouhier D (1977) Tube digestif et amyloïdose. Cah Med Lyon 2 : 2357-2359

Tête R, Boyer JD, Slaoui H, Mas R (1979) Diarrhée chronique avec malabsorption par amylose intestinale secondaire à une polyarthrite rhumatoïde au cours d'un diabète. Lyon Med 242 : 283-288

Vincent JP, Hardouin JP, Devars du Mayne JF (1979) Maladie amyloïde : revue générale. Rev Fr Gastroenterol 149 : 47-53

Pneumatosis cystoides intestinalis

Bocquet L, De Ranieri E, Charleux H, Moulle P, Léger L (1978) Pneumatose kystique de l'intestin grêle après court-circuit jéjuno-iléal pour obésité. Nouv Presse Med 7 : 545-548

Breiter J, Levine JB, Forouhar FA (1982) Pneumatosis cystoides intestinalis associated with refractory sprue. Am J Gastroenterol 77 : 322-325

Clements JL (1977) Intestinal pneumatosis, a complication of of the jejunoileal bypass procedure. Gastrointest Radiol 2 : 267-271

Ecker JA, Williams RG, Clay KL (1971) Pneumatosis cystoides intestinalis, bullous emphysema of the intestine. Am J Gastroenterol 56 : 125-136

Elidan J, Gimmon (Goldschmidt) Z, Schwartz A (1980) Pneumoperitoneum induced by pneumatosis cystoides intestinalis associated with volvulus of the stomach. Am J Gastroenterol 74 : 189-195

Frank PH, O'Connell DJ (1977) Pneumatosis cystoides intestinalis and obstructing intussusception in celiac disease. Gastrointest Radiol 2 : 109-111

Keats TE, Smith TH (1974) Benign pneumatosis intestinalis in childhood leukemia. AJR 122 : 150-152

Kleinman PL, King DR (1977) Ischemic jejunitis and pneumatosis intestinalis secondary to anastomotic obstruction following jejunal atresia repair. Gastrointest Radiol 2 : 113-115

Meyers MA, Ghahremani GG, Clements JL, Goodman K (1977) Pneumatosis intestinalis. Gastrointest Radiol 2 : 91-105

Olmsted WW, Madewell JE (1976) Pneumatosis cystoides intestinalis : a pathophysiologic explanation of the roentgenographic signs. Gastrointest Radiol 1 : 177-181

Samach M, Brandt LJ, Bernstein LH (1978) The radiology corner : spontaneous pneumoperitoneum with pneumatosis cystoides intestinalis in a patient with mixed connective tissue disease. Am J Gastroenterol 69 : 494-500

Vernacchia FS, Jeffrey RB, Laing FC, Wing VW (1985) Sonographic recognition of pneumatosis intestinalis. AJR 145 : 51-52

Wall LL, Linshaw MA, Bailie MD, Pierce GE (1982) Pneumatosis intestinalis in a pediatric renal transplant patient. J Pediatr 101 : 745-747

Yale CE (1975) Etiology of pneumatosis cystoides intestinalis. Surg Clin North Am 55 : 1297-1302

Food allergies

André C, André F, Cavagna S (1988) L'allergie alimentaire : mythe ou réalité. Acta Gastroenterol Belgica LI : 159-168

Buffard P, Crozet L (1964) Etude radiologique des manifestations allergiques du tube digestif. Rev Lyon Med, pp 189-200

Paraf A (1953) Sur l'allergie digestive. Sem Hop Paris 78 : 4148-4149

Polonovski C, Mougenot JF (1981) Flash sur 5 thèmes gastroentérologiques pédiatriques. Gastroenterol Pediatr 31 : 1143-1154

Schaffer HA, Eckard DA, De Lange EE, Ramakrishnan MR (1988) Allergy to baryum sulfate suspension with angioedema of the stomach and small bowel. Gastrointest Radiol 13 : 221-223

Tachev T, Hadjidekov G, Nedkova-Bratanova N, Yanev St (1967) Modifications radiologiques dans les entéropathies allergiques. Acta Gastroenterol Belgica 30 : 209-224

Henoch-Schönlein purpura

Allen DM, Diamond LK, Howell DA (1960) Anaphylactoid purpura in children (Schönlein-Henoch syndrome). Am J Dis Child 99 : 147-168, 833-854

Bernard J, Mathe G, Israël L, Chassigneux J (1957) Etudes cliniques et biologiques sur le syndrome de Schönlein-Henoch. Presse Med 65 : 759-764

Glasier CM, Siegel MJ, McAlister WH, Shackelford GD (1981) Henoch-Schönlein syndrome in children : gastrointestinal manifestations. AJR 136 : 1081-1085

Grossman H, Berdon WE, Baker DH (1964) Abdominal pain in Schönlein-Henoch syndrome. Am J Dis Child 108 : 67-72

Grossman H, Berdon WE, Baker DH (1965) Reversible gastrointestinal signs of hemorrhage and edema in the pediatric age group. Radiology 84 : 33-39

Handel J, Schwartz S (1957) The Schönlein-Henoch syndrome roentgenologic findings. AJR 78 : 643-652

Klein GL, Stafford S (1975) Unusual gastrointestinal manifestations of Henoch-Schönlein purpura. Am J Dis Child 129 : 1238-1239

Rodriguez-Erdmann F, Levitan R (1968) Gastrointestinal and roentgenological manifestations of Henoch-Schönlein purpura. Gastroenterology 54 : 260-264

Sahn DJ, Schwartz AD (1972) Schönlein-Henoch syndrome : observations on some atypical clinical presentations. Pediatrics 49 : 614-616

Schmutz G, Zeller Ch, Pauline D, Christmann C, Kempf F, Storck D (1982) Aspects radiologiques des localisations intestinales du purpura rhumatoïde de l'adulte, à propos de 6 observations. J Radiol 63 : 315-320

Siskind BN, Burrell MI, Pun H, Russo R, Levin W (1985) CT Demonstration of gastrointestinal involvement in Henoch-Schönlein syndrome. Gastrointest Radiol 10 : 352-354

Warter J, Storck D, Christmann D, Meyer F (1978) Syndrome de malabsorption à la phase initiale d'un purpura rhumatoïde sévère. Nouv Presse Med 8 : 1245-1248

Yentis I (1973) Henoch-Schönlein purpura mimicking acute appendicitis and Crohn's disease. Br J Radiol 46 : 555-556

Sarcoidosis

Chrétien J (1969) La sarcoïdose : bases anatomo-pathologiques, conceptions nosologiques et pathogéniques. Rev Prat XIX : 3530-3546

Ell RS, Franck PH (1981) Spectrum of lymphoid hyperplasia : colonic manifestations of sarcoidosis, infectious mononucleosis, and Crohn's disease. Gastrointest Radiol 6 : 329-332

Debray Ch, Darnaud Ch, Voisin R, Martin Et, Moreau G (1967) Les localisations sur le tube digestif de la maladie de Besnier-Boeck-Schaumann. Arch Fr Mal App Dig 56 : 253-273

Guérin JC, Alexandre C (1975) La sarcoïdose ou maladie de Besnier-Boeck-Schaumann (ou lymphogranulomatose bénigne). Cah Med Lyon 1 : 371-377

Janbon M, Bertrand L (1958) Sarcoïdose de l'intestin grêle, ses rapports avec l'iléite régionale de Crohn. Presse Med 66 : 1492-1494

Mitchell DN, Rees RJ (1971) Sarcoidosis and Crohn's disease. Proc R Soc Med 64 : 944-945

Popovic OS, Brkic S, Bojic P, Kenic V, Jojic N, Djuric V, Djordjevic N (1980) Sarcoidosis and protein losing enteropathy. Gastroenterology 78 : 119-125

Turiaf J (1974) Diagnostic de la sarcoïdose. Rev Prat XXIV : 4209-4213

Intraluminal foreign bodies

Beerman R, Nunez D, Wetli CV (1986) Radiographic evaluation of the cocaine smuggler. Gastrointest Radiol 11 : 351-354

Boyle TM, Agus SG, Bauer JJ (1987) Small intestinal obstruction secondary to obturation by a Garren gastric bubble. Amer J Gastroent 82 : 51-53

Brettner A, Euphrat EJ (1970) Radiological significance of primary enterolithiasis. Radiology 94 : 283-288

Javors BR, Bryk D (1983) Enterolithiasis : a report of 4 cases. Gastrointest Radiol 8 : 359-362

Kirby DF, Mills PR, Kellum JM, Messmer JM, Sugerman HJ (1987) Incomplete small bowel obstruction by the Garren-Edwards gastric bubble necessitating surgical intervention. Amer J Gastroent 82 : 251-253

Levin B, Shapiro RA (1980) Recurrent enteric gallstone obstruction. Gastrointest Radiol 5 : 151-153

Moriel EZ, Ayalon A, Eid A, Rachmilewitz D, Krausz MM, Durst AL (1983) An unusually high incidence of gastrointestinal obstruction by persimmon bezoars in Israeli patients after ulcer surgery. Gastroenterology 84 : 752-755

Pombo F, Arnal-Monreal F, Soler-Fernandez R, Alvarez-Fernandez JC, Carames J (1982) Multiple gastrointestinal atresias with intraluminal calcification. Br J Radiol 55 : 307-309

Renner W, Went J, McLean J, Plattner G (1982) Ultrasound demonstration of a non-calcified gallstone in the distal ileum causing small-bowel obstruction. Radiology 144 : 884

Rumley TO, Hocking MP, King CE (1983) Small bowel obstruction secondary to enzymatic digestion of a gastric bezoar. Gastroenterology 84 : 627-629

Sinner WN (1981) The gastrointestinal tract as a vehicle for drug smuggling. Gastrointest Radiol 6 : 319-323

Strauss S, Rubinstein ZJ, Shapira Z, Jacob ET (1977) Food as a cause of small intestinal obstruction, a report of · 5 cases without previous gastric surgery. Gastrointest Radiol 2 : 17-20

Acquired diverticula

Beal SL, Walton CB, Bodai BI (1987) Enterolith ileus resulting from small bowel diverticulosis. Amer J Gastroent 82 : 162-164

Dunn V, Nelson JA (1979) Jejunal diverticulosis and chronic pneumoperitoneum. Gastrointest Radiol 4 : 165-168

Freimanis MG, Plaza-Ponte M (1988) Radiologic diagnosis of jejunal diverticulitis. Gastrointest Radiol 13 : 312-314

Greenstein S, Jones B, Fishman EK, Cameron JL, Siegelman SS (1986) Small-bowel diverticulitis : CT findings. AJR 147 : 271-274

Krishnamurthy S, Kelly MM, Rohrmann CA, Schuffler MD (1983) Jejunal diverticulosis, a heterogenous disorder caused by a variety of abnormalities of smooth muscle or myenteric plexus. Gastroenterology 85 : 538-547

Salomonowitz E, Wittich G, Hajek P, Jantsch H, Czembirek H (1983) Detection of intestinal diverticula by double-contrast small bowel enema : differentiation from other intestinal diverticula. Gastrointest Radiol 8 : 271-278

Spiegel RM, Schultz RW, Casarella WJ, Wolff M (1982) Massive hemorrhage from jejunal diverticula. Radiology 143 : 367-371

Tisnado J, Konerding KF, Beachley MC, Mendez-Picon G (1979) Angiographic diagnosis of a bleeding jejunal diverticulum. Gastrointest Radiol 4 : 291-293

Pseudo-obstruction

Bain NH (1977) Ehlers-Danlos syndrome. Am J Gastroenterol 67 : 167-170

Boudin G, Barbizet J, Hillemand B, Lote J (1955) Le retentissement digestif de la sclérose latérale amyotrophique. Sem Hop Paris 1 : 7-14

Chinn JS, Schuffler MD (1988) Paraneoplastic visceral neuropathy as a cause of severe gastrointestinal motor dysfunction. Gastroenterology 95 : 1279-1286

Colombel JF, Parent M, Lescut D, Cortot A, Guillemot F, Plane C, Bonnière P, Lecomte-Houcke M, Paris JC (1988) Paraneoplastic intestinal pseudo-obstruction as the presenting feature of small-cell lung cancer. Gastroenterol Clin Biol 12 : 394-996

Etienne M, Pans A, Fridman V, Boniver J, Brassinne A (1987) Pseudo-obstruction intestinale idiopathique chronique. Acta Gastroenterol Belgica L : 425-434

Faulk DL, Anuras S, Christensen J (1978) Chronic intestinal pseudoobstruction. Gastroenterology 74 : 922-931

Franken EA, Smith WL, Smith JA (1980) Paralysis of the small bowel ressembling mechanical intestinal obstruction. Gastrointest Radiol 5 : 161-167

Gargouri M, Ayadi S, Ben Amor N (1979) Dilatation intestinale chronique et neuropathie. J Radiol 60 : 662

Haley HB, Leigh C, Bronsky D, Waldstein SS (1962) Ascite and intestinal obstruction in myxedema. Arch Surg 85 : 328-333

Karasick D, Karasick S, Mapp E (1982) Gastrointestinal radiologic manifestations of proximal spinal muscular atrophy (Kugelberg-Welander syndrome). J Natl Med Assoc 74 : 475-478

Legros A, Leconte D, Huguet C (1980) Pseudo-obstruction de l'intestin grêle par ganglioneuromatose, étude d'un cas. Gastroenterol Clin Biol 4 : 333-337

Lewicki AM, Kleinhaus U, Brooks JR, Membreno AA (1973) The small bowel following pyloroplasty and vagotomy. Radiology 109 : 539-544

Lorenzo Y, Losada H, Macri E, Nuchowitch M, Ravera JJ, Maggiolo J, Navarro A, Cervino JM, Mussio Fournier JC (1959) Etude radiologique de l'estomac, du duodénum et de l'intestin grêle dans le myxœdème de l'adulte. Sem Hop Paris, pp 2761-2764

Maldonado JE, Gregg JA, Green PA, Brown AL (1970) Chronic idiopathic intestinal pseudo-obstruction. Am J Med 49 : 203-212

McClelland HA, Lewis MJ, Naish JM (1962) Idiopathic steatorrhoea with intestinal pseudo-obstruction. Gut 3 : 142-144

Moadel E, Bryk D (1975) Idiopathic intestinal pseudo-obstruction. Am J Gastroenterol 63 : 162-165

Moss AA (1976) Postvagotomy unmasking of nontropical sprue. Gastrointest Radiol 1 : 173-175

Paul CA, Tomiyasu U, Mellin Koff SM (1961) Nearly fatal pseudo-obstruction of the small intestine, a case report and its relief by subtotal resection of the small bowel. Gastroenterology 40 : 698-704

Rohrmann CA, Ricci MT, Krishnamurthy S, Schuffler MD (1981) Radiologic and histologic differentiation of neuromuscular disorders of the gastrointestinal tract : visceral myopathies, visceral neuropathies, and progressive systemic sclerosis. AJR 143 : 933-941

Schuffler MD, Lowe MC, Bill AH (1977) Studies of idiopathic intestinal pseudoobstruction. Gastroenterology 73 : 327-338

Schuffler MD, Rohrmann CA, Templeton FE (1976) Intestinal pseudoobstruction. AJR 127 : 729-736

Snodgrass RW, Mellinkoff SM (1962) Idiopathic hypoparathyroidism with small-bowel x-ray features of sprue, without steatorrhea. Am J Dig Dis 7 : 273-280

Sullivan MA, Snape WJ, Matarazzo SA, Petrokubi RJ, Jeffries G, Cohen S (1977) Gastrointestinal myoelectrical activity in idiopathic intestinal pseudo-obstruction. N Engl J Med 297 : 233-238

Isolated transit time acceleration

Cattan D, Dervichian M, Gouerou H (1975) La diarrhée du cancer médullaire de la thyroïde. Arch Fr Mal App Dig 64 : 278-279

Friedman J (1954) Roentgen studies of the effects on the small intestine from emotional disturbances. AJR 72 : 367-379

Labayle D, Modigliani R, Matuchansky C, Rambaud JC, Bernier JJ (1977) Diarrhée avec accélération du transit intestinal, étude clinique, biologique, radiologique, histologique et étiologique de 56 cas. Gastroenterol Clin Biol 1 : 231-242

Matuchansky C (1975) La diarrhée du syndrome de Verner-Morrison. Arch Fr Mal App Dig 64 : 281-283

Prost A (1975) La diarrhée dans l'hyperthyroïdie. Arch Fr Mal App Dig 64 : 277-278

Vinnick IE, Kern F, Struthers JE (1962) Malabsorption and the diarrhea of diabetes mellitus. Gastroenterology 43 : 507-519

Fabry's disease

Le Bodic L, Le Bodic MF, Simon J, Lucas J, Welin J, Madec Y, Hamza H (1979) Manifestations digestives de la maladie de Fabry, présentation d'un cas avec étude histochimique et ultrastructurale de l'intestin grêle. Gastroenterol Clin Biol 3 : 541-548

Xanthomatosis

Beutler SM, Fretzin DF, Jao W, Desser R (1978) Xanthomatosis resembling scleroderma in multiple myeloma. Arch Pathol Lab Med 102 : 567-571

Gasster M, Golden R, Will D, Mellinkoff SM (1961) Xanthomatosis involving the colon and small intestine, report of a case. Am J Dig Dis 6 : 312-321

Pope TL, Shaffer H (1985) Small bowel xanthomatosis : radiologic-pathologic correlation. AJR 144 : 1215-1216

Mastocytosis

Clemett AR, Fishbone G, Levine RJ, James AE, Janower M (1968) Gastrointestinal lesions in mastocytosis. AJR 103 : 405-412

Debray C, Leymarios J, Cerf M, Bocquet L, Marche C, Boivin P, Kahn A, Husson JM (1973) Mastocytose diges-

Kellow JE, Phillips SF (1987) Altered small bowel motility in irritable bowel syndrome is correlated with symptoms. Gastroenterology 92 : 1885-1893
tive, présentation d'un cas et revue de la littérature. Arch Fr Mal App Dig 62 : 411-417
Legman P, Sterin P, Vallée C, Zag-Zag J, Levesque M, Richard JP (1982) Atteinte colique au cours d'une mastocytose systémique. Ann Radiol 25 : 167-170
Quinn SF, Shaffer HA, Willard MR, Ross S (1984) Bull's-eye lesions : a new gastrointestinal presentation of mastocytosis. Gastrointest Radiol 9 : 13-15
Robbins AH, Schimmel EM, Rao KCVG (1972) Gastrointestinal mastocytosis : radiologic alterations after ethanol ingestion. AJR 115 : 297-299

Abetalipoproteinemia

Gay G, Roche JF, Merlin P, Grégoire J (1987) Hypobétalipoprotéinémie : aspect endoscopique, intérêt diagnostique. Acta Endoscopica 17 : 79-81
Weinstein MA, Pearson KD, Agus SG (1973) Abetalipoproteinemia. Radiology 108 : 269-273
Willemin B, Coumaros D, Zerbe S, Weill-Bousson M, Annonier P, Hirsch E, Aby MA, Schmutz G, Bockel R (1987) Abétalipoprotéinémie. Gastroenterol Clin Biol 11 : 704-708

Hereditary angioneurotic edema

Ellis K, McConnell DJ (1969) Hereditary angioneurotic edema involving small intestine. Radiology 92 : 518-519
Pearson KD, Buchignani JS, Shimkin PM, Frank MM (1972) Hereditary angioneurotic edema of the gastrointestinal tract. AJR 116 : 256-261

Paroxysmal nocturnal hemoglobinuria

Hertz IH, Keller RJ (1981) Paroxysmal nocturnal hemoglobinuria : small bowel findings. AJR 136 : 204-205
Lee BCP (1973) Paroxysmal nocturnal haemoglobinuria presenting as an acute abdominal emergency. Br J Radiol 46 : 467-469

Degos' disease

Bilbao JI, Garcia Delgado F, Idoate M, Arejola JM, Aquerreta D, Otero M (1986) Maladie de Degos, atteinte intestinale mise en évidence par angiographie numérique, un cas. J Radiol 10 : 711-713
Moraga Lop FA, Gonzalez-Fernandez J, Gallart, Catala A, Cabre Piera J, Bosch Castane J, Huguet, Redecilla P, Bosch Banyeras JM (1980) Degos malignant atrophic papulosis. Ann Esp Pediatr 13 : 437-440

Extrinsic pathology

Several cases of small intestinal involvement by a neighbouring lesion are described in this chapter. The lesions can be tumoral, inflammatory or due to scar formation, excluding postoperative lesions (adhesions, textiloma, talcoma) and hematogenous bowel wall metastases, which are discussed in other chapters.

The spine, the full bladder, the aorta, the iliac vessels, the colon and, more importantly, the sigmoid loop and the liver produce normal indentations on the walls of the small bowel loops, which are deepened by hypotonia and compression.

Images of *displaced or compressed loops* (fig. 1) can be observed if an intra- or retroperitoneal organ is hypertrophied, often due to a tumour. The most common examples are unfolded loops or «void» images (lucent areas) around mesenteric adenopathy, pelvic loops displaced by a uterine fibroma, or a tumour of the ovary. Similar images can be observed with retroperitoneal pathology (hydronephrosis, renal tumour, aortic aneurysm, lumboaortic adenopathy). In most cases, the only abnormal feature is the position of the loops, which are still relatively mobile. The appearances of the exointestinal lesions vary during palpation or with changes in the patient's position.

This is also true for ascites (fig. 2 and 3). The unfolded loops are parallel to each other or crowded together in the midabdominal region. The interloop gap is regularly widened. Mobility is reduced in gelatinous ascites, this sign being associated with compression due to pseudomyxomas that are sometimes calcified.

External *hernias* containing loops of small intestine are readily identified, while internal hernias (fig. 4) are more misleading. In addition to the congenital and postoperative hernias described in other chapters, hernias (inguinal, crural or umbilical) may occur due to muscular weakness or to trauma (e.g. through the broad ligament). Several views can be useful to demonstrate the parallel position and relative stenosis of the loops in the neck of the hernia.

Linear *adhesions* can appear in a number of inflammatory diseases (appendicitis, pancreatitis, diverticulitis, etc.). SBFT reveals a linear compression across the intestinal lumen, fixing and deviating the loop. The appearance can be misleading, as a notch on the side of the loop may mimic extrinsic compression by a tumour.

A particularly interesting condition is the *«extrinsic parietal syndrome»* described by Régent. This syndrome is different from the appearance of compressed or displaced loops in that bowel wall involvement progresses from outside and is either confined to the serosa or is more extensive. Mesenteric and peritoneal lesions are its major causes. The intestinal abnormality occurs either if the visceral peritoneal layer is affected by a lesion of an intraabdominal organ or by a metastasis, or if infiltration caused by a retroperitoneal inflammatory focus or a tumor, or if mesenteric adenopathy extends into the mesentery. In the first case, the signs are mainly visible on the antimesenteric aspect of the loops. In the second, the signs are visible on the mesenteric aspect. Both processes often occur concomitantly.

The symptoms vary with the nature of the initial disease and most often include pain and signs

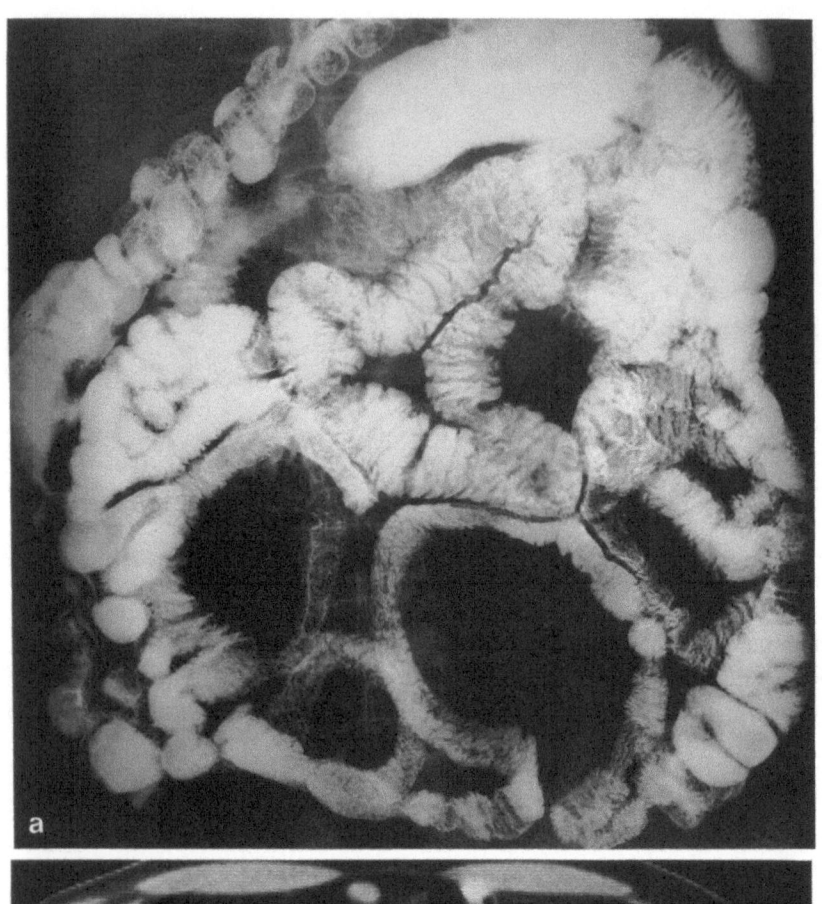

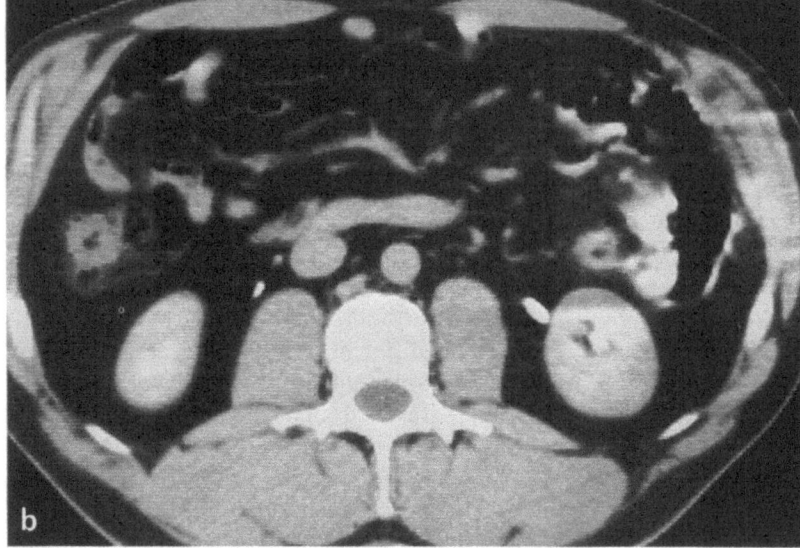

Fig. 1 a, b. Mesenteric lipomatosis. a SBFT : 3 ileal loops unfolded without wall abnormalities, b findings confirmed by computed tomography

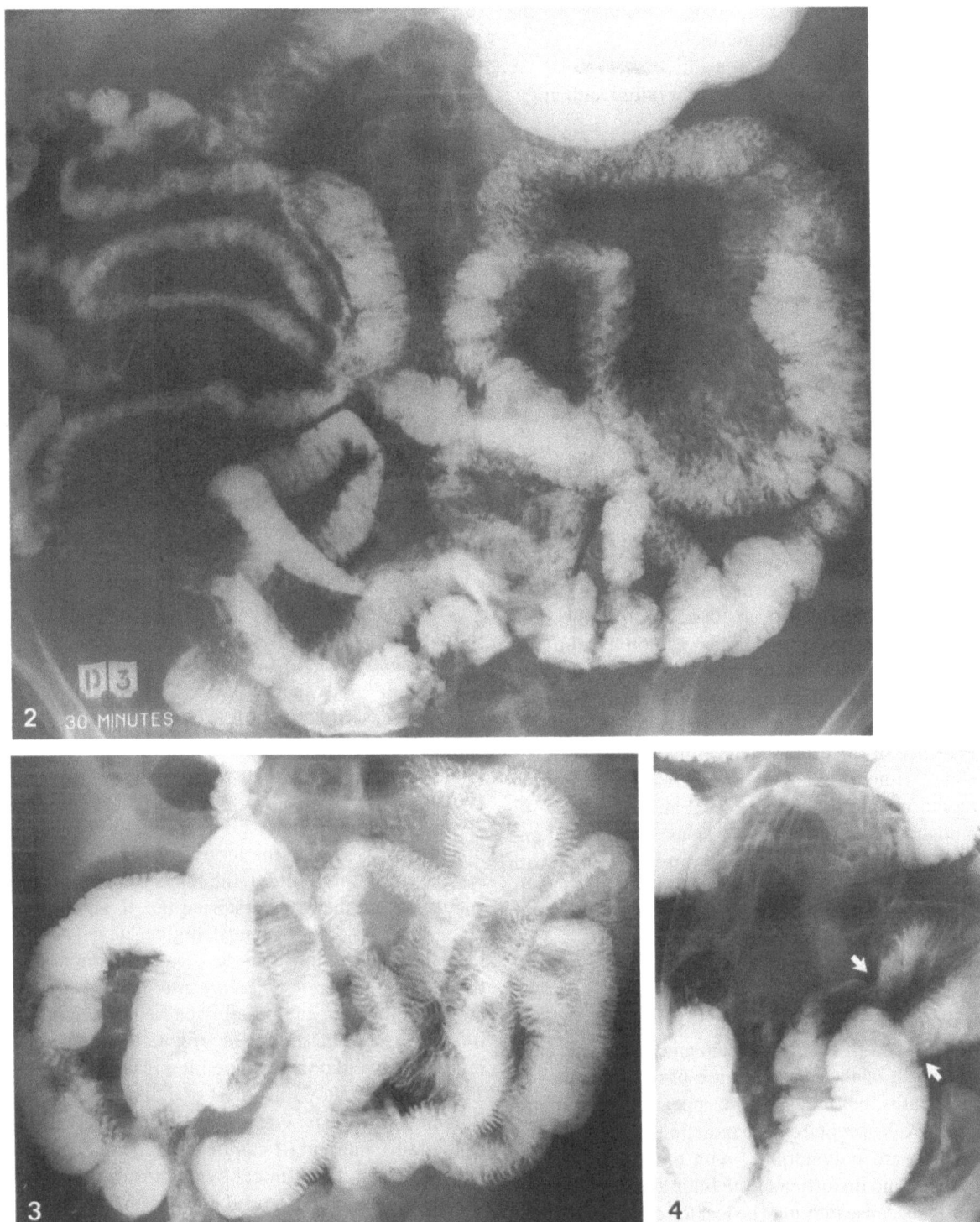

Fig. 2. Gelatinous ascites (pseudomyxoma peritonei). 51-year-old man. Skin fistula following the removal of an appendiceal mucocele with gelatinous ascites. SBFT : widened gaps between the ileal loops and unfolded loops

Fig. 3. Ascites. 30-year-old man. Abdominal pain. SBFT : unfolded jejunal loops with tall, rectilinear, parallel folds.

Fig. 4. Internal hernia (Courtesy of L Engelholm). 58-year-old man. Subocclusive syndrome. SBFT : fixed, narrowed and anguled ileal loop with proximal dilatation. Surgical findings : hernia through the sigmoid mesocolon

of obstruction. The radiological features of the extrinsic parietal syndrome include:
- fixity of the involved segments,
- abnormal position: disrupted curvature and, angulation,
- retraction and spiculation of one edge of the affected loops,
- stretched, parallel folds or folds converging into the retracted segment,
- asymmetric lesions,
- absence of ulceration.

Ultrasound and computed tomography play a very important part in the etiological diagnosis. In case of large tumours, arteriography is sometimes the only modality demonstrating the origin of the lesions.

Several clinical patterns can be distinguished according to the nature of the underlying disease. The parietal syndrome of *tumoral origin* (figs. 5 to 9) is almost always a consequence of the evolution of *malignant tumors*, most often metastases and rarely tumors of the neighbouring organs (ovaries, colon, kidneys, uterus, pancreas). In addition to the signs of neoplastic infiltration, the pathology shows a retractile connective tissue reaction. The clinical symptoms often include deterioration of the patient's general condition, a palpable tumor, or ascites. The evidence of the primary cancer may guide the diagnosis, without ruling out postoperative adhesions or radiation enteritis. Radiological studies mainly demonstrate the fixity of the lesions, their extent and their multiplicity. The lesions are associated with marginal notches, an often asymmetric stenosis with a smooth and gradual transition, areas of nodulation formed by small, juxtaposed elements, an interloop gap widened by infiltration of the neighbouring tissues or by ascites, as well as signs of ischemia (thickened wall and broadened, flattened folds). The lesions are mostly seen in the distal ileum and on the mesenteric aspect of the loops because of the frequency of metastases, but they can also appear in the jejunum. They are different from the radiation-induced lesions as they are polymorphic, with extensive notches, nodules and distortion of the folds and, more importantly, because they may be located outside the fields of radiation. Extrinsic tumoral invasion may be difficult to distinguish from adhesions, ischemia, endometriosis and even from a large intrinsic tumor or a tumor associated with extraluminal abnormalities (carcinoid tumor, lymphoma, Gardner's syndrome).

The only benign tumour likely to produce such an appearance is *endometriosis* (fig. 10). This disease is usually observed in women during their reproductive life but sometimes occurs after menopause. The involvement of the small intestine is rare, making up 1% of cases of operated gynecological endometriosis, while rectosigmoid involvement is observed in 10% of the cases. The lesion, single or multiple, is located in the pelvic loops and most often associated with gynecological endometriosis. It is sometimes encapsulated or infiltrating. It develops in the serosa and in the muscularis, which is hyperplastic, while the mucosa is congested and exceptionally ulcerated. Histology shows the infiltration of endometrial tissue containing small hemorrhagic areas. Some cases are clinically silent and are discovered incidentally at surgery. Pain sometimes follows the menstrual cycle and may be associated with constipation or subocclusion or with intestinal hemorrhage. The radiological appearance is similar to that of metastases, including mucosal notches, spiculation of one aspect of the loop, palisading folds in a pelvic loop that is fixed on palpation, and sometimes, the presence of an intramural nodule. The diagnosis is difficult if the more typical rectosigmoid involvement does not occur.

The *non-tumoral* extrinsic parietal syndrome (figs. 11 to 13) is mainly caused by postoperative adhesions described in another chapter. Inflammatory lesions, for instance salpingitis, pancreatitis, periappendiceal abscess formation, or Crohn's disease, are rare causes since the symptoms of the initial disease remain the major clinical findings. In addition to displacement of the loops and discrete inflammatory signs (large folds), the loops can be fixed or angulated and the folds distorted due to adhesions.

In cases other than postsurgical states, peritoneal dialysis, Crohn's disease, carcinoid tumours, or tuberculosis, *retractile mesenteritis* (figs. 14 and 15) may be idiopathic and possibly caused by trauma or infection. The mesentery is irregularly thickened, retracted, nodular and sometimes pseudotumoral. The pathology shows necrosis of adipocytes and inflammatory fibrosis. The compression of the vessels in the radix mesenterii can cause ischemia or lymphangiectasia. The clinical symptoms are not very specific, and include painful episodes, transit disorders and a palpable mass. Its course is most often benign. The SBFT demonstrates displaced, angulated loops and fixed strictures. The most typical appearance in mesenteric retraction is a star- or fan-shaped arrangement of several loops with their extremities bunched close together and fixed. Large, straight folds suggesting ischemia or micronodulation due to lymphangiectasia can be observed.

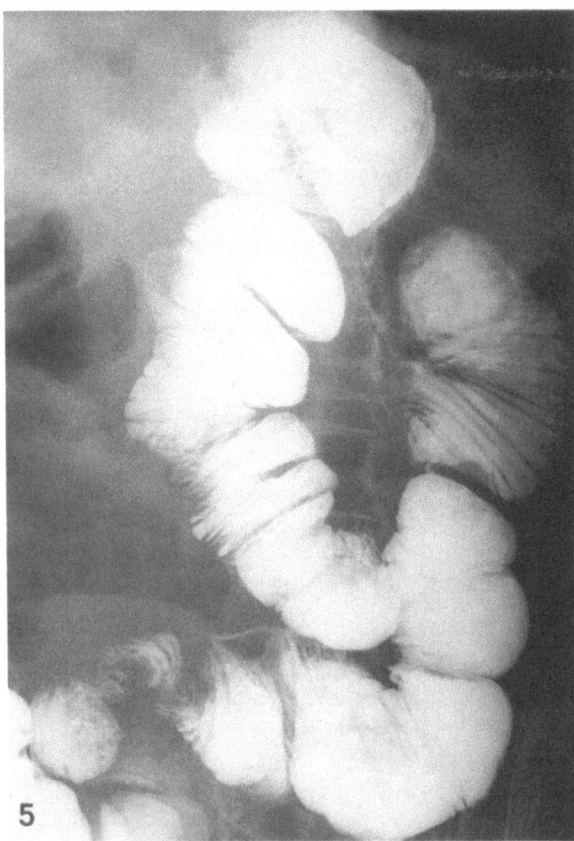

Fig. 5. Peritoneal carcinomatosis. 55-year-old man. Subocclusive syndrome one year after total gastrectomy for cancer. SBFT : stenosis and dilatation. Fixed staggered and angulated loops

Fig. 6. Peritoneal carcinomatosis. 65-year-old. Hiccup and diarrhea one year after total gastrectomy for adenocarcinoma. SBFT : abnormal position of the fixed and angulated midabdominal loops, alternating dilatation ans stenosis

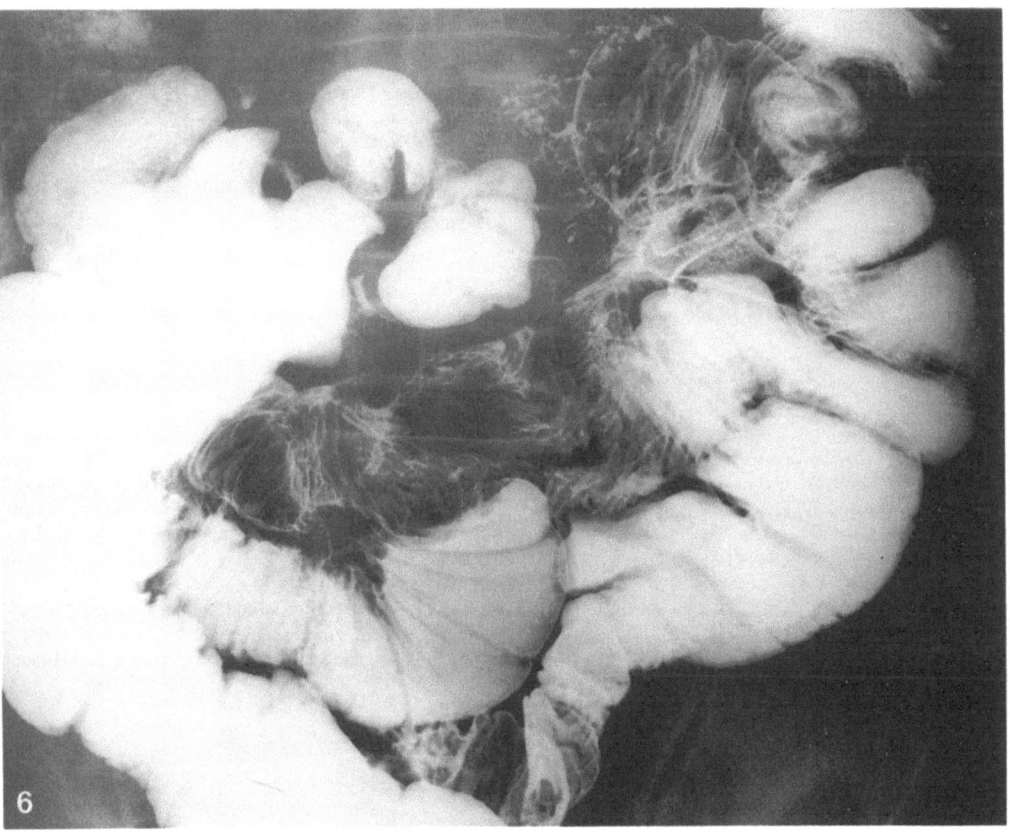

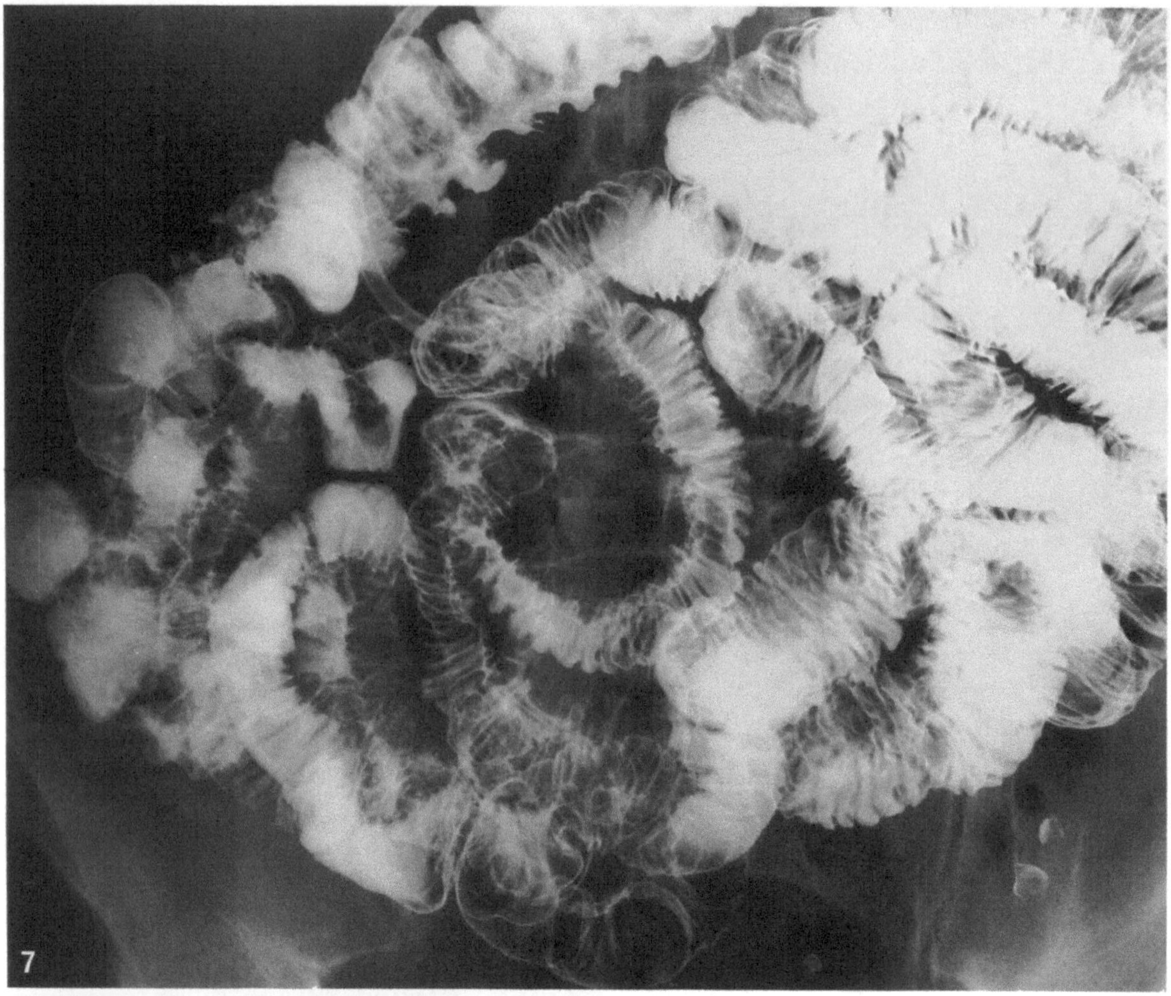

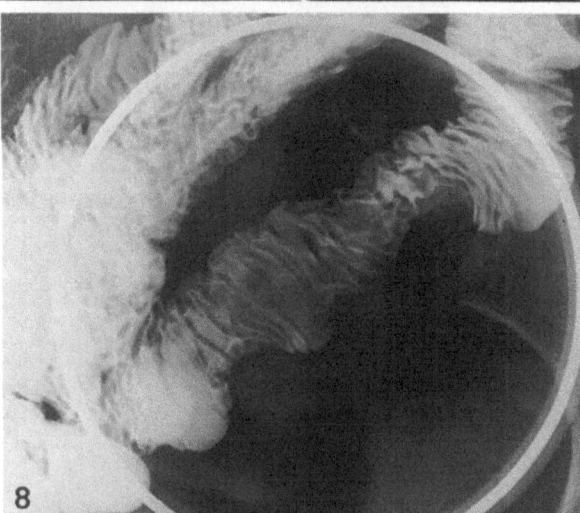

7

8

Fig. 7. Peritoneal carcinomatosis. 65-year-old man. Abdominal pain. Cancer of the bladder. SBFT : fixed ileal loops arranged concentrically with, in the right iliac foss, marginal spiculation along their mesenteric aspect

Fig. 8. Peritoneal metastases from an undifferentiated adenocarcinoma. 73-year-old woman. Anorexia. Weight loss, anemia. SBFT : marginal notches along the antimesenteric aspect of a jejunal loop

Computed tomography is very useful as it demonstrates the retractile hyperdensity of the mesentery, but the diagnosis is usually, nevertheless, only made at surgery.

In *tuberculous peritonitis* (fig. 16), the loops are fixed and angulated at several sites and are associated with ascites. In *peritonitis encapsulans* (figs. 17 and 18) of tuberculous origin, or secondary to long-lasting peritoneal dialysis, or to practotol therapy, most of the small intestinal loops are crowded in the centre of the abdomen to form a fixed, indissociable mass. The loops have an abnormal caliber and exhibit irregular margins. Computed tomography shows the peritoneal sac containing the loops, which are bordered by small areas of localized ascitic accumulations.

Practical conclusions

The extrinsic origin of small intestinal disease is suggested by abnormal position of loops (displaced, angulated), in particular when they are abnormally fixed, or if one side is retracted. This contrasts with the absence of mucosal ulcerations and the scarcity of nodulations.

References

Kidd R, Freeny PC (1982) Radiographic manifestations of extrinsic processes involving the bowel. Gastrointest radiol 7 : 21-28

Meyers M, Evans J (1973) Effects of pancreatitis on the small bowel and colon : spread along mesenteric planes. AJR 119 : 151-165

Régent D, Stines J, Claudon M, Soulard JM, Becker S, Treheux A (1986) Le syndrome pariétal extrinsèque du tube digestif. Feuillets de Radiologie 26 : 147-168

Malignant tumors

Wittich G, Salomonowitz E, Szepesi T, Czembirek H, Fruehwald F (1985) Small bowel double-contrast enema in stage III ovarian cancer. AJR 142 : 299-304

Yuhasz M, Laufer I, Sutton G, Herlinger H, Caroline DG (1985) Radiography of the small bowel in patients with gynecologic malignancies. AJR 144 : 303-307

Endometriosis

Boles RS, Hodes PJ (1958) Endometriosis of the small and large intestine. Gastroenterology 34 : 367-380

Counseller VS, Crenshaw JL (1951) A clinical and surgical review of endometriosis. Am J Gynecol 62 : 939-942

Fagan CJ (1974) Endometriosis clinical and roentgenographic manifestations. Radiol Clin North Am 12 : 109-124

Livolsi VA, Perzin KH (1974) Endometriosis of the small intestine, producing intestinal obstruction or simulating neoplasm. Digestive Diseases 19 : 100-107

Nitsch B, Ho CS, Cullen J (1988) Barium study of small bowel endometriosis. Gastrointest Radiol 13 : 361-363

Tavernier C, Jourde L, Dhamlencourt AM, Delafolie A (1980) Endométriose colique, diagnostic radiologique. J Radiol 61 : 437-445

Retractile mesenteritis

Aach RD, Kahn LI, Frech RS (1968) Obstruction of the small intestine due to retractile mesenteritis. Gastroenterology 54 : 594-598

Bendon JA, Poleynard GD, Bordin GM (1979) Fibrosing mesenteritis simulating pelvic carcinomatosis. Gastrointest Radiol 4 : 195-197

Caubria F, Cerf M (1973) Panniculites mésentériques et mésentérites rétractiles. RP 23 : 2827-2836

Clemett AR, Tracht DT (1969) The roentgen diagnosis of retractile mesenteritis. AJR 107 : 787-790

Gudinche F, Schnyder P (1987) Mesenteric panniculitis. Acta Radiol 28 : 727-729

Kopecky KK, Lappas JC, Baker MK, Madura JA (1988) Mesenteric panniculitis : CT appearance. Gastrointest Radiol 13 : 273-274

Maroy B, Bou G, Duroselle C (1985) Diagnostic radiologique pré-opératoire d'une mésentérite rétractile, efficacité prolongée d'une résection localisée. Ann Radiol 28 : 65-67

Maroy B, Benderbouz N, Tubiana JM, Aly Y, Leconte D, Parc R (1981) Occlusion régressive sur fibrose mésentérique en bande. Ann Radiol 24 : 647-650

Nouel O, Eugène C, Gilson J, Marche C (1975) Entéropathie exsudative et mésentérite rétractile. Arch Fr Mal App Dig 64 : 233-238

Seigel RS, Kuhns LR, Borlaza GS, McCormick TL, Simmons JL (1980) Computed tomography and angiography in ileal carcinoid tumor and retractile mesenteritis. Radiology 134 : 437-440

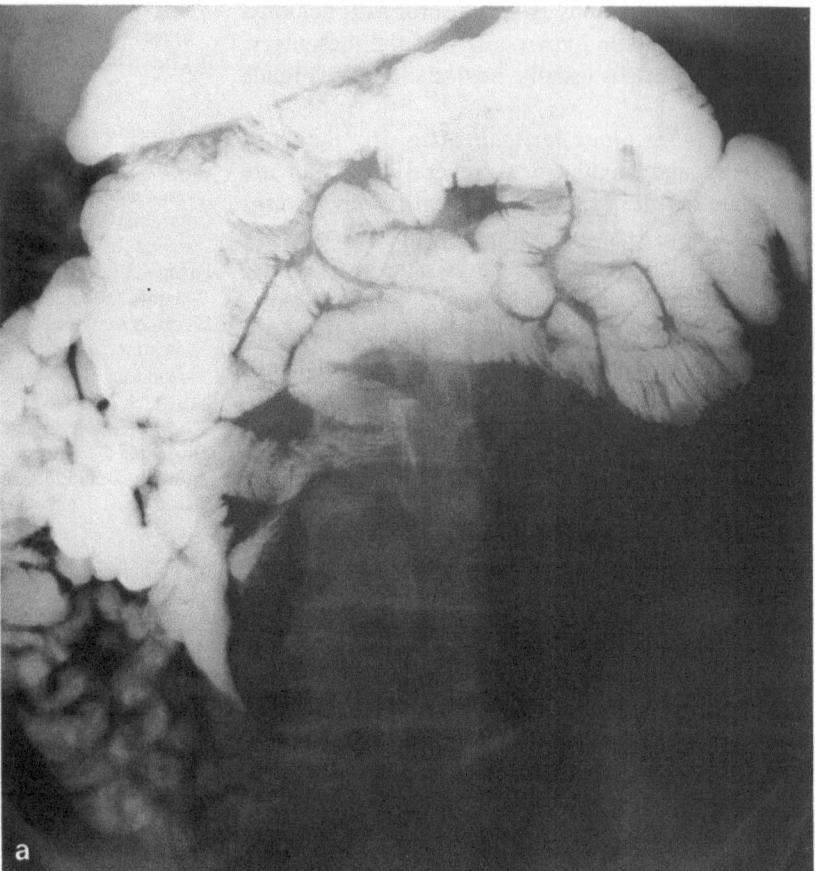

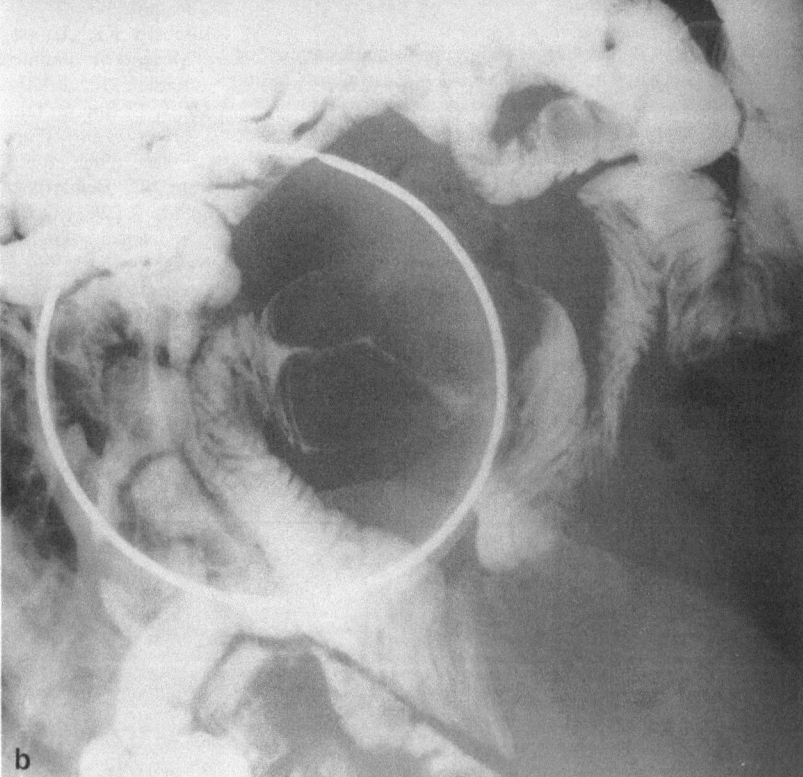

Fig. 9 a ,b. Invasion of a neighbouring cancer into a loop of small intestine. 43-year-old man. Mass in the left iliac fossa and poor general condition **a** SBFT : void image in the left iliac fossa, displacing the loops of small intestine **b** SBFT: flattened and nodulated jejunal loop

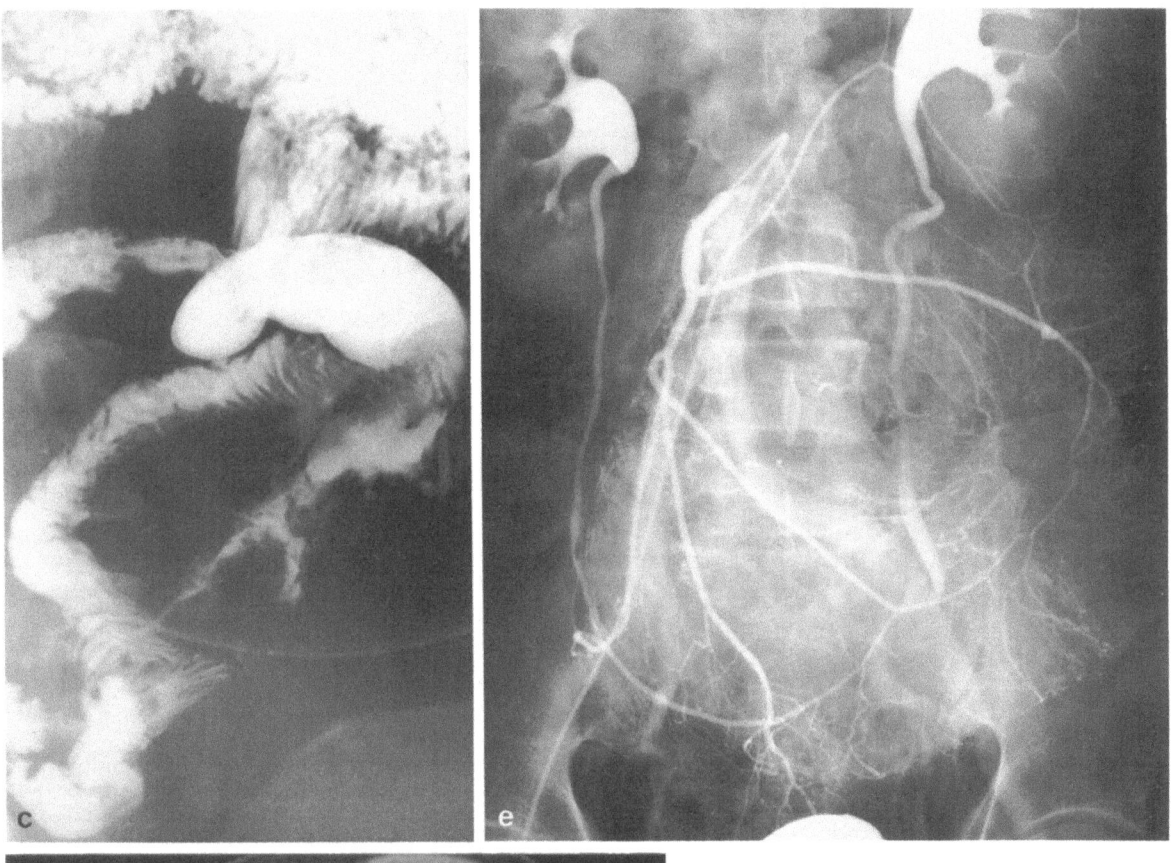

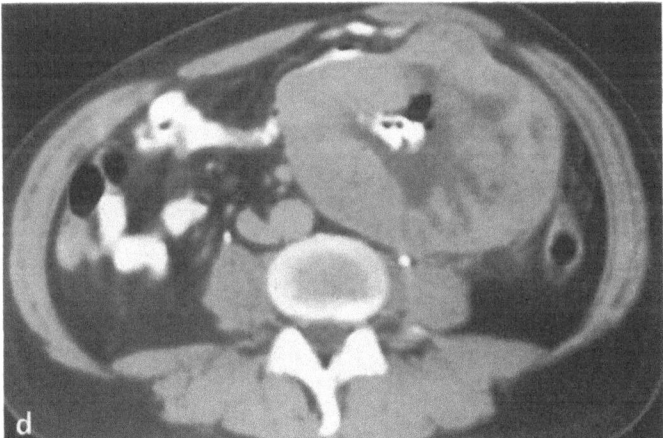

Fig. 9 c-e. c SBFT : barium pool between two jejunal loops, **d** computed tomography : necrotic mass in the left iliac fossa, with a central concentration of barium and gas, **e** mesenteric arteriography : hypervascular mass. Surgical findings : fibrohistiocytosarcoma of the sigmoid mesocolon

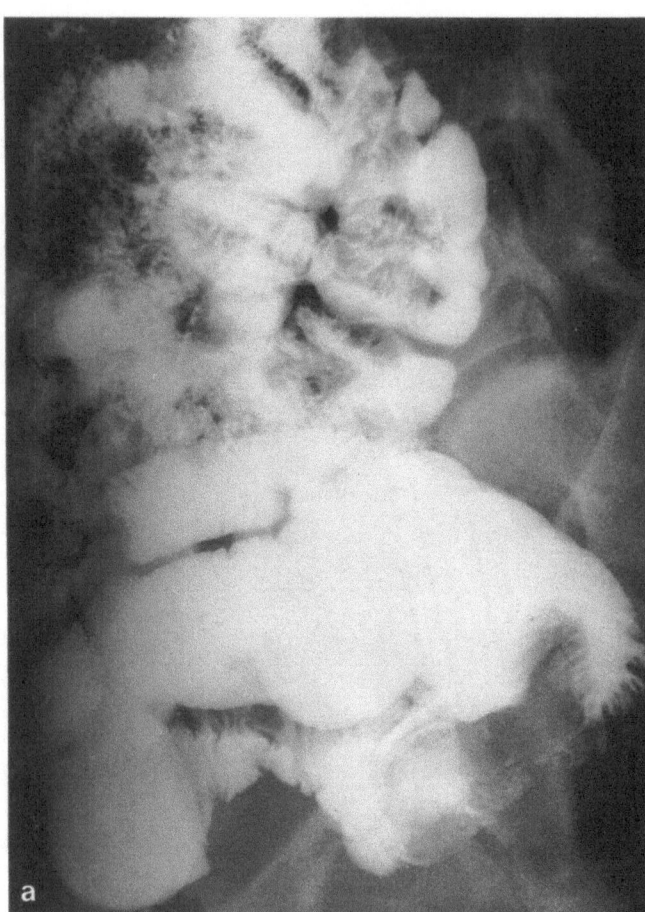

Fig. 10 a-c. Endometriosis. 33-year-old woman. Periodic low abdominal pain. SBFT : **a** stenosis of a pelvic loop with preserved mucosal folds, **b** marginal notches, gathered and spiculated margins of an ileal loop fixed in the right iliac fossa, **c** double contrast barium enema : identical appearance in the lower sigmoid loop

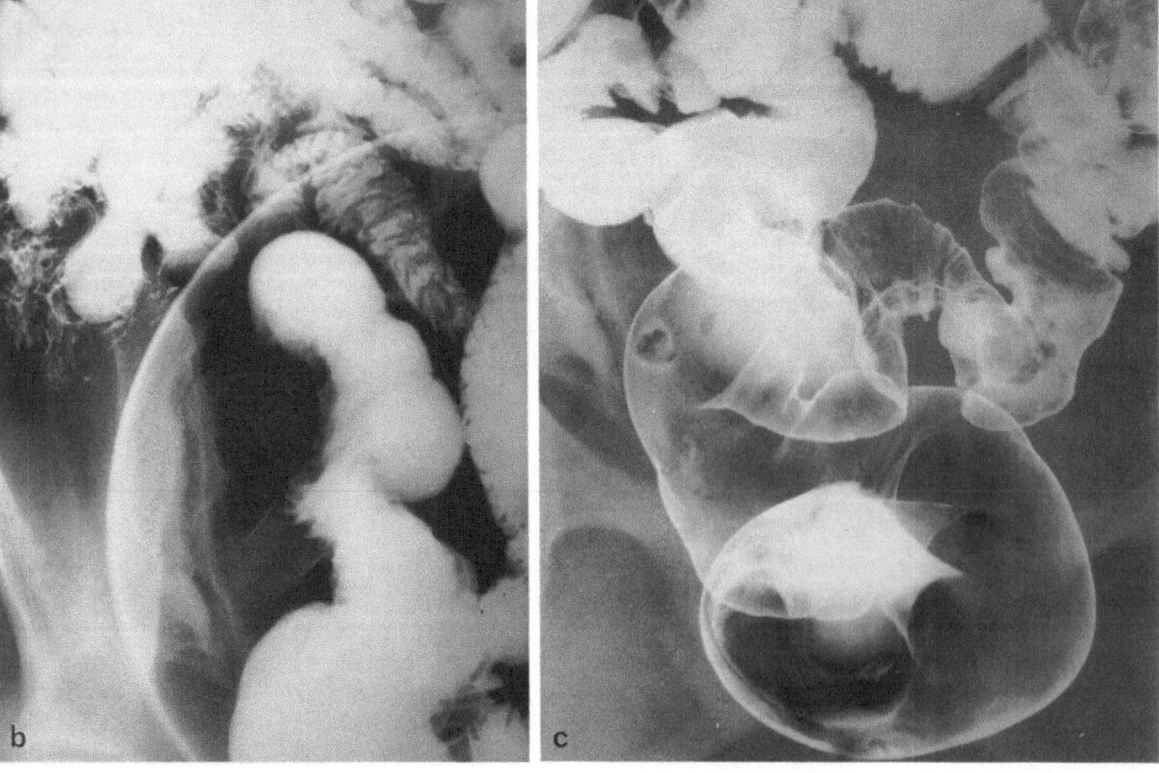

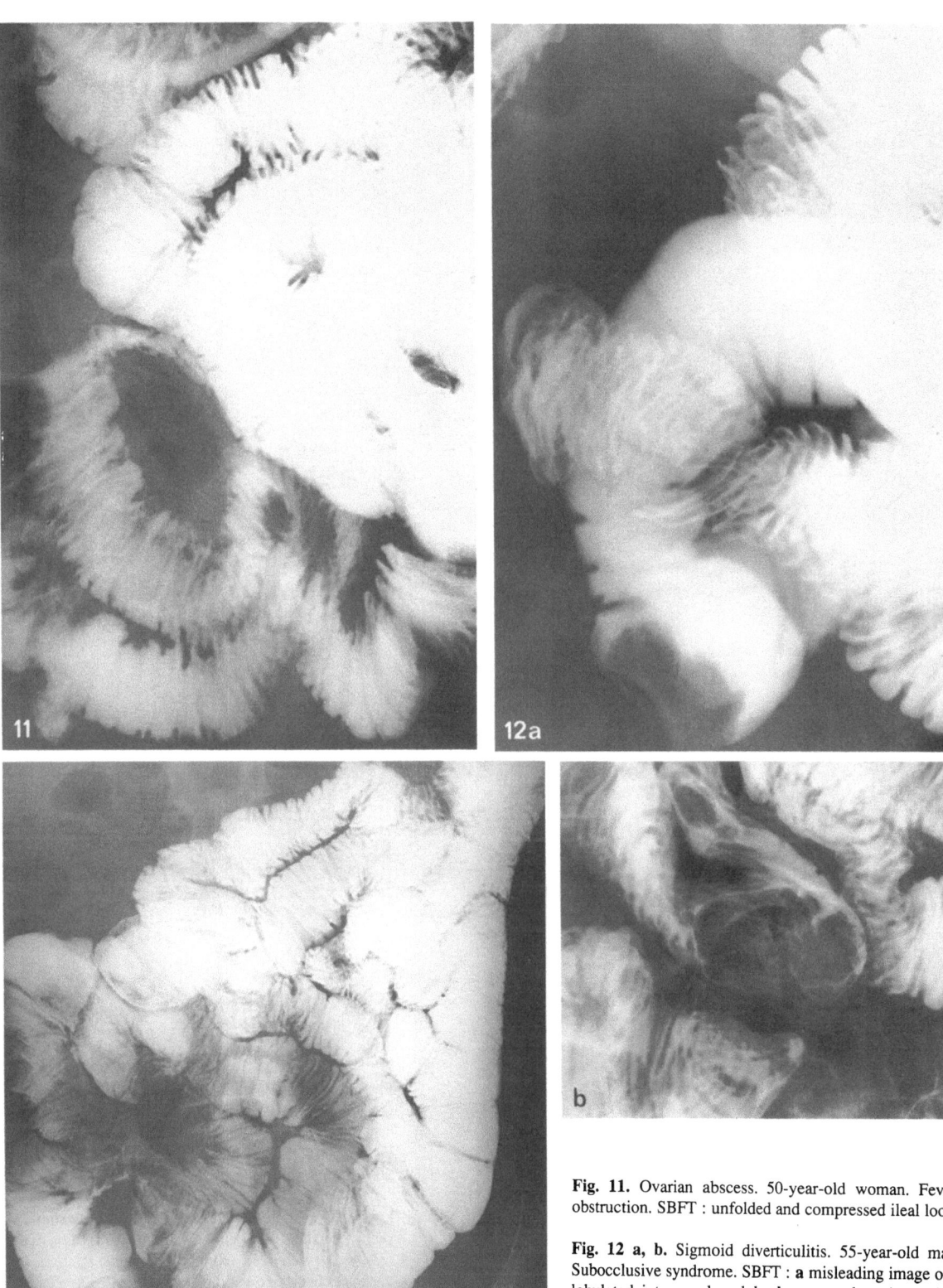

Fig. 11. Ovarian abscess. 50-year-old woman. Fever, obstruction. SBFT : unfolded and compressed ileal loop

Fig. 12 a, b. Sigmoid diverticulitis. 55-year-old man. Subocclusive syndrome. SBFT : **a** misleading image of a lobulated intramural nodule. **b** omega-shaped marginal notch. Surgical findings : ileosigmoid fistula

Fig. 13. Mesenteritis following pancreatitis. 32-year-old man. Episode of abdominal pain and diarrhea 6 months after edematous pancreatitis. SBFT : fixed, angulated ileal loops with marginal notches

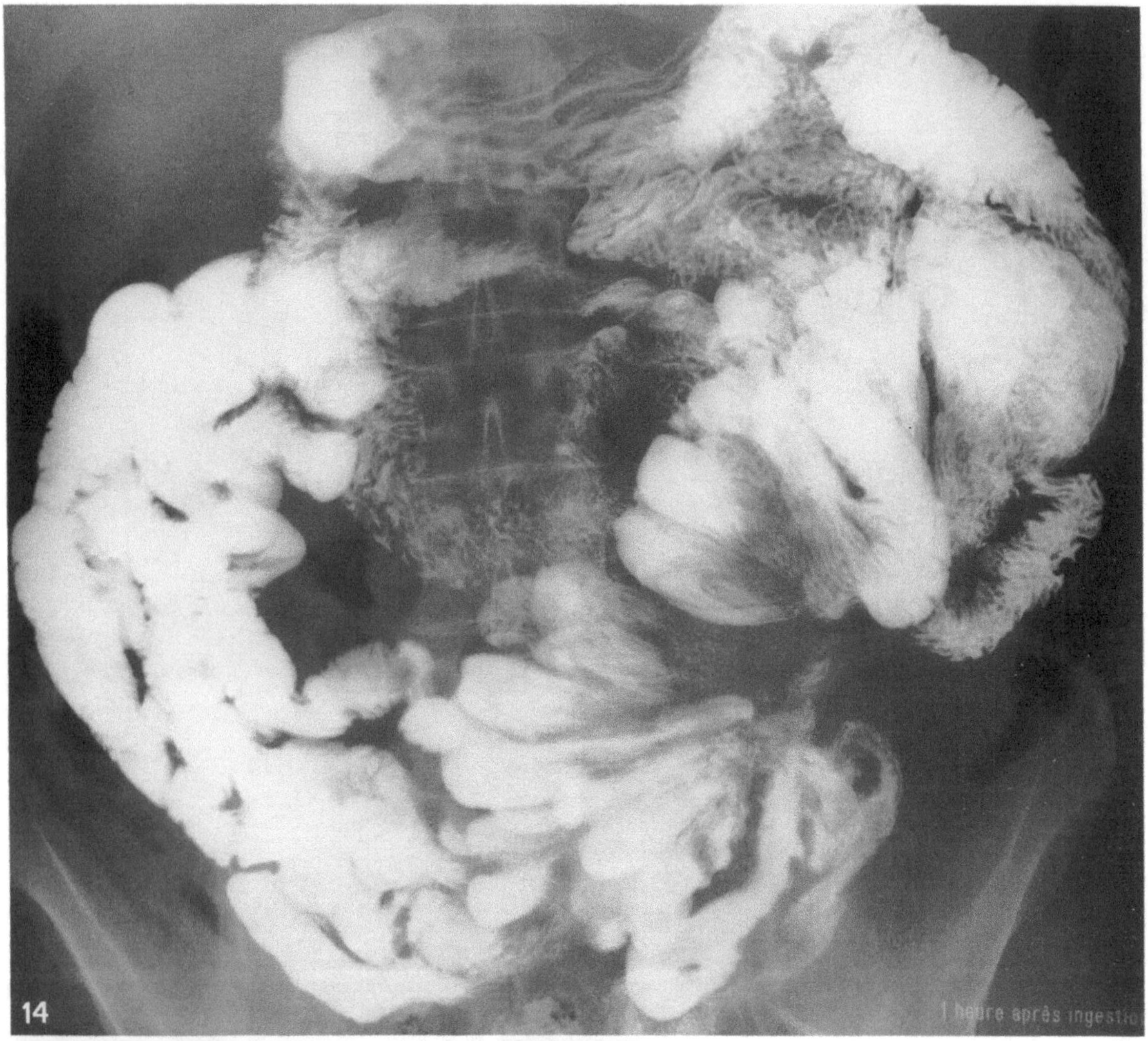

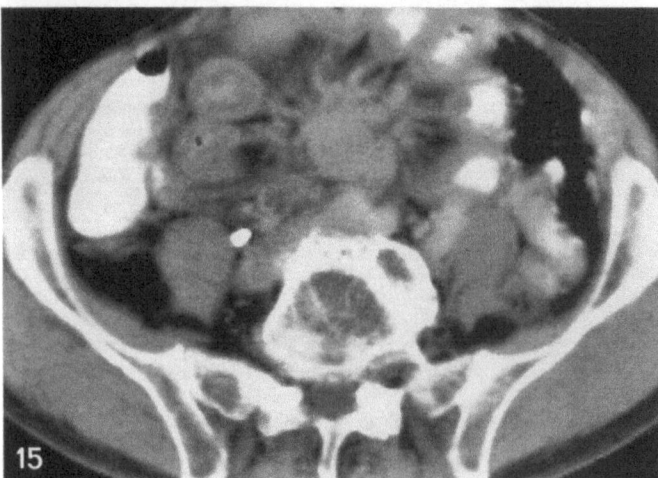

14

1 heure après ingestion

15

Fig. 14. Retractile mesenteritis. 62-year-old diabetic woman. Peritoneal dialysis during the past 2 years. Sub-occlusion. SBFT : star-shapped arrangement of the fixed distal jejunal loops, suggesting local mesenteric retraction with proximal distention

Fig. 15. Mesenteric retraction (Courtesy of M Piante). 78-year-old man. Long-lasting abdominal pain. Mass in the right side : carcinoid tumour. Computed tomography: thickened lines arranged in a star-shaped pattern caused by mesenteric retraction

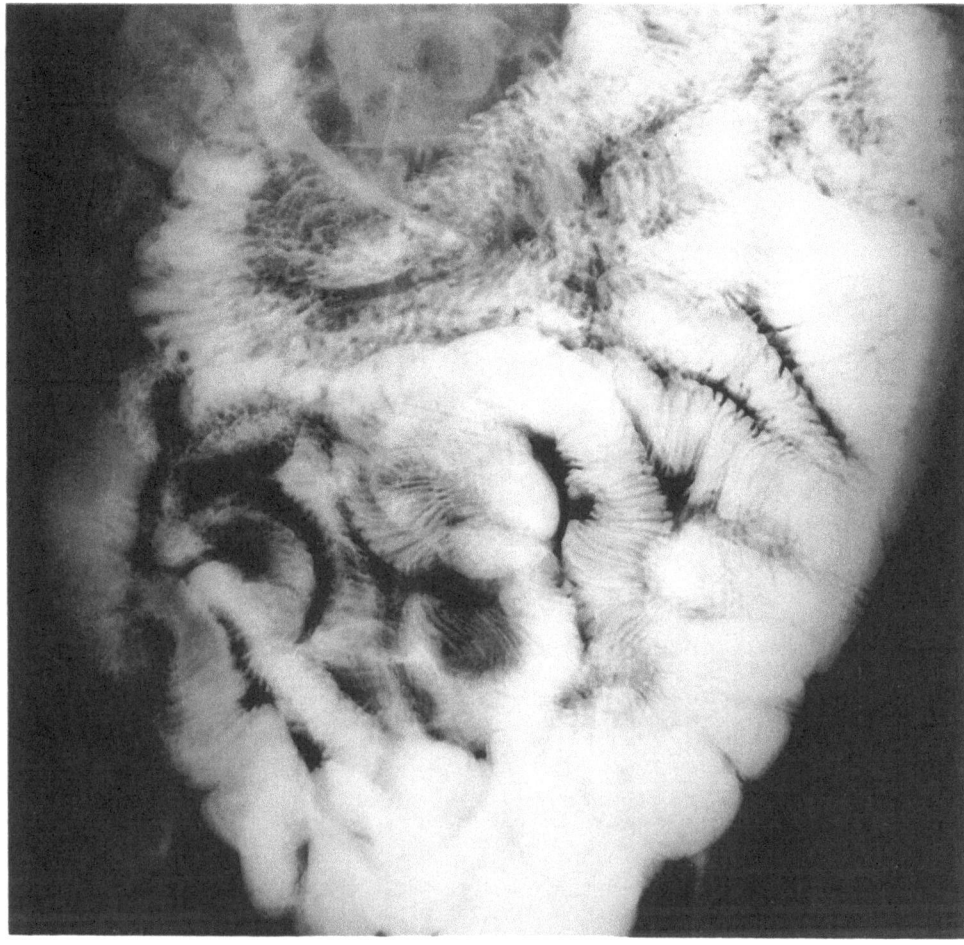

Fig. 16. Tuberculous peritonitis. 40-year-old : North African man. Poor general condition. Inflammatory syndrome. SBFT : unfolded, angulated ileal loops with marginal notches (adenopathy). Laparoscopy : peritoneal granulation (positive findings for Koch's bacillum)

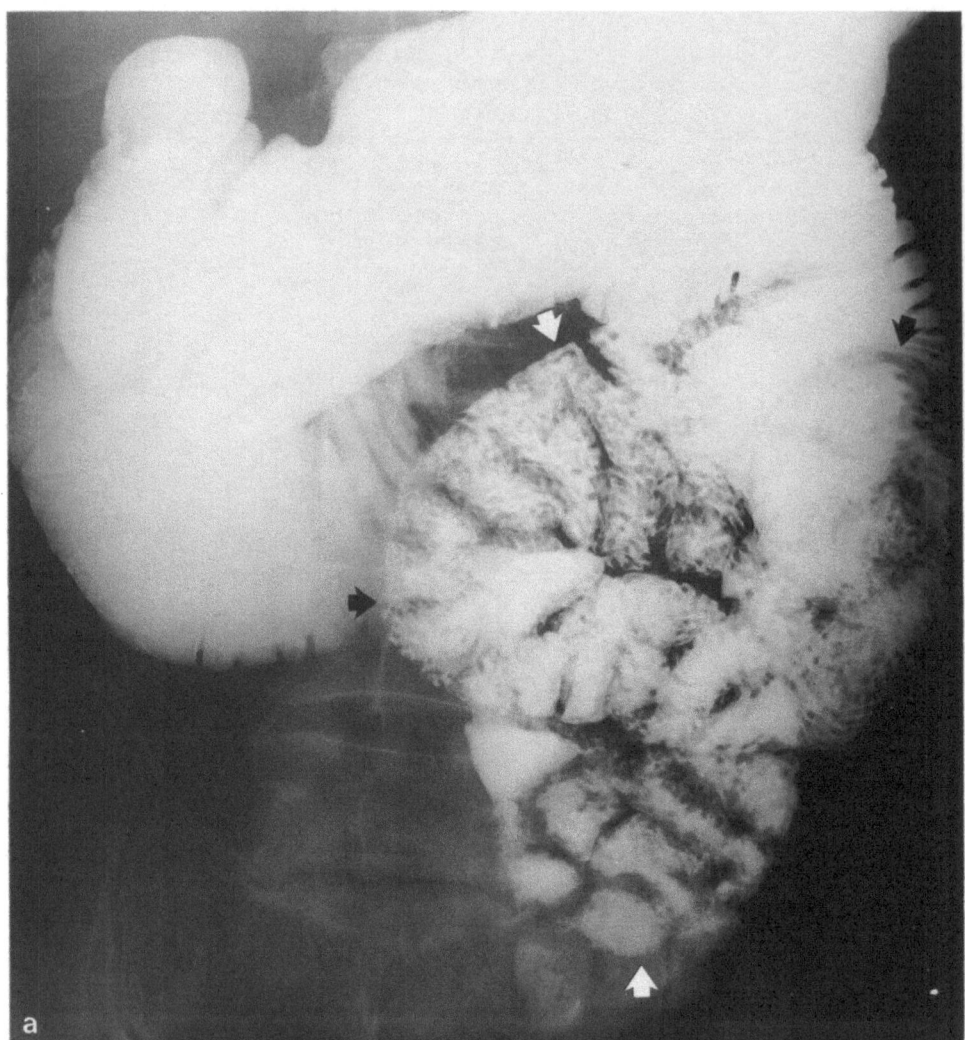

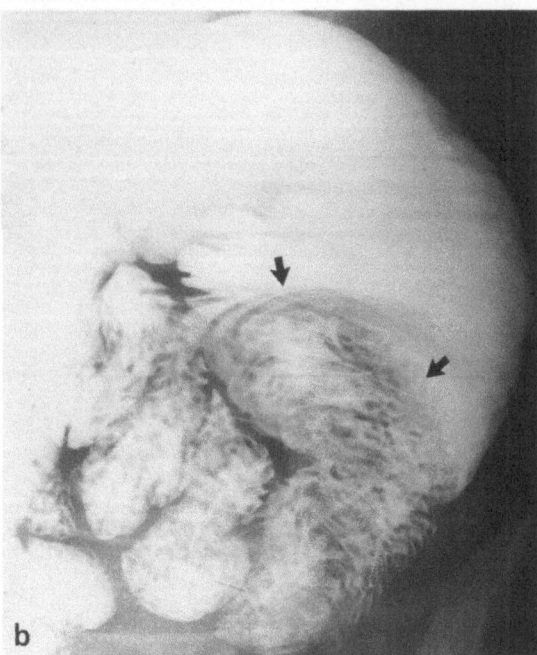

Fig. 17 a, b. Peritonitis encapsulans. 48-year-old man. Painful epigastric syndrome with weight loss. SBFT : **a** abnormal arrangement of the jejunal loops, which are grouped in a round cluster **b** duodenojejunal distention with early jejunojejunal intussusception

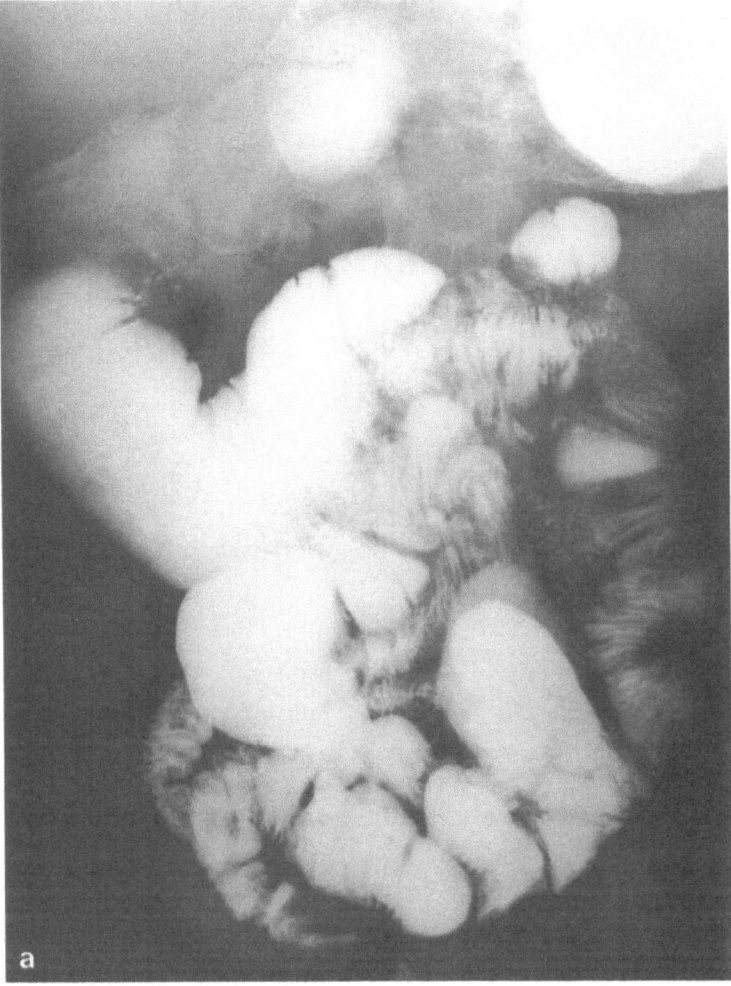

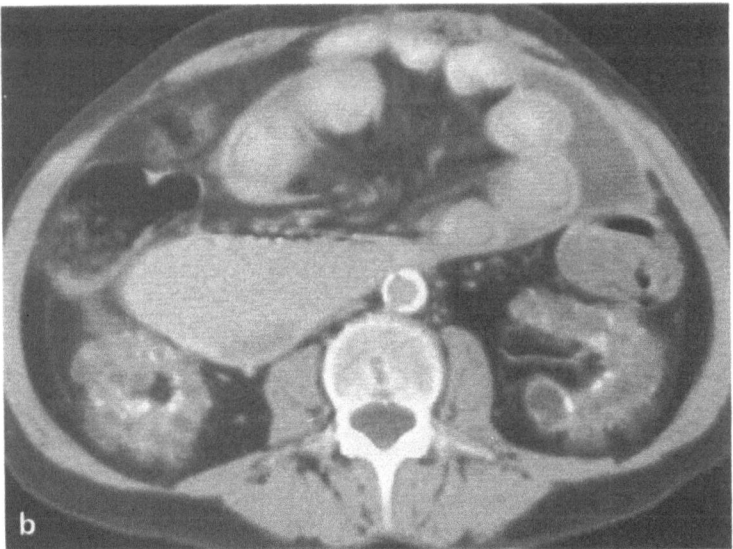

Fig. 18 a, b. Peritonitis encapsulans (Courtesy of D Fond). 62-year-old man. Peritoneal dialysis during the past 15 years . Abdominal pain and subocclusion. **a** SBFT : crowded jejunal loops forming a round cluster with alternating enlarged and narrowed segments. Proximal duodenal dilatation, **b** computed tomography : cluster of duodenal loops contained in a sac and bordered by fluid collection with proximal duodenal dilatation

The postoperative patient

For didactic reasons, we have studied first the normal and pathological appearances produced by small intestinal surgery, and then those observed after gastric surgery.

Postsurgical small intestine

Normal images

The treatment of short stenoses with jejunoplasty or ileoplasty produces local, more or less saccular expansions, sometimes angulated or folded and centered on longitudinal linear structures outlined by converging folds (fig. 1).

After the resection of one or several loops of small intestine for a segmental disease, the anastomosis is end to end as a rule. It may be difficult to detect if no metallic staples are visible. It is sometimes marked by a moderate annular narrowing or by small mucosal nodules of no pathological significance. The side to side, or side to end anastomoses (figs. 2 and 3) are only performed as palliative procedures nowadays, in cases of tumours or adhesions that cannot be excised. The ectatic image of the blind loop must not be confused with that of a diverticulum or with the barium pool appearance of a tumour.

The inversion of a loop of small intestine aimed at slowing down intestinal transit has practically ceased to be performed. Bypass surgery can be carried out in cases of extreme obesity. Payne's procedure consists of a side-to-end shunt preserving a 35 cm long segment of jejunum and a 10 cm long portion of ileum. The shunt is end-to-end in Scott's

procedure, with the excluded segment bypassing intestinal contents to the terminal or sigmoid colon.

The opacification of the intestinal tract during radiological studies must be continuous in order to assess transit time and the length of the remaining intestine. The loops can be enlarged and reach up to 5 or 6 cm in width. A microspiculated, punctated superficial appearance indicating compensatory villous hypertrophy (fig. 4) can be observed especially in the ileum after extensive resection.

After biliodigestive bypass surgery with a hepaticojejunal or choledocojejunal anastomosis, the anastomosis cannot always be demonstrated, especially after establishment of a roux-en-Y loop (fig. 5), in which reflux of barium is not always possible.

Anastomoses of the small intestine and colon, often in the form of ileotransversostomy with right hemicolectomy, are readily demonstrated because of the different calibers of both segments and of the differing appearance of the folds. The anastomosis is mainly end-to-end rarely side-to-side or sid- to-end anastomosis.

A continent ileostomy is currently performed when it is possible rather than a simple ileostomy following complete colectomy for ulcerative colitis or familial polyposis. The pouch is made up of an ileal loop opened longitudinally and sutured to form a «J» shape (fig. 6) or sometimes an «S» shape ; it is connected to the abdominal wall by an invaginated segment. The pocket has a capacity ranging from 200 to 500 cm3 and it can be opacified by SBFT or retrogradely, which permits the study of the folds, of the sutures and of the invaginated loop.

In the case of recurrent occlusion or of multiple adhesions, the loops of small intestine can be fixed by the Childs-Philips procedure (joining the

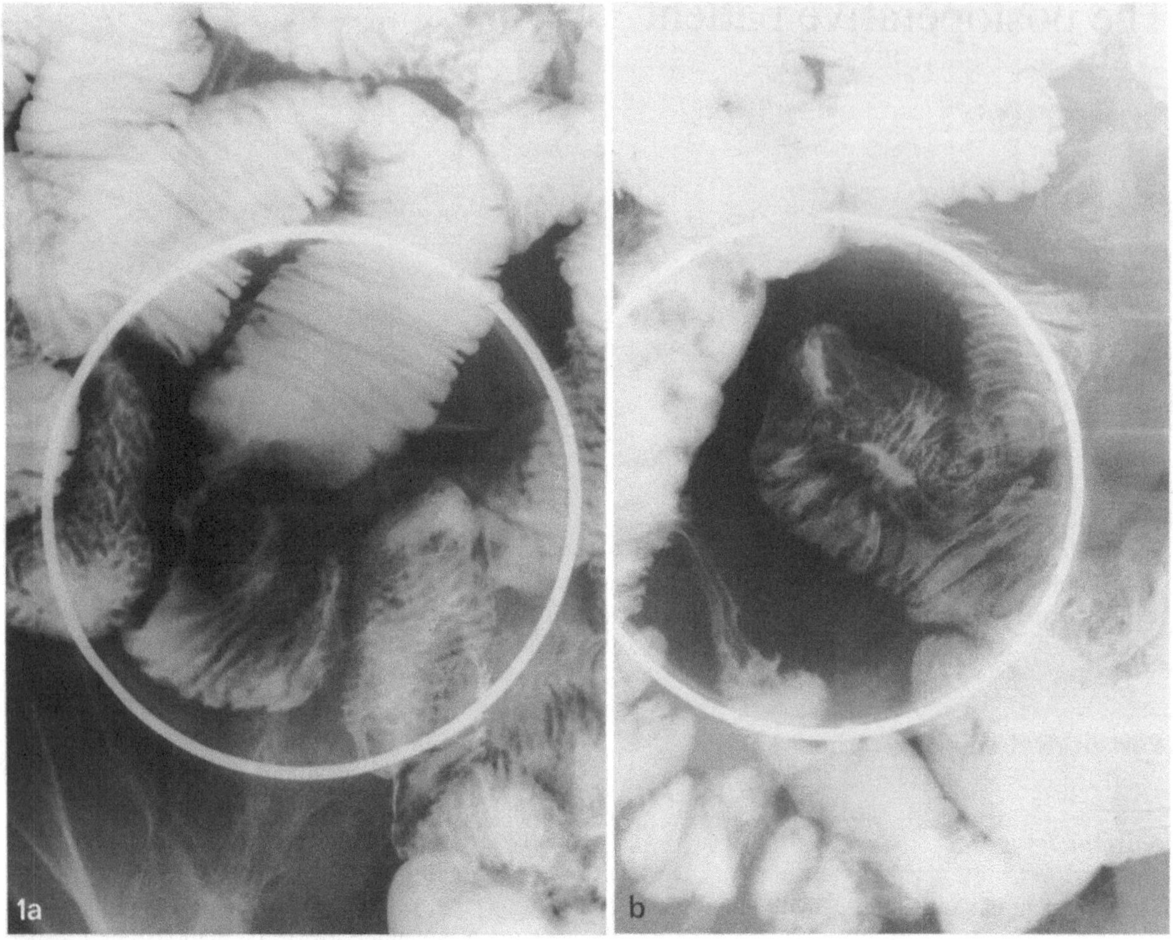

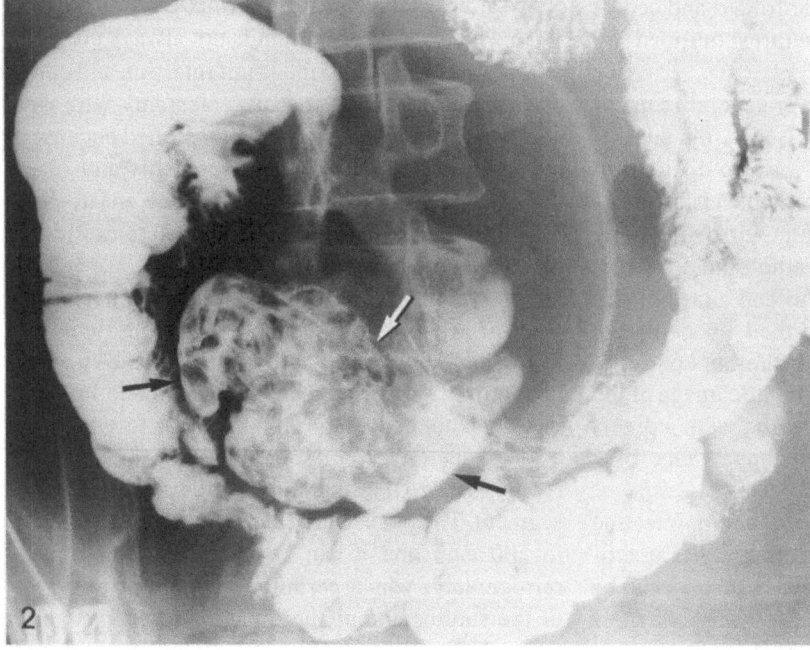

Fig. 1 a, b. Ileoplasty. SBFT : **a** ileal stenosis in Crohn's disease, **b** image following ileoplasty

Fig. 2. Blind loop following ileoileal anastomosis. 57-year-old man. Subocclusive syndrome 40 years after transient ileostomy for complicated appendicectomy. SBFT : diverticulum containing foreign bodies and connected to an ileoileal anastomosis

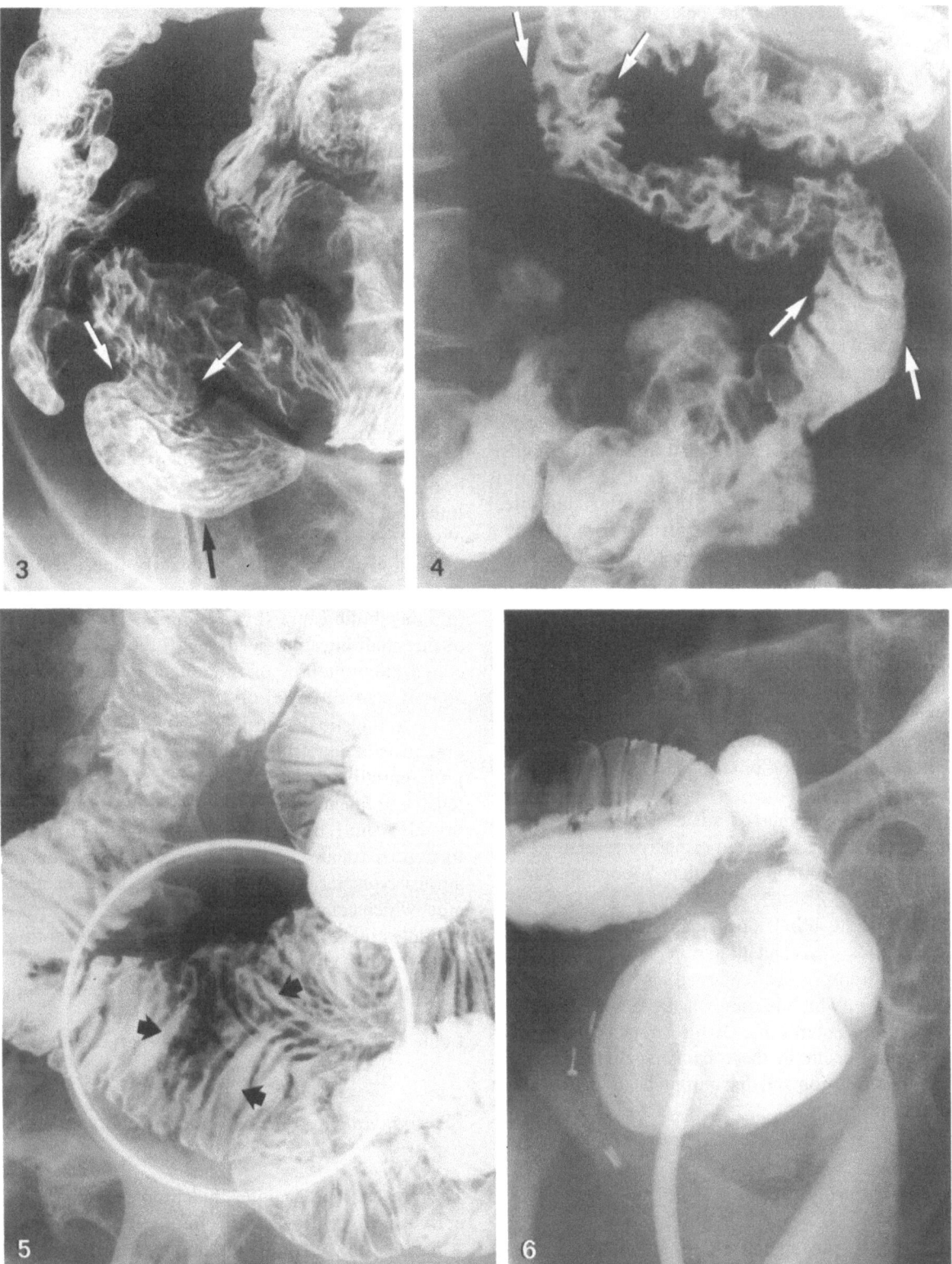

Fig. 3. Blind loop following side-to-end ileoileal anastomosis. 48-year-old man. Mild bowel habit changes and meteorism 11 years after appendicectomy having led to a subsequent intestinal resection. SBFT : postoperative diverticulum

Fig. 4. Villous hypertrophy following extensive ileal resection. SBFT : punctated superficial appearance and marginal microspiculation in the terminal ileum

Fig. 5. Biliodigestive anastomosis. SBFT : extremity of the anastomotic Roux-en-Y loop

Fig. 6. Ileoanal anastomosis. Barium enema : j-shaped ileal pouch

mesenteric layers by U-shaped sutures) or Noble's procedure (side to side suture of the loops) (fig. 7). Radiology shows parallel, transverse or fixed loops.

Complications

Functional abnormalities

Functional abnormalities can be caused by extensive resection or stasis. They occur as a diarrheic syndrome with malabsorption. When resection preserves less than one meter of the small intestine, absorption is no longer sufficient and it must be compensated for by chronic parenteral feeding. Some forms of selective malabsorption occur after short ileal resection. If an intestinal segment is bypassed by a side-to-side or end-to-side anastomosis, or if stasis occurs proximal to an area of anastomotic stenosis, bacterial overgrowth may cause malabsorption (anemia, hypoproteinemia, steatorrhea) and diarrhea, producing the «blind loop» syndrome. Disruption of the enterohepatic circulation of biliary salts aggravates diarrhea because of the laxative action of the biliary salts in the colon and can lead to specific complications including biliary and oxalic renal calculi formation.

The SBFT must permit assessment of the length of the intestine left after extensive resection. It is shorter than 100 cm if less than 5 loops are preserved.

In the blind loop syndrome, the SBFT demonstrates stasis and dilatation proximal to a narrowed anastomosis or an enlarged and hypotonic bypass segment in which barium stagnates with debris and sometimes enteroliths. Diffuse signs of malabsorption may occur in these cases, including contrast medium dilution and discontinuous dilatation of the intestinal loops.

Anastomotic lesions

In the early postoperative period, iodinated contrast media are used rather than barium to search for leakage.

Examinations with barium are performed later to detect complications such as stenosis, fistulae, abscesses, ulceration or an inflammatory polyp likely to bleed. The anastomosis must be carefully palpated because the lesion may be small. It is sometimes difficult to differentiate a normal anastomosis from a narrowed one. In Crohn's disease, ulcerations appearing on both ends of the anastomosis indicate recurrence (fig. 8).

Peritoneal adhesions (figs. 9 to 14)

Any abdominal operation can cause the formation of adhesions, either as layers of flexible connective tissue or hard sclerotic tissue, or as lines, several millimeters to one centimeter wide, often multiple. They can appear within a couple of days. The clinical signs of these complications are those of complete or partial small bowel obstruction. Plain radiographs demonstrate air-fluid levels. Obstruction must be differentiated from a postoperative paralytic ileus. Intestinal paresis without air-fluid levels is a normal physiological phenomenon lasting two or three days following surgery. An inflammatory ileus, also involving the entire colon, can occur later, rarely due to a metabolic cause (hypokalemia). The dilatation of the small intestine by air and fluid, without associated abnormalities of the colon, is therefore the sign of a small bowel obstruction.

If intestinal obstruction is incomplete or if the diagnosis is doubtful, a barium study is performed, preferentially with enteroclysis. The diagnosis of extensive or linear adhesions is easy if the examination reveals a short, tight stenosis with apparent fold distortion. A transverse notch or mucosal spiculation are also typical if associated with fixity in the abnormal area, which cannot be displaced by palpation. Proximal intestinal dilatation contrasting with the normal distal caliber is obviously important for diagnosis. The signs can be more discrete, with distended loops alternating with normal loops and fixity being difficult to demonstrate (retrovesical pelvic loops).

Internal and external hernias, eventration (fig. 15)

The presence of an intestinal loop in an external hernia or eventration is easily demonstrated as a rule. A fluoroscopic examination during efforts to cough or a tangential radiograph can be useful for the diagnosis.

When an internal hernia appears through a fissure in a mesocolon, the involved loops are crowded in a sac. They can be enlarged and contrast with the normal caliber of the distal loops. Dilatation sometimes appears in loops located proximal to the hernia.

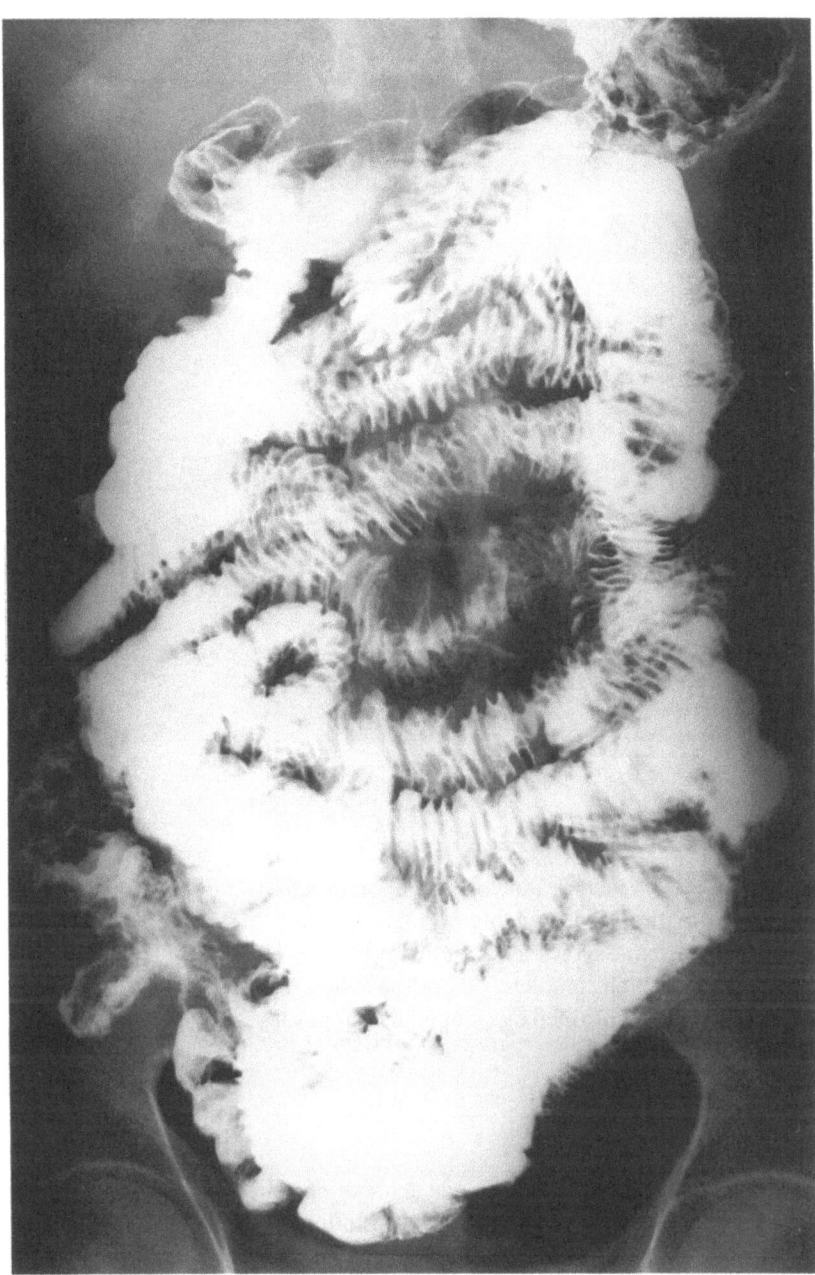

Fig. 7. Noble's procedure. SBFT : fixed, parallel midabdominal loops. Moderate disruption of folds pattern

Foreign bodies (figs. 16 to 19)

Inflammatory pseudotumours and granulomas (which histologically might suggest Crohn's disease if no bi-refringent crystals were seen) can be caused by talc on the surgical gloves. This explains why talc has been replaced by starch powder.

Significant surgical complications are caused by compresses, wads, operative fields and, more rarely, instruments left in the abdomen. The foreign body can cause an abscess or migrate into the lumen of a neighbouring loop through a fistula.

Plain films of the abdomen demonstrate the foreign body if it is radiopaque. A compress appears as an opacity punctated with light spots.

Barium studies reveal signs of mesenteric involvement with fixed loops and extrinsic compression. If the compress has migrated into an intestinal

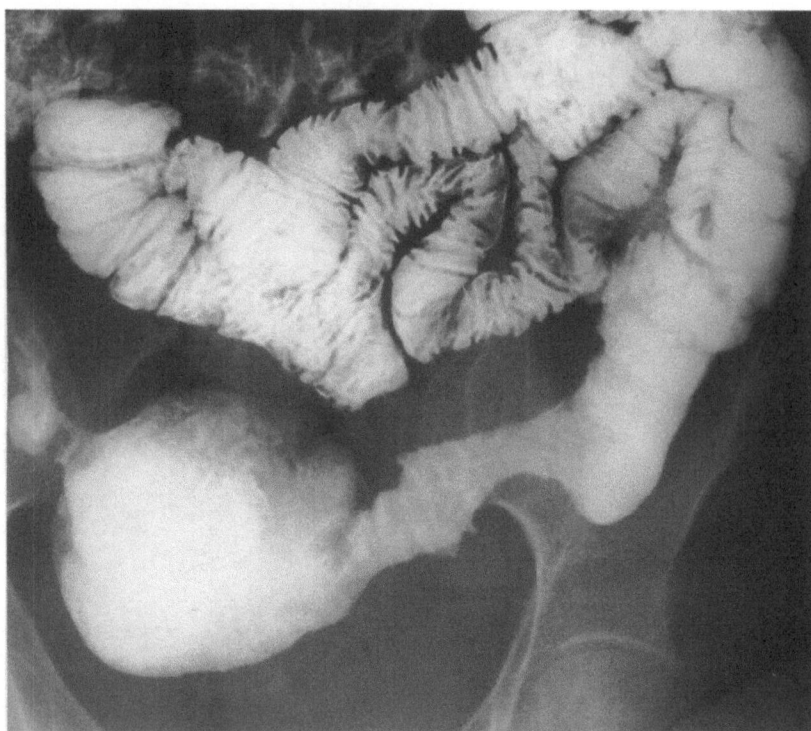

Fig. 8. Recurrence of Crohn's disease in a side to side ileoileal anastomosis. SBFT: stenosis of the terminal loop. Saccular dilatation of the superimposed pouches. Ulcerondonodular pattern proximally

loop, its appearance is that of an endoluminal fibrillar formation with variably regular contours.

Ultrasound shows a very typical hyperechogenic image which completely stops the echos. This finding may be confirmed by computed tomography.

Other complications

Early or late complications include acute or chronic ischemia (due to the perioperative obstruction of a blood vessel, to volvulus, to linear adhesions or to a hernia), intussusception or pneumatosis cystoides intestinalis.

Practical conclusions

Postoperative complications are searched for during the first week with plain radiographs and, if need be, by opacification with a water soluble iodinated contrast medium. Barium studies play an important part in the later search for complications, primarily extensive or linear adhesions, anastomotic lesions and residual foreign bodies.

The small intestine following gastric surgery

Normal images

Vagotomy, pyloroplasty, superior pole gastrectomy and gastrectomy with gastroduodenal anastomosis (Péan, Billroth I) can cause an increase in the jejunal caliber and sometimes intestinal hypotonia. Complete gastrectomy with esophagojejunal anastomosis exhibits similar effects. In addition to fistulae or loose sutures, which can occur in any type of operation, gastroenteroanastomosis and partial gastrectomy with gastrojejunostomy (Polya, Finsterer, Billroth II) cause specific complications.

A common appearance near the anastomosis is that of broadened folds or of increased height and density of the folds (palisading folds) without associated clinical symptoms.

Pathological images

Dumping syndrome

Observed in 5 to 10% of patients undergoing Polya-type surgery causes postprandial digestive discom-

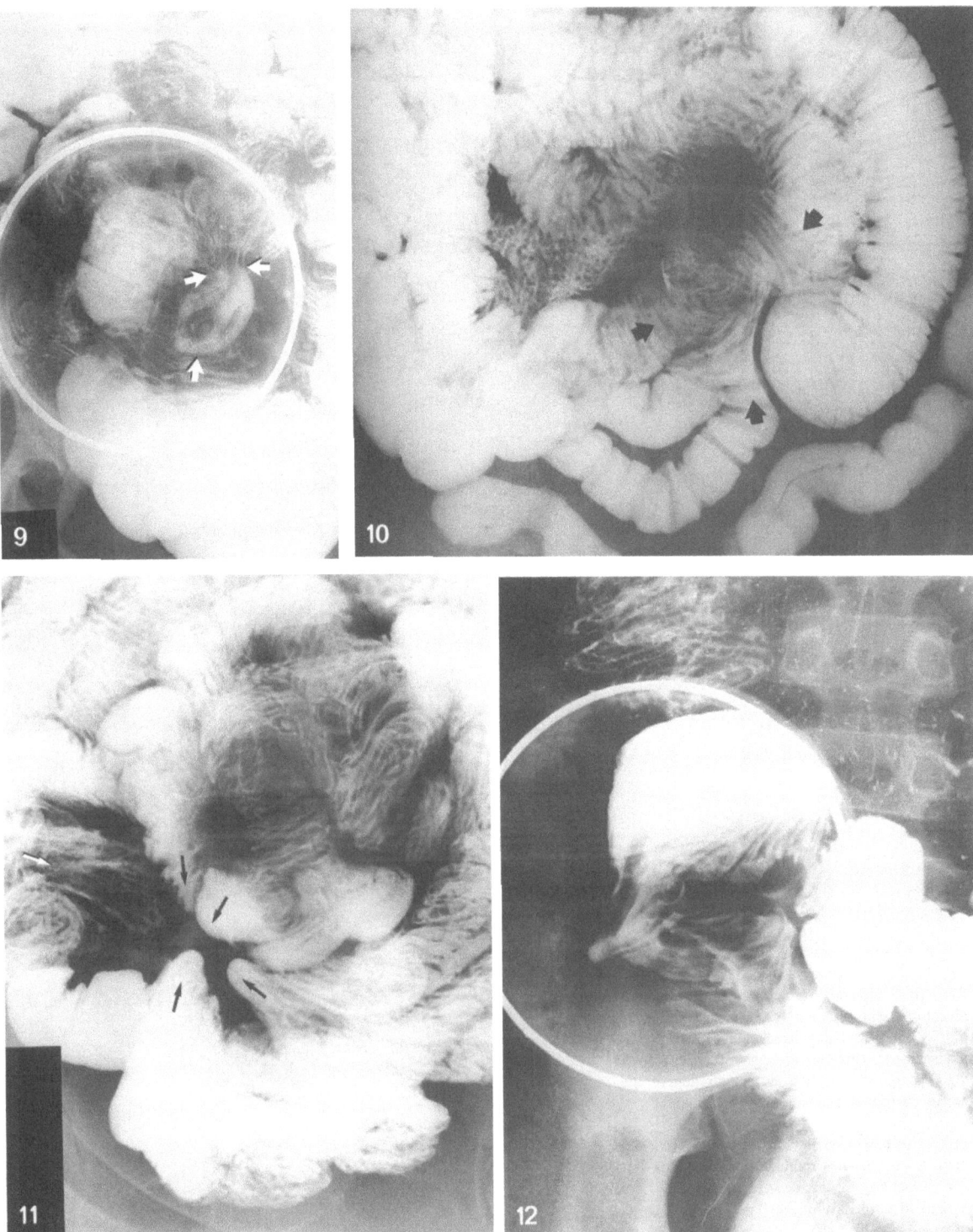

Fig. 9. Postoperative adhesion. 80-year-old man. Subocclusion, 7 years after sigmoidectomy for a villous tumour. SBFT : sacculation and folds radiating into a diverticular formation, which surgery identified as a cluster of ileal loops in the area of peritonization

Fig. 10. Postoperative adhesion. 60-year-old man. Hemorrhagic diarrhea and vomiting 2 months after resection of a Meckel's diverticulum with a leiomyoma. SBFT : two rigid, angulated ileal loops fixed to each other

Fig. 11. Postoperative adhesion. 45-year-old woman. Sigmoidectomy for a cancer. Failed attempt at restoring continuity due to fibrosing peritonitis. SBFT : angulated and fixed ileal loops arranged in a star-shaped pattern

Fig. 12. Postoperative adhesion. 13-year-old boy operated at 4 days of age for intestinal atresia. Subocclusive episode. SBFT : angulated and fixed ileal loop in the right iliac fossa

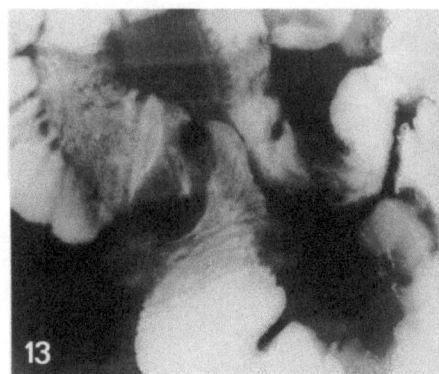

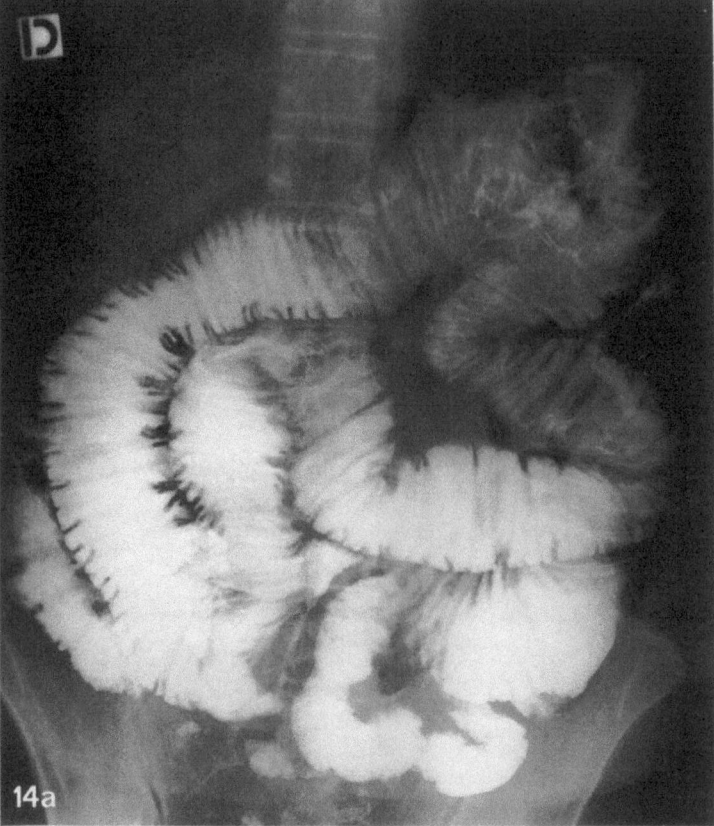

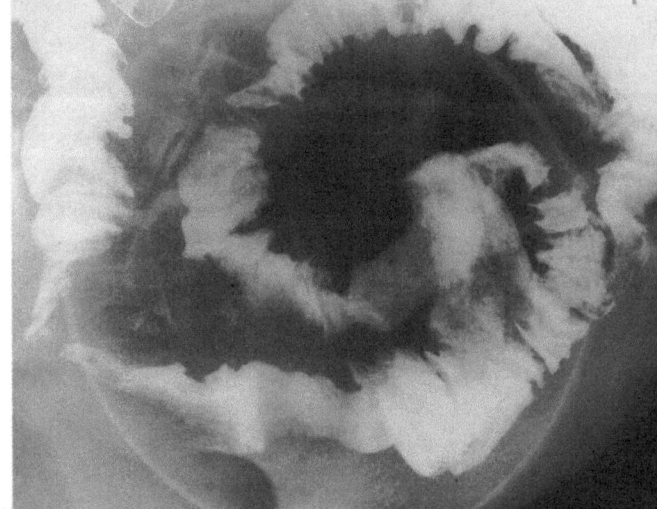

Fig. 13. Postoperative adhesion. 13-year-old girl. Right iliac pain and gurgling one year after appendicectomy with resection of a Meckel's diverticulum. SBFT : fixed, angulated and narrowed operated segment, centered on a small opaque spot, which surgery identified as an adhesion of the narrowed sutured segment to the omentum

Fig. 14 a, b. Postoperative adhesion. 57-year-old man. Subocclusive syndrome one year after left hemicolectomy for an adenocarcinoma. SBFT : **a** jejunal dilatation prominal to fixed angulated loops of irregular caliber (**b**)

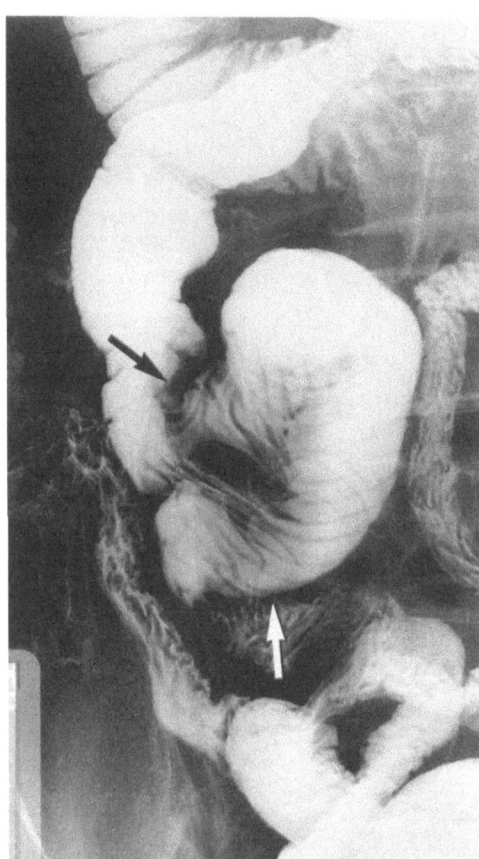

Fig. 15. Postoperative adhesion. 69-year-old woman. Multiple surgical procedures. Diarrhea. SBFT : U-shaped small intestinal loop in the right iliac fossa

fort associated with vasomotor disorders. It may be caused by the abrupt introduction of foods containing large quantities of carbohydrates into the jejunum. The radiological sign is one of hypotonia in the first jejunal loops, contrasting with the spastic appearance of the distal jejunum and of the ileum.

Peptic ulcer

Postoperative peptic ulcers (fig. 21) occur in 3% of operated patients. In addition to rare cases of pancreatic tumours producing ulcers (Zollinger-Ellison syndrome), they can be caused by incomplete vagotomy or gastric resection, or an excessively long afferent loop. The clinical symptoms include recurrence of pain and upper or lower gastrointestinal hemorrhage, requiring another operation.

Radiologic studies show the ulcer in the jejunum, less than 3 cm from the anastomosis. It becomes clearly visible when its diameter exceeds 5 mm and produces on frontal view a round, polygonal or star-shaped spot image, sometimes surrounded by edema or radiating folds, and an addition image on tangential view. It is sometimes concealed by inflammatory and spastic phenomena and may be difficult to distinguish from an interfold space if it is smaller than 5 mm. The ulcer can cause short jejunal stenosis and appear at some distance from the anastomosis. It can also produce a gastrojejunocolic fistula.

Jejunogastric intussusception (fig. 22)

Jejunogastric intussusception is often intermittent, so that its diagnosis may be difficult. The clinical symptoms include early postprandial cramps, sometimes relieved by vomiting. The presentation may be that of a high obstruction with complete food intolerance. This complication is specific for Polya-type gastrectomy. Intussusception is anterograde if located in the afferent loop and retrograde in the efferent loop.

The SBFT sometimes demonstrates the non-opacified jejunal loop and a nodular formation centered on the anastomosis. Protrusion of the intussus-

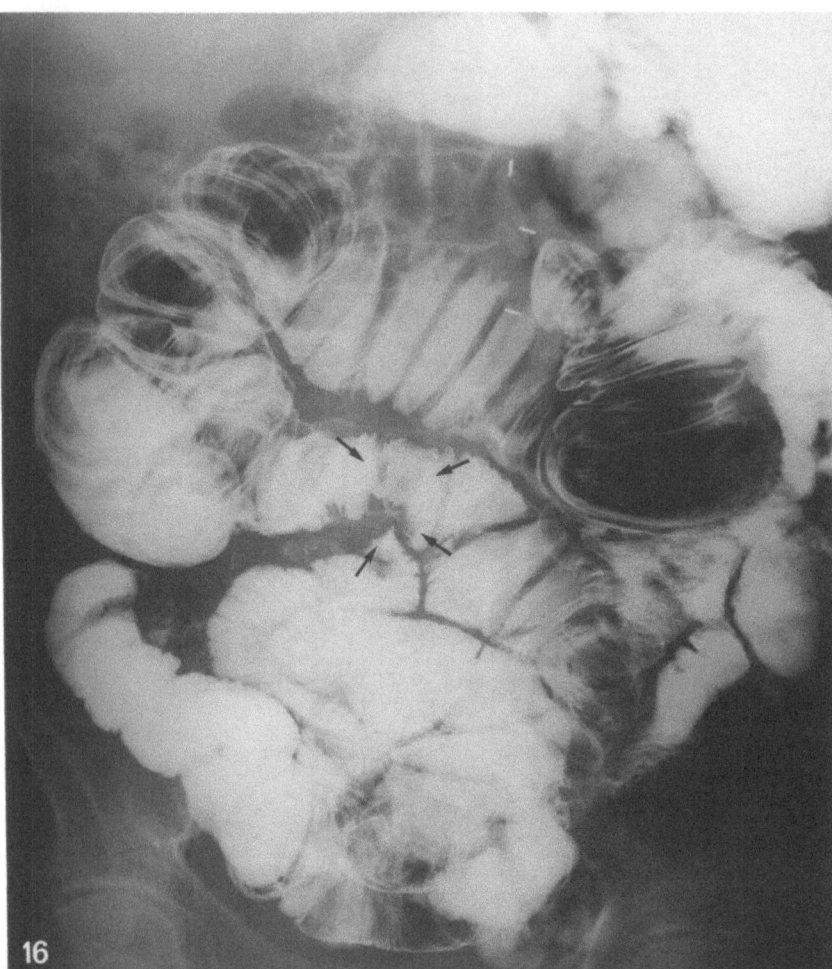

Fig. 16. Post-operative adhesion. 67-year-old man. Subocclusion 2 months after left nephrectomy for cancer with adrenal metastases. SBFT : distention of the jejunum proximal to a fixed midabdominal loop of irregular caliber. Surgical findings : linear omental adhesion. Histological findings : sclerolipomatosis and foreign-body granuloma formation (birefrengent material in polarized light)

Fig. 17 a, b. Postoperative talcoma. 28-year-old woman. Diarrhea, weight loss. Skin fistula following surgery for an abscess in the right iliac fossa secondary to previous appendicectomy. SBFT : **a** fixed, narrowed distal ileal loop with irregular course and caliber ; a fistula producing a pool image in its lower part is also seen. **b** marginal notch and modified folds in the upper part of the lesion. Surgical findings : foreign-body granuloma (talcoma)

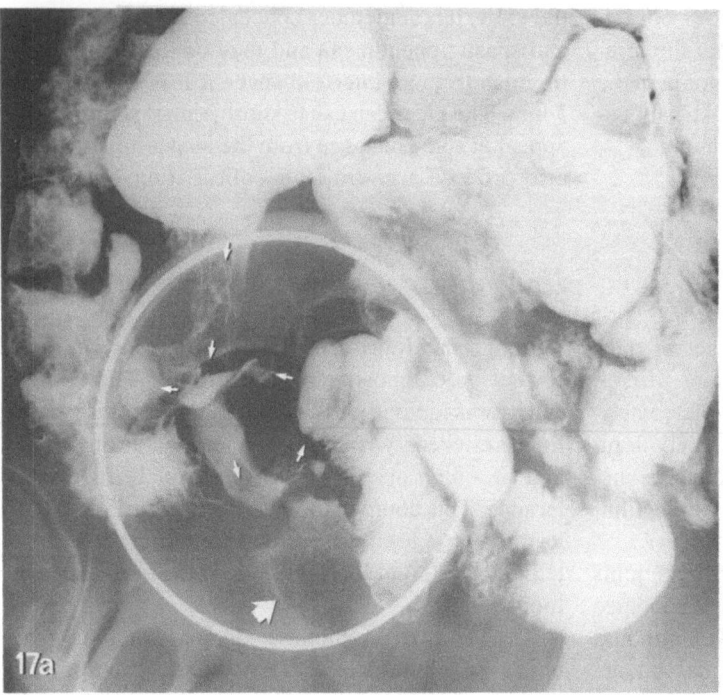

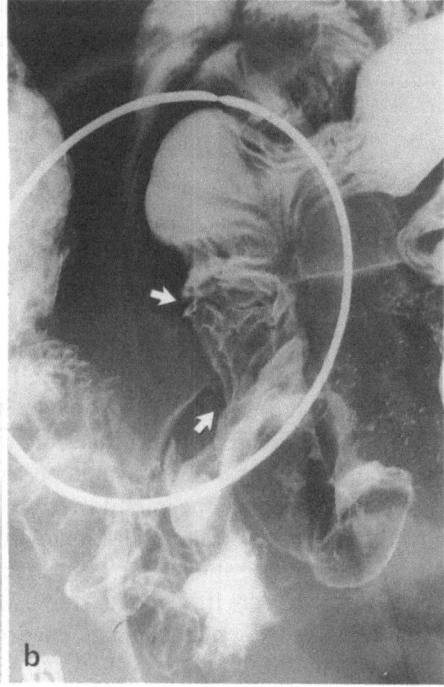

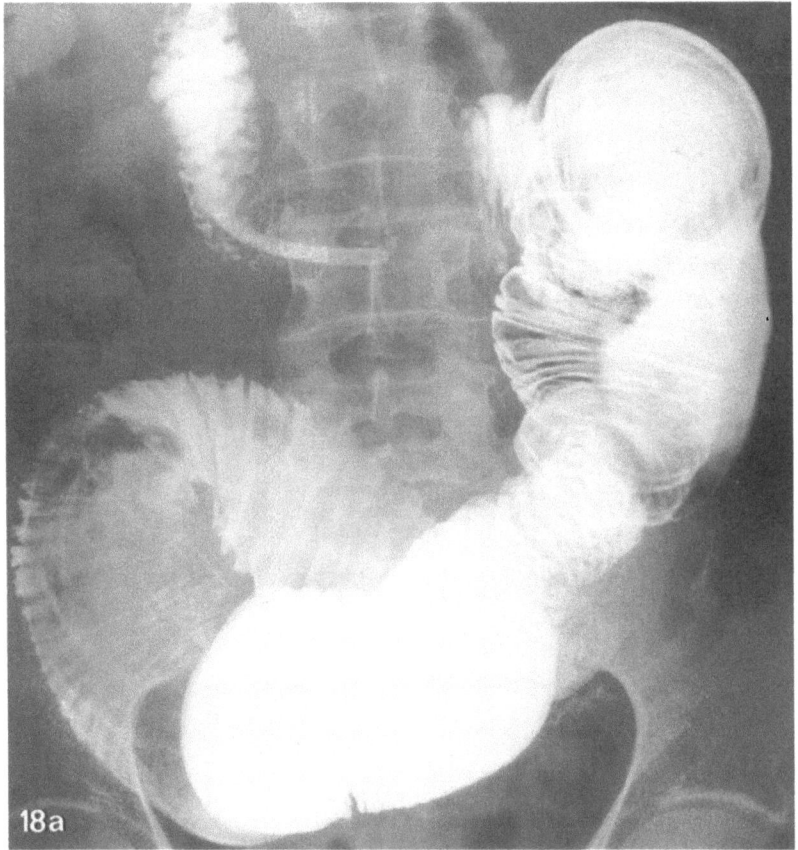

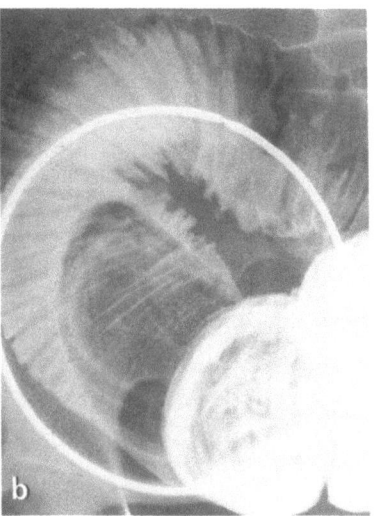

Fig. 18 a, b. Postoperative foreign body. 51-year-old woman. Right iliac pain and constipation 4 years after aortobifemoral bypass. SBFT : jejunal dilatation proximal to a large, heterogeneous nodular formation suggesting the presence of a compress

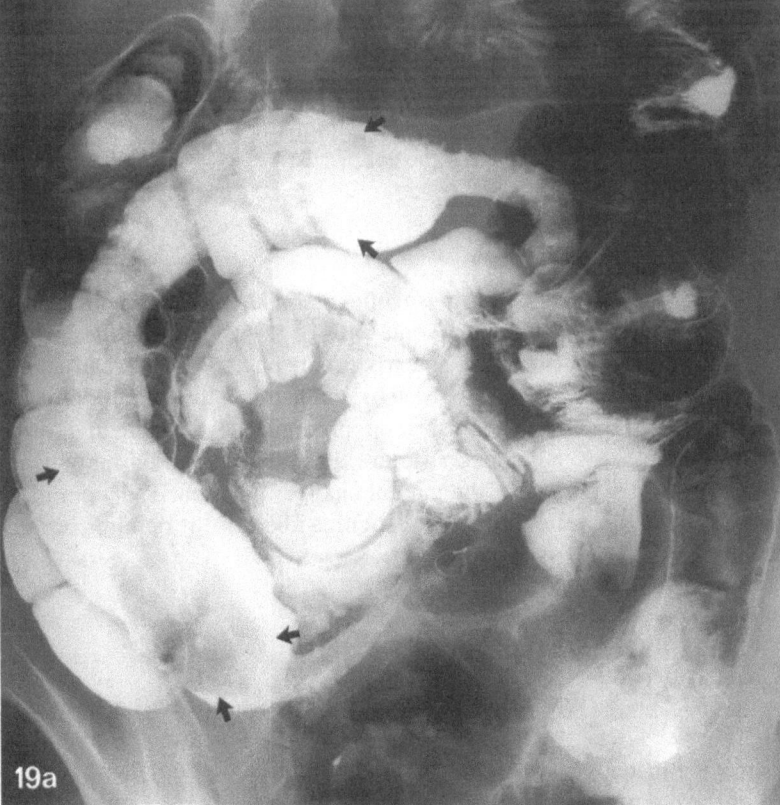

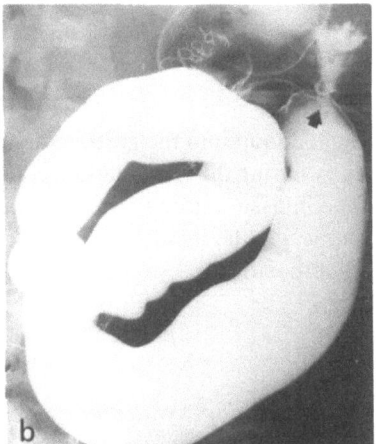

Fig. 19 a, b. Postoperative foreign body. 20-year-old woman. Hyperthermia, pain and vomiting 8 months after surgery for salpingitis with peritonitis. **a** SBFT : concentric midabdominal loops. Dilatation of the most lateral loop, which is narrowed at both ends. Heterogeneous appearance of the lumen (compress), **b** double-contrast barium enema : sigmoidoileal fistula

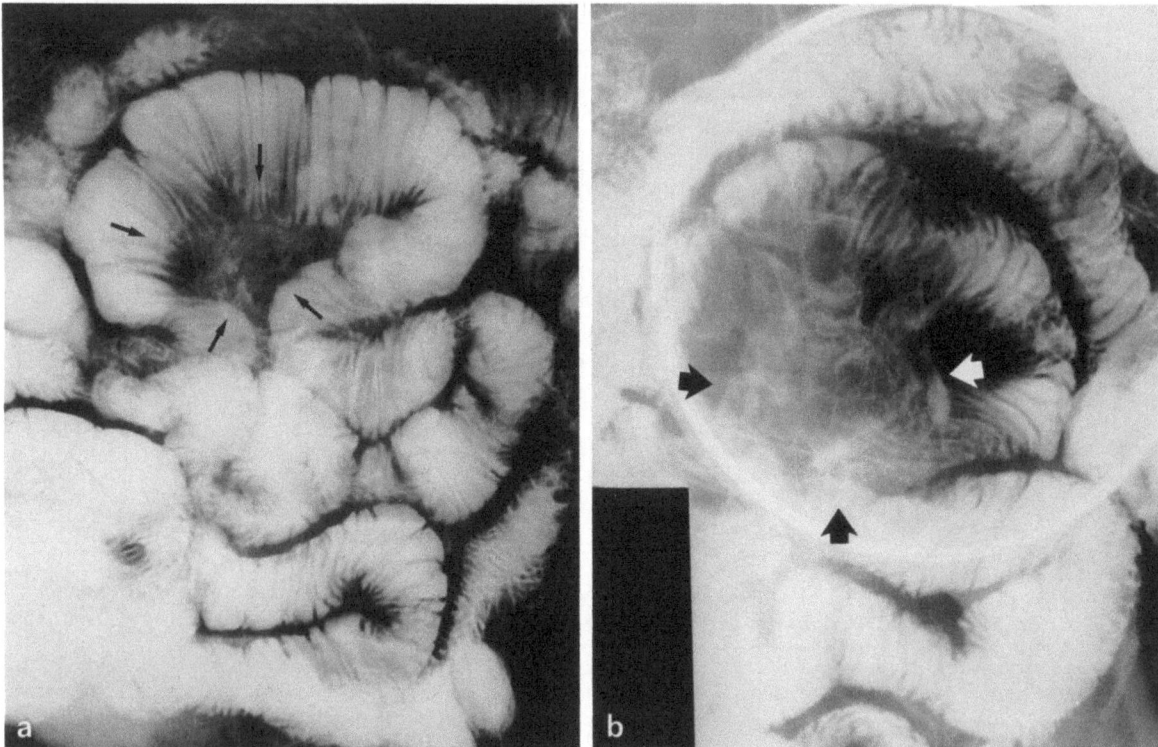

Fig. 20 a, b. Postoperative fistula. 56-year-old man. Cutaneous fistula following eventration secondary to repeated surgery for diverticular sigmoiditis. SBFT : **a** star-shaped arrangement of a group of jejunal loops, **b** with a barium pool image in the concavity of the upper loop : fistula on a Mersylene plate

cepted loop into the gastric stump, decreasing naturally during the examination, is sometimes observed. The intussusception must be demonstrated with two perpendicular incidences in order to rule out a simple superposition.

Afferent loop syndrome

The clinical symptoms of the afferent loop syndrome include a feeling of heaviness or pain in the right hypochondrium associated with relief by bilious vomiting. This syndrome is caused by the folding of the afferent loop due to defective assembly, or to adhesions. Surgery is necessary as bacterial overgrowth occurs in this stagnant loop and aggravates the digestive symptoms.

Radiological studies mainly show the distended afferent loop and the stagnation of the contrast medium. Selective intubation is sometimes needed to opacify the loop.

Internal hernia (fig. 23)

The transmesocolic internal hernia is a specific complication of some types of gastrojejunostomies, which can cause an early or late postoperative obstruction.

The SBFT demonstrates the dilatation of the first jejunal loop proximal to a fixed and often angulated stricture. Proximal dilatation may disappear if the patient changes position. This complication must be recognized because it requires corrective surgery.

Practical conclusions

In case of digestive disorders following gastrectomy, radiologists must search for mechanical complications or a peptic ulcer that endoscopy has failed to detect.

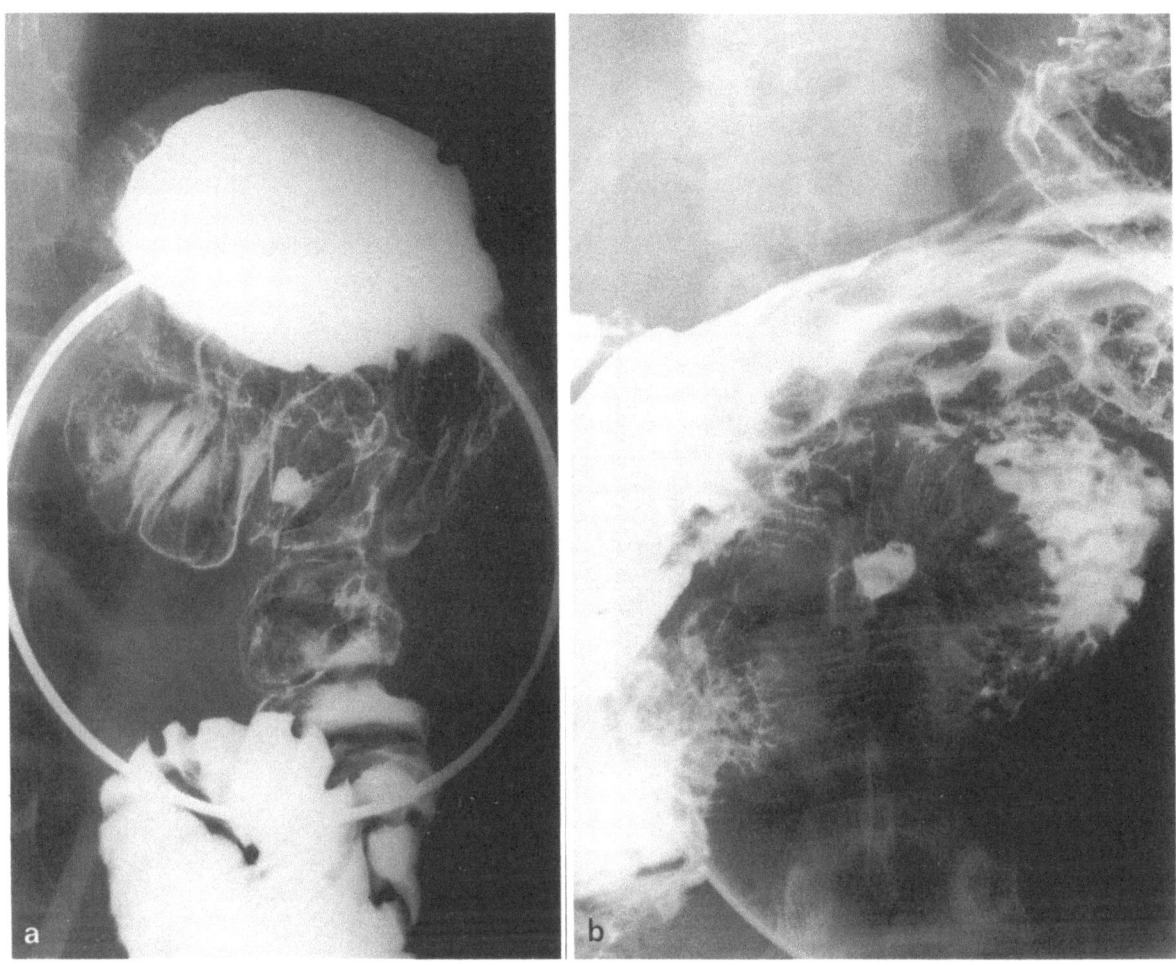

Fig. 21 a, b. Two examples of postoperative peptic ulcers. **a** following gastrectomy. **b** following gastroenteroanastomosis

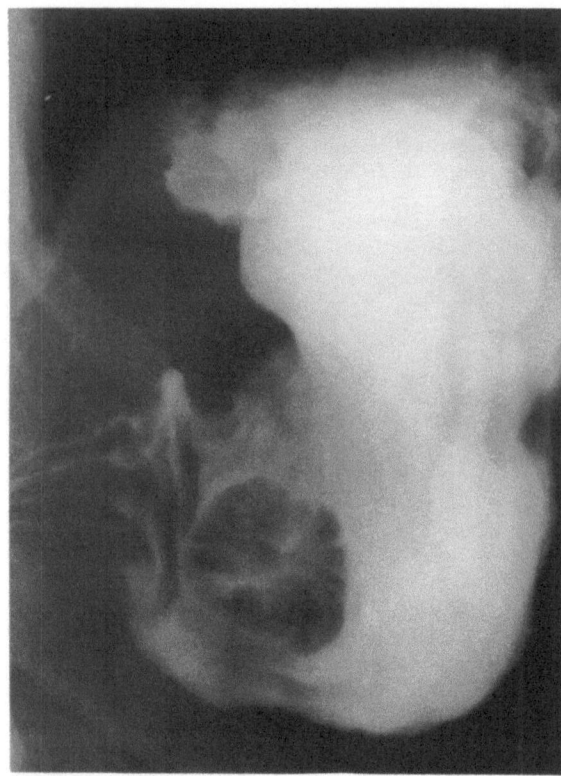

Fig. 22. Postoperative jejunogastric intussusception. 70-year-old man. Vomiting 10 days after gastroenteroanastomosis for cancer of the pancreas. SBFT : retrograde intussusception of the anastomotic loop into the stomach

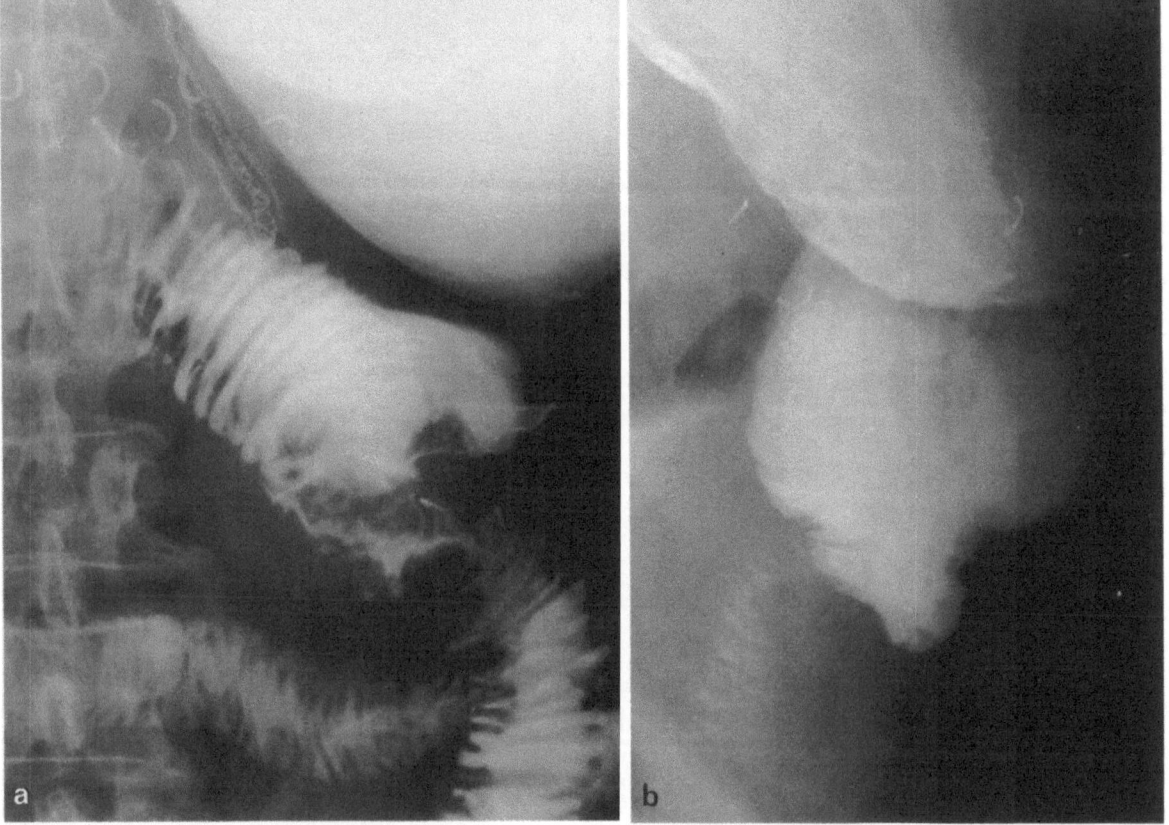

Fig. 23 a, b. Postoperative internal hernia. 82-year-old man. Regugitation 10 days after gastrectomy for an antral cancer. SBFT : **a** stenosis of the afferent loop along the mesocolic defect **b** increasing in the upright position

References

Postsurgical small intestine

Bartram CI (1980) The radiological demonstration of adhesions following surgery for inflammatory bowel disease. Br J Radiol 53 : 650-653

Baulieux J, Vuillard P, Venouil J, Fischer L (1971) Les occlusions post-opératoires précoces. Cah Med Lyon 47 : 4111-4117

Billimoria PE, Fabian TM, Schulz EE (1982) Computed tomography of intussusception in the bypassed jejunoileal segment. J Comput Assist Tomogr 6 : 86-88

Bocquet L, De Ranieri E, Charleux H, Moulle P, Léger L (1978) Pneumatose kystique de l'intestin grêle après court-circuit jéjuno-iléal pour obésité. Nouv Presse Med 7 : 545-548

Clements JL (1977) Intestinal pneumatosis, a complication of the jejunoileal bypass procedure. Gastrointest Radiol 2 : 267-271

Diner WC, Cockrill HH (1979) The continent ileostomy (Kock pouch) : roentgenologic features. Gastrointest Radiol 4 : 65-73

Dinstl K, Lechner G, Rield P, Schiessel R (1976) Spätergebnisse der Nobleschen Operation. Munch Med Wochenschr 118 : 941-944

Gourlay RH, Evans KG (1979) Jejunoileal bypass and the defunctioned bowel syndrome. Surg Gynecol Obstet 148 : 844-846

Grenier JF, Dauchel J, Marescaux J, Eloy MR, Schang JC (1977) Intestinal changes after jejuno-ileal shunt in obesity, a report of 2 cases. Br J Surg 64 : 96-99

Karasick D, Karasick S (1981) Obstructive and enteropathic syndromes after jejunoileal bypass surgery. Gastrointest Radiol 6 : 129-134

Kay VJ, Nolan DJ (1988) The small bowel enema in the patient with an ileostomy. Clin Rad 39 : 418-422

Kleinman PL, King DR (1977) Ischemic jejunitis and pneumatosis intestinalis secondary to anastomotic obstruction following jejunal atresia repair. Gastrointest Radiol 2 : 113-115

Lambert R, Marchat F (1975) Manifestations pathologiques de l'anse borgne. Concours Med 97-46 : 7474-7483

Lewicki AM, Kleinhaus U, Brooks JR, Membreno AA (1973) The small bowel following pyloroplasty and vagotomy. Radiology 109 : 539-544

Chandrasoma P, Wheeler D, Randall Radin D (1985) Traumatic neuroma of the intestine. Gastrointest Radiol 10 : 161-162

Lo G, Fisch AE, Brodey PA (1981) CT of the intussuscepted excluded loop after intestinal bypass. AJR 137 : 157-158

Mabille JP, Faivre J, Leflot A (1980) Pseudo-diverticule post-opératoire du grêle : cause méconnue d'hémorragie digestive. J Radiol 61 : 541-543

Maglinte DDT, Miller RE, Lappas JC (1984) Radiologic diagnosis of occult incisional hernias of the small intestine. AJR 142 : 931-932

Sava G, Marescaux J, Grenier JF (1979) Les diarrhées consécutives aux interventions chirurgicales. Ann Gastroenterol Hepatol 15 : 209-220

Woelfel GF, Campbell DN, Penn I, Reichen J, Warren GH (1983) Inflammatory polyposis in an ileal blind loop. Gastroenterology 84 : 1020-1024

The small intestine following gastric surgery

Nahum J, Fekete F (1976) Radiographie de l'appareil digestif opéré. Masson, Paris, pp 41-66

Fontaine R, Warter P, Sibilly A, Bridier JJ, Jary CI (1966) Les complications de la chirurgie gastro-duodénale et leur traduction radiologique. J Radiol Electrol 47 : 105-117

Burhenne HJ (1973) The postoperative stomach. In : Alimentary Tract Roentgenology. Margulis AR, Burhenne HJ (eds). Mosby, Saint-Louis, pp 740-783

Acute conditions

All diseases of the small intestine can cause acute abdominal involvement at a given stage of their evolution. This acute condition associates general clinical symptoms and signs as well as digestive disorders. The general signs are variable but they can include shock with cardiovascular collapse and agitation. The location and degree of the digestive disorders are also variable. The symptoms include shooting or colic-like pains, nausea, vomiting and changes in bowel habits (constipation or, on the contrary, diarrhea, which is sometimes bloody). The clinical findings can be absent, but they more often reveal muscular rigidity, or local or diffuse abdominal guarding painfull areas, rebound, abdominal distension, or absent bowel sounds. Rectal examination may yield blood and cause pain in contact with Douglas' pouch. The laboratory abnormalities may include: anemia, leucocytosis, metabolic acidosis or hyperamylasemia.

Once the initial stabilisation of the patient has occurred, three major outcomes may be differentiated, according to the patient's presentation:
- A highly precarious clinical condition and significant abdominal signs may be present, surgery must then rapidly be performed with or without rapid, non invasive imaging modalities, i.e. plain radiography or ultrasound.
- If a stable clinical condition with marked clinical signs exists, then the diagnosis can be rapidly confirmed and the decision to operate taken after a full radiological assessment which may include plain radiography, ultrasound examination, exam with iodinated contrast media, computed tomography, angiography.
- If moderate systemic signs without alarming abdominal signs predominate, barium studies may then be considered in addition to the other aforementioned imaging modalities.

Therefore three tiers of imaging modalities can be considered: first plain radiography and abdominal ultrasonography, they are the basic examinations. Second angiography and abdominal computed tomography, and thirdly complementary barium examinations if the clinical situation is least urgent.

Plain abdominal radiography

Plain abdominal radiographs include at least two large views (36x43), one in the supine and the other in the upright position. If the patient cannot stand, a film is taken in the left lateral decubitus position with a horizontal X-ray beam. Complementary views are taken if required, including films of the abdomen in prone positions and images centered on the domes of the diaphragm with the patient standing upright or on the sides with the patient in the supine position.

In addition to calcific opacities (vesicular, pancreatic, nodal, tumoral or vascular), three major types of signs are searched for:
- air-fluid levels,
- abnormal lucencies and
- abnormal opacities.

The association of air-fluid levels, air in the bile ducts and calcific opacitie on the intestinal area suggets gallstone ileus.

Air-fluid levels in cases other than a diarrheic syndrome suggest an intestinal obstruction. The location of these levels is a reliable criterion to determine the site of the obstruction. The loops of small

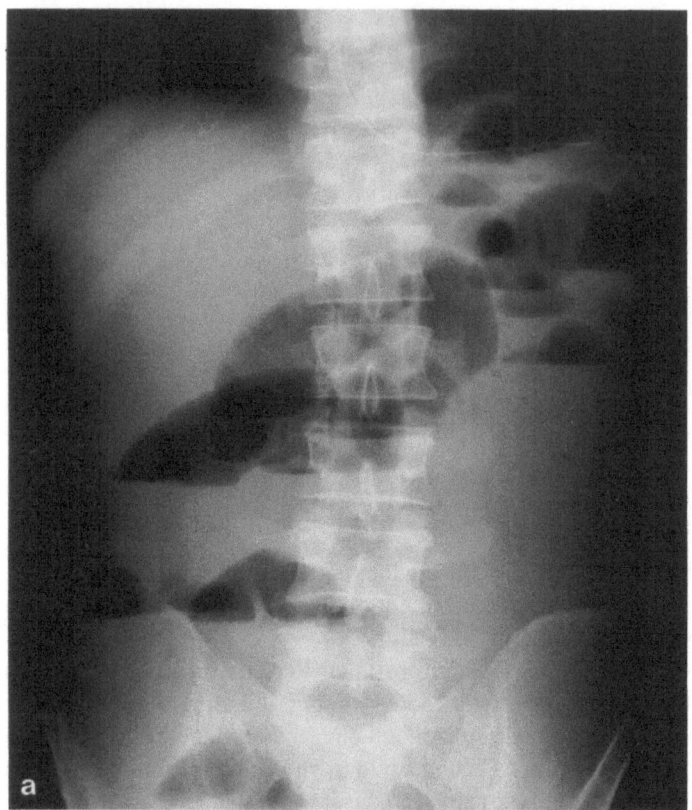

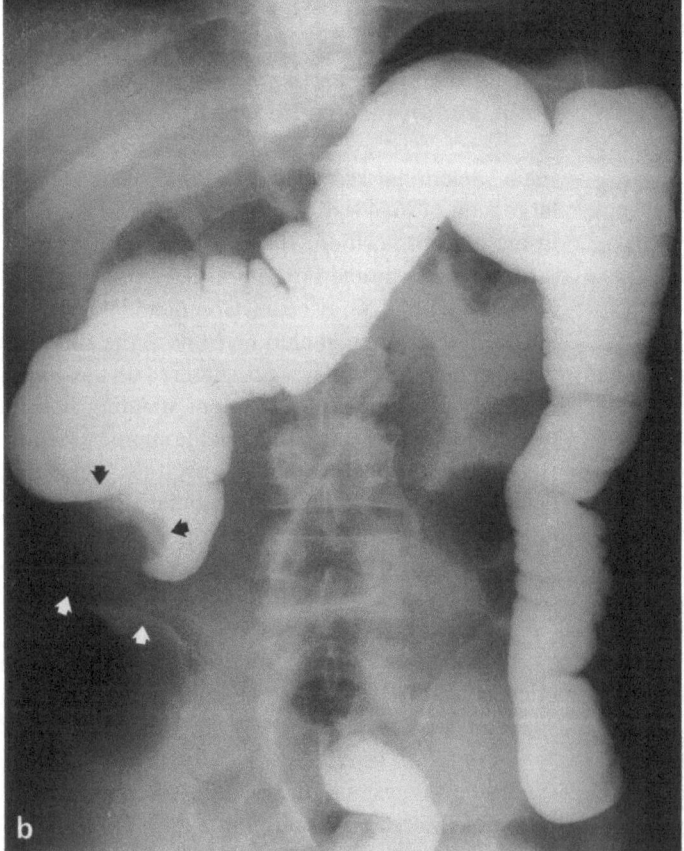

Fig. 1 a, b. Acute intestinal obstruction. 41-year-old man. Acute intestinal obstruction following several episodes of subocclusion. Weight loss. **a** Plain abdominal upright films : several staggered air-fluid levels in the periumbilical region, **b** barium enema : filling defect in the cecum with an early intussusception in the upper pole of the obstruction. Surgical findings : adenocarcinoma near the ileocecal valve

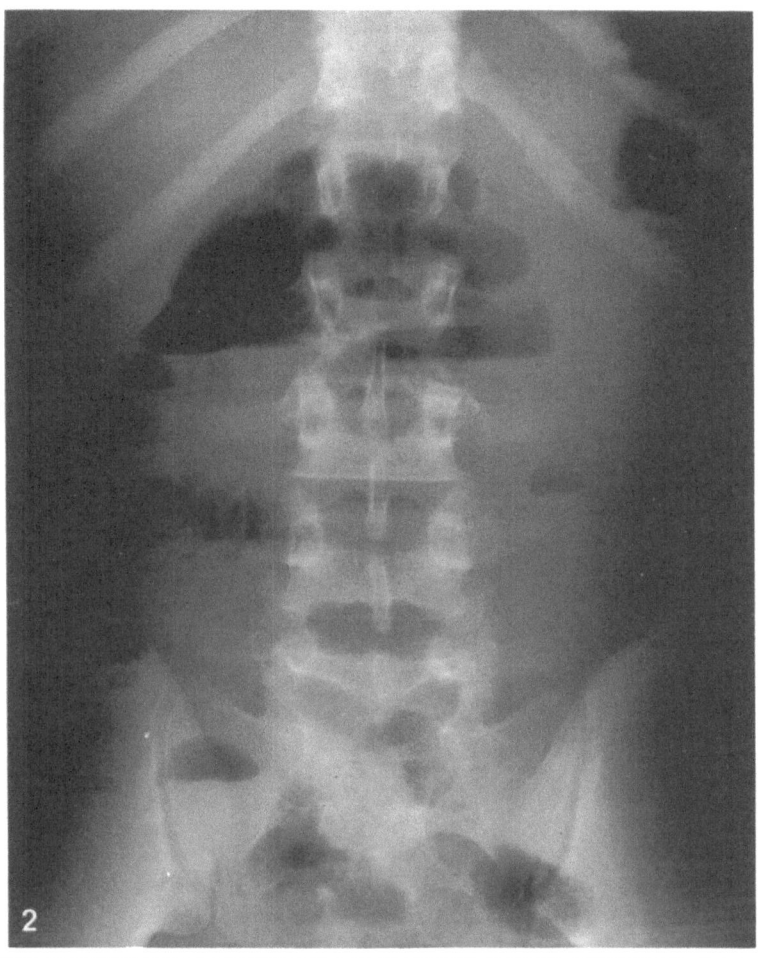

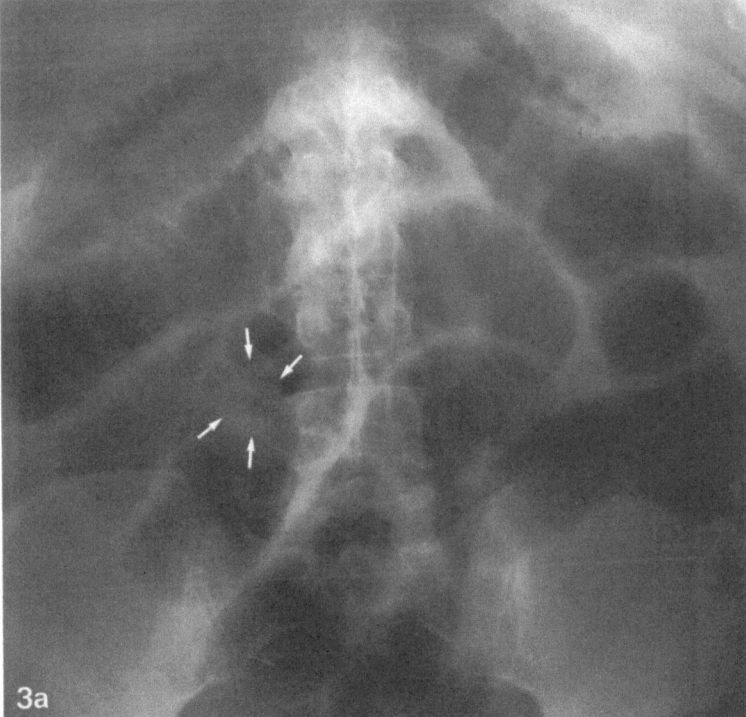

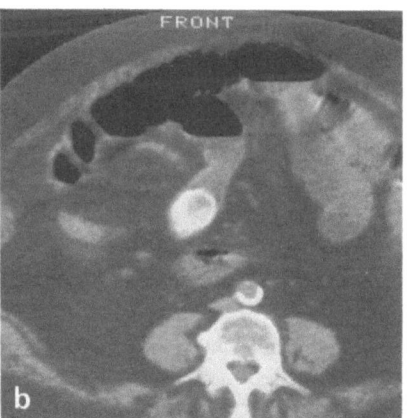

Fig. 2. Acute diarrhea. SBFT : air-fluid levels

Fig. 3 a, b. Gallstone ileus. 70-year-old woman. Acute intestinal obstruction. **a** Plain abdominal supine films : diffuse distention of the small intestine by air, 2 cm slightly radiopaque calculus projecting to the right of the 4th lumbar vertebra. No air in the bile ducts, **b** computed tomography : image confirming the findings

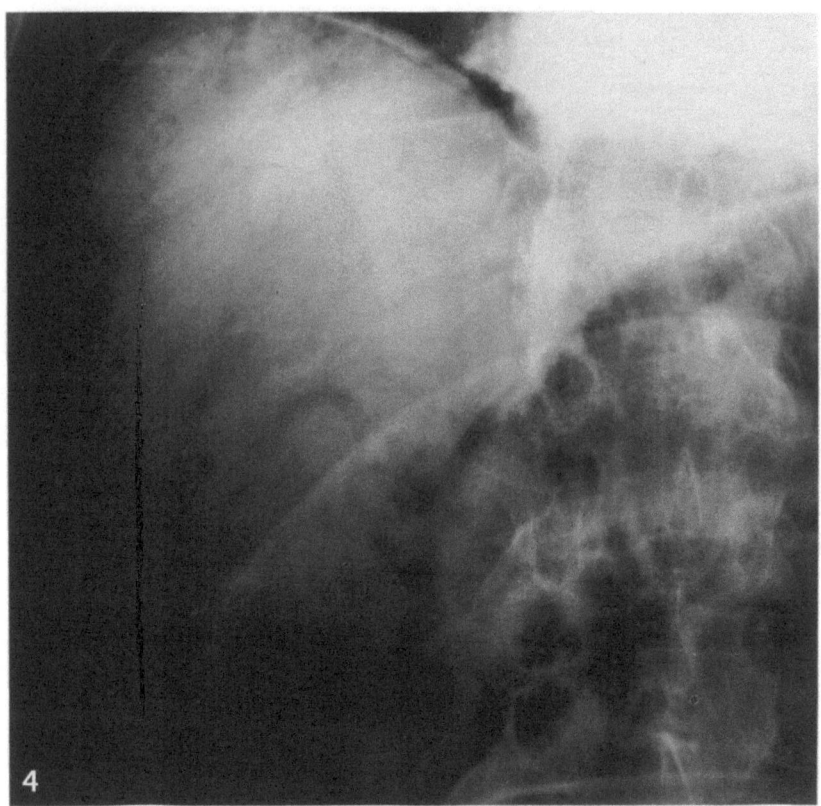

Fig. 4. Acute ischemia. 76-year-old male cardiac patient. Abdominal pan, bloody diarrhea followed by subocclusion. SBFT: dilatation of the intestine by air and gas in the portal vein

intestine lie in a central position on supine films. The morphology of the folds outlining the air-filled loops can help differentiate colonic from small bowel obstruction. The valvulae conniventes are thin, several millimeters apart and project across the entire intestinal lumen. The colonic haustral folds are short with a thickened free margin and do not extend across the intestinal lumen. These distinctive features are not always observed: the ileum can have a smooth appearance, without valvulae conniventes, the distended loops of the small intestine can present with the appearance of pseudohaustration, and colonic dilatation can flatten the haustrations.

Functional and organic obstructions must be distinguished. The former causes simultaneous distention of the small intestine and of the colon with a large quantity of gas.

Abnormal lucencies can be found in the intestinal lumen, in the intestinal wall or outside the intestine alltogether. The presence of small quantities of air is normal in the small intestine. It can be increased and permit visualization of the intestinal mucosal pattern, which can be irregular with thickened valvulae conniventes and marginal notches, and is sometimes associated with a decrease in the intes-

tinal caliber. The presence of air in the intestinal wall eventually produces long, lucent stripes, or strings of small bubbles. According to the clinical signs, necrotizing enterocolitis or pneumatosis cystoides intestinalis will be the cause. Extraintestinal air can be found in the peritoneal cavity, the bile ducts (aerobilia), the portal vein or within a tumoral opacity. If no laparotomy, laparoscopy or celioscopy have been performed recently, a pneumoperitoneum indicates the perforation of a hollow viscus. Exceptionally, it may be caused by pneumatosis cystoïdes. Perforation of the small intestine may be due to drug-induced ulcers, ischemic necrosis, abdominal trauma or tumors such as a malignant non-Hodgkin's lymphoma. A pneumoperitoneum presents as unilateral or bilateral subphrenic gas crescents on abdominal upright films. On left lateral decubitus views, this crescent is located under the right lateral abdominal wall in front of the opaque liver. The falciform ligament of the liver is outlined on supine films, as are the intestinal walls. If there has been no previous biliary surgery, air in the bile ducts sugges bilioenteric fistula. The appearance of air in the portal vein is different from the latter condition as the lucent lines are more peripheral. It is usually caused by ischemic involvement of the intestinal mucosal barrier. An excavated, lucent gaseous appearance different from a colonic segment and from the loops of small intestine within an opacity suggests a tumoral lesion communicating with the digestive tract. (e.g. malignant lymphoma) or an abcess.

Abnormal opacities are produced by intraperitoneal fluid accumulations or tumors. The radiological detection of intraperitoneal effusion has given rise to a number of signs, whose utility has significantly decreased since the advent of ultrasound. Three signs of intraperitoneal fluid accumulation have been described, i.e. opacity of the lateral recesses of the bladder, enlarged paracolic gutters and widely separated intestinal loops. A full bladder permits the visualization of two lateral recesses outlined by retroperitoneal fat. Intraperitoneal fluid collects in these recesses and produces the «dog ear» appearance described by Frimann-Dahl. A liquid-filled loop of the small intestine can produce a similar picture. The paracolic gutters are opacities several millimeters thick which separate the lucent outline of colonic gas from the properitoneal fat stripe. This linear opacity is broadened in presence of ascites. On supine abdominal films, contiguous intestinal loops containing gas should be no more than 2 mm apart. This gap increases in the presence of intraperitoneal fluid.

Abdominal ultrasonography

Abdominal ultrasonography plays an increasingly important part in the study of acute abdominal conditions because it is easily performed, even in bedridden patients.

Ultrasound rules out extraintestinal lesions likely to cause a paralytic ileus (pyelocaliceal dilatation, cholecystitis, pancreatitis, etc.). In the small intestine, it permits to identify obstructive lesions by demonstrating liquid-filled, dilated loops with a diameter exceeding 3 cm. The valvulae conniventes are clearly visible as transverse, hyperechogenic stripes. Peristalsis is sometimes increased. The obstructing lesion, which may be a tumour, an inflammatory stricture, a gallstone, an intraluminal foreign body or intussusception, is visible in some cases.

Ultrasound is very sensitive for the detection of ascites.

Computed tomography

Computed tomography provides similar information. The quality of its images is not dependent upon the presence of intestinal gas as is ultrasound. Moreover, contrast medium injection permits the study of the vascularity of the small intestine and of its possible lesions.

Iodinated enema

The iodinated enema can indicate an obstruction on the colon. It sometimes allows the radiologist to localize an obstruction on the last ileal loops.

Celiomesenteric arteriography

Arteriography is performed at once in cases of gastrointestinal bleeding or if the suspicion of an ischemic intestinal lesion arises. It can reveal a hypervascular tumour (angioma, leiomyoma, etc.) in case of abundant hemorrhage of the lower digestive tract when colonoscopy is negative. Hemorrhagic ulcers due to a Meckel's diverticulum are less easily visualized. If a mesenteric vascular accident is suspected, arteriography can demonstrate an atheromatous stenosis, an arterial embolism or venous thrombosis, which require surgery. A decrease in the peripheric vascular supply, disappearing after the injection of vasodilators, is sometimes noted. Angiography can be negative, even in the case of an ischemic lesion.

Barium studies

A SBFT is only performed in emergency cases when an intestinal perforation and bowel infarction have been ruled out.

A solution with a short barium index is not effective as contrast medium becomes diluted and fragmented in the hypotonic or enlarged loops and therefore satisfactory opacification of the intestine cannot be obtained. No cases of intestinal subocclusion progressing to complete obstruction due to the ingestion of large quantities of diluted barium have been reported in the literature.

Emergency SBFT must be performed preferably with enteroclysis. Duodenal intubation permits a satisfactory filling of the loops of small intestine and does not cause vomiting. Gastric and duodenal aspiration can be performed at the end of the examination if the duodenal tube is left in place.

Iodinated studies are useful if surgery has to be performed a short time after examination, since large quantities of barium can be bothersome for the surgeon. Hyperosmolar products have to be avoided because hypertonia causes contrast medium dilution. It also creates an electrolyte and water imbalance which may be dangerous for children. New products less osmolar can be used at a dose of 100 or 200 ml. Some authors have stated that these products may improve occlusion due to adhesions.

Practical conclusions

A global approach to the acute abdomen is necessary. The primary imaging modalities are plain radiography and abdominal ultrasonography, the results of which must be confronted with the clinical and laboratory findings.

On the basis of this first assessment, treatment may be determined. If not, computed tomography, angiography iodinated or barium studies can be undertaken.

References

Balthazar EJ, Hulnick D, Megibow AJ, Opulencia JF (1987) Computed tomography of intramural intestinal hemorrhage and bowel ischemia J Comput Assist Tomogr 11 : 67-72

Benson M, Bree RL, Schwab RE, Ouimette M (1985) Computed tomographic studies of the painful abdomen radiology 155 : 443-444

Gammill SL, Nice CM (1972) Air fluid levels : their occurrence in normal patients and their role in the analysis of ileus. Surgery 71 : 771-780

Laerum F, Stordahl A, Aase S (1988) Water soluble contrast media compared with barium in enteric follow-through. Acta Radiol 29 : 603-610

Nelson SW, Christoforidis AJ (1968) The use of barium sulfate suspensions in the diagnosis of acute diseases of the small intestine. AJR 104 : 505-521

Peetz DJ, Gamelli RL, Pilcher DB (1982) Intestinal intubation in acute, mechanical small bowell obstruction. Arch Surg 117 : 334-336

Saegesser F (1981) « Abdomens aigus » d'origine vasculaire, chez les adultes et les vieillards. Schweiz Rundsch Med Prax 70 : 7-30

Saegesser F (1981) The acute abdomen. Clin Gastroenterol 10 : 123-175

Schmutz G, Jahn Ch, Benhaim M, Drape JL, Chapuis A, Vaxman F (1987) Intérêt du transit du grêle par entéroclyse dans les syndromes obstructifs de l'intestin grêle. A propos de 212 examens. J Radiol 68 : 23-29

Simpson A, Sandemand, Nixon SJ (1985) The value of an erect abdominal radiograph in the diagnostic of intestinal obstruction. Clin Radiol 36 : 41-42

Stordahl A, Laerum F, Gjolberg T, Enge I (1988) Water-soluble contrast media in radiography of small bowel obstruction. Acta Radiol 29 : 53-56

Practical conclusions

The current technique for the examination of the small intestine is based on filling of the loops (with small bowel follow-through or enteroclysis) and palpation (preferably with hypotonia) of all intestinal loops under fluoroscopy.

The study of the films must be methodical and accomplished in an orderly fashion. The authors have not always followed this order in describing the signs of each disease in this book, since they have chosen for some, to discuss their most important findings first, in order to emphasize these.

The number of pages dealing with each disease is not proportional to their frequency. If it was, Crohn's disease would fill more than half this book, followed by celiac disease, lymphomas, Meckel's diverticula, ischemia and iatrogenic complications. Some of the other diseases are very uncommon and would deserve one or two lines only.

Some appearances are specific for given diseases. Others are specific enough to suggest the diagnosis. Others still are nonspecific, and the diagnosis cannot be made without also resorting to concomitant clinical and laboratory tests.

The clinical and laboratory findings should guide the radiological examinations, as only what is searched for is eventually found. However, the examination must be performed systematically in order to detect possible unsuspected abnormalities.

Index

Achevé d'imprimer à Clamecy
par l'imprimerie Laballery
en novembre 1989

Dépôt légal : novembre 1989
N° d'éditeur : 231 / N° d'imprimeur : 909049